Comprehensive cardiac care

A TEXT FOR NURSES, PHYSICIANS, AND OTHER HEALTH PRACTITIONERS

Comprehensive cardiac care

A TEXT FOR NURSES, PHYSICIANS, AND OTHER HEALTH PRACTITIONERS

Edited by

KATHLEEN GAINOR ANDREOLI, B.S.N., M.S.N., D.S.N., F.A.A.N.

Executive Director of Academic Services and Professor of Nursing,
The University of Texas Health Science Center at Houston,
Houston, Texas

VIRGINIA KLINER FOWKES, F.N.P., M.H.S.

Director, Primary Care Associate Program,
Regional Co-Director, Stanford Area Health Education Center,
Division of Family Medicine, Stanford University School of Medicine,
Stanford, California

DOUGLAS P. ZIPES, M.D.

Professor of Medicine, Indiana University School of Medicine;
Krannert Institute of Cardiology, Indianapolis, Indiana

ANDREW G. WALLACE, M.D.

Professor of Medicine, Chief Executive Officer, Duke Hospital;
Associate Vice President of Health Affairs,
Duke University, Durham, North Carolina

FIFTH EDITION

with **1111** *illustrations*

The C. V. Mosby Company

ST. LOUIS • TORONTO • LONDON   1983

MOSBY

A TRADITION OF PUBLISHING EXCELLENCE

Editor: Michael R. Riley
Assistant editor: Sally Gaines
Manuscript editor: Stephen Dierkes
Book design: Kay M. Kramer
Cover design: Suzanne Oberholtzer
Production: Linda R. Stalnaker, Barbara Merritt, Ginny Douglas

FIFTH EDITION

Previous editions copyrighted 1968, 1971, 1975, 1979

Printed in the United States of America

The C.V. Mosby Company
11830 Westline Industrial Drive, St. Louis, Missouri 63141

Library of Congress Cataloging in Publication Data

Main entry under title:

Comprehensive cardiac care.

    Includes bibliographies and index.
    1.   Cardiovascular disease nursing. 2.   Coronary
care units. I.   Andreoli, Kathleen G. [DNLM:
1. Coronary care units. 2.   Heart diseases—
Nursing.   WY 152.5 C737]
RC674.C65 1983   616.1'2   82-12570
ISBN 0-8016-0265-3

GW/VH/VH 9 8 7 6 5 4 3 2 1   03/B/313

CONTRIBUTORS

KATHLEEN GAINOR ANDREOLI, B.S.N., M.S.N., D.S.N., F.A.A.N.

Executive Director of Academic Services and Professor of Nursing, The University of Texas Health Science Center at Houston, Houston, Texas

JAMES A. BLUMENTHAL, Ph.D.

Assistant Professor of Medical Psychology, Duke University Medical Center, Durham, North Carolina

MARTHA E. BRANYON, M.S.N.

Associate Professor of Nursing, The University of Alabama School of Nursing, University of Alabama in Birmingham, Birmingham, Alabama

EDWIN G. DUFFIN, Jr., Ph.D.

Medtronic, Inc., Minneapolis, Minnesota

VIRGINIA KLINER FOWKES, F.N.P., M.H.S.

Director, Primary Care Associate Program, Regional Co-Director, Stanford Area Health Education Center, Division of Family Medicine, Stanford University School of Medicine, Stanford, California

GREGORY C. FREUND, B.S.

Research Associate, Division of Cardiology, Medical School, The University of Texas Health Science Center at Houston, Houston, Texas

FREDERIC W. HAFFERTY, Ph.D.

Research Associate, Division of Family Medicine, Stanford University School of Medicine, Stanford, California

JAMES J. HEGER, M.D.

Assistant Professor of Medicine, Division of Cardiology, Indiana University School of Medicine, Indianapolis, Indiana

PAULA HINDLE, R.N., M.S.N.

Nurse Leader, Adult Medicine, New England Medical Center, Boston, Massachusetts

MARGUERITE R. KINNEY, D.N.Sc.

Professor of Nursing, The University of Alabama School of Nursing, University of Alabama in Birmingham, Birmingham, Alabama

F. PAUL KOISCH, B.A., B.S.

Administrative Director, DUPAC, Duke University Medical Center, Durham, North Carolina

BRENDA LEWIS, R.N., C.C.R.N.

Knoll Pharmaceuticals, Whippany, New Jersey

HELENE MAU, R.N.

Staff Nurse, DUPAC, Duke University Medical Center, Durham, North Carolina

LINDA J. MIERS, M.S.N.

Assistant Professor of Nursing, The University of Alabama School of Nursing, University of Alabama in Birmingham, Birmingham, Alabama

MIRIAM C. MOREY, M.A.

Exercise Physiologist, DUPAC, Duke University Medical Center, Durham, North Carolina

DONNA ROGERS PACKA, M.S.N.

Associate Professor of Nursing, The University of Alabama School of Nursing, University of Alabama in Birmingham, Birmingham, Alabama

ERIC N. PRYSTOWSKY, M.D.

Assistant Professor of Medicine, Division of Cardiology, Indiana University School of Medicine, Indianapolis, Indiana

LAWRENCE A. REDUTO, M.D., F.A.C.C.

Attending Cardiologist, St. Francis Hospital, Roslyn, New York

ELIZABETH WAGNER, R.N.

Staff Nurse, DUPAC, Duke University Medical Center, Durham, North Carolina

ANDREW G. WALLACE, M.D.

Professor of Medicine, Chief Executive Officer, Duke Hospital; Associate Vice President of Health Affairs, Duke University, Durham, North Carolina

JENNIFER WILLIAMS, P.A.

DUPAC, Duke University Medical Center, Durham, North Carolina

R. SANDERS WILLIAMS, M.D.

Assistant Professor of Medicine, Staff Cardiologist, Duke University Medical Center, Durham, North Carolina

DOUGLAS P. ZIPES, M.D.

Professor of Medicine, Indiana University School of Medicine; Krannert Institute of Cardiology, Indianapolis, Indiana

PREFACE

The fifth edition of *Comprehensive Cardiac Care* continues the mission of the former editions, that is, to bring readers advances in cardiac research, technology, and patient care in relation to coronary artery disease. Recognizing the magnitude and complexities of this growing body of knowledge, we invited a multidisciplinary group of experts to contribute chapters. Nineteen contributing authors participated in the first team effort to produce *Comprehensive Cardiac Care*. The team consists of cardiologists, exercise physiologists, clinical nursing specialists, family nurse practitioners, physician assistants, psychologists, medical sociologists, researchers, and health administrators from academic medical centers. This national group of authors is from the east, west, midwest, and southwest areas of the United States.

A number of changes appear in this edition. The general format has been changed to incorporate the appendix of former editions into the body of the text. The number of chapters has expanded from eight to fifteen, and six of these are completely new. The remaining chapters have dramatic revisions. Chapters 1 and 2 on anatomy and physiology of the heart and pathogenesis of coronary artery disease reflect these changes. A new Chapter 3 presents the important role of prevention of coronary artery disease with an emphasis on risk factor reduction and health promotion. Patient assessment has been divided into three chapters in order to give full coverage to the process, procedure, and implications of data collection through the history and physical examination (Chapter 4), laboratory studies (Chapter 5), and electrocardiography (Chapter 6).

The problems associated with the onset of coronary artery disease are covered in the next three chapters as complications (Chapter 7), arrhythmias (Chapter 8), and sudden death (Chapter 9). Numerous new examples of arrhythmias appear in Chapter 8, and Chapter 9 brings an important dimension to the book.

Therapeutic approaches to the patient with coronary artery disease are included in the updated Chapter 10 on cardiovascular drugs, a new Chapter 11 on artifical cardiac pacemakers, and an updated Chapter 12 on care of the cardiac patient.

The last three chapters are new and broaden the therapeutic perspective of the patient experiencing acute myocardial infarction. For example, in former editions the psychologic and rehabilitative considerations for cardiac patients were incorporated into the nursing care chapter. The importance of these areas influenced their conversion to single units, Chapters 13 and 14, respectively. Furthermore, the area of death and dying, briefly mentioned in former editions, was recognized as deserving of full coverage in Chapter 15.

Although the chapters follow a reasonable sequence for learning about patients with coronary artery disease, it is important to note that each chapter can serve as an independent resource for learning or reinforcement in that subject area. Throughout the book the reader is referred to supplementary relevant information in other sections.

The fifth edition of *Comprehensive Cardiac Care* represents a meaningful combination of the old and the new. The style and pertinent information from former editions have been retained, but new authors, content, illustrations, and tables have been carefully selected and added.

Organizing this multidisciplinary project was challenging, and we extend our sincere thanks to all who helped in the production—contributing authors, typists, illustrators, and especially you, our readers. Your support and feedback continues to inspire us to move forward.

Kathleen Gainor Andreoli
Virginia Kliner Fowkes
Douglas P. Zipes
Andrew G. Wallace

CONTENTS

1

ANATOMY AND PHYSIOLOGY OF THE HEART

Miriam C. Morey
F. Paul Koisch

This chapter briefly reviews the anatomy and physiology of the heart. It is intended not to be a detailed discussion but merely to serve as a general background.

Anatomy

The heart is a muscular pump that propels blood into the arterial (delivery) system and receives blood from the venous (return) system. As illustrated schematically in Fig. 1-1, the heart is divided into anatomically separate right and left sides. Each side has a receiving chamber (atrium) and a pumping chamber (ventricle). The right atrium receives unoxygenated venous blood from three sources: the inferior vena cava, which drains blood from the lower half of the body, the superior vena cava, which drains blood from the upper half of the body, and the coronary sinus, which drains blood from the heart muscle. The blood flows from the right atrium through the tricuspid valve to the right ventricle. The three leaflets of the tricuspid valve are attached by chordae tendineae to the papillary muscles that lie in the floor of the ventricle. Contraction of the papillary muscles prevents the leaflets from everting into the right atrium during ventricular contraction (systole). During ventricular systole, blood is ejected by the right ventricle through the pulmonary valve into the pulmonary artery and then into the lungs. The blood returning from the lungs enters the left atrium through four pulmonary veins. It passes from the left atrium through the mitral valve to the left ventricle. The two leaflets of the mitral valve are attached to the wall of the left ventricle by chordae tendineae, which connect to the papillary muscles. The left ventricle ejects blood through the aortic valve into the aorta, and the aorta distributes this cardiac output to peripheral tissues. Cardiac output (normally 3 L/minute/square meter) is the volume of blood pumped by the heart per minute.[1]

The right side of the heart collects blood from the systemic circulation and distributes it to the pulmonary circulation. As blood passes through the pulmonary capillaries, red blood cells exchange carbon dioxide for oxygen within pulmonary alveoli in preparation for returning to the systemic circulation. The left side of

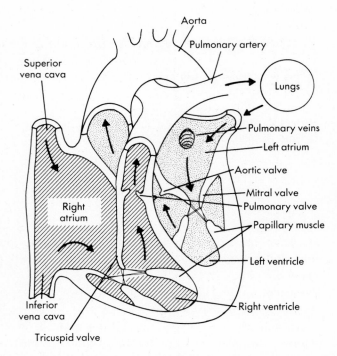

Fig. 1-1. Internal anatomy of the heart. (Modified from Guyton, A.C.: Function of the human body, ed. 3, Philadelphia, 1969, W.B. Saunders Co.)

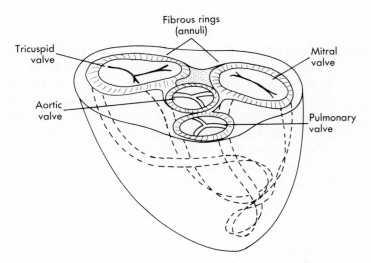

Fig. 1-2. Fibrous rings connecting the four heart valves.

the heart collects blood from the pulmonary circulation and distributes it to the systemic circulation. As blood passes through the systemic capillary bed, which joins peripheral arteries and veins, the red blood cells surrender their oxygen to metabolizing tissues and accumulate carbon dioxide.

The heart has a skeleton made up of four fibrous rings (annuli) and nonconductive tissue that connects them into a single framework (Fig. 1-2). Each annulus is the supporting structure for one of the four valves of the heart and the connecting site of the muscular network that comprises the four chambers. Because the fibrous skeleton is nonconductive, the musculature of the atria normally is separated electrically from ventricular muscle. The specialized conduction system that coordinates the rhythm of atria and ventricles, the atrioventricular node and bundle of His, passes through the fibrous connective tissue.

Physiology

The major physiologic roles of the circulatory system are to deliver oxygen and other essential substrates to the tissues of the body, and to remove carbon dioxide and other products of cellular metabolism. Many of the substances carried to and from the tissues dissolve in plasma, and their transport depends on the volume of flow. Oxygen and carbon dioxide, however, are transported partially or almost entirely by red blood cells. The transport of these gases to and from tissues is affected not only by flow volume but also by the metabolic needs of specific tissues or organs at a given time; this is referred to as the local rate of metabolism. During exercise, for example, blood flow increases in areas involved in the activity—such as specific muscle groups and the skin—and decreases in areas of little metabolic activity—such as the kidneys, stomach, and intestines. Brain blood flow remains nearly the same at rest or during exercise. The local rate of metabolism is probably the most important determinant in the distribution of cardiac output.

Systemic circulation

The systemic circulation is the continuous passage of blood from the heart through the arteries, arterioles, capillaries, venules, veins, and back to the heart. Its continuity depends largely on the different pressures, resistances, and rates of blood flow through the different portions of the systemic circuit.[2]

Pressure is highest at the arterial level. It progressively decreases until the blood reaches the right atrium. When blood is pumped from the left ventricle into the aorta, the aorta distends and creates a high arterial pressure. Depending on the pumping action of the heart, arterial pressure normally fluctuates between approximately 120 mm Hg (systolic pressure) and 80 mm Hg (diastolic pressure).

The arteries begin branching off at the arch of the aorta and continue branching until they become small arterioles. The arterioles have muscular walls that can dilate or constrict considerably, thus controlling the blood flow into the capillary bed. Vasodilatation or vasoconstriction is usually dictated by the needs of the tissues for oxygen or other nutrients. Vascular resistance is highest at this arteriolar level in the systemic circuit, causing a drop in pressure so that the blood entering the capillaries has a pressure of only about 30 mm Hg.[3]

Once the blood is inside the capillary bed, its rate of blood flow is at its slowest. This allows sufficient time for the blood and the interstitial spaces of tissues and organs to exchange fluid, gases, and nutrients. Capillary walls are very thin, and most exchanges occur by diffusion. The total surface area of the capillary walls is extensive enough to ensure adequate perfusion of all organs and tissues.

Blood flows from the capillaries into venules, which converge to form larger veins. At this level of the systemic circuit, pressure is very low (about 5 to 10 mm Hg) so as not to impede the return of the blood to the heart. Venous walls are thin and muscular, which allows them to accommodate their capacity to variations in total blood volume based on the needs of the body. The final step in the systemic circuit is the passage of blood from the largest veins, the superior and inferior venae cavae, into the right atrium.

Pulmonary circulation

The pulmonary circulation, like the systemic circulation, consists of a continuous circuit of blood flow. Blood flows from the right ventricle to the lungs through the pulmonary arteries, which branch off into pulmonary capillaries, where oxygen is absorbed into the blood and carbon dioxide is released from the blood. The pulmonary capillaries converge into pulmonary veins and return oxygenated blood to the left atrium.

Gas exchange between the pulmonary capillaries and the alveoli takes place through a thin tissue called the pulmonary membrane. The pores of the pulmonary membrane are large enough to ensure rapid diffusion of oxygen and carbon dioxide but small enough to prevent blood proteins from leaking out of the capillaries. When the body is at rest, blood usually traverses the pulmonary capillaries in about 1 second. When oxygen demand increases, the increased rate of blood flow through the pulmonary capillaries can shorten the diffusion time to less than half a second. The pulmonary circulation adjusts to the increased blood flow by opening additional capillaries to ensure adequate aeration.

An important feature of pulmonary circulation and distribution is the ability of the pulmonary blood vessels to regulate blood flow through the lungs. Since gas exchange is the major reason blood flows through the lungs, the pulmonary blood vessels must ensure that blood flows only through adequately ventilated areas. Therefore, if certain alveoli become blocked or damaged, the local pulmonary vessels normally constrict and force the blood through a properly aerated area of the lungs.

The pulmonary blood vessels are expansile and thin walled; these two characteristics allow fluctuating volumes of blood to flow freely into the lungs. The volume of blood flowing through the lungs is the same as the systemic blood volume (because the two circulations are in series). The lungs must therefore be prepared to accept as much as a fivefold increase in blood volume during strenuous exercise without putting additional strain on the right ventricle. A slightly elevated pulmonary arterial pressure, about 20 mm Hg, enhances blood flow into the lungs by stimulating pulmonary vessel expansion. The pressure gradually decreases as blood flows through the pulmonary capillaries and completes its circuit into the left atrium.

Coronary arteries

The function of the coronary artery system is to maintain an adequate blood supply to the heart muscle (myocardium). Impairment of the coronary circulation by atherosclerosis constitutes the most frequent cause of heart disease.

Two major coronary arteries, the left and right, arise from the aorta immediately behind their respective cusps of the aortic valve.[4] The left coronary artery divides into two branches shortly after its origin (Fig. 1-3), the anterior descending and the circumflex. The anterior descending branch passes down the groove between the two ventricles on the anterior surface of the heart. From it arise diagonal branches that supply the left ventricular wall, and septal perforating branches that supply the anterior portion of the interventricular septum and the anterior papillary muscle of the left ventricle. The anterior descending artery usually supplies the entire apical portion of the interventricular septum before turning at the apex to terminate in channels anastomotic with the posterior descending coronary artery. The circumflex branch of the left coronary passes posteriorly and to the left in the groove between the left atrium and left ventricle. It gives off several small and one or two large marginal branches that supply the lateral aspects of the left ventricle.

The right coronary artery passes around the right atrioventricular (AV) groove, giving off branches to the right ventricle, and then turns at the crux of the heart to descend in the posterior interventricular groove. The posterior descending artery supplies the posterior aspect of the septum and the posterior left ventricular papillary muscle before terminating in channels anastomotic with the anterior

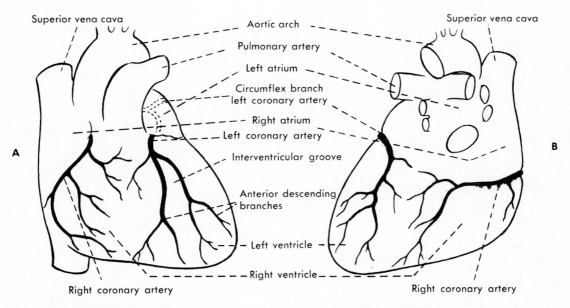

Fig. 1-3. A, Coronary arteries supplying the anterior aspect of the heart. **B,** Coronary arteries supplying the posterior aspect of the heart.

descending branch of the left coronary artery. The right coronary artery gives off important branches, which supply the sinoatrial (SA) node in 50% to 60% of human hearts and the AV node in 90% of human hearts. If the right coronary artery turns at the crux and supplies the posterior aspect of the left ventricle and interventricular septum, the coronary circulation is said to be *dominant right*. About 80% to 90% of the population have a dominant right coronary circulation. When the posterior aspect of the ventricle is supplied by the left circumflex artery, coronary circulation is then referred to as *dominant left* circulation.[5]

Conduction system

The normal cardiac impulse arises in the specialized pacemaker cells of the SA node, located about 1 mm beneath the right atrial epicardium at its junction with the superior vena cava (Fig. 1-4). The impulse then spreads over the atrial myocardium to the left atrium via Bachmann's bundle and to the region of the AV node via the anterior, middle, and posterior internodal tracts connecting the sinus and AV nodes. These represent the usual routes of spread, but are not specialized tracts analogous to the Purkinje system. When the impulse reaches both atria, they depolarize electrically, producing a P wave on the electrocardiogram (ECG), and then contract mechanically, producing the A wave of the atrial pressure pulse and propelling blood forward into the ventricles.

Conduction slows markedly when the impulse reaches the AV node, allowing sufficient time for blood to flow from the atria into the ventricles. After the impulse emerges from the AV node, conduction resumes its rapid velocity through the

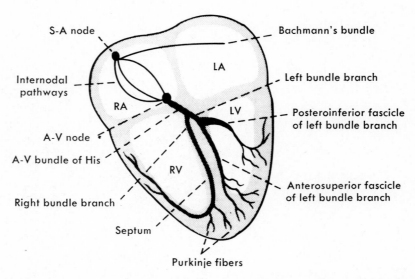

Fig. 1-4. Transmission of the cardiac impulse from the sinoatrial (SA) node over atrial myocardium, Bachmann's bundle, and internodal pathways, then through the AV node and bundle of His and down the left and right bundle branches, emerging into the Purkinje fibers, which distribute the impulse to all parts of the ventricle.

His bundle and down the left and right bundle branches. The left bundle divides into anterosuperior, middle, and posteroinferior divisions. Left and right bundle branches supply the inner shells (endocardium) of their respective ventricles with a profusely branching terminal network called Purkinje fibers. These fibers allow almost simultaneous depolarization of both ventricles by distributing the impulse rapidly throughout the ventricular endocardium.

All conduction prior to an impulse leaving the Purkinje fibers takes place between atrial and ventricular contractions (PR interval) on the ECG recording. When the impulse emerges from the Purkinje fibers, ventricular depolarization occurs, producing the QRS complex on the ECG and the mechanical contraction of the ventricles that propels the blood forward into the pulmonary artery and aorta. Considering the many different parts of the specialized conduction system, it is interesting that only atrial depolarization (P wave), ventricular depolarization (QRS complex), and ventricular repolarization (T wave) appear in the standard ECG recording.[6]

Regulation of cardiac function

Many factors contribute to the regulation of the heart. One of the major control systems is the autonomic nervous system; it plays an important role in the rate of impulse formation, the speed of conduction, and the strength of cardiac contraction.[7] It regulates the heart through two different sets of nerves: the sympathetic and the parasympathetic (Fig. 1-5). The sympathetic nerve fibers supply all areas of the atria and ventricles. Vagal nerve fibers primarily innervate the SA

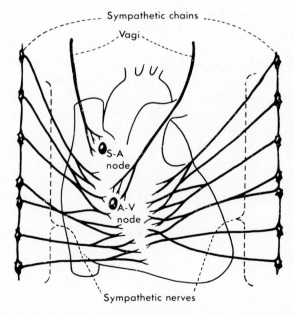

Fig. 1-5. Connections of parasympathetic nerves (vagi) and sympathetic nerves with the heart. (Adapted from Guyton, A.C.: Function of the human body, ed. 3, Philadelphia, 1969, W.B. Saunders Co.)

node, atrial muscle fibers, and the AV node. They supply the ventricular myocardium also, but the density of innervation there is less than in the atrium, and the physiologic consequences of vagal innervation of the ventricles are uncertain. Recent data suggest, however, that vagal innervation may affect ventricular electrophysiology more than has been previously thought.

Within the postganglionic nerve fibers are located neurotransmitters—acetylcholine in the vagus nerve and norepinephrine in the sympathetic nerves. Electrical impulses traveling down the postganglionic nerve fibers release the neurotransmitters, which in turn mediate the influence of the autonomic nerves on the heart by binding to specific receptors on the surface membrane of myocardial cells.

Vagal nerve stimulation has the following effects on the heart: decreased firing rate of the SA node, decreased contractile force of atrial (and probably ventricular) muscle, and decreased impulse conduction speed through the AV node, which lengthens the delay period between atrial and ventricular contraction (PR interval). Vagal stimulation also speeds conduction through the atrial muscle and shortens the atrial repolarization period. Sympathetic nerve stimulation has several effects on the heart: increased heart rate, increased conduction speed through the AV node, a shortened ventricular (and probably atrial) repolarization period, and increased vigor of cardiac contraction. Vagus nerve and sympathetic nerve stimulations have essentially opposite effects on the heart.

Autonomic nerve activity can be modulated by the central nervous system (such as reflexes triggered by fear or pain) or by reflex changes caused by stimulation of sensors that detect changes in pressure (pressoreceptors).[8] Pressoreceptors are located in the aortic arch and carotid arteries and are connected to the vasomotor center in the medulla by way of the vagus and glossopharyngeal nerves. Sudden elevation of blood pressure within the aorta or the carotid sinus (for example, by a hypertensive drug or by carotid sinus massage) stimulates the pressoreceptors in these vessels. This stimulates the cardioinhibitory center, which in turn inhibits the accelerator center. Conversely, a sudden drop in blood pressure within the aorta or carotid sinus stimulates pressoreceptors less intensely. The cardioinhibitory center is stimulated less, producing less depression of the accelerator center and consequently less reflex acceleration of the heart. This phenomenon becomes apparent during hypotension.[9]

The heart also has several intrinsic autoregulatory mechanisms and can operate without nervous influence. The major intrinsic mechanism is described by Starling's law, which states that within limits the more the heart is filled during diastole, the greater will be the force of contraction and resulting work during systole. Striated muscle, such as cardiac muscle, characteristically contracts with greater force when stretched. Thus the heart automatically adapts to different incoming blood volumes by changing its force of contraction.

Another mechanism that regulates cardiac function is based on the rate of metabolism in peripheral tissues. The blood flow to various organs is influenced by each organ's metabolic rate, which in turn influences systemic vascular resistance, a determinant of cardiac output. Thus, with anxiety, fever, and exercise, cardiac output increases because peripheral resistance drops.

Other factors that can affect the control mechanism of the heart rate include the levels of oxygen and carbon dioxide in the blood, electrolyte disorders, and the presence of certain drugs in the body.

The effects of aging

The heart and circulatory system are known to change with age, although the changes and rate of changes vary considerably in different cultural settings.[10] After age 35 the heart's ability to circulate blood diminishes gradually and continuously. The expected consequence of a compromised cardiac output is a reduction in the amount of oxygen available for tissue use. In actuality, however, the working muscle is able to extract a higher percentage of oxygen; so the decrease in work capacity, although significant, is much less than expected. The mechanisms that contribute to the reduced cardiac output in the aging heart include a lower heart rate for any work level and an increasingly noncompliant cardiac muscle. The more resistant the heart muscle is to contraction, the less blood is ejected with each heartbeat.

The decrease in heart rate, cardiac output, and stroke volume with advancing age contributes to a reduction in work capacity.[10] There is considerable debate as to the pathophysiology that changes the heart's response to work or stress. Current evidence indicates that the effects that aging can exert on the heart can be minimized by life-style adjuncts such as undertaking vigorous exercise, following a low-fat and low-sodium diet, and not smoking.

Atherosclerosis has been viewed in the past as an age-correlated change in the coronary arteries. Although it is true that aging coronary arteries demonstrate an increase in tortuosity, atherosclerosis is not a universal complication in the aged. The causes of atherosclerosis are under investigation, and there is little apparent evidence that age is the precipitating factor.

REFERENCES

1. Rushmer, R.F.: Structure and function of the cardiovascular system, ed. 2, Philadelphia, 1976, W.B. Saunders Co.
2. Katz, A.M.: Physiology of the heart, New York, 1977, Raven Press.
3. Guyton, A.C.: Textbook of medical physiology, ed. 5, Philadelphia, 1976, W.B. Saunders Co.
4. James, T.N.: Anatomy of the coronary arteries in health and disease, Circulation **32:**1020, 1965.
5. Braunwald, E., Ross, J., and Sonnenblick, E.H.: Mechanisms of contraction of the normal and failing heart, ed. 2, Boston, 1976, Little, Brown & Co.
6. Wellens, H.J.J., Lie, K.I., and Janse, M.J.: The conduction system of the heart, Leiden, 1976, Hyman, Stenfort Kroese & Zoon, N.V.
7. Abbond, F.F., and others: Reflex control of the peripheral circulation, Prog. Cardiovasc. Dis. **18:**371, 1976.
8. Hirsch, E.F.: The innervation of the human heart, Arch. Pathol. **75:**378, 1963.
9. Heymans, C., and Neil, E.: Reflexogenic areas of the cardiovascular system, London, 1968, Churchill Livingstone.
10. Caird, F.I., Dall, J.L.C., and Kennedy, R.D.: Cardiology in old age, New York, 1980, Raven Press.

2
CORONARY ARTERY DISEASE

Jennifer Williams
Andrew G. Wallace

Pathogenesis

Coronary artery disease and its complications are currently the leading cause of death in Europe and the Western hemisphere, responsible for 1.5 million heart attacks and 600,000 deaths in the United States each year.[1] Coronary artery disease and arteriosclerotic heart disease are essentially synonymous.

Arteriosclerosis means a chronic disease of the arteries characterized by abnormal thickening and hardening of the vessel walls resulting in loss of elasticity. Since there are several possible causes of the arteriosclerotic process, its manifestations differ according to the type of vessel involved and the site and extent of the disease within the vessel. It is convenient to categorize the disease into the following types:

Type I: Intimal atherosclerosis. This form of arteriosclerosis affects the internal membranes (intima) of arteries and consists of irregular thickening and plaque formation. Plaques consist of lipid, proliferating smooth muscle cells, and variable amounts of collagen. Intimal atherosclerosis affects primarily the large vessels, may begin at a very young age, and to some degree is almost universally present in people over the age of 20 years.[2]

Type II: Medial sclerosis. This process consists of calcification and hypertrophy of the muscular portion of the artery (media). It affects medium-sized blood vessels such as the brachial artery and the femoral artery, which become thickened, rigid, and tortuous. It is not necessarily associated with any reduction in the caliber of the involved vessel.[2]

Type III. Arteriolar sclerosis. This type of the disease affects small blood vessels and is characterized by hypertrophy of the muscular media and thickening of the intima; it is usually seen in patients with long-standing hypertension. It often affects the small vessels in the fundus of the eye and in the kidney.[2]

Although these three types of arteriosclerosis may exist separately, there is in fact considerable overlap. Type I, or intimal atherosclerosis, is the cause of most coronary artery disease but may be aggravated or accelerated by coexisting hypertension.

The natural history of coronary artery disease has three phases. The first phase begins with injury to the intimal endothelium, which may either heal or progress to the second phase. The second phase is the response to injury: blood platelets and other plasma constituents adhere to the site of injury, inducing proliferation of smooth muscle cells, and lipid accumulates abnormally in the arterial intima. At the earliest (and still reversible) part of this stage only a fatty streak may be produced. With more severe involvement, however, massive amounts of lipid, extensive smooth muscle proliferation, and the influx of cells such as macrophages and collagen-producing fibroblasts may combine to produce a full-blown atherosclerotic plaque. Although mature atherosclerotic lesions may occasionally regress, the usual course is a variable progressive encroachment upon the lumen of the affected artery. The third phase in the natural history of coronary artery disease is the production of clinically manifest symptoms, either angina pectoris, myocardial infarction, or, all too frequently, sudden cardiac death.[3]

Different factors may contribute to the development of clinically evident heart disease during each of these three phases. For example, homocysteine, which accumulates in patients with congenital homocystinuria, a genetic disorder characterized by the early onset of severe and diffuse atherosclerosis, has been shown to produce diffuse sites of endothelial injury. Carbon monoxide inhaled during cigarette smoking may work through similar mechanisms. On the other hand, excessive levels of β-lipoprotein probably produce accelerated atherosclerosis by increasing the accumulation of lipid at the sites of endothelial injury. Finally, other poorly identified factors must exist to explain the tremendous variability in longevity and clinical symptoms among subjects with equivalent amounts of coronary artery disease.

A number of pathologic events, either gradual or sudden, may affect the clinical course of coronary artery disease. Usually a plaque enlarges slowly and gradually as fat is deposited and scar tissue develops. Sometimes blood vessels that grow into the fibrous plaque rupture, producing small hemorrhages. Such subintimal hemorrhages increase the size of the plaque and are frequently followed by scarring and fibrosis, which further enlarge the lesion. Rupture of blood vessels within the plaque also could cause a sudden major obstruction of the lumen of the vessel. The intima covering a plaque may break, causing a small clot to form on the surface, which adds to the building obstruction of the vessel's lumen. The clot or plaque also may embolize and occlude the vessel where the lumen becomes narrow.

In addition to compromising blood supply by obstruction, the atherosclerotic process may cause weakening of the arterial wall and aneurysm formation. Thus obstruction and aneurysm may coexist in the same artery.

Gross pathology and prognosis

Atherosclerotic lesions usually form at branch points in the arterial tree. In the carotid and iliac arteries the disease is most prevalent at the bifurcation. Coronary arteries are particularly susceptible to atherosclerosis. Although it is unusual to have peripheral vascular disease without coronary artery involvement, coronary disease without involvement of peripheral arteries is not rare. In the coronary circulation, the atherosclerotic process is confined to the portions of the vessels that lie on the epicardial surface, sparing the arteries. Such a pattern of distribution suggests that turbulence of flow at branch points and rhythmic torsion of untethered vessels may contribute to the genesis of the lesion.

Several factors affect the prognosis of patients with coronary atherosclerosis, and the most important is the number of major coronary vessels with obstructions exceeding 75% of the vascular lumen. Persons with only one involved vessel have annual mortality rates of only 1% to 3%, whereas death rates approach 10% to 15% in persons with three-vessel disease, and up to 25% to 30% in persons with a high-grade obstruction of the left main coronary artery.[4] Coronary artery disease occurs most frequently in the left anterior descending artery, less in the right coronary artery, and less frequently (although not rarely) in the circumflex artery. Narrowing tends to be most severe in the proximal 2 to 3 cm of each artery, but distal involvement, particularly of the right coronary artery, is not uncommon. The site of vessel obstruction is clinically important, since proximal lesions are much more amenable to therapy by saphenous vein grafting or by percutaneous transluminal coronary angioplasty with balloon-type catheters. In almost all cases of myocardial infarction examined pathologically, the vessel supplying the infarcted area demonstrated a lesion of 95% or greater. Thus significant disease of the right coronary artery is found in patients with inferior myocardial infarction and disease of the left anterior descending artery in patients with anterior infarction.[5]

A second factor with prognostic importance for the patient with coronary artery disease is the contractile function of the left ventricle, which is determined largely by the amount of muscle tissue damaged by previous myocardial infarction. Subjects with good ventricular function have a much better prognosis than those with impaired function and equivalent degrees of coronary obstruction. Exceptions to these general rules include disabling angina pectoris, myocardial infarction, or sudden cardiac death in subjects with only single-vessel disease and severe three-vessel involvement in mostly asymptomatic persons.

Insidious at its onset, coronary atherosclerosis may be without symptoms for many years until the disease process produces a degree of obstruction that interferes with the arterial blood supply to the myocardium. If the obstruction progresses gradually over a period of years, intercoronary collateral circulation may develop, and clinical evidence of disease may be deferred or never occur. Despite marked obstructive disease, the myocardial cells may receive adequate oxygen regardless of demands. On the other hand, when an artery is partially obstructed and sufficient collateral circulation has not yet developed, the obstruction may impair blood flow during conditions of increased demand, producing symptoms of intermittent vascular insufficiency.

Incidence, prevalence, morbidity, and mortality

In 1979 the American Heart Association estimated that 4.19 million persons in the United States had coronary artery disease. Of the nearly 40 million Americans with some form of cardiovascular disease, coronary artery disease ranked second to hypertensive heart disease in prevalence. Of the approximately 600,000 who die annually from heart attacks, sudden death is the first clinical manifestation in 20% to 25% of the first events and is responsible for 50% to 60% of all heart attack deaths. Of those who die 25% are under the age of 65. Furthermore, two thirds of the deaths from heart attack occur outside of the hospital and within the first 2 hours of an acute attack.[1]

Risk factors

The mortality for coronary heart disease increased steadily in the 1950s, reached a plateau in the 1960s, and has steadily decreased 16% to 20% since 1968.[6] An important reason for this decline has been recognition and increased public awareness of cardiovascular risk factor. These have been identified in recent years by large-scale epidemiologic studies as factors that contribute to the development of coronary artery disease and that presumably contribute to atherosclerosis. Because several apparently unrelated risk factors can exist in a person, coronary atherosclerosis is most likely a multifactorial disease, which probably develops when more than one factor exists over a long period of time. In this context risk is viewed as the probability of developing coronary heart disease, and that probability is determined by the number of risk factors in any given individual, by the level of each factor (that is, the level of blood pressure, cholesterol, etc.) and by time (that is, age). The cumulative nature of risk factors is important to consider in the clinical evaluation of the patient. For example, a person who smokes and is hypertensive has approximately twice the risk as one who smokes and is normotensive.[7]

Risk factors are either primary or secondary. Primary factors are those that are thought to contribute to the development of coronary atherosclerosis, and secondary factors are those that are thought to enhance the risk of any specific manifestation of the disease (that is, arrhythmias, myocardial infarction, and so forth) in those who already have coronary atherosclerosis. Cigarettes and cholesterol clearly appear to be both primary and secondary risk factors. The likelihood of developing coronary heart disease is influenced by and can be predicted from many primary risk factors.

AGE, SEX, AND RACE

Atherosclerosis is more prevalent in older people. It is, however, a major cause of death in men of age 35 to 45 and causes 40% of the deaths in men of ages 55 to 64. In the United States the death rate is nearly six times higher in white men between 35 and 55 years of age than in white women of the same age. After menopause, however, the incidence of the disease in women rapidly approaches that in men. Prior to 1968 nonwhite males had lower death rates than white males. Since that time, however, nonwhite males have shown higher mortality up to the age of 65. Nonwhite females have higher mortality than white females.[8]

BLOOD PRESSURE

In the coronary heart disease study in Framingham, Massachusetts, middle-aged men with arterial pressures in excess of 160/95 showed a fivefold increase in the incidence of ischemic heart disease, compared with that in subjects having blood pressures of 140/90 or less.[9] A man with a systolic pressure over 150 has more than twice the risk of heart attack compared with a man with systolic pressure under 120. Both systolic and diastolic pressure elevations correlate positively with ischemic heart disease; systolic blood pressure often increases with age, but elevated systolic blood pressure is still a risk factor in the elderly.[8]

HYPERLIPIDEMIA AND DIET

The lipids in the plasma that are of general importance are cholesterol, triglycerides, and free fatty acids. Cholesterol has been measured more extensively than the other lipids and, when its level is elevated, it is associated with increased incidence of coronary heart disease.[10] Cholesterol and triglycerides are insoluble in plasma and therefore must be transported by lipoproteins, which are soluble. These lipoproteins can be separated and measured. In the fasting state very low–density lipoproteins (VLDL) carry mostly triglyceride and lesser amounts of cholesterol. Low-density lipoproteins (LDL) are derived from the metabolism of VLDL and carry most of the cholesterol in plasma. High-density lipoproteins (HDL) are mostly protein and carry about 35% cholesterol. Recent epidemiologic studies[11] have shown that the relationship between total serum cholesterol and risk of coronary atherosclerosis is even stronger if LDL cholesterol levels are high. A high ratio of HDL to LDL conveys protection against vascular disease. The significance of these associations is heightened by pathophysiologic studies that have shown that high levels of LDL cholesterol damage the endothelial lining of vessels and promote a proliferation of both smooth muscle cells and other components of the atherosclerotic lesion.[12] Among patients with premature atherosclerosis the two most common patterns of hyperlipidemia are type IV (elevated level of triglycerides with a normal or only slightly elevated level of cholesterol) due to increased VLDL, and type II (elevated levels of cholesterol with normal or only slightly elevated levels of triglyceride) due to increased LDL. Dietary and pharmacologic methods are moderately effective in lowering serum cholesterol and triglyceride.

Only recently have the effects of treatment on HDL and LDL been explored in detail. Population studies have shown a relationship between the fat content of the diet and serum lipids, both in individuals and whole countries. In 1979 the twenty-nation study[13] examined the relationship between the calories from fat and high-cholesterol animal products and the risk of coronary heart disease mortality for whole countries. The United States, Finland, New Zealand, Australia, and the United Kingdom led the list of countries consuming the most calories from these products and have the most deaths from coronary heart disease. Conversely, Japan had the least fat-related calories and the lowest mortality. Studies are currently underway to determine if lowering serum lipids in humans causes regression of or prevents atherosclerosis, but conclusive results are not yet available.

SMOKING

The relationship between cigarette smoking and the development of coronary heart disease is clear. Statistical evidence supports a mean increase of about 75% in the death rate from coronary artery disease in middle-aged men who smoke one pack of cigarettes per day when compared with nonsmokers.[6] This percentage decreases with advancing age, and the relationship is less firm in women. Pipe and cigar smokers do not have an increased risk, probably because they do not inhale. The chief effects of nicotine upon the cardiovascular system are cardiac stimulation and peripheral vasoconstriction. The former results in an increase in heart rate, stroke volume, cardiac output, and cardiac work. The peripheral vasoconstriction caused by nicotine is not greater in patients with vascular disease than in normal persons, but the resultant decrease in blood flow is more conspicuous in the patient with circulatory impairment and enhances the ischemia already present. With smoking, carbon monoxide levels of possibly 5% or more accumulate in the blood. The chief effects of carbon monoxide are interference with oxygen binding to hemoglobin and decrease in the threshold for ventricular fibrillation. It has also recently been found to be associated with a decrease of HDL.

GLUCOSE INTOLERANCE

Coronary heart disease is more prevalent in patients with adult onset diabetes mellitus, although the precise mechanism is unclear. It may be that insulin reacts to lipid metabolism or modifies the response of the artery to its environment. Diabetic patients have an increased tendency toward degeneration of connective tissue, which may make them more prone to atheroma formation. Men with a glucose intolerance have a 50% greater risk of developing coronary artery disease than those without it.[8]

PHYSICAL INACTIVITY

Many studies in the past have suggested that physical inactivity is associated with an increased risk of coronary heart disease. However, the strength of the relationship was low and, after correcting for other inequalities between active and inactive subjects, physical inactivity was generally regarded as a minor risk factor. One problem with most of these studies was the lack of a precise method to measure activity. More recently, a careful study[14] of California longshoremen demonstrated a strong inverse relationship between energy expenditure at work (excessive calorie expenditure) and the incidence of fatal and nonfatal heart attacks. The reduced risk was evident in all age groups, but was most striking in the young and was still evident after correcting for excess weight, smoking patterns, and serum cholesterol. The most significant finding of this study of over 3000 men was that habitual expenditure of about 1800 calories per day above basal level through physically demanding work reduced by nearly 50% the incidence of fatal heart attacks compared with those who expended less than 1000 calories per day above basal level. The Harvard alumni study in 1978 extended the longshoremen data, finding a progressive decrease in risk with increased activity up to 2000 calories per week despite other risk factors.[15]

PERSONALITY FACTORS

For many years coronary heart disease has been thought to be more prominent among individuals subject to chronic anxiety or stress. Subsequently a personality type related to coronary heart disease, called type A, was identified. The characteristics of the type A behavioral pattern include: aggressiveness, ambition, competitive drive, and chronic sense of urgency (see Chapter 13). The report of a western collaborative study showed that the incidence of coronary heart disease was two times higher in type A individuals than in type B (having these traits to a lesser degree) even after correcting for other risk factors.[16] These observations are of considerable interest, but a link between the type A personality and the pathophysiology of coronary atherosclerosis remains to be defined. Furthermore, it remains to be shown that modification of behavioral patterns will be possible or effective in altering risk.

OBESITY

Although this is a controversial issue, most epidemiologic studies show a positive relationship between obesity (any weight greater than 20% over ideal weight) and morbidity and mortality from coronary heart disease. It has been primarily considered as a risk in conjunction with its effects on other characteristics such as hypertension; but current data suggest that obesity makes an independent contribution to coronary heart disease risk, at least up to 50 years of age.[8]

OTHER RISK FACTORS

Additional factors associated with increased risk of coronary heart disease are electrocardiographic abnormalities at rest and in response to exercise and hyperuricemia. Some major risk factors may be determined by familial or genetic factors. The tendency toward development of hypertension, diabetes, and hyperlipidemia may be inherited in a familial manner. Also, certain life-styles such as smoking, overeating, and lack of exercise may be passed down in a family. There also may be other inherited traits, currently immeasurable, that affect one's risk. It is vitally important to recognize that risk is multifactorial, that the influence of two or more factors may be synergistic, and that risk is influenced by any given factor's degree of abnormality—not just its presence or absence. The emphasis for the future is on primary prevention, which includes risk factor education, basic research support, and acceptance by the public of responsibility for their own health maintenance. See Chapter 3 for discussion of preventive strategies. Secondary risk factors, including myocardial infarction and arrhythmias, will be discussed in subsequent chapters.

REFERENCES

1. American Heart Association: Heart facts, 1979, American Heart Association.
2. McGill, H.C.: The geographic pathology of atherosclerosis, Lab. Invest. **18**:463, 1968.
3. Wolintsky, H.: A new look at atherosclerosis, Cardiovasc. Med. **1**:41, 1976.
4. Stamler, J.: Epidemiology of coronary heart disease, Med. Clin. North Am. **1**:1973.
5. Roberts, W.C.: Coronary arteries in fatal acute myocardial infarction, Circulation **45**:215, 1972.
6. Levy, R.I.: Progress toward prevention of cardiovascular disease—a 30-year retrospective, Circulation **60**:1555, 1979.
7. Kannel, W., and Gordon, T.: Evaluation of cardiovascular risk in the elderly: the Framingham Study, Bull. N.Y. Acad. Med. **54**:573, 1978.
8. Levy, R.I., and Feinleib, M.: Risk factors for coronary artery disease and their management. In Braunwald, E., editor: Heart disease: a textbook of cardiac medicine, Philadelphia, 1980, W.B. Saunders Co.

9. Kannel, W.: Coronary risk factors: the Framingham Study, J. Occup. Med. **9:**611, 1967.

10. Kannel, W.W., and others: Serum cholesterol, lipoproteins, and the risk of coronary heart disease: the Framingham Study, Ann. Intern. Med. **74:**1, 1971.

11. Gordon, T., and others: High density lipoprotein as a protective factor against coronary heart disease, Am. J. Med. **62:**707, 1977.

12. Goldstein, J.L., and Brown, M.S.: The low-density lipoprotein pathway and its relation to atherosclerosis, Annu. Rev. Biochem. **46:**897, 1977.

13. Stamler, J.: Research related to risk factors, Circulation **60:**1575, 1979.

14. Paffenbarger, R.S.: Physical activity and fatal heart attack: protection or selection. In Amsterdam, E., and others, editors: Exercise in cardiovascular health and disease, New York, 1977, Yorke Medical Books.

15. Paffenbarger, R.S., and others: Physical activity as an index of heart attack risk in college alumni, Am. J. Epidemiol. **108:**161, 1978.

16. Friedman, M., and others: The relationship of behavior pattern A to the state of the coronary vasculature, Am. J. Med. **44:**525, 1968.

3

PREVENTIVE STRATEGIES FOR CORONARY ARTERY DISEASE

Kathleen Gainor Andreoli
Virginia Kliner Fowkes

One of the most serious problems facing the American health care delivery system is the continuously rising cost of health care. Between 1965 and 1978 this cost escalated at an annual rate of 10% to 14%.[1] In 1965, $43 billion were spent for health purposes, representing 6.2% of that year's gross national product (GNP). By contrast, in 1980 health care consumed almost 10% of the GNP, or $240 billion.[2] If current trends continue, the health costs will rise to $1 trillion, or about 12% of the GNP, by the year 2000.[3] Clearly, steps must be taken to curb this inflationary phenomenon.

Since the greatest proportion of the health care bill belongs to hospitals and medical services, it appears that cost-effective results may be obtained more by preventing the development of disease or disability than by managing the consequences. In the United States the major causes of death and disability in adults are chronic diseases, in particular the cardiovascular diseases and cancer (Fig. 3-1). Heart disease is the greatest cause of permanent disability claims among workers under 65 and is responsible for more days of hospitalization than any other single disorder. It is the principal cause of limited activity for about 2.5 million Americans under the age of 65.[4] Premature ischemic heart disease is overall the most costly and common of the complications of atherosclerosis.[5]

The methods of preventing coronary heart disease may be categorized into primary and secondary approaches, both involving specific strategies to reduce the *risks* of developing disease.

Primary preventive strategies are those implemented before overt manifestations of disease occur in normal or high-risk individuals. Examples of this group include behavior changes such as ceasing to smoke or beginning an exercise program. Also included are therapeutic strategies for high-risk persons, such as administering cholestyramine to an individual with hypercholesterolemia.

Secondary strategies are used after the onset of disease. These may include Coronary Care Unit therapy and/or use of a beta blocking agent following myocardial infarction to reduce further risk. The enormous health, social, and economic dimensions of coronary artery disease call for serious and urgent consideration of measures necessary to prevent atherosclerosis. Since the cause of this

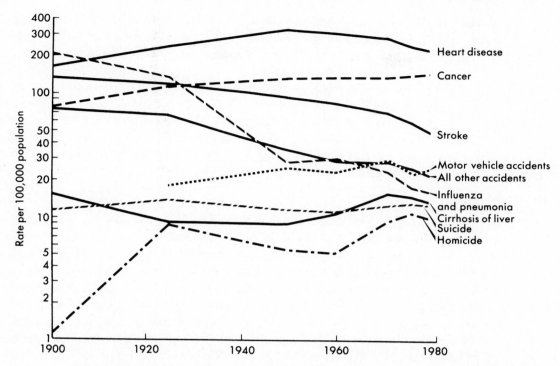

Fig. 3-1. Trends in age-adjusted death rates from selected causes: selected years, 1900-1978. (Rate per 100,000 population.) The selected years are 1900, 1925, 1950, 1960, 1970, and 1978. (Based on data from DHHS, Healthy people: the Surgeon General's report on health promotion and disease prevention, 1979; NCHS, Special report on diabetes, vol. 43, no. 12, 1956; NCHS, Vital statistics special report, vol. 43, no. 3, 1956.)

disorder is not known, the focus of a preventive program must begin with the human characteristics associated with its onset.

This chapter focuses on primary preventive strategies for the general population. Later chapters address secondary level programs.

Health

In American society, health and illness have become symbols for many positively and negatively valued social, cultural, and metaphysical phenomena.[6] For example, it is not unusual to hear a circumstance described as a "healthy state of affairs" or a "sick system." The concept of health invokes a reality that is regarded as eminently desirable. When one is in good health, it is not even noticed; when one is not, it is desperately desired.[7]

It seems to be taken for granted that everyone knows the meaning of "health." Attempts have been made, however, to define the term. For example, the World Health Organization has defined it as "a state of complete physical, mental, and social well-being and not merely the absence of disease or infirmity." The emphasis in this definition on "complete" puts health care providers and society in the untenable position of being required to attain the impossible.[7] Instead, health should be seen as an individual phenomenon related to a person's ability to adapt to biologic, psychologic, and social changes in a manner which allows the individual to function at an optimal level of well-being in his or her environment. Wellness is a dynamic state in which an individual progresses toward a higher level of functioning, thus maximizing his or her potential in the environment.

Factors that determine or affect health include environment, behavior, medical care, and heredity.[8] The concept of health has intellectual, emotional, physical, social, occupational, and spiritual dimensions. The balance between health and illness depends upon both strength of individual resistance and the stressors encountered. Stressors can be physical or psychologic, including the lack of adequate nutrition, physical exercise, or a meaningful purpose and value in life.[9]

Health promotion

According to Knowles,[10] over 99% of American people are born healthy and suffer premature death and disability as a result of personal misbehavior and environmental conditions. If American health is to be maintained at its optimal level, then it is clear that individuals will have to recognize unhealthy habits and adopt life-styles that will assist them in adapting to change and functioning at an optimal level of well-being in the environment. Health promotion is directed toward people who are basically healthy; it seeks to develop individual and community measures that facilitate the development of life-styles that can enhance and maintain the state of well-being.[4] Methods of health promotion include both passive and active strategies. Passive approaches are public health measures, such as water and sewage sanitation, by which the individual passively benefits. In contrast, active measures persuade the individual to adopt a given program of health promotion, which may include exercise or a stress management plan.[9] Health promotion efforts designed to prevent the onset of premature coronary artery disease consider the genetic endowment of the individual and include health protection services and health education.

HEALTH PROTECTION SERVICES

There are periodic preventive health services designed for different age and risk groups that provide screening for risk factors in addition to health education and counseling for well persons. The Lifetime Health Monitoring Program[11] is one model for preventive care that could be incorporated into existing patterns of health care practice. The program divides the population into 10 groups based upon different life-styles, health needs, and problems from infancy to old age. For each group overall health goals and professional services are prescribed that relate to the accomplishment of the goals. The health goal is optimal total functioning, and the services offered identify specific health measures as well as education and counseling. An example of health screening practices for selected groups is a test for detection of hyperlipidemia in all persons between 20 and 30 years of age, especially in young persons who have family histories of premature ischemic heart disease.[5] Routine blood pressure surveillance may be performed on women taking oral contraceptives, black males, and the elderly.

The periodic health examination may have a health risk appraisal, a technique which compares an individual's health-related behaviors and characteristics to mortality statistics and epidemiologic data to estimate his or her chance of dying by some specified future time.[12] Frequently, the appraisal includes a calculation of the amount of risk that can be eliminated by making appropriate behavioral changes. These estimations of risk and the potential benefits of changes in behavior are presented to the individual to stimulate his or her participation in activities aimed at changing life-style and improving health. The health risk appraisal has become popular recently for several reasons: (1) it provides the health educator with a rationale and teaching aid to focus discussions on health and behavior; (2) it identifies and measures health risk for the individual with potential for use in behavioral change; (3) it relies on self-administered questions, simple physiologic measurements, and computer-assisted calculations, making its application to large groups feasible, efficient, and, relative to a program in which health professionals administer the questionnaire, inexpensive.[12] It must be pointed out, however, that health hazard appraisal should be viewed with circumspection, since there is a paucity of evidence regarding its effectiveness on health-related behaviors, morbidity, and mortality.[13]

HEALTH EDUCATION

Health education is any combination of learning experiences designed to predispose the public toward, make available the means of, and reinforce the voluntary adaptation of behavior conducive to good health.[14] Consumers participate under their own direction in determining their health practices. Although health behavior is considered a voluntary activity, there are circumstances in which health behavior is mandated, as in "smoking" and "no smoking" sections of public places. When a behavior is judged by society to be hazardous to the common good, curtailment of individual choice is warranted.[14]

Health education programs aim to maintain positive health behavior or interrupt a behavioral pattern that is linked to increased risks, such as smoking cigarettes. Such programs must take into consideration the beliefs, values, attitudes, socioeconomic resources, educational levels, support systems, and availability of health care for a given population. The success of such a program is more likely to occur when the educator and client follow fundamental steps of planning such as the following: (1) assessing the client's present risk status for premature onset of coronary artery disease; (2) establishing mutual goals with the client for reducing risks, (3) reviewing and educating about the predisposing factors, (4) identifying the enabling factors that appear to exist, (5) assisting in the mobilization factors that reinforce the client's healthful behavior, (6) evaluating the effectiveness of the program, and (7) modifying the program on the basis of program evaluation data.

Risk reduction of cardiovascular disease
RISK FACTORS AND THE PREVENTION OF ATHEROSCLEROSIS

Certain conditions and habits appear more frequently in individuals who develop atherosclerosis than in the general population. These characteristics are considered risk factors and are discussed in detail in Chapter 2. Risk estimates are determined by comparing the frequency of death or illness from a specific cause in the population having some specific trait (risk factor) with the frequency in another population not having that trait, or in the population as a whole.[4] A single significant risk, such as lack of immunization, can be attributed to some diseases. Conversely, other diseases may involve many contributing factors, as exemplified by coronary artery disease and its contributing risks: uncontrolled hypertension, hyperlipidemia, diet, smoking, glucose intolerance, physical inactivity, stress, obesity, and others. A person with at least one risk factor is more likely to develop a clinical atherosclerotic event, and to do so earlier, than a person with no risk factors.[5] Risk factors add up, and risk increases. The development of atherosclerosis is accelerated by the presence of multiple risks. Recent evidence indicates that risk factor reduction appears to lessen the incidence of coronary artery disease.

Although an effective preventive program for atherosclerosis has not been established, enough is known to guide health professionals and the public both in the identification of persons at high risk for disease and in the development of measures to reduce that risk. For example, there is evidence that changes in life-style, such as following a few simple good health habits, can affect significantly the duration and quality of a person's life. In a series of studies[15,16] in Alameda County, California, findings showed substantial increases in the life spans of people who exercised regularly and vigorously, maintained normal weight, ate breakfast, did not snack between meals, avoided smoking, limited alcohol consumption, and slept at least 7 hours a night. A 45-year-old man who followed three or fewer of these seven routines could, on the average, expect to live to age 67. If he followed six or seven, he could expect to live to age 78. Also, women who practiced such habits lived longer than women who did not.

Other studies report that the incidence of certain risk factors declined during the same period that mortality rates for heart disease dropped. Between 1968 and 1978, the age-adjusted death rates for heart disease declined by 22.7%, and stroke deaths declined by 36.5%[17] (Fig. 3-1). The actual cause of the unprecedented decline in heart disease in the last decade is not entirely understood. According to Stern,[18] the available evidence implies that a portion of the decline may be due to improvements in diet with concomitant declines in serum cholesterol concentration, decreased cigarette smoking, improved hypertension control, and increased leisure-time physical exercises.

Although the role of diet in the development of coronary artery disease is not clear, it is interesting to note that during the twentieth century the consumption of animal fat decreased modestly while the consumption of vegetable fat increased dramatically.[19] The average serum cholesterol level in the United States has declined about 10 to 20 mg/dl during the last 10 to 15 years.[20] Moreover, during this same period there was a consistent decline of cigarette smoking in males with an overall decline from 53% to 37%.[21] For women less consistent declines were noted.

The results of the Hypertension Detection and Follow-up Program[22] initiated in 1973 showed a significant decline in mortality from all causes and showed clearly the benefits of treatment for persons with mild as well as moderate to severe high blood pressure.[17] This study involved 14 clinical centers and nearly 11,000 black and white hypertensive males and females between 30 and 69 years of age. These patients were randomly assigned to clinical centers for therapy, or they were referred to their usual sources of care. Considering deaths from all causes, the results revealed 5-year mortality reductions for those treated by the clinical centers as compared with those experiencing customary sources of treatment for hypertension.

According to Levy,[23] before the National Institutes of Health launched a National High Blood Pressure Education Program in 1972, only half of all Americans with high blood pressure knew they had it. Today, in certain communities surveyed, an estimated 70% are aware of their hypertension. Furthermore, patient visits for high blood pressure have increased since 1972 by 50%, suggesting that more people with hypertension are now being treated.

The foregoing discussion implies that reduction of the risk factors associated with the onset of coronary artery disease is possible and probably has healthful results. This information serves as an incentive to initiate a primary prevention program on a national scale to reduce the incidence of this costly disorder.

LIFE-STYLE CHANGE

Behavior modification is complex and may require a long period of time to be successful. Although many people are aware of the positive and negative predicted outcomes of personal health behavior, they often lack the readiness to act on that knowledge. For example, in spite of a rigorous public health education program on the hazards of smoking, many people continue to smoke cigarettes. Evidence suggests that 95% of smokers who successfully quit do so without outside pressure.[4] Four factors seem to contribute to this success: (1) health concerns (including symptoms), (2) a desire to set an example for others, (3) a desire for self-control, and (4) esthetic reasons such as breath odor and loss of taste for food. Motivation is a key to risk reduction, and the factors that move people to accept responsibility for reducing risks should be advertised in health education programs.

The most common examples of desirable life-style changes are these: (1) reduction of overweight, (2) increase of physical activity, (3) cessation of smoking, (4) moderation of alcohol consumption, (5) better nutrition, and (6) more effective stress management.[9]

A variety of educational methods and resources are available to support people in making life-style changes. These can be tailored for specific programs that are individualized, group, or public. Green and associates[14] provide a list of recommended teaching strategies including lectures, individual instruction, programmed learning, skill development, inquiry learning, peer-group discussions, modeling, behavior modification, simulations and games, audiovisual aids, educational television, social planning, and organizational change.

Achieving change in life-style involves a process of sequential stages. First, the person must become aware of the risk and accept that the behavior is harmful personally. Second, this knowledge must be integrated into the person's self-image. Finally, effort must be made to change and apply the new knowledge in sustaining the change in behavior.[9]

Health care providers should become knowledgeable about the process of promoting behavioral change and the professional and community resources available to support this effort. A few specific strategies follow.

STRESS MANAGEMENT

The relationship of stress to the development or progression of cardiovascular disease is not well established. The type A behavior pattern and other psychosocial and behavioral precursors of coronary disease are described in Chapter 13. Stress is an aggravating factor contributing to a number of risks. For example, many people smoke in response to stress. Stress is experienced in a variety of ways, including muscle tightness, stomach discomfort, feelings of tension and anxiety, or physical symptoms such as tachycardia or diaphoresis. Managing one's stress can be helpful in weight reduction and cessation of smoking, and it may facilitate control of blood pressure.

Farquhar[24] describes an approach to management of stress and other lifestyle changes as a six-step process:

1. Identify the kinds of stress one experiences and explore the barriers to change. This involves deciphering the process, its effect on the body, and any attitudes or beliefs that may interfere with change.
2. Build confidence and commitment to change. This includes goal-setting and self-contracts to modify behavior.
3. Become increasingly aware of the sources of stress and responses to them. Keep a careful record of the stress experienced, the time of day, in which circumstances it occurred, and the feelings and responses it precipitated.
4. Develop a stress management plan (such as the one outlined on the opposite page). This involves practicing deep muscle and mental relaxation exercises once or twice daily. Visualization techniques such as imagining a quiet, peaceful place or sensation of warmth and light are helpful in achieving a relaxation for all body areas.
5. Evaluate the stress management plan. Compare progress against goals and adjust them as necessary.
6. Maintain the management of stress through daily exercise and practice. Relaxation exercises, such as those described, have been found to lower the blood pressure. The blood pressure remains lowered for the duration of the program, but a lasting effect has yet to be determined. There are no long-term studies available to document the effect of relaxation on blood pressures.[25] Most individuals perceive an increased sense of well-being and find activities of daily life more enjoyable and easier to handle.

EXERCISE

Evidence of the relationship between exercise and reduced cardiovascular risk comes from a study of 17,000 Harvard alumni.[4] Regular, vigorous exercise was found to reduce the risk of heart disease regardless of other risk factors such as cigarette smoking or high blood pressure. The effects of exercise on cardiovascular health are discussed in Chapter 14. Briefly, regular exercise facilitates weight control, increases HDL, and lowers blood pressure. Individuals who exercise regularly are more likely to have other healthy habits that lower risk, such as eating less, coping more effectively with stress, and avoiding smoking.

Aerobic exercise or sustained physical activity for a minimum of 15 to 20 minutes three or four times each week contributes to cardiovascular conditioning.

Deep muscle relaxation drill

1. Find a quiet environment. Lie on your back in a comfortable position or sit comfortably. Close your eyes.
2. For right-handed people, begin by physically tensing the right hand for an instant, then relaxing it and letting it go loose. Tell your hand to feel heavy and warm. Continue with the rest of the right side of the body, moving up to forearm, upper arm, shoulder, then down to the foot, lower leg, and upper leg. Next, follow the same procedure on the left side of the body. (If you are left-handed, begin the procedure with the left hand and continue.) The hands, arms, and legs should feel relaxed, heavy, and warm. Wait for these feelings. After mastering the technique, you will not need to tense your muscles before relaxing them.
3. Next, relax the muscles of the hips and let a wave of relaxation pass up from the abdomen to the chest. Do not tense these muscles. Tell them to feel heavy and warm. Your breathing will come more from the chest and will be slower. Wait for this breathing change.
4. Now let the wave of relaxation continue into the shoulders, neck, jaw, and the muscles of the face. Pay special attention to the muscles controlling the eyes and forehead. Finish the drill by telling your forehead to feel cool.

Mental relaxation drill

After entering a state of deep muscle relaxation, you are ready to begin the mental process that deepens the relaxation state. Your eyes are closed and your forehead is cool.

1. Enter a passive state; let thoughts flow through your head.
2. If thoughts recur, respond by saying "no" under your breath.
3. Imagine a calm sky or sea or any blue area or object without detail (with your eyes closed). Try to see the color blue (which has been found to be a particularly relaxing color).
4. Become aware of your slow, natural breathing. Follow each breath as you inhale and exhale.
5. If you still do not feel calm and rested, you may find it helpful to use a repeated, soothing word (such as "love" or "God") or a less symbolic word (such as "now" or "breath"). If you find that using a word distracts you, try a sound (such as "ah"). Think of the word or sound silently, preferably during exhalation. Always remind yourself to keep the muscles of the face, eyes, and forehead loose; and to keep your forehead cool.

These exercises are usually done together to achieve relaxation.

Reprinted from THE AMERICAN WAY OF LIFE NEED NOT BE HAZARDOUS TO YOUR HEALTH by John W. Farquhar, M.D., by permission of W.W. Norton & Company, Inc. Copyright © 1978 by John W. Farquhar.

Aerobic exercise may be done with brisk walking, dancing, jogging, running, swimming, cross-country skiing, bicycling, or tennis.[24]

In assessing readiness for an exercise program, Farquhar[24] recommends that individuals over 40 years of age have a physical examination and exercise ECG. Following assessment and readiness, the same six steps described under stress management can be modified for the development of an exercise program.

DIET

Typical American eating habits also contribute to health risks. The average American consumes 12 g of salt each day, despite the fact that studies have demonstrated that high salt intake contributes to an elevated blood pressure and that reduction of salt intake can lower the blood pressure. High cholesterol levels have been associated with intake of saturated fats. The overconsumption of sugar also is deleterious; refined sugar increases the blood triglyceride levels and requires an increased amount of insulin. Foods with high sugar content also have high calorie concentration and contribute to weight increase. On the other hand, diets high in fiber content are associated with low incidence of cardiovascular disease as well as certain cancers,[24] and the fat-modified diet is recommended for patients with hypercholesterolemia. National recommendations for dietary goals come from the Select Committee on Nutrition and Human Needs of the United States Senate.[26] They are summarized as follows:

Reduce fat consumption to 30% of total calories.

Reduce saturated fat consumption to 10% of total calories.

Balance monounsaturated and polyunsaturated fat intake to 10% of total calories.

Reduce cholesterol intake to about 300 mg daily.

Increase complex carbohydrate consumption to 48% of total calories.

Reduce sugar consumption to 10% of total calories.

Reduce salt consumption to 5 g daily.

Again, the same six-step process discussed under stress management can be adapted to an individual to modify eating habits.

SMOKING

Smoking has been established firmly as a risk factor in cardiovascular disease (Chapter 2). Cessation of smoking reduces the risk, since the cardiovascualr damage caused by smoking is reversible.[24]

To assist in stopping smoking, the six-step process may again be employed. Careful attention to one's patterns of smoking develops awareness of one's need to smoke. Substitutes, tapering, and other support can then be used to assist in cessation.

Health promotion in the community

Preventive strategies can be implemented singularly or in combination in a number of settings such as the home, school, and work site, and through community and national health information programs.

HOME

Early health habits are learned and health values are developed at home. Behavior learned there includes eating habits, exercise, smoking, use of alcohol, attitudes that relate to self-confidence and to society, management of stress, involvement with others, and decision-making abilities.[27] If parents set examples conducive to health, children are more likely to assume a healthy life-style than if the opposite is true.

An example of the importance of the home influence can be illustrated in the development of eating habits. Approximately one third of today's obese adults were overweight children.[4] Furthermore, an obese child is at least three times more likely than a normal-weight child to be an obese adult. Since obesity is more difficult to correct in adults than in children, major preventive efforts initiated in the home must be directed toward children. In apparently healthy teenagers there is evidence of coronary atherosclerosis that had its beginnings in childhood.[4] Limiting animal fat consumption and encouraging exercise in children may contribute to the reduction of blood fat levels and therefore reduce the likelihood of developing premature coronary artery disease.

Smoking has deleterious effects in the home. Children of smoking parents are more likely to have upper respiratory tract infections. Since children spend most of their young lives under the influence of home and school, there should be an overlap between the two settings in contributing to the development of children's healthful behavior patterns.

SCHOOLS

More than 40 million children and young people spend a large part of their time in school.[27] Thus schools are a natural focal point for health education and health practice; required enrollment creates a large captive audience.[28] Instead, for the most part, schools neglect health instruction. According to Knowles,[10] the current state of student health programs at all levels—elementary, high school, and institutions of higher education—leaves much to be desired:

> Student health programs are abysmal at best, confining themselves to preemptory sick calls and posters on brushing teeth and eating three meals a day; there are no examinations to determine if anything's been learned. Awareness of danger to body and mind is not acquired until the mid-twenties in our culture. . . . Children tire of 'scrub your teeth', 'don't eat that junk', 'leave your dingy alone', 'go to bed', and 'get some exercise.' By the time they are sixteen, society says that they should have cars, drink beer, smoke, eat junk at drive-ins, and have a go at fornication. (p. 60)

Frequently, when health education is provided in schools, it is treated as an afterthought tacked onto another subject such as biology or physical education. Exercise is centered on organized team sports rather than on individual activities that children can carry into adult life. Some school systems have abandoned these time-worn approaches to health education and have begun to treat healthful behavior as a positive force in the students' lives, but this is the exception rather than the rule.

Inasmuch as lifelong behavior patterns and development of chronic disease both have their roots in childhood, health education in schools is an essential component of primary prevention for premature coronary artery disease. Children and young people should learn to appreciate the body as their greatest natural resource in life, uniquely owned by themselves, and influenced by the choices they make throughout life.

The onset of puberty is an especially vulnerable time for children, since developmentally they are establishing their independence. Peer pressure becomes a way of life. Young students exposed to older students experience more frequent opportunities to smoke or drink and a social environment that favors these acts as symbols of adulthood and freedom.[29] To resist pressure successfully and overcome susceptibilities, young people need training in social and psychologic skills.

Schools could provide assertiveness training, including role playing and social reinforcement, to teach adolescents verbal and cognitive strategies for handling situations in which they might be pressured to assume unhealthful behavior.[29]

Through education children also can learn how to analyze critically television programs and commercials, which are prominent sources of inaccurate health information. Furthermore, schools should provide physical fitness and exercise programs that emphasize activities for all persons rather than just competitive sports. Children should be educated not only about how to achieve and maintain health for themselves, but also about how to work for a healthier community. Personal and social health is an aspect of good citizenship.

There are notable programs[27] promoting health for school-age children. The Opendoor Health Enrichment Project at the University of South Carolina is a peer education program designed to raise health awareness among students, using peer educators, health awareness seminars, self-help mutual support groups, and other strategies to help students achieve high-level health. The American Nurses' Foundation in Kansas sponsors a "you-the-scientist" approach to teach students to measure their own risk factors and learn how to control them. The Wayne County Cancer Society has involved over 250,000 children and young people in primary and secondary grades in a program in which high school students educate the younger children about the dangers of smoking and teach sound health habits.

WORK SITE

A safe assumption is that employers will always be interested in high employee productivity, increased work attendance, reduction in workers' compensation claims, and improved "health age" of their workers. Since complications of coronary artery disease occur for the most part in adults, and more than 97 million adult Americans are at work each day,[27] the work site becomes an ideal setting for offering preventive health service and health education programs aimed at the prevention of coronary artery disease.

Many employers have initiated work site health promotion programs involving health education, stress management, physical fitness, weight control, smoking cessation, risk appraisal, and the like. Some companies provide high blood pressure detection and treatment service at the work site with a systematic program for follow-up.

There are several good examples of work site health promotion programs.[27] The Ford Motor Company sponsors a cardiovascular risk reduction and intervention program at its world headquarters in Dearborn, Michigan. This program includes testing, assessment of risk, and group sessions to motivate employees to take steps to lower their risk factors. National ChemSearch in Dallas, Texas, has a program for employee fitness, which includes walking, jogging, cross-country running, swimming, aerobic dancing, weight training, and advice on stress, nutrition, and the like. The Model Wellness Project for employees at the University of South Carolina is a pilot project using health hazard appraisal, physical assessment, wellness seminars, self-help groups, and social activities to bring about weight loss, improved fitness, stress reduction, increased productivity, and self-esteem. The Government Employees Insurance Company of Washington, D.C., awards a day off with pay to any employee who does not gain weight during a 6-month period.[28]

COMMUNITY

The future health of people of the United States will not depend upon individualized health plans, but rather on plans that involve communities, where health changes are seen as vital statistics. A major problem in community health, however, is how to reach those most in need of health counseling, that is, the underserved people characterized by poverty and poor education. There are 34 million people in the United States who are classified as underserved; half of these live in urban settings, the rest in rural areas.[30] These people, marked by higher mortality and morbidity, fare much worse than the rest of the population.[31]

There are some community primary prevention programs that have been successful. For example, the Health Education Center in Pittsburgh, a United Way agency, serves a 10-county region and fulfills two major functions in health education: (1) communications and information through telephone tapes on health topics, and (2) health education programs for schools, YMCAs, and workplaces.

The Stanford Health Disease Prevention Program[32,33] was a 2-year experiment in three northern California communities to determine whether an intensive education campaign could reduce cigarette smoking, blood cholesterol levels, and high blood pressure. Two communities were exposed to a mass media campaign designed to influence adults to change their living habits in ways that could reduce the risk of heart attack and stroke. In one of these towns, the media campaign was supplemented with intensive face-to-face instruction for people identified as high risk. A third community, which was relatively isolated from the media shared by the other two communities, served as a control.

After 2 years the overall risk of cardiovascular disease in the control community increased about 7%, whereas in the other two towns there was a substantial (15% to 20%) decrease in risk. In the community that had the media campaign plus personal instruction, the initial improvement was greater than in the other experimental town, and health education was more successful in reducing cigarette smoking. At the end of the second year the decrease in risk was roughly the same in both experimental communities. The conclusions were that intensive face-to-face instruction and counseling seem important for changing such behaviors as smoking and inadequate diet; however, where resources are limited, mass media education campaigns are an effective influence in reducing the risk of cardiovascular disease.

Reaching everyone in the community on a face-to-face basis is not always possible or desirable from a cost effective viewpoint. Thus considerable interest has developed in the area of educational media, on the premise that media programs can usually reach more learners at less cost than the traditional methods. This is an excellent way to reach people in rural and inner-city communities.

Communities need a well-designed motivational media program in combination with follow-up by a health educator to answer questions, discuss ideas, and share experiences. An excellent way to introduce health information into homes with an after-the-show phone and personal follow-up is through cable television with a patient education channel.[34] The media have a strong influence on the way Americans behave and perceive the world, since they reach into almost every home and are accessible at any hour. The media not only push attitudes and products, they also reflect community feelings, and they will transmit healthier messages if they learn the community is interested.[27]

NATIONAL HEALTH INFORMATION PROGRAMS

Both the government and the private sector have important responsibilities in national health education. As discussed previously, the government-sponsored National High Blood Pressure Education Program increased awareness about hypertension and may have influenced hypertensive people to seek medical care for their disease. There are about 70 private organizations affiliated with the National Health Council, the majority of which are engaged in some type of health education aimed at broad segments of the population.[35] The National Clearinghouse on Smoking and Health has implemented a rigorous educational program for smoking cessation, and legislation has promoted consumer choice by labeling foods for sodium and caloric content as well as by labeling cigarettes as health hazards. Voluntary organizations such as the American Heart Association have been notable in their sponsorship of primary prevention programs for coronary artery disease. Thus the informed consumer becomes the moving force in a successful health promotion program. What impact healthful life-style changes will have on the public's health, however, remains to be determined through research.

Costs

The role of third party payers in the reimbursement of preventive health promotion services is critical to widespread application of these concepts. Over the past 4 years there has been an increasing trend to reimburse for preventive services; however, this varies among insurers.

In the current health care delivery system, which is dominated by a fee-for-service mode, health maintenance organizations are the only system with built-in incentives to emphasize preventive services. However, traditional approaches such as multiphasic screening have not proven cost-effective, and even though the rhetoric exists, there has not been widespread utilization of preventive services.[36]

In the absence of national policy on disease prevention or health promotion, and given a national system of resource allocation,[35] these services must be couched within other acute or primary care regimens. The costs and benefits to the consumer or community as a whole must be weighed carefully. Services for the treatment of disease currently control the greater portion of the health care dollar. Health promotion services need the same trial evaluation to determine the most cost-efficient and effective measures to prevent morbidity. Costs need to be evaluated in terms of expense to the consumer, payer, and public and measured against long-term results achieved by the specific intervention.

Research needs in health promotion

A comprehensive approach to health promotion has been decribed as an essential part of a primary prevention program directed against premature onset of coronary artery disease. Given the acceptance of disease prevention and health promotion by the American people, the scientific base upon which these concepts rest must be strengthened; program evaluation techniques must be refined; ways must be found to allocate resources fairly; the needs of special populations must be accommodated; new organizational structures must be developed—all these, and many more issues, must be carefully and intelligently considered for all levels of society.[27]

Preventive strategies must be tested through longitudinal, multidisciplinary, invasive studies of the intersection of high-risk groups and high-risk situations against control groups.[37] Research is also needed to identify the developmental determinants of unhealthful behavior during childhood and adolescence. For example, if it were possible to identify individuals whose genetic constitution makes them more susceptible to the harm associated with unhealthful behavior, then efforts to change behavior could be focused on persons at greatest risk, rather than on society at large.[38]

Many of the ramifications of health education are still unknown, such as its impact on health practices and outcomes. There are questions needing study. What kinds of national education models will work most effectively on the heterogeneous U.S. population? Will benefits accrue rapidly or slowly? Will they be temporary or permanent? Will they occur in the general population or only in high-risk groups?[39] Unfortunately, there are still continuing weaknesses in the evaluation of patient education: oversimplification of the behavior and causes of behavior that must be influenced by patient education; failure to make explicit the theoretical or assumed connection between educational interventions and behavioral or health results; and limited analyses of data, which leave many questions untouched.[40]

The approach to evaluation of patient education must present a theoretical rationale for the strategy, a conceptual model in the practice of patient education, and the education program itself.[41] For example, the theoretical rationale for self-management should focus on a set of learnable skills for processes brought together to influence a specific behavior. This reciprocal interaction theory involves three factors: (1) persons with individual goals, perceptions, emotions, and values, (2) the environment, with influences from peer group and family, and customs and standards, and (3) action taken by the person to change behavior. Another important point is that evaluation of patient education usually takes place in real life situations, not in social science laboratories or other artificial environments.[42]

Clearly, successful health education programs offer great promise; consumers will assume more responsibility for adopting health practices that protect health and prevent illness or complications, and they will make more timely and appropriate use of health resources.[43] Such changes should result in increased patient satisfaction, an improved sense of quality of life, better use of health care provider time, fewer hospital admissions, and shorter hospital stays. These predicted results would contribute to the control of rising health care costs. The truth in the predictions would be learned through research.

REFERENCES

1. McCarthy, C.: Financing for health care. In Jonas, S., editor: Health care delivery in the United States, New York, 1981, Springer Publishing Co., Inc.
2. Ashworth, R.B., and Simmons, H.E.: Medicine and management, World, Spring 1981.
3. Califano to medical schools: cut back class size, Science **202**:726, 1978.
4. Department of Health, Education, and Welfare, Healthy people: the Surgeon General's report on health promotion and disease prevention, Public Health Service Pub. No. 79-55071, Washington, D.C., 1979, U.S. Government Printing Office.
5. Bierman, E.L.: Atherosclerosis and other forms of arteriosclerosis. In Isselbacher, K.J., and others, editors: Harrison's principles of internal medicine, ed. 9, New York, 1980, McGraw-Hill Book Co., Inc.
6. Fox, R.C.: The medicalization and demedicalization of American society. In Knowles, J.H., editor: Doing better and feeling worse: health in the United States, New York, 1977, W.W. Norton & Co., Inc.
7. Callahan, D.: Health and society: some ethical imperatives. In Knowles, J.H., editor: Doing better and feeling worse: health in the United States, New York, 1977, W.W. Norton & Co., Inc.
8. Blum, H.L.: Social perspective on risk reduction, Fam. Commun. Health **3**:41, 1982.
9. Milsum, J.H.: Health risk factor reduction and lifestyle change, Fam. Commun. Health **3**:2, May 1982.
10. Knowles, J.H.: The responsibility of the individual. In Knowles, J.H., editor: Doing better and feeling worse: health in the United States, New York, 1977, W.W. Norton and Co., Inc.
11. Breslow, L., and Somers, A.R.: The lifetime health-monitoring program, N. Engl. J. Med. **296**:601, 1977.
12. Beery, W., and others: Description, analysis and assessment of health hazards/health risk appraisal programs: executive summary/final report, Contract No. 233-79-3008, submitted to the Department of Health and Human Services, Public Health Service, Hyattsville, Md., March 13, 1981.
13. Sacks, J.J., and others: Reliability of the health hazard appraisal, Am. J. Public Health **70**:730, 1980.
14. Green, L.W., and others: Health education planning: a diagnostic approach, Palo Alto, Calif., 1980, Mayfield Publishing Co.
15. Belloc, N.B., and Breslow, L.: Relationship of physical health status and health practices, Prev. Med. **1**:409, 1972.
16. Belloc, N.B.: Health practices and mortality, Prev. Med. **2**:67, 1973.
17. Prevention '80: U.S. Department of Health and Human Services, Public Health Service Pub. No. 81-50157, Washington, D.C., 1980, Office of Disease Prevention and Health Promotion.
18. Stern, M.P.: The recent decline in ischemic heart disease mortality, Ann. Intern. Med. **91**:630, 1979.
19. Board of Agriculture and Renewable Resources, Commission on Natural Resources and Food and Nutrition Board, and Assembly of Life Sciences: Fat content and composition of animal products, Washington, D.C., 1976, National Academy of Sciences.
20. Stamler, J.: Population studies. In Levy, R.I., and others, editors: Nutrition, lipids, and coronary heart disease: a global view, New York, 1979, Raven Press.
21. Bureau of Health Education: Adult use of tobacco (1975), Atlanta, 1976, Center for Disease Control.
22. Hypertension detection and follow-up program cooperative group: blood pressure studies in 14 communities, a two-stage screen for hypertension, J.A.M.A. **237**:2385, 1977.
23. Levy, R.I.: Presentation at the National Conference on High Blood Pressure Control, April 1978, Los Angeles, Calif.
24. Farquhar, J.W.: The American way of life need not be hazardous to your health, New York, 1978, W.W. Norton and Co., Inc.
25. Benson, H.: Systemic hypertension and the relaxation response, N. Engl. J. Med. **296**:1152, 1977.
26. Select Committee on Nutrition and Human Needs, U.S. Senate: Dietary goals for the United States, ed. 2, Washington, D.C., 1977, U.S. Government Printing Office.
27. Promoting health: a source book, regional forums on community health promotion, U.S. Office of Health Information and Health Promotion Pub. No. 282-78-0060, Department of Health, Education, and Welfare, Washington, D.C., Spring 1980.
28. Lehman, P.: Health education. In Healthy people: the Surgeon General's report on health promotion and disease prevention, Department of Health, Education, and Welfare, Public Health Service Pub. No. 79-55071A, Washington, D.C., 1979, U.S. Government Printing Office.
29. McAlister, A.C.: Tobacco, alcohol, and drug abuse: onset and prevention. In Healthy people: the Surgeon General's report on health promotion and disease prevention, Department of Health, Education and Welfare, Public Health Service Pub. No. 79-55071A, Washington, D.C., 1979, U.S. Government Printing Office.
30. Institute of Medicine: Physicians and new health practitioners: issues for the 1980s, Washington, D.C., 1979, National Academy of Sciences.
31. Kalisch, B.J.: The promise of power, Nurs. Outlook, Jan. 1978, p. 42.
32. Farquhar, J.W., and others: Community education for cardiovascular health, Lancet **1**:1192, 1977.
33. Maccoby, J., and others: Reducing the risk of cardio-

vascular disease: effects of a community-based campaign on knowledge and behavior, J. Commun. Health **3**(2):100, 1977.

34. Hecht, R.: Considerations on the use of media in patient education. In Squyres, W.D., editor: Patient education: an inquiry into the state of the art, vol. 4, New York, 1980, Springer Publishing Co., Inc.

35. Task Force on Consumer Health Education, National Institutes of Health, American College of Preventive Medicine: Promoting health: consumer education and national policy, Germantown, Md., 1976, Aspen Systems Corp.

36. Peddecord, K.M.: Competing for acute care dollars: the economics of risk reduction, Fam. Commun. Health **3**:25, 1980.

37. Levi, L.: Psychosocial factors in preventive medicine. In Healthy people: the Surgeon General's report on health promotion and disease prevention, Department of Health, Education, and Welfare, Public Health Service Pub. No. 79-55071A, Washington, D.C., 1979, U.S. Government Printing Office.

38. Institute of Medicine: Policy issues in the health sciences, Washington, D.C., 1977, National Academy of Sciences.

39. Green, L.W.: Evaluation and measurement: some dilemmas for health education, Am. J. Public Health **67**:155, 1977.

40. Squyres, W.D.: Inquiry into action: what are the next steps? In Squyres, W.D., editor: Patient education: an inquiry into the state of the art, vol. 4, New York, 1980, Springer Publishing Co., Inc.

41. Ormiston, L.: Self-management strategies. In Squyres, W.D., editor: Patient education: an inquiry into the state of the art, vol. 4, New York, 1980, Springer Publishing Co., Inc.

42. Green, L.W., and others: What do recent evaluations of patient education tell us? In Squyres, W.D., editor: Patient education: an inquiry into the state of the art, vol. 4, New York, 1980, Springer Publishing Co., Inc.

43. D'Onofrio, C.N.: Evaluating patient education: purposes, politics, and a proposal for practitioners. In Squyres, W.D., editor: Patient education: an inquiry into the state of the art, vol. 4, New York, 1980, Springer Publishing Co., Inc.

4

PATIENT ASSESSMENT: HISTORY AND PHYSICAL EXAMINATION

Virginia Kliner Fowkes
Kathleen Gainor Andreoli

People who have coronary artery disease enter the health care system at varying stages of disease progression. Thus, to determine the individual goals of care and complementary management plans, a clinical data base must be generated. This information can be procured systematically through an interview with the patient and through a complete physical examination, plus pertinent laboratory and physiologic tests. This begins the process of identifying and solving patient problems, a process that continues throughout the therapeutic relationship. As plans are developed and implemented toward resolving each problem, subjective and objective data are collected to evaluate the success of the plan and determine the necessity of management revision.

The intent of this chapter is to focus on the data collection process as it pertains to the patient's cardiovascular status. It is important to remember, however, that other body systems may affect, or be affected by, cardiac disease, and other systems may be involved in disease processes that secondarily affect the heart. Consequently, any patient who develops a new problem should have a complete evaluation.

The discussion that follows includes the patient interview, physical examination, recording of data, and assessment of common symptoms and risk factors. This process of data gathering can be used to explore a patient's problem in an outpatient clinic, to develop a patient care plan in the coronary care unit, or to acquire further information about a new or acute problem.

Clinician's ability in assessment

Patient assessment is a complicated, detailed, and orderly process that should incorporate physical, psychologic, and social dimensions. Its objective is to achieve a comprehensive view of the patient as a person in the context of his or her family, occupation, physical and psychologic health, and immediate needs to mobilize appropriate care interventions. Obviously, most clinicians have mastered the skills of simple data gathering and recording. What is more difficult in the often hurried clinical encounter is to absorb less obvious information, for example, an appreciation of the patient's feelings.

Each examiner brings to the clinical encounter personal attitudes, beliefs, biases, and feelings of the moment. This includes such things as cultural experiences, limitations, and even (with a number of patients waiting to be seen) feelings of pressure. Furthermore, settings such as the coronary care unit are replete with technologic equipment which may easily distract the clinician from focusing on the patient as a person. For example, the examiner may focus on the arterial line or monitoring equipment and miss the fact that the patient is afraid or in pain. Or, the examiner under pressure of time may convey a hurried presence, which intimidates the patients and makes them refrain from sharing their worries or feelings.

The key to comprehensive assessment is to be wholly involved with the patient during the encounter. This means employing whatever tools one uses to relax, concentrate, and focus—perhaps deep breathing in the midst of a hurried schedule. It also entails maximizing for the moment one's skills in listening, touching, and observing quietly and carefully. An openness to learn and an ability to be sensitive to individual attitudes and needs enhance the quality of practitioner-patient interaction and the information received.

Patient interview

The patient interview is the first step in the data collection process. Its purpose is to gather pertinent information about the patient's present complaint or problem, health history, and family and social history. The accuracy and completeness of the subjective data gathered during this interaction depend on the examiner's ability to establish effective communication and rapport with the patient. A gentle, confident approach will help anxious patients describe their illness. Structure can be provided by the interviewer through simple, open-ended questions, and the patient's facial expression and attitude should be observed to make sure the patient understands the questions. Listening to the patient is essential in learning about the disease as well as about the patient as a person.

PATIENT'S PRESENT COMPLAINT OR PROBLEM

The patient's chief problem, whether it be chest pain, shortness of breath, or palpitations, among others, precipitates contact with the health care system. It is the chief concern and therefore the first subject of the interview. As the patient expresses his perceived physical and/or mental changes, the interviewer should reorganize the patient's words into a clinical format to help identify the bodily or mental processes underlying each symptom. This reorganization is accomplished by employing seven basic characteristics or descriptors that differentiate a symptom of one disease from that of another.

Descriptors

Location. Where did the symptom originate? Did it radiate? To what site? It is helpful if the patient indicates the location of the symptom and the radiation pattern with his hand.

Quality. How did the symptom feel to the patient? It may be described as being like something else. For example, the chest pain of myocardial infarction is often compared to "being squeezed in a vise." Other qualifiers include "choking," "burning," and "constricting."

Quantity. How intense is the symptom? Is it mild, moderate, severe, or unbearable?

Course. When did the symptom first occur? Was its onset sudden or gradual? How long did it last in terms of minutes, hours, or days? Over time, has the symptom stayed the same or become better or worse?

Setting. Describe the circumstances when the symptom first occurred. Look for associations between the symptom and the patient's physical activity, emotional status, and personal interactions.

Aggravating and alleviating factors. Are the symptoms influenced by certain activities or physiologic processes? What produces relief—resting, avoiding food, medication? What aggravates the problem—exertion, eating, body position, coughing?

Associated symptoms. Rarely is a disease process present with only one symptom. Therefore the presence or absence of symptoms commonly associated with cardiovascular conditions should be noted. The patient should be asked specifically about each of these, and affirmative responses should be characterized and described as stated in the six previous steps. Questions for eliciting this information should explore whether or not the patient is experiencing any of the following: (1) chest pain or discomfort, (2) unexplained weakness or fatigue, (3) weight loss or gain, (4) swelling of ankles (*edema*), (5) shortness of breath on exertion (*dyspnea*), (6) shortness of breath while sleeping that wakens the patient (*paroxysmal nocturnal dyspnea*), (7) a need to sleep on more than one pillow to breathe comfortably (*orthopnea*), (8) dizzy or fainting spells (*syncope*), (9) coughing at night, (10) coughing up blood (*hemoptysis*), (11) rapid heart beat or palpitations, (12) a need to get up several times during the night to urinate, and (13) pain or cramps in the legs while walking that is relieved by rest (*intermittent claudication*). Finally, asking the patient generally about his daily activities and any self-imposed restrictions on these can provide clues as to the severity of the problem.

PATIENT'S HEALTH HISTORY

The patient's health history may contribute to defining the problem and planning interventions. The patient is asked about general health status and stability of weight. Allergies such as food, contact, or drug are noted. Additional queries are made about past infectious diseases, immunizations, surgical procedures, hospitalizations, injuries, major illnesses, allergies, obstetric history, and psychologic conditions.

The patient is asked specifically about previous heart problems, including heart enlargement, heart failure, murmurs, heart attacks, rheumatic fever, hypertension, elevated cholesterol or triglyceride levels, and diabetes. Information is recorded chronologically, with dates and other pertinent details.

PATIENT'S FAMILY HISTORY

The patient's family background and social profile also may contribute important information to the assessment. The age, sex, and health of parents, siblings, children, and spouse and the age and cause of death of deceased members are relevant. In addition, certain familial diseases that grandparents and close relatives may have had are pertinent. These include hypertension, coronary artery disease, rheumatic fever, stroke, kidney disease, diabetes, thyroid disease, cancer, blood disease, asthma, glaucoma, and gout.

PATIENT'S PERSONAL AND SOCIAL HISTORY

This section of the data base provides information about the patient's life situation and lends perspective to an assessment of his or her ability to cope with the illness. This information is critical in planning care that considers home conditions and family resources. Knowledge of patient habits and life patterns aids in planning hospital routine.

Information is collected about the patient's place of birth, education, military affiliation, position in the family, and state of satisfaction with life situation. Inquiries about habits or patterns such as sleep, exercise, nutrition, alcohol consumption, use of tobacco, coffee or tea, and medications are important. When asking about medication and diet history, it is useful to ask the patient to pick a typical day and describe all drugs (physician- and self-prescribed) taken from morning until bedtime. This approach to diet is useful in giving the practitioner a complete picture of nutrition, including snacks, which the patient may neglect to mention otherwise.

The medication history is particularly necessary with the elderly, who may see more than one health care provider and consume a series of drugs that have synergistic or mutually inhibitory effects.

The home conditions, nature of family relationships, economic resources, including source of income and insurance, satisfaction with sexual relationship, religious affiliation, and occupation are other areas important to assess.

Review of systems

The review of systems is done as a part of the initial assessment and is a record of the patient's past and present health in each system. Questions covered in the review of systems are detailed on page 38.

Physical examination

The cardiovascular physical examination is performed to collect objective data about the patient's complaint, symptoms, or illness. The information that has been obtained from the patient interview is then correlated with the physical findings as the next step in the evaluation process. Often a sufficient and accurately obtained history establishes the nature of the problem prior to the physical examination.

The examiner evaluates the cardiovascular system in an orderly fashion, using the techniques of inspection, palpation, percussion, and auscultation, as appropriate.

inspection examining visually the parts of the system. It includes whatever the examiner can see, such as pulsations, deformities, color, manner of breathing, and so forth.
palpation feeling or pressing with the fingers or hands to locate possible vibrations, thrills (blood flowing past an obstruction), impulses, grating sensations, and so on.

percussion tapping the patient's body surface to determine, through touch and hearing, the relative amount of air or solid material underneath the skin.

auscultation listening with or without the stethoscope to internally produced sounds. Such sounds include breath sounds, heart sounds, bruit (murmur over a peripheral vessel), friction rubs, and heart murmurs.

The physical examination actually begins when the patient meets the examiner. At this time the examiner makes general observations about the patient regarding apparent age versus stated age, grooming, speech, posture, gait, nutritional state, attitude, color, and degree of distress, if any. The collection of objective data begins with the recording of the patient's vital signs, including temperature, pulse, respiration, and blood pressure.

REVIEW OF SYSTEMS

General	State of health, appetite, weight, fatique
Skin	Temperature, rashes, growths, sun sensitivity, itching, texture, change in pigment and color, excessive dryness or sweating
Head	Headaches
Eyes	Diplopia, acuity, blurring, spots, lacrimation, itching, photophobia, pain, infection, discharge
Ears	Hearing, infections, earaches, discharge, tinnitus, vertigo
Nose	Discharge, obstruction, sinus, sense of smell, epistaxis
Mouth and throat	Sore throats, hoarseness, dysphagia, bleeding or sore gums
Neck	Pain, stiffness, lumps
Cardiopulmonary	Chest pain, dyspnea, palpitations, cough, hemoptysis, night sweats, edema, history of murmur, paroxysmal nocturnal dyspnea, orthopnea, wheezing, stridor, syncope
Gastrointestinal	Food intolerance, pyrosis, nausea, vomiting, abdominal pain, bloody stools or vomitus, diarrhea, constipation, melena, bowel habits (change in frequency, consistency, or color), jaundice
Genitourinary	Dysuria, polyuria, oliguria, urgency, frequency, hesitation, nocturia, hematuria, pyuria, urethral discharge, incontinence, sexual problems Male: prostate problems Female: menarche, last menstrual period, usual menstrual period (duration, amount, and interval), dysmenorrhea, hypermenorrhea (amount), polymenorrhea (intermenstrual bleeding), menopause (date, if any), vaginal bleeding or discharge, pelvic inflammatory disease, birth control measures, gravida, para, abortions, complications of pregnancy
Musculoskeletal	Muscle pain or cramps, joint pain, swelling or stiffness of joints; weakness, coldness, and discoloration of extremities, back pain
Nervous	Paresthesias, balance, numbness, paralysis, tremor, nervousness, depression (symptoms), hallucinations, therapy
Hematopoietic	Easy bleeding or bruising
Endocrine	Temperature intolerance, polydipsia

TEMPERATURE

A temperature elevation above the normal level of 98.6° F or 37° C is common during the first few days following acute myocardial infarction. The fever is usually less than 101° F and is associated with necrosis of cardiac muscle. Prolonged, high, or late development of fever suggests other complications. Although fever may indicate the onset of infectious processes, it may also be the first sign of thrombophlebitis, pulmonary embolism, pericarditis, or atelectasis. Moreover, prolonged temperature elevation in the patient with a myocardial infarction may be harmful, since it causes a rise in the metabolic rate of body tissues and therefore a demand for increased circulation and oxygenation. This, in turn, increases the myocardial oxygen demands, a threatening situation in the face of infarction.

Temperature assessment is therefore a part of routine examination and daily monitoring activities for critically ill patients. The temperature is taken orally, rectally, or in the axilla for a period of 3 minutes. Rectal temperatures are the most accurate. In the past the taking of rectal temperatures was avoided in patients with myocardial infarctions as a precaution against undue vagal stimulation. However, recent studies suggest that taking rectal temperatures is quite safe.

Temperature is measured on a Fahrenheit or centigrade scale. The formula for converting centigrade measurement to Fahrenheit and vice versa follows:

$$\text{Fahrenheit} = 1.8\ (°C) + 32$$
$$\text{Centigrade} = \frac{°F - 32}{1.8}$$

PULSE

Arterial pulse. The arterial pulse is a propagated wave of arterial pressure resulting from left ventricular contraction. The pulse wave begins in the aorta with the opening of the aortic valve and the ejection of blood from the left ventricle (Fig. 4-1). The pressure in the aorta rises sharply, since blood enters the vessel more rapidly than it runs off to the peripheral vessels. A notch may appear during the sharp rise in the central arterial pressure curve. This is called the *anacrotic notch* and is generally absent from peripheral pulse recordings but may be prominent in valvular aortic stenosis. After peak pressure has been reached, aortic pressure decreases, ventricular ejection slows, and blood continues to flow to peripheral vessels. As the ventricles relax, there is a brief reversal of flow (from the central arteries back toward the ventricle) and the aortic valve closes. This produces the *dicrotic notch* on the peripheral pressure pulse tracing, corresponding to the *incisura* recorded centrally. Following this, aortic pressure increases slightly and then decreases as diastole continues and blood flows to the periphery, a result of energy imparted to the elastic tissue in the great vessels during systole. In the graphic recording of aortic pressure in Fig. 4-1 the peak of the pulse wave represents systolic pressure and the lowest point on the wave represents diastolic pressure.

The pulse wave changes in shape as it travels to the periphery. The height, or amplitude, of the wave (the systolic reading) increases as it moves from the

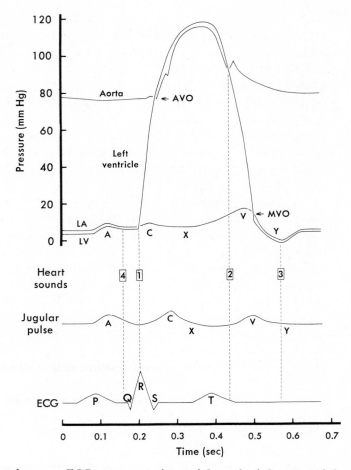

Fig. 4-1. Simultaneous ECG, pressures obtained from the left atrium, left ventricle, and aorta, and the jugular pulse during one cardiac cycle. For simplification, right-sided heart pressures have been omitted. Normal right atrial pressure closely parallels that of the left atrium, and right ventricular and pulmonary artery pressures time closely with their corresponding left-sided heart counterparts, only being reduced in magnitude. The normal mitral and aortic valve closure precedes tricuspid and pulmonic closure, respectively, whereas valve opening reverses this order. The jugular venous pulse lags behind the right atrial pressure.

During the course of one cardiac cycle, note that the electrical events (*ECG*) initiate and therefore precede the mechanical (*pressure*) events, and that the latter precede the auscultatory events (*heart sounds*) they themselves produce. Shortly after the P wave, the atria contract to produce the wave; a fourth heart sound may succeed the latter. The QRS complex initiates ventricular systole, followed shortly by left ventricular contraction and the rapid buildup of left ventricular (*LV*) pressure. Almost immediately LV pressure exceeds left atrial (*LA*) pressure to close the mitral valve and produce the first heart sound. When LV pressure exceeds aortic pressure, the aortic valve opens (*AVO*), and when aortic pressure is once again greater than LV pressure, the aortic valve closes to produce the second heart sound and terminate ventricular ejection. The decreasing LV pressure drops below LA pressure to open the mitral valve (*MVO*) and a period of rapid ventricular filling commences. During this time a third heart sound may be heard. The jugular pulse is explained under the discussion of the venous pulse. (Modified with permission from Hurst, J.W., and others: The heart: arteries and veins, ed. 3, New York, 1974, McGraw-Hill Book Co.)

aortic root to the peripheral arteries, with a slight decrease in the diastolic pressure. The ascending part of the wave becomes steeper and the peak becomes sharper.

The competency of the arterial system is assessed through blood pressure measurement, inspection of the carotid artery, palpation of the arteries, and auscultation of the arteries. Blood pressure is discussed in a subsequent section.

Examination. The arterial pulses are palpated to evaluate patency, heart rate and rhythm, and character of the pulse. This examination covers the carotid, brachial, radial, femoral, popliteal, dorsalis pedis, and posterior tibial pulses. These pulses can best be evaluated with the patient in a reclining position and the trunk of the body elevated about 30 degrees. If diffuse atherosclerosis in an elderly patient has resulted in absence of the dorsalis pedis or posterior tibial pulse, this observation should be noted on initial examination so that the hospital staff do not interpret this finding as a new catastrophic event, such as arterial embolus, at a later time during the patient's hospitalization.

Although the radial pulse is commonly used in determining heart rate, the carotid pulse best correlates with central aortic pressure and reflects cardiac function more accurately than peripheral vessels. Furthermore, if the patient develops marked vasoconstriction, the radial pulse may be difficult to palpate. However, caution must be exercised in palpating the carotid pulse to avoid pressure on the carotid sinus, since palpating at that site may result in severe bradycardia.

The pulse is examined for *rate and rhythm, equality of corresponding pulses, contour*, and *amplitude*. The pulses should be palpated on both sides and simultaneously at the brachial and femoral arteries. To obtain information about *cardiac rate and rhythm*, the pulse should be palpated for 30 seconds in the presence of a regular rhythm and for 1 to 2 minutes in the face of an irregular rhythm. If an irregularity exists, an apical pulse should be recorded. The term *peripheral pulse deficit* indicates that the heart rate counted at the apex by auscultation exceeds the heart rate counted by palpation of the radial pulse. A deficit means that not every cardiac systole is forceful enough to produce a palpable radial pulse and may occur in the presence of premature extrasystoles or atrial tachyarrythmias, such as atrial fibrillation. Bilateral, simultaneous palpation of the radial and pedal pulses is helpful in determining whether the pulses arrive without delay and provides information about the peripheral arterial blood supply.

The *character of the arterial wall*, which normally feels soft and pliable, is noted by palpation. With significant atherosclerotic disease the vessel may be resistant to compression and feel much like a rope.

The pulse *contour* may be assessed by extending the patient's arm and palpating the radial or brachial pulse or the carotid pulse in the neck. The artery should be compressed lightly with a finger while the examiner ascertains the contour of the pulse wave. Variations in the contour of the arterial pulse are depicted in Fig. 4-2.

The *normal arterial pulse* (Fig. 4-2, *A*) has a pulse pressure of about 30 to 40 mm Hg; the systolic pressure measures the peaks of the waves, and the

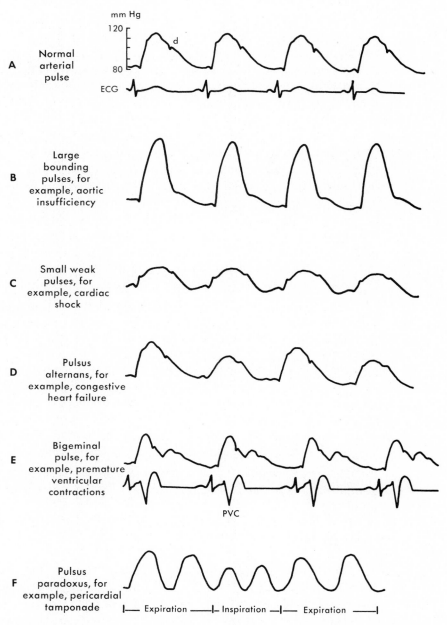

Fig. 4-2. Variations in contour of the arterial pulse with correlated ECGs for the normal arterial pulses (*A*) and bigeminal pulse (*E*). See text for description.

diastolic pressure measures the troughs. One can feel a sharp upstroke and a more gradual downstroke (the dicrotic notch of the descending slope of the wave is too weak to be palpable). The contour of the normal pulse is smooth and rounded.

With *large bounding pulses* (Fig. 4-2, *B*), the pulse pressure is increased and one feels a rapid upstroke, a brief peak, and a fast downstroke. This type of pulse wave is encountered most often in conditions termed *hyperkinetic circulatory states*. These states include exercise, anxiety, fear, hyperthyroidism, anemia, patent ductus arteriosus, aortic regurgitation, and complete heart block with bradycardia and hypertension. It is also found as a result of generalized arteriosclerosis and rigidity of the arterial system in old people.

Small weak pulses (Fig. 4-2, *C*) are characterized by diminished pulse pressure and pulse contour that is felt as a slow gradual upstroke, a delayed systolic peak, and a prolonged downstroke. This pulse is found in severe cases of left ventricular failure as a result of decreased stroke volume and in moderate or severe cases of aortic stenosis as a result of slow ejection of blood through the narrowed orifice.

Pulsus alternans (Fig. 4-2, *D*) refers to a pulse pattern in which the heart beats with a *regular* rhythm, but the pulses alternate in size and intensity. When this alternation is present in lesser degrees, the difference may not be palpable, but it can be readily detected by measuring blood pressure by auscultation.

As the sphygmomanometer cuff is slowly deflated from a pressure above the systolic level, the sounds from the alternate beats are heard first. Then one hears the alternating loud and soft sounds or a sudden doubling of the rate as the cuff pressure declines. Pulsus alternans often accompanies left ventricular failure and can masquerade as a bigeminal pulse.

The *bigeminal pulse* (Fig. 4-2, *E*) is usually produced by a premature ventricular extrasystole that occurs regularly following a normally conducted beat. The stroke volume of the premature beat is less than that of the normal beat, since contraction occurs before complete ventricular filling. The rhythm is *irregular,* since the time between the normal beat and the premature beat is shorter than the time between the pairs. The irregularity may be consistent. Simultaneous arterial palpation and cardiac auscultation assist in diagnosing this cardiac irregularity.

The *amplitude* of pulses is categorized into levels in the following code and compared bilaterally:

    0 = Not palpable
+1 = Barely palpable
+2 = Decreased
+3 = Full
+4 = Bounding

In patients with significant vascular disease it is useful to draw a small stick figure and label the amplitude of pulses accordingly.

Pulsus paradoxus (Fig. 4-2, *F*) refers to the phenomenon in which the pulse diminishes perceptibly in amplitude during normal inspiration. Although the differences in pulse volume can be palpated, they can be more precisely demonstrated with sphygmomanometry. Under normal conditions of rest the systolic blood pressure ordinarily decreases by 3 to 10 mm Hg. The procedure for detecting pulsus paradoxus is as follows:

1. Have the patient breath *normally*.
2. Pump up the sphygmomanometer, then lower the pressure until the first sound (systolic) is heard.
3. Observe the patient's respirations. The systolic sound may disappear during normal inspiration.
4. Slowly deflate the cuff until all systolic sounds are heard, regardless of phase in the respiratory cycle. The change (in millimeters of mercury) from the point at which systolic sounds were first heard to the point where they are heard during the entire respiratory cycle represents the millimeters of paradox observed. A paradox greater than 10 mm Hg is usually abnormal.

To be significant, a paradoxical pulse must occur during normal cardiac rhythm and with respirations of normal rhythm and depth. In short, it is an exaggeration of a normal response during respiration. Pulses paradoxus is found in cases of pericardial tamponade, adhesive pericarditis, severe lung disease, advanced heart failure, and other conditions.

Auscultation of arteries. Arteries are normally silent when auscultated with the bell or diaphragm of the stethoscope, which is placed lightly over them. Occlusive arterial disease, such as arteriosclerosis, will interfere with normal blood flow through the artery, resulting in a blowing sound called a *bruit*. Auscultation of the carotid arteries should be done with the patient holding the breath so that the bruits can be distinguished from the sounds of respiration. Often these abnormal arterial vibrations can be *felt* as *thrills*. Auscultation is also done over the abdominal aorta and femoral arteries to detect the presence of bruits.

Venous pulse. Examination of the neck veins provides diagnostic information about the dynamics of the right side of the heart. For this clinical evaluation, one must study the waveform of the venous pulsations, correlate them with the cardiac rhythm, and determine the venous pressure.

The character of the venous pulse is determined by four factors: (1) the rate at which blood is returned from the peripheral tissues to the venous system, (2) the amount of resistance to flow presented by the right atrium and ventricle during different phases of the cardiac cycle, (3) the pressure-volume properties of the segment of the vein, and (4) in part, the nature of the tissues overlying the veins at the focus of observation. Elevations in venous pressure occur with right ventricular failure, rapid blood flow due to exercise, fever or hyperthyroidism, fluid overload, constriction of the heart from pericarditis, pericardial effusion or cardiac tamponade, and tricuspid valvular disease.

Examination. The examination begins with observation of the external and internal jugular veins on both sides of the neck as well as of the venous pulsations that may be present in the supraclavicular fossae or in the suprasternal notch. For accurate evaluation of the venous waveform the *right internal jugular vein*

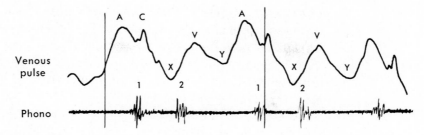

Fig. 4-3. Relationship of the jugular venous pulse to right atrial activity.

is usually selected, although one of the other veins may be preferred and is just as revealing. If the venous pressure is relatively normal, the patient can assume a comfortable recumbent position with the head and trunk elevated to about a 30-degree angle without flexing the neck. If the venous pressure is greatly elevated, the pulses can be examined better with the patient in a completely upright position so that the pulsations appear at the jugular level.

The patient's head should be gently rotated away from the examiner. A light shined tangentially across the area being examined may help detect a slightly distended vein. A series of undulant waves that are more clearly seen than felt characterize the venous pulse, a graphic recording of which is shown in Fig. 4-3. These pulsations are evaluated in relation to the cardiac cycle and therefore the carotid pulse or heart sounds can be used for timing them.

a WAVE. The a wave is produced by right atrial contraction and the retrograde transmission of the pressure pulse to the jugular veins. It occurs at the time of the fourth heart sound, preceding the first heart sound. The a wave can be easily identified by placing the index finger on the carotid pulse opposite the side being inspected. Because of the compliance of the great veins and the low pressures in the right side of the heart, the a wave will be seen to start just slightly before the carotid pulse is palpated in the neck. The a wave is absent during atrial fibrillation. Giant a waves reflect an elevated right atrial pressure and may be seen in such conditions as pulmonary hypertension and pulmonic and tricuspid stenosis. *Cannon a waves* are an exaggerated form of the giant a wave. In this situation the right atrium contracts during ventricular systole, when the tricuspid valve is closed, and the blood regurgitates into the neck veins. *Regular* cannon waves may occur during AV junctional (nodal) rhythm when the atria and ventricles contract almost simultaneously. *Irregular* cannon waves may occur during an AV dissociation of any cause and during ectopic beating.

c WAVE. The c wave begins shortly after the first heart sound and may result from impact of the carotid artery on the adjacent jugular vein or from the retrograde transmision of a positive wave in the right atrium, generated by the bulging tricuspid valve during right ventricular systole. The c wave is often difficult to visualize by inspecting the neck veins.

v WAVE. Continued atrial filling during ventricular systole produces the v wave, which peaks just after the second heart sound, when the tricuspid valve opens. Tricuspid insufficiency causes a very large v wave.

x DESCENT. The x descent is the downslope of the a and c waves and results from right atrial diastole, plus the effects of the tricuspid valve being pulled downward during ventricular systole. Tricuspid insufficiency blunts or eliminates the x descent, whereas elevated right ventricular output and constrictive pericarditis may enhance it.

y DESCENT. The y descent represents the fall in the right atrial pressure from the peak of the v wave following tricuspid valve opening and occurs during the period of rapid atrial emptying in early diastole. Impedance to right atrial emptying, caused by tricuspid stenosis or atresia or by a right atrial myxoma, dampens the y descent. Constrictive pericarditis produces a speedy y descent and prominent trough, followed by a rapid y ascent as the ventricular, atrial, and venous pressures promptly rise when the nondistensible right ventricle becomes filled with blood.

• • •

Respiration alters the venous pulse. Deep inspiration lowers the level of the venous pressure pulsation (actual amplitude of the pulse waves may be increased) by a decrease in intrathoracic pressure. This increases venous return, reduces central venous pressure, and increases right-sided heart filling to lower the level of the venous pulse in the neck and collapse the neck veins. Expiration produces reversed effects. The *Valsalva maneuver,* that is, forced expiratory straining against a closed glottis, elevates the venous pressure by obstructing flow into the chest.

KUSSMAUL'S SIGN is a paradoxical rise in venous pressure and neck vein disten- during inspiration and is seen in the patient with severe right heart failure or pericardial constriction. The limited capacity of the right ventricle to receive the increased volume of venous return generated by inspiration results in a backing up of blood into the superior vena cava and distention of the neck veins.

HEPATOJUGULAR REFLUX is a sustained rise in the level of venous pressure during abdominal compression when the patient is breathing normally. As the liver or splanchnic vessels are compressed, the volume of venous blood returning to the right side of the heart is thought to increase. The normal heart accepts this extra load easily. During right-sided heart failure, constrictive pericarditis, or hypervolemia the venous pressure rises because the right ventricle is unable to accommodate the increased blood volume. The prominent v wave of tricuspid insufficiency may be exposed by this maneuver. Manual abdominal compression may cause discomfort resulting in muscular guarding. This muscle tension may increase intraabdominal pressure (Valsalva maneuver) and give a falsely positive hepatojugular reflux.

RESPIRATION

The rate and character of the patient's respiration should be carefully observed. Under normal conditions the adult should breathe comfortably about 16 to 20 times per minute. Variations in the normal rate and character of respirations include the following:

tachypnea rapid shallow breathing that may indicate pain, cardiac insufficiency, anemia, fever, or pulmonary problems.

bradypnea slow breathing as a result of opiates, coma, excessive alcohol, and increased intracranial pressure.

hyperventilation simultaneous rapid, deep breathing found in extreme anxiety states, in diabetic acidosis, and after vigorous exercise.

Cheyne-Stokes respiration periodic breathing with *hyperpnea* (increase depth of breathing) alternating with *apnea* (cessation of breathing), encountered in cardiac failure and central nervous system disease.

sighing respiration normal respiratory rhythm interrupted by a deep inspiration, followed by a prolonged expiration accompanied by an audible sigh. This variation is often associated with emotional depression.

dyspnea concious difficulty or effort in breathing. When the patient assumes an elevated position of the trunk at rest to breathe more comfortably, this is called *orthopnea*. Dyspnea is a cardinal sign of left ventricular failure and may also occur in certain lung disorders.

obstructive breathing (air trapping) In obstructive pulmonary diseases such as emphysema and asthma, it is easier for air to enter the lungs than for it to leave. During rapid respiration, sufficient time for full expiration is not available and air becomes trapped in the lungs. The patient's chest overexpands and his breathing becomes more shallow. Expiratory wheezes may be present. Further examination of lung function is discussed later in this chapter.

BLOOD PRESSURE

Arterial blood pressure. Cardiac contraction maintains blood pressure in both arteries and veins. The arterial blood pressure is an overall reflection of the function of the ventricles as pumps. Blood pressure in the arterial system is represented by the peak systolic and diastolic levels of the pressure pulse and is modified by cardiac output, peripheral arteriolar resistance, distensibility of the arteries, amount of blood in the system, and viscosity of the blood. Accordingly, changes in blood pressure reflect changes in these measurements. For example, the decrease in vessel distensibility in the elderly lowers diastolic pressure and increases systolic pressure to produce systolic hypertension. Increments in blood volume may raise both systolic and diastolic components.

Normal blood pressure in the aorta and large arteries, such as the brachial artery, varies between 100 and 140 mm Hg systolic and between 60 and 90 mm Hg diastolic. Pressure in the smaller arteries is somewhat less, and in the arterioles, where the blood enters the capillaries, it is about 35 mm Hg. However, wide variation of normal blood pressure exists, and a value may fall outside the normal range in healthy adults. The normal range also varies with age, sex, and race. A pressure reading of 100/60 may be normal for one person but hypotensive for another.

Observing changes in blood pressure and in pulse pressure (the difference between systolic and diastolic pressures and normally 30 to 50 mm Hg) is important in the care of a patient with an acute myocardial infarction. A reduction in blood pressure from a prior level of 150/100 mm Hg to 115/70 after myocardial infarction may indicate impending cardiovascular decompensation, such as congestive heart failure or shock. Tachycardia and pericardial tamponade also may reduce arterial pressure and narrow pulse pressure.

Measurement. Arterial blood pressure can be measured directly or indirectly. The *indirect* method is performed with a sphygmomanometer. It is a simple procedure and accurate enough for most determinations. With this method systolic pressures may be slightly below and diastolic pressures slightly above directly obtained values. Rather than measuring one complete beat, the indirect method measures the systolic pressure of some beats and the diastolic pressure of other beats; it does not measure a mean pressure.

For routine indirect blood pressure measurements the patient may be either sitting or reclining. In some cases blood pressure may change with body position, and in this situation the pressure should be recorded with the patient in reclining, sitting, and standing positions. To obtain a realistic measurement the patient should have the opportunity to relax for a while.

The collapsed cuff should be affixed snugly and smoothly to the patient's arm, with the distal margin of the cuff at least 3 cm above the anticubital fossa. The patient's arm should be rested on a table or a bed, and the examiner should palpate for the location of the brachial artery pulse. Pressure in the cuff is then rapibly increased to a level about 30 mm Hg above the point at which the palpable pulse disappears. As the cuff is deflated, observations may be made by either palpation or auscultation. The point at which the pulse can be felt is recorded from the manometer as the palpatory systolic pressure. The auscultatory method is usually preferred; with this method, vibrations from the artery under pressure, called *Korotkoff sounds*, are used as indicators.

For auscultatory blood pressure measurement the bell or diaphragm of the stethoscope is pressed lightly over the brachial artery while the cuff is slowly deflated, and pressure readings begin at the time the sounds first become audible. As the cuff is deflated further, the sounds become louder for a brief period; then they become muffled and finally disappear. The systolic blood pressure is the point at which sounds become audible, and the diastolic blood pressure is the point at which the sounds cease to be heard. If sounds continue to zero pressure, as they may at times in aortic regurgitation and thyrotoxicosis, three values may be recorded: the first value is the point of audibility of sounds; the second value is when sounds become muffled; and the third value is zero, when sounds disappear. The second value should be accepted as the diastolic pressure, since a diastolic pressure of zero is impossible.

Although the sounds may disappear at a certain reading on the sphygmomanometer, one should continue to listen at zero pressure to detect the possible presence of the *auscultatory gap*. In this situation the examiner may first detect systolic sounds at a high level, only to have them suddenly disappear and then reappear at a lower level. For example, sounds may be heard first at 180 mm Hg, disappear at 160 mm Hg, and then reappear at 120 mm Hg. This phenomenon is depicted in Fig. 4-4. One can appreciate the problem only by inflating the cuff to 150 mm Hg. In this instance the patient might be considered normotensive when actually he is hypertensive.

The patient's blood pressure should be checked in both arms, and any difference should be noted. A difference of 5 mm Hg may exist. If the patient has hypertension or reduced pulses in the lower extremities, blood pressure readings are also taken in the legs. In this situation the cuff is placed around the lower third of the thigh and the stethoscope is applied to the popliteal artery. In the event that the thigh is too thick for cuff placement the examiner may place the cuff around the calf and palpate the dorsalis pedis or posterior tibial pulse. The

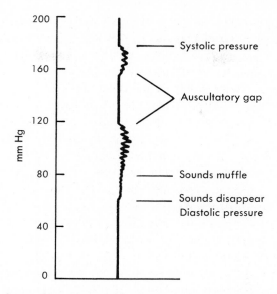

Fig. 4-4. Detection of auscultatory gap in blood pressure measurement. The systolic sounds are first heard at 180 mm Hg. They disappear at 160 mm Hg and reappear at 120 mm Hg; the silent interval is called the auscultatory gap. The Korotkoff sounds muffle at 80 mm Hg and disappear at 60 mm Hg. The blood pressure is recorded as 180/60, noting the presence of the auscultatory gap.

blood pressure in the leg should be equal to or slightly greater than that in the brachial artery. If the patient has hypertension, is taking medication that may affect blood pressure, or is just beginning to ambulate following a period of bed rest, it is also important to check the blood pressure in the standing, sitting, and supine positions.

Direct measurement of arterial pressure may be indicated for the patient in shock whose blood pressure is too low to be determined accurately by the cuff method. It also may be useful in managing patients who have a low blood volume or who are being treated with drugs for hypertension or hypotension. An arterial catheter, in addition to directly measuring blood pressure, provides continuous recording without disturbing the patient and allows frequent blood sampling to determine blood gas levels and arterial pH during the management of patients with cardiogenic shock or respiratory insufficiency and those using mechanical ventilators.

For direct measurement of arterial blood pressure, a needle or catheter is inserted into the brachial, radial, or femoral artery. A catheter may be advanced centrally into the aorta or even into the left ventricle. A catheter in the central aorta permits accurate assessment of the diastolic and mean aortic pressures and is very important for the patient who has a myocardial infarction because these pressures may significantly affect coronary blood flow. Catheters should not remain in the left ventricle or ascending arch of the aorta proximal to the origin of the cephalic arteries because of the risk of embolization. They may be maintained safely in the subclavian artery or the descending thoracic aorta for several hours or even several days with proper attention.

A plastic tube filled with heparinized saline solution connects the catheter to a pressure-sensitive device or a strain-gauge transducer. This device converts the mechanical energy that the blood exerts on the recording membrane into changes in electrical voltage or current that can be calibrated in millimeters of mercury. The electrical signal can then be transmitted to an electronic recorder and an oscilloscope, which continually record and display the pressure waves. The transducer and oscilloscope method is more accurate than the sphygmomanometer method and yields an electrically integrated mean pressure.

On the oscilloscopes, the arterial pressure waveforms for the brachial and radial arteries appear identical. The more distal the catheter is from the aorta, the higher the systolic pressure, resulting from the amplification effect in the arterial system during systole. The normal arterial waveform should be clearly discernible, reflecting a rapid upstroke to the peak of systolic pressure, followed by a more gradual downslope. Approximately at the end of ventricular systole, a secondary smaller upstroke, termed the *dicrotic notch* and caused by a rebound against the closing aortic valve, occurs (see Fig. 4-2, *A*). The accuracy of intraarterial pressure readings depends on accurate catheter placement, solid connections between the parts of the system, and arterial line patency. Further discussion of arterial monitoring can be found in Chapter 7.

Venous blood pressure. In addition to evaluating the contour of the jugular venous pulse, one can obtain further information about the right side of the heart by determining the level of venous pressure. Venous pressure refers to the pressure exerted within the venous system by the blood. It is highest in the venules of the extremities and lowest at the point where the vena cava enters the heart. Venous blood flow is continuous rather than pulsatory. In the arm, venous pressure normally ranges from 5 to 14 cm H_2O and in the inferior vena cava, from 6 to 8 cm H_2O. Blood volume, tone of the vessel wall, patency of veins, competence of venous valves, function of the right heart, respiratory function, and force of gravity all influence venous pressure. The veins most commonly used in this estimation are the hand and arm veins, the internal jugular veins, and the external jugular veins.

Measurement. When the examiner is using the veins on the dorsum of the hand to determine venous pressure, the patient should be sitting with his hand held sufficiently below the level of the heart to permit venous distention. As the arm is slowly raised, one can observe the level at which venous collapse occurs. Normally this occurs when the dorsum of the hand reaches a point just above the sternal notch. In cases of elevated venous pressure, the vertical distance above the sternal notch at which the veins collapse provides a rough estimate of the venous pressure.

The *external jugular vein* is commonly used because of its easy accessibility. It is considered less reliable in determining venous pressure than the internal jugular veins, since it is smaller and takes a less direct route to the superior vena cava. To evaluate the pressure in the external jugular vein, the examiner should have the patient recline with the trunk elevated at an angle of 30 to 60 degrees and the head rotated slightly away from the vein being examined. Slight elevation is important because the external jugular veins are normally collapsed above the level of the suprasternal notch when the person is upright. The examiner gradually elevates the head of the bed or table until venous distention is visible. The

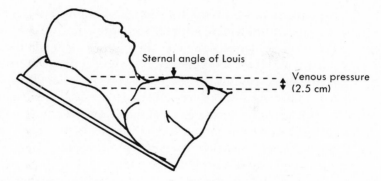

Fig. 4-5. Sternal angle of Louis as a reference point for measuring venous pressure. The height of the distended fluid column in the external jugular vein is less than 3 cm above the sternal angle.

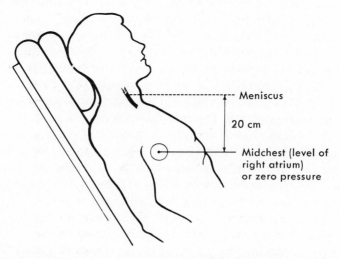

Fig. 4-6. Estimation of venous pressure accomplished by elevating the head until the meniscus is visualized. The venous pressure is measured as the vertical distance between the meniscus and midchest, or right atrial level, in this case, 20 cm and elevated above normal.

examiner then occludes the external jugular vein by pressing the neck just above and parallel to the clavicle. After waiting approximately 20 seconds for the vein to fill, the examiner quickly withdraws the finger and observes the height of the distended fluid column within the vein. If visible at all, the level will normally be less than 3 to 5 cm above the sternal angle of Louis (Fig. 4-5).

As previously mentioned, the *internal jugular vein* is the most reliable indicator of indirect venous pressure as well as venous pulse waveform. The patient's trunk should be elevated to the optimum angle for the observation of venous pulse. The highest point of visible pulsation of the internal jugular vein is determined and the vertical distance between this level and the level of the sternal angle of Louise is recorded. The angle of elevation of the patient should also be recorded.

It is important to note that the sternal angle is used as a bedside reference point for the sake of convenience. The ideal reference level for venous pressure measurement is the midpoint of the right atrium. This level is established by running an imaginary anteroposterior line from the fourth interspace halfway to the back. A horizontal plane through this point is the zero level for the measurement of venous pressure. The vertical distance from this plane to the head of the blood column, or the meniscus, approximates the venous pressure (Fig. 4-6). Elevations of pressure above 10 cm H_2O are considered abnormal.

Central venous pressure. The direct measurement of central venous pressure (CVP) becomes important if there is a doubt about the value obtained by indirect measurement, or when monitoring a critically ill patient, a situation in which CVP is considered an important sign to follow.

The CVP indicates right arterial pressure, which primarily reflects alterations in right ventricular pressure and only secondarily reflects changes in the pulmonary venous pressure or the pressure in the left side of the heart. The CVP provides valuable information with regard to blood volume and adequacy of central venous return.

The CVP can be obtained by inserting a polyethylene catheter into the external jugular, antecubital, or femoral vein and threading it into the vena cava. The medical antecubital veins are used more commonly than the others. The catheter offers a method of CVP measurement as well as an intravenous route for drawing blood samples, administering fluid or medications, performing phlebotomy, and possibly inserting a pacing catheter.

The procedure for setting up the CVP system is as follows:

1. Using a three-way stopcock, attach the catheter to a water manometer and an intravenous infusion line. When the venous pressure is not being read, the stopcock is adjusted so that the intravenous fluid will run through the catheter and keep it patent.
2. Mount the manometer on a pole by placing the zero marking at the level of the right atrium. The level of the right atrium can be determined by placing the patient flat and measuring 5 cm down from the top of the chest at the fourth interspace. Run a yardstick from the patient's chest to the baseline of the manometer.
3. Flush the line as necessary to maintain patency.
4. To prevent infection, place an antibiotic ointment and a 2 × 2 inch dressing over the catheter insertion site.

The procedure for measuring CVP is as follows:

1. Place the patient flat in bed and be certain that the zero point of the manometer is at the level of the right atrium.
2. Determine patency of the catheter by opening the intravenous infusion line briefly to a rapid flow rate.
3. Turn the stopcock to allow the intravenous solution to run into the manometer to a level of 10 to 20 cm above the expected pressure reading.
4. Turn the stopcock to allow the intravenous solution to flow from the manometer into the catheter. The fluid level in the manometer falls rapidly and fluctuates during respiration, decreasing with inspiration and increasing with expiration. Ventilatory assistance should be stopped during the measurement.

5. When the fluid level is constant, read the CVP. Some fluctuation occurs during respiration.
6. After the reading has been obtained, return the stopcock to the intravenous infusion position.

The normal CVP range is 4 to 10 cm H_2O. The CVP may be measured either in centimeters of water or in millimeters of mercury. The value in centimeters of water may be converted to milimeters of mercury by dividing the former by 1.36, since 1 mm Hg = 1.36 cm H_2O.

Abnormal CVPs must be interpreted according to the clinical situation and other considerations—urine output, skin turgor, temperature, systemic blood pressure, heart rate, and so on. An elevated CVP (above 10cm H_2O) may indicate right ventricular failure secondary to left-sided heart failure, pulmonary disease such as pulmonary hypertension or embolism, or cardiac tamponade. A low CVP (below 4 cm H_2O) may indicate hypovolemia or peripheral blood pooling, as in septic shock. Taking a single CVP value is less useful than noting repeated measurements, particularly after administering a challenge volume load. Further discussion of this measurement appears in Chapter 7.

INSPECTION AND PALPATION OF THE HEART

The anterior part of the chest is inspected with the patient in a supine position and the trunk elevated to about a 30-degree angle. The approach should be made from the patient's right side. Certain landmarks on the anterior chest wall are useful as points of reference in describing the location of the heart. The heart rests on the diaphragm and is located beneath and to the left of the sternum. The base of the heart is situated approximately at the level of the third rib; the apex of the heart lies approximately at the level of the fifth rib in the midclavicular line. The anterior surface of the heart proceeding from the examiner's left to right, facing the patient, is composed of the right atrium, right ventricle, and left ventricle (Fig. 4-7). The anterior surface of the chest closest to the heart and aorta is called the *precordium*.

Inspection begins by observing the precordium for abnormal pulsations. Tangential lighting may be helpful in detecting these pulsations. Any visible impulse medial to the apex and in the third, fourth, or fifth interspace generally originates in the right ventricle and is usually abnormal. In pronounced right ventricular enlargement, one can usually see the lower sternum heave with the heartbeat. It is important to determine when the movements occur by correlating them with the heart sounds or carotid artery pulsations.

Following inspection, palpation of the precordium is performed to confirm the findings of inspection and to locate further impulses and thrills. The palmar bases of the fingers are used, since this area is most sensitive to feeling vibrations. First palpate the areas where pulsations are visible, then feel specific areas of the precordium systematically (Fig. 4-8).

Aortic area. The second interspace to the right of the sternum is felt for a pulsation, thrill, or vibration of aortic valve closure. Abnormal pulsations may be produced by dilatation of the ascending aorta. A vibratory thrill is associated with aortic stenosis, and an accentuated aortic valve closure is felt in patients with

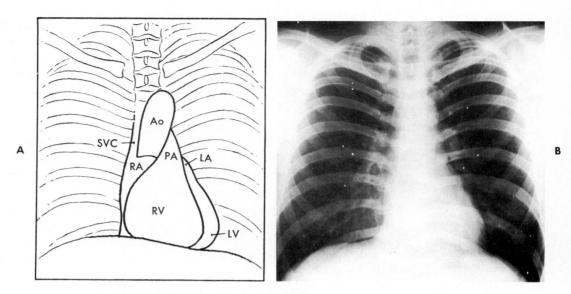

Fig. 4-7. A, Schematic illustration of the parts of the heart whose outlines can be detected in **B.** *Ao,* Aorta; *SVC,* superior vena cava; *RA,* right atrium; *PA,* pulmonary artery; *LA,* left atrium; *RV,* right ventricle. *LV,* left ventricle. **B,** Frontal projection x-ray film of the normal cardiac silhouette.

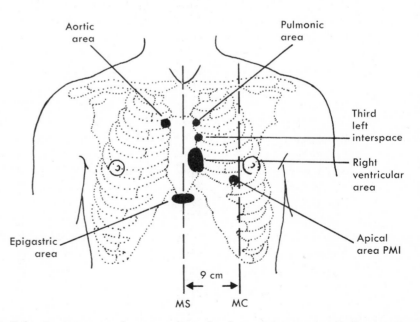

Fig. 4-8. Palpation areas on the precordium for detecting normal and abnormal cardiac pulsations. See text for description.

arterial hypertension. Thrills at the base can best be palpated with the patient sitting up and leaning forward.

Pulmonic area. The second and third left interspaces are evaluated for abnormalities in the pulmonary artery or valve. A relatively slow, sustained, and forceful pulsation of the pulmonary artery may be felt in mitral stenosis and primary pulmonary hypertension. A palpable sustained pulse and a thrill are associated with pulmonary stenosis.

Right ventricular area. The lower left sternal border, incorporating the third, fourth, and fifth intercostal spaces, is palpated. Abnormal pulsations here are most commonly found in conditions associated with right ventricular enlargement. When the sternum can be felt to move anteriorly during systole, this movement is termed a *substernal heave* or *lift*. Furthermore, a thrill in this area may be palpated in patients who have a ventricular septal defect.

Apical area. The fifth intercostal space at or just medial to the left midclavicular line is palpated for the *point of maximum impulse* (PMI) and the thrills of mitral valve disease. The PMI is evaluated for its location, diameter, amplitude, and duration. In normal adults the PMI is located at or within the left midclavicular line in the fifth intercostal space (Fig. 4-8). The impulse is normally less than 2 cm in diameter and often is smaller. It is felt as a light tap, beginning approximately at the time of the first heart sound, and is sustained during the first one third and one half of systole.

When the PMI is displaced lateral to the midclavicular line, it indicates left ventricular enlargement. A weak PMI may be palpated and may indicate inadequate stroke volume or reduced left ventricular contraction. This finding is difficult to detect in a muscular or obese chest or in patients with emphysema. A sustained or forceful apical impulse usually indicates left ventricular enlargement, such as that associated with aortic stenosis or arterial hypertension. A diffuse systolic thrill may be found in patients with mitral regurgitation, whereas a localized diastolic thrill generally is associated with mitral stenosis. Thrills at the apex are best felt with the patient in the left lateral decubitus position. This maneuver helps one find the impulse, but since this position displaces the PMI, no assessment can be made about location.

Epigastric area. The upper central region of the abdomen can have visible or palpable pulsations in some normal individuals. Abnormally large pulsations of the aorta may be produced by an aneurysm of the abdominal aorta or by aortic valvular regurgitation. In right ventricular hypertrophy right ventricular pulsations may also be detected in this area, which may be the best location to palpate the apical impulse in a patient with a distended chest, as in emphysema. To distinquish aortic from right ventricular pulsations, the palm of the hand should be placed on the epigastric area, sliding the fingers up under the rib cage. The palmar surface feels the aorta pulsating as the fingertips feel the impulses of the right ventricle.

AUSCULTATION OF THE HEART

Listening over the precordium with a stethoscope remains the most useful physical examination technique for providing information about heart function. Since the examiner depends on the stethoscope to register normal and abnormal sounds for interpretation, attention must be given to selection of the proper instrument. The stethoscope should have properly fitting earpieces, double tubes that are approximately 12 inches long and ⅛ inch in internal diameter, a bell, and a diaphragm. The bell accentuates the lower frequency sounds, such as diastolic gallops and the rumbling murmur of mitral stenosis, and filters out high-pitched notes. It should be placed very lightly on the skin, with just enough pressure to seal the edge of the unit. More pressure on the bell will cause the skin itself to act as a diaphragm, accentuating high-frequency sounds. Since the diaphragm brings out high-pitched sounds, it should be pressed very firmly against the skin. This will make high-frequency murmurs, such as the murmurs of aortic or mitral insufficiency, audible.

The environment and the patient's position also play important parts in the auscultation procedure. The room should be quite and the patient should be on a table or bed that will accommodate him comfortably when he is asked to lie flat, sit up, or roll to one side.

Finally, auscultation of the heart should not be performed as an isolated event. The findings should be correlated with the other results of the physical examination, such as the arterial pulse contour, venous pulse waves, and precordial movements, to understand the altered cardiac physiology and anatomy.

Auscultation of the heart requires selective listening for each component of the cardiac cycle as the examiner inches the stethoscope over the five main topographic areas for cardiac auscultation (Fig. 4-9). Note that these auscultatory areas do not correspond to the anatomic locations of the valves, but rather to the sites at which the particular valve sounds are best heard. Accordingly, one listens with the stethoscope over the following areas:

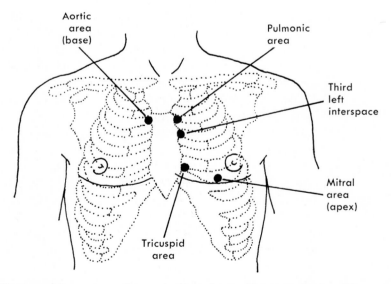

Fig. 4-9. Topographic areas on the precordium for cardiac auscultation. The auscultatory areas do not correspond to the anatomic locations of the valves but rather to the sites at which the particular valves are heard best. See text for description.

1. *Aortic area* at the base of the heart in the second intercostal space close to the sternum
2. *Pulmonic area* at the second left intercostal space close to the sternum
3. *Third left intercostal space* where murmurs of both aortic and pulmonic origin may be heard
4. *Tricuspid area* at the lower left sternal border
5. *Mitral area* at the apex of the heart in the fifth left intercostal space just medial to the midclavicular line

Auscultation is conducted in a systematic fashion. By beginning the process at the aortic area, one can determine the cardiac cycle time by identifying the first and second heart sounds. This will serve as a frame of reference as the examiner moves to other auscultatory areas of the precordium. The diaphragm of the stethoscope is used first to evaluate the high-pitched sounds, S_1 and S_2. The bell is used to detect lower-pitched sounds such as S_3 and S_4. At each site the procedure is as follows:

1. Listen to the first heart sound, noting its intensity and splitting.
2. Listen to the second heart sound, noting its intensity and splitting.
3. Note extra sounds in systole, identifying their timing, intensity, and pitch.
4. Note extra sounds in diastole, identifying their timing, intensity, and pitch.
5. Listen for systolic and diastolic murmurs, noting their timing, intensity, quality, pitch, location, and radiation.
6. Listen for extracardiac sounds, such as a pericardial friction rub.

If an abnormal sound is detected, the surrounding area is carefully explored to evaluate the distribution or radiation of the sound. The patient's position should be changed for better evaluation of abnormal sounds. For example, an aortic murmur may be heard best by having the patient sitting, leaning forward, exhaling, and holding the breath. Or an initial murmur or an S_4 may be heard by positioning the patient on his or her left side and listening to the apical area. Changes with respiration or during Valsalva maneuver may be important.

Changes in the intensity of heart sounds may be clinically significant. The intensity of valve sounds is probably related to the speed and force of the valve closure, the excursion of leaflets during closure, and the physical condition of the cusps. Intensity is modified by the proximity of the valve to the chest wall and by the nature of the tissues interposed between valve and stethoscope. Accordingly, the first sound heard at the mitral area (apex) may not only become softer at the aortic area (base), but may also seem shorter and have a different quality, which is caused by the dampening effect of the interposed soft tissues. Similarly, the second sound loses intensity as the stethoscope is moved toward the apex. The diagrams in Fig. 4-10 indicate the intensity and splitting of the first and second heart sounds, their relationship to the third and fourth heart sounds, and the auscultatory areas where these sounds can be heard best.

First heart sound (S_1). S_1 is associated with the closure of the mitral and tricuspid valves. It is synchronous with the apical impulse and corresponds to the onset of ventricular systole (Fig. 4-11). It is louder, longer, and lower pitched than the second sound at the apex (Fig. 4-10, *A*). As the ventricles begin to contract and pressure rises within, the tricuspid and mitral valves close. Valvular

HEART SOUNDS   AREA HEARD BEST

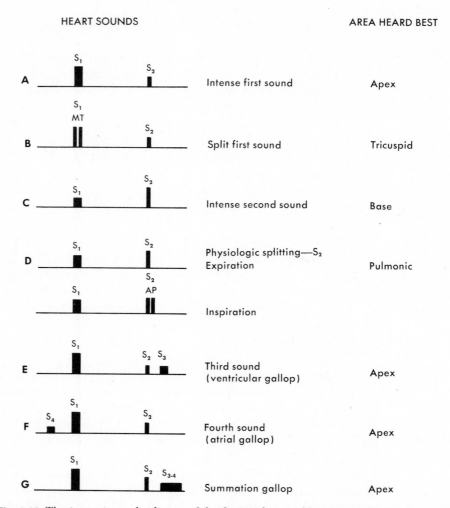

Fig. 4-10. The intensity and splitting of the first and second heart sounds, their relationship to the third and fourth heart sounds, and the auscultatory areas where these sounds are heard best.

sounds of the left side slightly precede those of the right and are of higher intensity; the mitral valve closes from 0.02 to 0.03 second before the tricuspid valve. *Splitting* of the first sound may therefore be heard, particularly in the tricuspid area (Fig. 4-10, *B*). Tricuspid closure is normally inaudible to the examiner's ear. The intensity of S_1 relates to the relative position of atrial contraction with respect to ventricular contraction, that is, PR interval. When the PR interval is prolonged, the intensity of the first heart sound is decreased, and when the PR interval shortens up to a point, the S_1 is increased. During AV dissociation the intensity of the first sound varies as the PR interval varies.

As the pressure within the ventricles continues to rise and exceeds the pressure within the pulmonary artery and aorta, the pulmonic and aortic valves open. Opening of these valves is usually inaudible. If opening of the aortic valve is heard, this is called an aortic ejection sound or click. The same is true for the

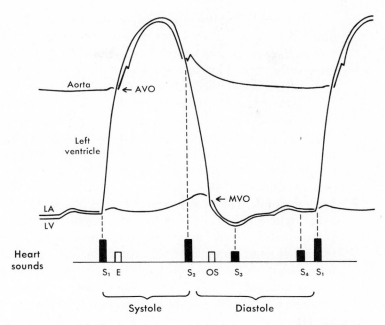

Fig. 4-11. Normal and abnormal heart sounds during one complete cardiac cycle as correlated with left-sided heart pressure waves. Right-sided heart pressures have been omitted for simplification. At the onset of ventricular systole, left ventricular (*LV*) pressure exceeds left atrial (*LA*) pressure to close the mitral valve, producing S_1 (in association with tricuspid valve closure). When LV pressure exceeds aortic pressure, the aortic valve opens (*AVO*). With valvular disease and hypertension, aortic valve opening may be audible and heard as an early ejection click (E). When aortic pressure exceeds LV pressure, the aortic valve closes to produce S_2 in association with pulmonic valve closure. When LV pressure drops below LA pressure, the mitral valve opens (*MVO*). With thickening of the mitral valve as a result of rheumatic heart disease an opening snap (*OS*) is produced in early diastole. During rapid ventricular filling an S_3, or ventricular gallop, is produced in patients with myocardial failure. Late in diastole an S_4, or atrial gallop, is produced in association with atrial contraction, owing to increased resistance to ventricular filling.

pulmonic valve. *Early systolic ejection clicks* occur shortly after S_1, as depicted in Fig. 4-11. Aortic ejection clicks are associated with aortic stenosis, dilatation of the aorta, and hypertension and are heard at both the base and the apex. Pulmonary ejection clicks are associated with pulmonary stenosis, dilatation of the pulmonary artery, and pulmonary hypertension and are heard in the pulmonic area. A common syndrome is the single or multiple midsystolic click that initiates a late systolic murmur of mitral insufficiency, caused by prolapse of the mitral valve. The click in this instance is a nonejection click.

Second heart sound (S_2). S_2 is associated with the closure of the aortic and pulmonic valves. With the completion of ventricular contraction the pressure within the ventricles and great vessels decreases. The ventricular pressure decreases more rapidly than the pressures within the aorta and pulmonary arteries, causing the aortic and pulmonic valves to close. This is followed by the start of ventricular diastole. At the aortic area, or base, the second sound is almost always louder than the first sound (Fig. 4-10, *C*).

The aortic component is widely transmitted to the neck and over the precordium. It is, as a rule, entirely responsible for the second sound at the apex. The pulmonary component is softer than the aortic and is normally heard only at and around the second left interspace (pulmonic area). Splitting of the second sound is therefore usually heard best in this region.

Again, events of the left side of the heart occur before those on the right, and aortic valve closure slightly precedes that of the pulmonic valve. Transient *splitting* of the second sound may be demonstrated in most normal people during inspiration. Closure of the aortic and pulmonary valves during expiration is synchronous or nearly so because right and left ventricular systoles are approximately equal in duration. With inspiration, venous blood rushes into the thorax from the large systemic venous reservoirs. This action increases venous return and prolongs right ventricular systole by temporarily increasing right ventricular stroke volume, which delays pulmonary valve closure. At the same time, venous return to the left heart diminishes because of the increased pulmonary capacity during inspiration, which decreases left ventricular stroke volume and shortens left ventricular systole. Thus the aortic valve tends to close earlier. These two factors combine to produce transient *physiologic splitting* of the second sound (Fig. 4-10, *D*).

As the pressure in the ventricles decreases below the pressure in the atria, the atrioventricular valves open. The opening of these valves is characteristically silent. However, when either the mitral or the tricuspid valve is thickened or otherwise altered, as by rheumatic heart disease, it produces an *opening snap* in early diastole (Fig. 4-11). The opening snap of the mitral valve is differentiated from a third heart sound at the apex because it occurs earlier, is sharper and higher pitched, and radiates more widely.

Third heart sound (S_3). S_3 occurs early in diastole during the phase of rapid ventricular filling, about 0.12 to 0.16 second after S_2 (Fig. 4-11). It is a low-pitched sound, heard best with the bell of the stethoscope pressed lightly over the apex and the patient in the left lateral decubitus position (Fig. 4-10, *E*). When S_3 is heard in healthy children and young adults, it is called a *physiologic third heart sound* and usually disappears with age. When an S_3 is heard in an older peron with heart disease, it usually indicates myocardial failure and is called a *ventricular gallop*. In patients with cardiac disease, one should search carefully for the presence of a ventricular gallop, since it is a key diagnostic sign for the presence of congestive heart failure from any cause.

Fourth heart sound (S_4). S_4 occurs late in diastole, prior to S_1, and is related to atrial contraction (Fig. 4-11). It is a low-pitched sound heard best at the apex with the bell (Fig. 4-10, *F*). It is uncommon to hear this sound in normal individuals. S_4, or *atrial gallop*, is associated with increased resistance to ventricular filling and is frequently heard in hypertensive cardiovascular disease, coronary artery disease, myocardiopathy, and aortic stenosis. It is a common finding in patients who have had a myocardial infarction. An S_4 may also be heard in patients with AV block where there is a delayed conduction between the atria and the ventricles.

Summation gallop. In adults with severe myocardial disease and tachycardia, summation of S_3 and S_4 may occur, producing the so-called summation gallop (Fig. 4-10, *G*).

Murmurs. Although the physical principles governing the production of murmurs are complex, from a practical point of view murmurs are related to three main factors, which are as follows:
1. High rates of flow, either through normal or abnormal valves
2. Forward flow through a constricted or deformed valve or into a dilated vessel or chamber
3. Backward flow through a regurgitant valve

The identification of murmurs may contribute important information to the recognition and diagnosis of heart disease. Accordingly, murmurs should be carefully evaluated and described in a manner that provides maximum information. Murmurs are usually characterized in relation to the following criteria:

1. *Timing.* Does the murmur occur during systole, during diastole, or continuously through both? A murmur may be easily differentiated as systolic or diastolic by palpating the pulse. If the murmur occurs simultaneously with the pulse, it is systolic; if it does not, it is diastolic. If a murmur occupies all the time period measured, it is described as holosystolic (pansystolic) or holodiastolic (pandiastolic).
2. *Intensity.* How loud is the murmur? A graded point system is generally accepted to describe the intensity of murmurs, as follows:

    > *Grade 1:* Softest audible murmur
    > *Grade 2:* Murmur of medium intensity
    > *Grade 3:* Loud murmur unaccompanied by thrill
    > *Grade 4:* Murmur with thrill
    > *Grade 5:* Loudest murmur that cannot be heard with the stethoscope off the chest
    > *Grade 6:* Murmur audible with the stethoscope off the chest

3. *Quality.* What is the tonal characteristic of the murmur? Is it harsh? Musical? Blowing? Rumbling? The configuration or shape of a murmur further defines its quality. It may be a crescendo (increasing intensity), decrescendo (decreasing intensity), or crescendo-decrescendo (diamond-shaped) type. Fig. 4-12 depicts these configurations.
4. *Pitch.* What is the sound frequency of the murmur? Is it high? Medium? Low?
5. *Location.* Over what area on the precordium is the murmur heard best? The aortic area? The pulmonic area? The triscuspid area? The mitral area?
6. *Radiation.* Is there transmission of the murmur elsewhere in the body? Does it radiate across the chest? Into the axilla? Into the neck? Down the left sternal border?

In addition, each of these characteristics is further evaluated as it is influenced by the patient's position and respiration. Certain other maneuvers may be used to define murmurs further, including Valsalva's maneuver, which decreases cardiac output and stroke volume during the strain and increases flow after release. Also, amyl nitrite can be administered, with resultant peripheral vasodilatation and increased cardiac output. Changes in the intensity and character of murmurs with these maneuvers aid in determining the type of lesion involved. For instance, with the administration of amyl nitrite, murmurs associated with stenotic lesions usually become louder, whereas regurgitant murmurs decrease in intensity.

Systolic murmurs. Systolic murmurs are the most common murmurs and generally are either ejection or regurgitant murmurs. *Functional* or innocent systolic murmurs are commonly heard in young people and should be distinguished from

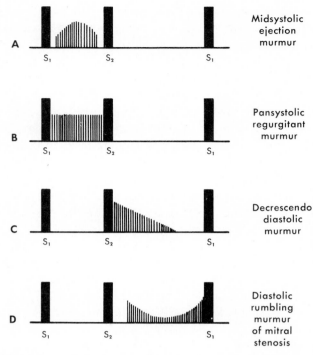

Fig. 4-12. Configuration of murmurs. **A,** Aortic and pulmonic stenosis produce systolic ejection murmurs that begin after the S_1, swell to a crescendo in midsystole, then decrease in intensity (decrescendo), and terminate before the S_2. **B,** Tricuspid and mitral regurgitation and ventricular septal defects produce pansystolic (holosystolic) murmurs that last throughout ventricular systole; usually no interval can be heard between S_1 and S_2. **C,** Aortic and pulmonic regurgitation produce murmurs that begin early in diastole immediately after the S_2 and then diminish in intensity (decrescendo). **D,** Mitral and tricuspid stenosis produce murmurs that begin during early diastole, have a rumbling or rolling quality, and terminate in late diastole with a crescendo effect.

those murmurs that represent valvular heart disease. Functional murmurs occur during ejection, are short (less than two thirds of systole), are grade 2 or less in intensity (they may become inaudible if the patient raises from a supine to a sitting position), and are heard best over the pulmonary outflow tract. It is important to remember that functional murmurs are intensified by fever, anxiety, anemia, and pregnancy. Therefore the patient should be reexamined under normal conditions.

Midsystolic (ejection) murmurs. *Aortic stenosis* and *pulmonic stenosis* produce systolic ejection murmurs that begin after the first sound, swell to a crescendo in midsystole, then decrease in intensity, and terminate before S_2, generated by closure of the appropriate valve (Fig. 4-12, *A*). The murmur may be harsh or musical and is usually high pitched because of the high velocity of blood flow. Aortic valve murmurs frequently radiate from the second right interspace to the cardiac apex and the carotid arteries. A systolic thrill may be present. Characteristically, pulmonic stenosis murmur is heard better at the second left interspace. Atrial septal defects increase pulmonary flow to produce a pulmonary ejection murmur.

Holosystolic (regurgitant) murmurs. Holosystolic murmurs last throughout ventricular systole (Fig. 4-12, *B*) and no interval can be heard between S_1 and S_2. *Tricuspid* and *mitral regurgitation* and *ventricular septal defects* produce holosystolic murmurs owing to the backflow of blood from the ventricle (high pressure) to the atrium (low pressure) through an incompetent tricuspid or mitral valve or from a high-pressure ventricle (left) to a low-pressure ventricle (right). Unlike the production of ejection murmurs, when a holosystolic murmur is produced one chamber maintains a greater pressure than the other throughout *all* of systole, causing regurgitant blood flow (and the murmur) to last through the entire systolic period. Murmurs caused by ventricular septal defects may seem louder during early systole and those of mitral regurgitation louder during late systole. The murmurs may be blowing, musical, or harsh and are often high pitched. The tricuspid regurgitation murmur is best heard along the lower left sternal border, and the intensity commonly increases during inspiration. Mitral regurgitation is best heard at the apex with the patient lying on his left side and often radiates to the left axilla or back. Some forms of mitral regurgitation do not produce holosystolic murmurs. Ventricular septal defects are loudest at the third and fourth left interspaces along the sternal border; often a systolic thrill accompanies the murmur in that area.

During the acute phase of myocardial infarction the *interventricular septum* may *rupture*. Although uncommon, the resulting ventricular septal defect produces a loud systolic murmur, as described previously. The onset of this murmur is sudden, and it may be accompanied by a thrill and the features of left and right-sided heart failure.

Myocardial infarction may also produce *papillary muscle rupture*, with subsequent mitral insufficiency and predominantly left-sided heart failure. The onset of the murmur is abrupt and may be difficult to distinguish from that of the perforated interventricular septum, since the features of both catastrophes overlap. Mitral valve dysfunction, without actual rupture of the papillary muscle or chordae tendineae, may establish less severe mitral insufficiency. Abnormalities of the chordae tendineae may produce clicking sounds that occur in the middle of ventricular systole and are referred to as *midsystolic clicks*. These may occur with or without a late systolic murmur. *Ventricular aneurysms* secondary to myocardial infarction may produce muffled heart sounds, gallop rhythms, and both systolic and diastolic murmurs; often a prominent systolic impulse may be palpated over the left precordium.

Diastolic murmurs. Diastolic murmurs generally can be classified into two types: the high-pitched decrescendo murmurs of aortic and pulmonic regurgitation and the lower-pitched murmurs of mitral and tricuspid stenosis.

Murmurs of aortic and pulmonic regurgitation begin early in diastole, immediately after the S_2, and then diminish in intensity (decrescendo), as shown in Fig. 4-12, *C*. They are high pitched and blowing and may vary in intensity roughly according to the size of the leak. The murmur of aortic regurgitation may be heard best at the second right or third left interspace along the left sternal border with the patient holding his breath in expiration while leaning forward. The murmur of pulmonic regurgitation is heard at the upper left border of the sternum and cannot be distinguished from its aortic counterpart by auscultation

Table 4-1. Characteristics of types of valvular heart disease

Condition	Causes	Description of murmurs					Other signs
		Time	Quality	Pitch (frequency)	Location of maximum intensity	Radiation or transmission	
Aortic stenosis (narrowing of valve)	Rheumatic Calcification Congenital	Systolic (ejection)	Crescendo-decrescendo (diamond shaped) Harsh Rough	Variable pitch	Second interspace (aortic area)	Radiates to carotid arteries and apex	Slow rising "anacrotic" Sustained pulse Left ventricular lift Systolic thrill Ejection "click" Diminished aortic closing sound
Aortic regurgitation (blood flows back from aorta into left ventricle)	Rheumatic Syphilitic Calcification Cystic medial necrosis	Diastolic	Blowing loudest just after S_2—diminishes during diastole decrescendo	High pitch	Second right interspace; third left interspace or along left sternal border with patient leaning forward and holding breath		Wide pulse pressure Left ventricular lift Brisk, quick pulses (water hammer) Tambour aortic closing sound
Mitral stenosis (narrowing of valve; blood flows through valve during diastole)	Rheumatic Congenital Tumor (myxoma)	Diastolic	Rumbling, presystolic accentuation in sinus rhythm	Low pitch	Well localized to apex, best heard in left lateral decubitus position		Atrial fibrillation often develops Loud S_1 Opening snap
Mitral regurgitation ("leaky" valve—blood reenters left atrium from left ventricle during systole)	Rheumatic Congenital Papillary muscle dysfunction/rupture Chordae tendineae dysfunction/rupture Heart failure associated with left ventricular dilation from any cause	Holosystolic	Blowing	High pitch	Apex, best heard in left lateral decubitus position	Axilla and back	S_3 common

alone. The pitch, timing, quality, and location of these murmurs are similar, although the murmur of pulmonic regurgitation tends to be more localized in the pulmonic area.

Mitral stenosis characteristically produces a low-pitched, localized apical, diastolic rumble, which may be accentuated in late diastole (Fig. 4-12, *D*) when atrial systole causes increased flow across the narrowed mitral valve. A sharp mitral "opening snap" frequently initiates the murmur in early diastole. In addition, a loud, sharp S_1 and accentuation of the S_2 often accompany mitral stenosis. The murmur of mitral stenosis is usually confined to the apex and may be enhanced by mild exercise or by the patient's lying on his left side. The *tricuspid stenosis* murmur is heard near the tricuspid area and is often accentuated along the left sternal border by inspiration.

Continuous murmurs. Murmurs audible in both systole and diastole are usually caused by connections between the arterial and venous or systemic and pulmonary circulations. A patent ductus arteriosus produces such a murmur. Table 4-1 summarizes the characteristics of the most common heart murmurs.

A benign sound heard at the lower border of the sternocleidomastoid muscle in some normal adults in the sitting position is called a *venous hum*. Although continuous, the venous hum is loudest in diastole and radiates to the first and second interspaces, with a soft to moderate intensity. It has a roaring quality, is low pitched, and can be obliterated by pressure on the jugular veins.

Pericardial friction rub. An extracardiac sound that may be detected during the auscultation procedure is the pericardial friction rub. It is a sign of pericardial inflammation, and in its complete form it exhibits three components. One is associated with ventricular systole, the second with the phase of rapid ventricular filling early in diastole, and the third with atrial systole. If only the systolic component of the rub is present, it may be misinterpreted as a scratchy murmur. With the patient lying flat on his back the pericardial friction rub is best heard in the third or fourth interspace to the left of the sternum, although the location may be variable. There is little radiation, and the quality of the sound is a leathery, high-pitched, multiphasic, scratchy rub, which sounds like two pieces of sandpaper being rubbed together.

EXAMINATION OF THE LUNGS

Disorders of the lungs may alter or be altered by cardiac conditions. Consequently, in assessing the cardiovascular status of a patient, one must also evaluate lung function. Examination of the anterior, lateral, and posterior aspects of the chest is best accomplished with the patient in the sitting position. This may be done immediately following or just prior to the cardiac examination, before the patient assumes the supine position.

Understanding the anatomy of the lungs is essential to conducting a proper examination, since each bronchopulmonary lobe must be evaluated. The schematic illustrations of the lung lobes in anterior, posterior, and right and left lateral views in Fig. 4-13 may be helpful.

The lungs rest in the thorax, with the apex of each lung rising about 2 to 4 cm above the inner one third of the clavicles. The inferior border of the lungs runs from approximately the sixth rib at the midclavicular line to the eighth rib

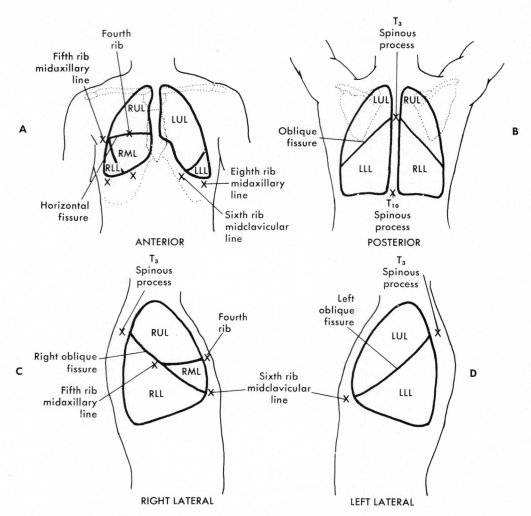

Fig. 4-13. The lung lobes and their anatomic landmarks in anterior, **A,** posterior, **B,** and right and left lateral, **C** and **D,** views. See text for description.

at the midaxillary line anteriorly and along the level of the tenth thoracic spinous process posteriorly. The lungs are divided by fissures into lobes, the left lung into two lobes, the right lung into three lobes. The locations of the fissures are identified by corresponding surface sites. On the anterior chest wall the horizontal fissure of the right lung runs from the fifth rib at the midaxillary line to the level of the fourth rib. On the lateral chest wall the spinous process of the third thoracic vertebra and the sixth rib at the midclavicular line denote the direction of the right and left oblique fissures. When a patient holds up his arms, the oblique fissures are close to the vertebral borders of the scapulae on the posterior chest wall.

The following discussion briefly covers the physical findings gathered during inspection, palpation, percussion, and auscultation of the chest with reference to the lungs.

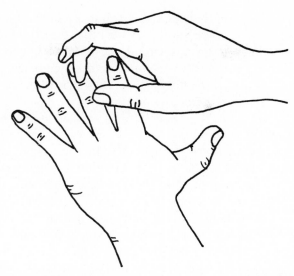

Fig. 4-14. Position of the hands in percussion. The distal two phalanges of the middle finger of the left hand for a right-handed examiner are placed firmly against the patient's chest in the intercostal space parallel to the ribs. The palm and other fingers of the left hand do not touch the chest wall. Then, as shown here, the examiner *quickly* strikes the distal phalanx of the stationary finger with the tip of the middle finger of the right hand.

Inspection and palpation. As discussed earlier in the chapter, the examiner observes the rate and pattern of respiration, the expansion of the chest with breathing, and the symmetry of the thorax. Normally the entire rib cage uniformly moves laterally and upward with respiration. Palpation refines assessment of the degree and symmetry of expansion in respiration, detects any areas of tenderness, and permits the examiner to feel *fremitus* (sound vibrations) when the patient speaks. Fremitus is most prominent over areas where the bronchi are relatively close to the chest wall and can be elicited by asking the patient to repeat words such as "one-one-one" or "ninety-nine." Fremitus increases as the intensity of the voice increases and its pitch drops; conversely, it decreases as the intensity of the voice decreases and the pitch rises. Fremitus may also decrease or be absent with an obstructed bronchus, pneumothorax, or pleural effusion. If the chest wall is markedly thick, as in obesity, fremitus may be diminished. Increased fremitus is produced by consolidation of the lung in the presence of an intact airway.

Percussion. Percussion is performed to determine the relative amount of air or solid material in the underlying lung and to delineate the boundaries of organs or the portions of the lung that differ in structural density. The procedure of percussion involves placing the distal two phalanges of the middle finger of the right hand (for right-handed examiners) firmly against the patient's chest in the intercostal space parallel to the ribs. The palm and other fingers of the left hand should not touch the chest wall. Then with the tip of the middle finger of the right hand, *quickly* strike the distal phalanx of the stationary finger, as shown in Fig. 4-14. One or two rapid strikes in succession with a loose wrist action produces the desired percussion note. (To learn the technique of percussion, it may be helpful to percuss a wall in a room and note the difference in sound over the beams when compared with that over the hollows.)

The anterior and lateral chest walls are percussed in a top-to-bottom, side-to-side fashion while comparing the symmetry of sound and feeling. Similarly, the posterior lung fields are percussed, working down to the level of the diaphragm and comparing percussion notes.

The sounds produced by percussion should be evaluted with respect to four qualities:

1. *Resonance*. Resonance is the percussion note elicited over the normal lung. Although it may vary with the thickness of the chest wall, resonance projects a clear, low-pitched, and well-sustained note. A hyperresonant note, in general, is associated with hyperaeration of the lungs, as in pneumothorax or obstructive emphysema.

2. *Tympany*. The tympanic note is normally heard in the left upper quadrant of the abdomen over the air-filled stomach or over any hollow viscus. The note is loud, musical, and well sustained, with a high-pitched, clear, hollow, and drumlike quality.

3. *Dullness*. Dullness is produced when the air content of the underlying tissue is decreased and its solidity increased, as in pneumonia or pleural effusion. The dull sound is soft, short, and high pitched, with a thudding quality. It lacks the vibratory quality of the resonant note. A dull note is elicited normally over the heart or over bone. Of particular importance is the phenomenon of shifting dullness, that is, a change in the site of abdominal percussion dullness with a change in posture, since it suggests free fluid in the pleural cavity.

4. *Flatness*. Flatness is produced when no air is present in the underlying tissue. It is absolute dullness. The flat note is short, high pitched, and feeble. Normally the flat sound is percussed over the muscles of the arm and thigh and over the liver.

Diaphragmatic excursion can be measured by determining the distance between the levels of dullness on full expiration and full inspiration, normally about 5 cm. High levels of dullness over the posterior aspect of the chest are associated with pleural effusion, atelectasis, or an elevated diaphragm.

Auscultation. Auscultation of the lung fields permits the examiner to make determinations about the state of bronchial patency of various lung divisions, to assess the quality and intensity of breath sounds, and to note any abnormal sounds. The patient should be asked to breathe somewhat more deeply than usual, with the mouth open. Auscultation is then accomplished in a sequence similar to that or percussion, beginning with the upper lung fields; one side is listened to, then the other, and then both are compared down to the level of the diaphragm. All portions of the lung fields—posterior, anterior, and lateral—must be systematically auscultated.

Normal breath sounds. Normal breath sounds can be categorized as vesicular, bronchial, and bronchovesicular. *Vesicular* breath sounds occur over most of the lungs and have a prominent inspiratory component and a brief expiratory phase. *Bronchial* breath sounds, also called tracheal breath sounds, are normally heard over the trachea and main bronchi. These sounds are hollow, tubular, and harsh and are heard best during expiration. *Bronchovesicular* breath sounds are heard over the main stem of the bronchi and represent an intermediate stage between bronchial and vesicular breathing.

Abnormal breath sounds. Normal breath sounds in one area may be pathologic when heard somewhere else. For example, bronchial and bronchovesicular breath sounds are heard over a consolidated, compressed, or fibrosed lung. Furthermore, diminished breath sounds occur with local or diffuse bronchial obstruction and with pleural disease associated with the presence of fluid, air, or scar tissue. With airways narrowed, the breath sounds are characteristically wheezing and whistling in nature, with a prolonged expiratory and a short inspiratory phase, as heard in patients with asthma.

Rales are abnormal sounds that occur when air passes through bronchi that contain fluid of any kind. They are subdivided into interrupted crackling sounds, termed *moist rales*, and continuous coarse sounds, called *rhonchi*. Rhonchi suggest a pathologic condition in the trachea or larger bronchi, whereas moist medium and fine rales imply bronchiolar and alveolar disease. *Fine rales* are short and high pitched and can be simulated by rubbing a strand of hair between the thumb and forefinger next to the ear. *Medium rales* are louder and lower pitched.

In left ventricular failure the presence of rales is one of the earliest physical findings. Rales occur as a result of the transudation of edema fluid into the pulmonary alveoli. At first the alveolar fluid is dependent in location, and rales are present at the base of the lungs. As the failure becomes increasingly severe, the rales become more generalized. The rales of left ventricular failure are typically fine and crepitant, but as failure progresses, they may become moist and coarse. The findings may be difficult to differentiate from those caused by pulmonary infiltrations of an inflammatory nature. Rales from left ventricular failure often develop first at the right lung base but are frequently bibasilar.

Pleural friction rub. Inflammation of the visceral and parietal pleurae may result in loss of lubricating fluid so that apposing pleural surfaces rub together, producing a low-pitched, coarse, grating sound with respiration. When the patient holds his breath the rub disappears.

Finally, one should be wary of the adventitious sounds produced when a stethoscope is not held firmly against the chest. Body hair can rub across the instrument during respiration and produce an annoying crackling sound.

Assessment of common symptoms and signs

A number of symptoms are commonly associated with heart disease. Most individuals with coronary heart disease or hypertension are asymptomatic. When symptoms or signs do appear, either they relate to complications from the disease, or the disease state is well advanced.

Patients who have heart disease should be queried specifically about the presence or absence of the following conditions. Each symptom, if present, should be evaluated and described carefully using the descriptors on pp. 35 to 36.

1. *Dypsnea.* Dypsnea is labored or difficult breathing; it accompanies a number of cardiac conditions and is a manifestation of congestive heart

failure. Commonly, this occurs with strain and may be affected by position. Dypsnea varies in degree. The amount of exertion required to cause it and the amount of rest necessary to relieve it should be quantitated carefully. *Paroxysmal nocturnal dypsnea* occurs at night; the patient awakens with a terrifying sensation of suffocating. The distress diminishes after sitting up for a few minutes. *Orthopnea* is associated with congestive heart failure; the patient has difficulty breathing when lying flat in bed and requires two or more pillows for sleep.

2. *Cardiac asthma.* Cardiac asthma refers to wheezing caused by pulmonary congestion.

3. *Palpitations.* Palpitations occur with premature beats or other rhythm disturbances and are perceived by the patient as abnormal sensations of the heartbeat, a skipped beat, or a flutter.

4. *Syncope.* Syncope is a temporary loss of consciousness due to inadequate oxygen supply to the brain. Heart block, cardiac asystole, severe sinus bradycardia or arrest, or ventricular tachyarrhythmias may be causes.

5. *Fatigue, mental confusion, failure to thrive.* These and other vague symptoms may be associated with coronary complications and are particularly common in elderly patients.

6. *Hemoptysis.* Hemoptysis, or coughing up blood, may be associated with pulmonary edema or pulmonary embolus.

7. *Edema.* Edema or fluid in the form of edema tends to accumulate in the dependent areas of the body: the hands and feet in the ambulatory patient and the sacral area of the bedridden patient. Edema accompanies right-sided heart failure. Edema is assessed by firmly indenting the skin with the fingertips. The degree of pitting that occurs should be quantitated and described with the following scale:

> 0 = None present
> +1 = Trace—disappears rapidly
> +2 = Moderate—disappears in 10 to 15 seconds
> +3 = Deep—disappears in 1 to 2 minute
> +4 = Very deep—present after 5 minutes[2]

In examining the bedridden patient for edema it is important to press over the sacrum, buttocks, and posterior thighs. Sudden weight gain may be a sign of edema.

8. *Cyanosis.* Cyanosis is a bluish discoloration appearing in the extremities and lips caused by poor circulation. It is brought on by cold temperatures or some severe dysfunction, such as pulmonary disease or shock. The examiner should observe the color of earlobes, lips, fingernail beds, and mucous membranes. *Central cyanosis* occurs with low arterial oxygen saturation associated with congenital right-to-left shunts or pulmonary diseases such as pneumonia. It is observed in the mucous membranes such as the conjunctiva and the inside of the lips and cheeks. With *peripheral cyanosis* the arterial oxygen saturation may be normal, but the oxygen within the peripheral vascular bed is inadequate. This may occur with heart failure and shock.

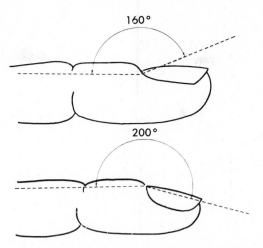

Fig. 4-15. Profile sign. Early clubbing sometimes evidence by a nail-to-nailbed angle of more than 180 degrees. Top view is normal and bottom view is abnormal. (From Thompson, D.A.: Cardiovascular assessment: guide for nurses and other health professionals, St. Louis, 1981, The C.V. Mosby Co.)

9. *Clubbing* is a condition of the nail bed associated with certain pulmonary or cardiac diseases (Fig. 4-15).
10. *Hypoxemia (hypoxia).* This is an insufficient supply of oxygen in the blood. Signs of hypoxia include increased pulse rate, irritability, restlessness, disorientation, and cyanosis.
11. *Chest pain.* Chest pain is a complaint associated with a reasonably large number of clinical problems, in addition to angina and acute myocardial infarction. To differentiate between myocardial ischemia and these other causes of chest pain requires a systematic evaluation of the patient's symptoms. The descriptors associated with angina and myocardial infarction are described in Chapter 7. Table 4-2 summarizes distinguishing features of other conditions commonly appearing in settings of cardiac care.

Problem-oriented patient record

The problem-oriented record is a method of organizing and recording the patient's health history, throughout which specific problems are defined, numbered, and referred to by number.

The problem-oriented record includes an *initial data base* consisting of the patient's health history, a complete physical examination, and laboratory data. The *problem list* consists of medical, social, and psychologic problems derived from the initial data base. The dates of onset and resolution of these problems (both active and inactive) are recorded and the problems numbered. Each problem retains its original number. The problem list usually is at the beginning of the record and serves as an index. Each problem has a plan that includes diagnostic measures, therapeutic approaches, and patient education.

This problem-oriented approach is useful in the process of nursing assessment

Table 4-2. Assessment of chest pain

Condition	Location	Quality	Severity	Course	Aggravating or relieving factors	Symptoms or signs
Angina	Retrosternal region; radiates to neck, jaw, epigastrium, shoulders or arms—left common	Pressure, burning, squeezing, heaviness, indigestion	Moderate to severe	< 10 minutes	Aggravated by exercise, cold weather, emotional stress, or after meals; relieved by rest or nitroglycerin; atypical (Prinzmetal's) angina may be unrelated to activity and caused by coronary artery spasm	S_4, paradoxical split S_2 during pain
Intermediate syndrome or coronary insufficiency	Same as angina	Same as angina	Increasingly severe	> 10 minutes	Same as angina, with gradually decreasing tolerance for exertion	Same as angina
Myocardial infarction	Substernal, and may radiate like angina	Heaviness, pressure, burning, constriction	Severe, sometimes mild (in 25% of patients)	Sudden onset 30 minutes or longer but variable; usually goes away in hours	Unrelieved	Shortness of breath, sweating, weakness, nausea, vomiting, severe anxiety
Pericarditis	Usually begins over sternum and may radiate to neck and down left upper extremity	Sharp, stabbing knifelike	Moderate to severe	Lasts many hours to days	Aggravated by deep breathing, rotating chest or supine position; relieved by sitting up and leaning forward	Pericardial friction rub, syncope, cardiac tamponade, pulsus paradoxus (Kussmaul sign)
Dissecting aortic aneurysm	Anterior chest; radiates to thoracic area of back; may be abdominal; pain shifts in chest	Tearing	Excruciating, tearing knifelike	Sudden onset lasts for hours	Unrelated to anything	Lower blood pressure in one arm, absent pulses, paralysis, murmur of aortic insufficiency; pulsus paradoxus, stridor: myocardial infarction can occur

	Location	Quality	Severity	Duration/Onset	Aggravating factors	Associated findings
Pulmonary embolism (most pulmonary emboli do not produce chest pain)	Substernal "anginal"	Not pleuritic unless infarction exists	Can be severe	Sudden onset; minutes to <hour	May be aggravated by breathing	Fever, tachypnea, tachycardia, hypotension, elevated jugular venous pressure, right ventricular lift, accentuated P_2, occasional murmur of tricuspid insufficiency and right ventricular S_4; with infarction usually in the presence of congestive heart failure, rales, pleural rub, hemoptysis, clinical phlebitis present in minority of cases
Pulmonary hypertension	Substernal	Pressure; oppressive	Variable		Aggravated by effort	Pain usually associated with dyspnea; right ventricular lift, accentuated P_2
Spontaneous pneumothorax	Unilateral	Sharp, well localized		Sudden onset, lasts many hours	Painful breathing	Dyspnea, hyperresonance, and decreased breath and voice sounds over involved lung
Pneumonia with pleurisy	Localized over area of consolidation	Pleuritic, well localized	Moderate		Painful breathing	Dyspnea, cough, fever, dull to flat percussion, bronchial breathing, rales, occasional pleural rub
Gastrointestinal disorders	Lower substernal area, epigastric, right or left upper quadrant	Burning, colicklike aching			Precipitated by recumbency or meals	Nausea, regurgitation, food intolerance, melena, hematemesis, jaundice
Musculoskeletal disorders	Variable	Aching		Short or long duration	Aggravated by movement, history of muscle exertion	Tender to pressure or movement
Neurological disorders (herpes zoster)	Dermatomal in distribution			Prolonged period of time; Unassociated with external events		Rash appears in area of discomfort with herpes
Anxiety states	Usually localized to a point	Sharp burning, commonly location of pain moves from place to place	Mild to moderate	Varies; usually very brief	Situational anger	Sighing respirations, often chest wall tenderness

and the documentation of nursing care and may be used to assess and describe the behavioral dimensions of care unique to the concern of nursing practice.

Patient assessment should be an orderly process whereby subjective and objective data are gathered and synthesized, assessment of the problem is made, and finally a plan is formulated for each problem identified.

Subjective information includes information obtained from the patient about the health history and present complaint, as well as the time interval since the last entry. Objective information includes information gathered by the health provider during the physical examination and laboratory studies. The assessment identifies one or more situations or problems and is stated in those terms until a firm diagnosis is made. The assessment includes the practitioner's analysis of the subjective and objective data relating to the etiology of the problem, the course of the problem, the patient's response to therapy and coping ability, the patient's participation in and reaction to the plans, and probable outcomes. A plan is formulated for each problem. The plan may include diagnostic studies, medication or other treatment, or health education, such as working with the patient to stop smoking.

PROGRESS NOTES

Progress notes include subjective (S), objective (O), assessment (A), and plan (P) components. The acronym SOAP refers to the format for recording progress notes.

S = subjective information from the patient's history
O = objective information including the physical examination and results of laboratory studies
A = assessment or analysis of the observations
P = plans for further treatment, diagnostic procedures or patient education

Assessment of risk factors

Risk factors have been discussed in Chapters 2 and 3. The management of risk factors is an important clinical strategy in the care of patients who have coronary heart disease. It is therefore important to possess an orderly process of patient assessment to identify risk factors. The SOAP process can be applied as a reminder in completing a total risk assessment with the patient and planning interventions or modifications in life-style. The procedure for gathering and recording information is as follows:

1. *Subjective data* obtained from patient history, such as heredity, smoking, occupation, and exercise
2. *Objective data* obtained from physical examination and laboratory studies, such as age, sex, race, weight, blood pressure, cholesterol level, triglyceride level, and blood sugar level
3. *Assessment* of patient's risk
4. *Plan* or interventions

Using this process of health assessment gives the practitioner and patient a good perspective on quantitative and qualitative aspects of individual risk and facilitates planning for behavioral change.

SUGGESTED READINGS

Bates, B., and Hoekelman, R.A.: Physical examination, ed. 2, Philadelphia, 1979, J.B. Lippincott Co.

DeGowin, E.L., and DeGowin, R.L.: Bedside diagnostic examination, ed. 3, New York, 1976, Macmillan Publishing Co., Inc.

Fowkes, W.C., and Hunn, V.K.: Clinical assessment for the nurse practitioner, St. Louis, 1973, The C.V. Mosby Co.

Fowler, N.O.: Inspection and palpation of venous and arterial pulses. Examination of the heart. Part 2, New York, 1972, American Heart Association.

Harris, A., Sutton, G., and Towers, M., editors: Physiological and clinical aspects of cardiac auscultation, Philadelphia, 1976, J.B. Lippincott Co.

Hobson, L.B.: Examination of the patient, New York, 1975, McGraw-Hill Book Co.

Hurst, J.W., et al., editors: The heart, ed. 4, New York, 1978, McGraw-Hill Book Co.

Hurst, J.W., and Schlant, R.C.: Inspection and palpation of the anterior chest. Examination of the heart. Part 3, New York, 1972, American Heart Association.

Judge, R.D., and Zuidema, G.D., editors: Methods of clinical examination: A physiologic approach, ed. 3, Boston, 1974, Little, Brown & Co.

Leatham, A.: Auscultation of the heart and phonocardiography, ed. 2, London, 1975, Churchill Livingstone.

Leonard J.J., and Croetz, F.W.: Auscultation. Examination of the heart. Part 4, New York, 1967, American Heart Association.

Lesser, L.M., and Wenger, N.K.: Carotid sinus syncope, Heart Lung **5:**453-456, 1976.

Luckman, J., and Sorenson, K.C.: Medical surgical nursing, Philadelphia, 1974, W.B. Saunders Co.

Ravin, A., et al.: Auscultation of the heart, ed. 3, Chicago, 1977, Year Book Medical Publishers, Inc.

Sanan, J., and Judge, D.: Physical appraisal methods in nursing practice, Boston, 1975, Little, Brown & Co.

Schroeder, J.P., and Daily, E.K.: Techniques in bedside hemodynamic monitoring, St. Louis, 1976, The C.V. Mosby Co.

Silverman, M.E.: The clinical history. Examination of the Heart. Part 1, New York, 1975, American Heart Association.

Thompson, D.A.: Cardiovascular assessment: guide for nurses and other health professionals, St. Louis, 1981, The C.V. Mosby Co.

Thorn, G.W., et al., editors: Harrison's principles of internal medicine, ed. 8, New York, 1977, McGraw-Hill Book Co.

Walker, H.K.: The problem-oriented medical system, J.A.M.A. **236:**2397-2398, 1976.

Weed, L.: Medical records that guide and teach, N. Engl. J. Med. **278:**593-600, 1968.

Winslow, E.H.: Visual inspection of the patient with cardiopulmonary disease, Heart Lung **4:**421-429, 1975.

5

PATIENT ASSESSMENT: LABORATORY STUDIES

Gregory C. Freund
Brenda Lewis
Lawrence A. Reduto

Over the past several years, major advances have occurred in the development of various noninvasive laboratory techniques designed to aid in the diagnosis and management of the patient who has coronary artery disease. These noninvasive techniques supplement traditional laboratory tools and provide new insights into the pathophysiology of myocardial ischemia and infarction. Laboratory techniques such as two-dimensional echocardiography and radionuclide angiocardiography can now reliably assess global and regional ventricular performance noninvasively, thus providing a major advantage over invasive techniques such as cardiac catheterization.

The purpose of this chapter is to acquaint the reader with these diagnostic techniques and their application to the patient who has coronary artery disease. In addition, traditional laboratory tools used to evaluate the patient who has coronary artery disease, such as cardiac catheterization and blood chemistries, will be reviewed.

Exercise stress testing

The treadmill exercise stress test is the most commonly used noninvasive technique to detect coronary artery disease. In the patient who has a fixed coronary obstruction, myocardial ischemia is typically precipitated by physical or emotional stress, which results in an imbalance between myocardial oxygen demands and available supply. During the exercise stress test, an attempt is made to provoke and electrocardiographically document exercise-induced myocardial ischemia and to correlate these electrocardiographic changes with the patient's symptoms.

The treadmill stress test is performed as follows. A baseline ECG, heart rate, and blood pressure are obtained and are monitored during exercise. Although stress testing may be performed supine or upright during a bicycle exercise, it is performed most commonly in the upright position on a moving belt or treadmill. The rate and incline at which the patient exercises on the treadmill are progressively increased at 3-minute intervals until the patient achieves a *target* heart rate. This target heart rate may be ≥85% of the predicted maximum heart rate for the patient's age and sex or some predetermined heart rate. The exercise

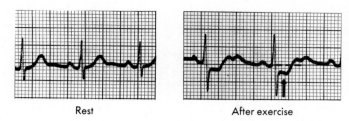

Rest   After exercise

Fig. 5-1. Exercise stress ECG in a patient with triple-vessel coronary artery disease. Arrow indicates 2 mm of downsloping ST segment depression in the postexercise ECG. This degree of ST segment depression at a heart rate of only 75 beats/min would strongly suggest a diagnosis of ischemic heart disease in this patient.

stress test may be terminated before the target heart rate is achieved due to the development of hypotension, malignant ventricular arrhythmias, marked ST segment depression, or chest pain.[1]

A positive exercise stress test is defined as ≥1 mm of horizontal or down sloping ST segment depression (Fig. 5-1). In addition, the magnitude of ST segment depression and the level of exercise at which ST segment depression occurs provide an index of the severity of the coronary artery disease.[2] For example, 3 mm of downsloping ST depression developing at a heart rate of only 100 beats/minute would suggest multivessel coronary artery disease or left main coronary artery stenosis. The development of ventricular arrhythmias during exercise is less specific as a marker of coronary artery disease than the development of ST segment abnormalities.[3] Additional criteria for a positive stress test include hypotension, inverted U waves on this ECG, and chest pain.[4]

The most frequent use for the treadmill exercise stress test is to evaluate the patient who has atypical chest pain that is suggestive of angina. In this setting an attempt is made to induce the patient's symptoms during exercise and to correlate these symptoms with electrocardiographic evidence of myocardial ischemia. An additional frequent use for the exercise stress test is to screen individuals for latent coronary artery disease. However, this has lately been discouraged, since the probability is very high that a stress test in this population is likely to have a false positive result.[5] Since the initial and only manifestation of coronary disease in many individuals is sudden death or acute myocardial infarction, the exercise stress test is often utilized as a means of screening individuals with high-risk factors for coronary artery disease in an attempt to diagnose and treat those patients who have ischemic heart disease. The exercise stress test also is an excellent tool for objectively evaluating an individual's overall physical condition by measuring the maximal heart rate, blood pressure, and duration of exercise achieved. This application of the stress test is especially important for the patient who has angina or valvular heart disease because the patient's functional status may determine the timing of surgical intervention. Exercise testing also is used in conjunction with cardiac rehabilitation programs for the patient who has stable coronary artery disease or in serially assessing the cardiovascular effects of exercise. Finally, stress testing may provide information regarding adequate drug therapy with antiarrhythmic or beta-adrenergic blocking agents in the treatment of exercise-induced arrhythmias or angina, respectively.

Radionuclide techniques
THALLIUM 201 MYOCARDIAL IMAGING

Thallium 201 is a radionuclide whose biologic activity closely parallels that of potassium in normal myocardium. When thallium is injected into the bloodstream, it is concentrated in heart muscle in a ratio that is proportional to regional coronary blood flow. In addition to adequate coronary blood flow, myocardium must be viable to extract thallium from the blood. Thus the major factors determining thallium uptake in myocardium are coronary blood flow and cellular viability.[6] Normal thallium images in the anterior and left anterior oblique projections are displayed in Fig. 5-2. As shown, normal images appear in a horseshoe or doughnut configuration representing thallium uptake in the walls of the left ventricle.

Myocardial imaging with thallium 201 is used primarily in conjunction with exercise stress testing. In response to exercise, coronary blood flow normally increases to a level four to five times that of resting values. Coronary blood flow cannot increase to these levels during exercise in the presence of a significant coronary artery stenosis. Thus, since thallium uptake is proportional to coronary blood flow, myocardial segments supplied by a stenotic coronary artery demonstrate a perfusion defect compared with normal segments (Fig. 5-3). Since both

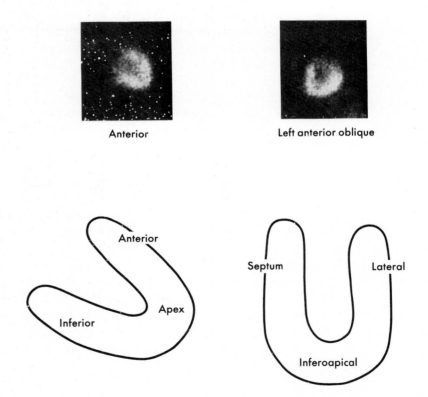

Fig. 5-2. Normal study of thallium 201 myocardial perfusion images in the anterior and left anterior oblique projections. Diagrams below images depict the corresponding left ventricular wall segments.

coronary flow and tissue viability are necessary for myocardial uptake of thallium, either exercise-induced ischemia or previous myocardial infarction with nonviable scar could cause a perfusion defect. Thus, a single thallium 201 myocardial perfusion image cannot reliably distinguish transient myocardial ischemia from old myocardial infarction. To distinguish transient ischemia from myocardial infarction, a redistribution myocardial image is typically obtained 4 hours after the exercise.[7] Within 4 hours after exercise, ischemic viable myocardium demonstrates an increase in thallium content despite the presence of a severe coronary artery stenosis. This phenomenon occurs because there is a constant exchange of thallium between viable myocardium and the blood pool.[8] Therefore, as blood flow in normal and stenotic coronary arteries becomes equivalent, regional myocardial uptake of thallium in normal and transiently ischemic myocardium also will equilibrate. Exercise-induced ischemia typically exhibits perfusion of the previously noted defect while myocardial infarction, with resulting scar formation, continues to result in a perfusion defect during redistribution. It is also important to remember that in patients who are suspected of having acute myocardial infarction, thallium imaging cannot distinguish acute infarction from old myocardial injury.

Myocardial perfusion imaging with stress testing offers a number of advan-

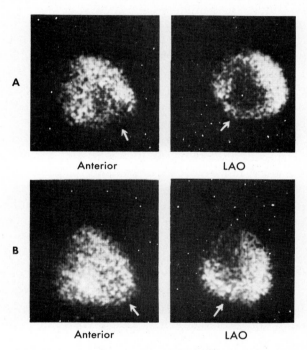

Anterior   LAO

Anterior   LAO

Fig. 5-3. Myocardial perfusion images with thallium 201 at exercise **(A)** and redistribution **(B)** in a patient with exercise-induced ischemia. The arrow in the anterior view indicates apical and inferoapical perfusion defects during exercise; in the left anterior oblique (LAO) view the arrow indicates septal and inferoapical perfusion defects. Redistribution myocardial perfusion images obtained 4 hours after exercise show an increase in thallium uptake in the segments with previous perfusion defects. This improvement in redistribution study suggests exercise-induced ischemia of the apex and inferoapical and septal regions of the left ventricle.

tages over the conventional exercise stress test. First, the sensitivity and specificity of thallium 201 myocardial imaging during exercise in detecting significant coronary artery disease are 80% to 85% and 90% to 95% respectively compared with only a 60% to 65% sensitivity and an 80% to 85% specificity with the conventional treadmill exercise stress test.[9] Second, myocardial perfusion imaging provides a means of detecting ischemia in the patient in whom left bundle branch block, digitalis, or left ventricular hypertrophy may hamper interpretation of the ECG recorded during stress testing. Although myocardial perfusion imaging with stress testing cannot predict the number of diseased coronary vessels, it can be helpful in evaluating the significance of a given coronary artery lesion. For example, in the patient who has exertional chest pain and a coronary stenosis at arteriography that appears to have borderline significance, the demonstration of an exercise-induced defect helps to prove the hemodynamic significance of the coronary stenosis.

MYOCARDIAL INFARCT IMAGING

The demonstration that certain radiopharmaceuticals such as technetium 99m pyrophosphate concentrate in acutely necrotic myocardium has provided the clinician with an additional means of detecting acute myocardial infarction that supplements traditional laboratory tools such as the ECG and serum enzyme measurements. There are a number of clinical settings in which a diagnosis of acute myocardial infarction may be difficult to establish by these traditional laboratory methods. For example, the ECG identification of acute myocardial infarction may be impossible in the patient who has a left bundle branch block or pacemaker rhythm. Similarly, the enzymatic criteria for acute myocardial infarction may be complicated by the presence of shock, cardioversion, surgical procedures, and so forth.

Technetium 99m pyrophosphate begins to accumulate in acutely necrotic myocardium about 12 to 16 hours after the onset of infarction, and maximal uptake of radiotracer by infarcted myocardium occurs 24 to 72 hours after the onset of infarction (Fig. 5-4). Myocardial uptake of technetium 99m pyrophosphate becomes progressively less intense so that by 10 to 14 days after infarction, pyrophosphate imaging is typically negative. Pyrophosphate uptake in acutely infarcted myocardium is believed to be caused by binding of the radiopharmaceutical to calcium within damaged myocardial cells.[10] It is important to remember that technetium 99m pyrophosphate concentrates in bones and acutely infarcted myocardium: normal myocardium does not concentrate pyrophosphate. This contrasts with thallium 201 perfusion imaging, in which normal myocardium concentrates the radionuclide while areas of infarction are indicated by decreased thallium activity.

Technetium 99m pyrophosphate imaging has a sensitivity of about 90% and a specificity of about 85% in the detection of acute myocardial infarction.[11] There are, however, a number of clinical situations that can result in false positive uptake of pyrophosphate. Repeat cardioversion, chest wall trauma, and rib fractures are potential causes of extracardiac uptake of technetium 99m pyrophosphate. Imaging with multiple projections will show whether the area of pyrophosphate

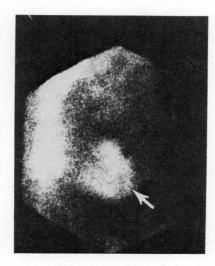

Fig. 5-4. Technetium 99m pyrophosphate scan in a patient with acute myocardial infarction and cardiogenic shock. Arrow indicates area of pyrophosphate uptake in acutely infarcted, necrotic myocardium. Note that in contrast thallium imaging, pyrophosphate is visualized in sternum and ribs.

uptake lies within the myocardium. Calcified valve structures, left ventricular aneurysm, or cardiac tumors also may result in a false positive pyrophosphate uptake.

RADIONUCLIDE ANGIOCARDIOGRAPHY

One of the most useful applications of nuclear medicine techniques for the patient who has coronary artery disease has been in the evaluation of ventricular performance. The clinician currently has at his disposal a reproducible, accurate laboratory tool for the assessment of global and regional left ventricular performance. These radionuclide techniques are noninvasive, requiring only an intravenous injection of radionuclide, and can be performed at the bedside, allowing evaluation of the critically ill patient in the Intensive Care Unit. A single injection of radionuclide allows sequential measurements of ventricular performance for several hours, thus providing a means of evaluating the effects of therapeutic interventions with factors such as inotropic agents and afterload reduction.

Typically radionuclide angiocardiography measures the overall left ventricular systolic performance in what is termed *ejection fraction*. Although affected by changes in afterload (ventricular output resistance), preload (ventricular input pressure), and contractility, ejection fraction remains the most commonly employed measure of ventricular pump performance. A left ventricular ejection fraction is angiographically calculated from the following formula:

$$\text{Ejection fraction (\%)} = \frac{\text{End-diastolic volume} - \text{End-systolic volume}}{\text{End-diastolic volume}} \times 100$$

The numerator of the above equation is the stroke volume. With radionuclide techniques, the ejection fraction is calculated from changes in radioactive counts within a cardiac chamber rather than changes in volume. This is an important advantage that radionuclide techniques have in assessing ventricular performance in patients with coronary artery disease and regional dysfunction, since ejection fraction measurements are independent of ventricular shape—unlike measurements by angiography or M-mode echocardiography.

The most commonly utilized radionuclide technique for assessing ventricular performance is gated cardiac blood pool imaging. In this technique the patient's red blood cells are labeled in vivo with technetium 99m. Changes in radioactive counts are therefore proportional to changes in blood volume within a cardiac chamber.[12] The patient's ECG provides a gate, or physiologic marker, of when end-diastole and end-systole occur within the cardiac cycle. The RR interval on the patient's ECG is typically divided into 16 to 30 intervals by a computer, and the gamma camera records counts within the left or right ventricle during each of these intervals. This information is obtained over a period of 200 to 300 heartbeats, and then the individual beats are added together to create a representative cycle of the patient's ventricular performance.

In addition to measuring either left or right ventricular ejection fraction, gated cardiac blood pool imaging provides an excellent means of evaluating left ventricular regional wall motion.[13] Thus one can determine if a wall of the left ventricle is hypokinetic or akinetic, or if a left ventricular aneurysm is present. Relative cardiac chamber size and dilatation of the aorta or pulmonary artery also can be qualitatively assessed with this technique.

Radionuclide angiocardiography with gated cardiac blood pool imaging also can be utilized in conjunction with exercise stress. Normal patients demonstrate an increase in left ventricular ejection fraction during exercise stress.[14] In contrast, most patients with coronary artery disease who develop ischemia during exercise either fail to increase ejection fraction or actually demonstrate a decrease in ejection fraction during exercise (Fig. 5-5). In addition to an abnormal response of ejection fraction, the patient with exercise-induced ischemia may also develop abnormalities in regional wall motion that can localize the site of exercise-induced

Rest   Exercise

A   B

Fig. 5-5. Radionuclide angiocardiogram at rest **(A)** and exercise **(B)** in a patient with coronary artery disease. The end-systolic image is displayed within the end-diastolic ring. The aorta is seen at the top of each image. At rest, left ventricular ejection fraction (57%) and wall motion are normal. Exercise-induced ischemia results in a fall in ejection fraction (34%) and the development of anteroapical and inferior hypokinesis. At coronary angiography the patient had triple-vessel coronary artery disease.

ischemia. For example, a patient with a significant stenosis of the left anterior descending coronary artery may develop hypokinesis or akinesis of the anterior wall or apex during exercise. Gated cardiac blood pool imaging with stress therefore provides an alternative radionuclide technique for the detection of coronary artery disease and has a sensitivity comparable to myocardial perfusion imaging with thallium 201.

Echocardiography

Echocardiography uses the techniques of ultrasound to visualize the cardiac structures and assess the motion and function of these structures. This allows for the diagnosis of a variety of cardiac abnormalities with virtually no ill effects for the patient.

TECHNIQUES

There are currently two techniques by which an echocardiogram can be obtained: M-mode echocardiography and two-dimensional or cross-sectional echocardiography. Both techniques employ the transmission of high-frequency sound waves into the chest. These sound waves are reflected back to the transmitter (which also serves as a receiver) from the cardiac structures. The resultant signals are recorded either on a strip chart recorder or videotape.

M-mode echocardiography utilizes a single ultrasound beam. This beam is swept across the cardiac structures, and the resulting time-motion information is displayed on a strip chart recording with the ECG of the patient.

Two-dimensional or cross-sectional echocardiography is a more recently developed technique. As opposed to the single beam of ultrasound transmitted with M-mode echocardiography, cross-sectional echocardiography utilizes a planar beam of ultrasound. The ultrasound can be transmitted by a single crystal that oscillates or rotates throughout a given plane or by a series of crystals with each crystal transmitting ultrasound through a different point on the chest. The resulting "echo" information is recorded on videotape for subsequent interpretation.

The M-mode and two-dimensional approaches to echocardiography both have advantages and disadvantages, which will be discussed further. It is important to understand that although two-dimensional echocardiography is a more recent development, it is not a replacement for M-mode echocardiography but rather an additional technique providing unique information valuable in the care and diagnosis of the patient who has heart disease.

APPLICATIONS

The normal heart. Normal M-mode and two-dimensional echocardiograms in two different patients are shown in Figs. 5-6 and 5-7. Of importance are the relative sizes and positions of the cardiac chambers and the motion of the cardiac valves during systole and diastole.

Pericardial disease. Pericardial disease can be easily assessed with echocardiography. The existence of a pericardial effusion is easily determined by the presence of an echo-free space between the pericardium and the heart (Fig. 5-8). Furthermore, assessment of ventricular wall motion in the presence of a pericardial effusion yields useful information regarding the possibility of cardiac

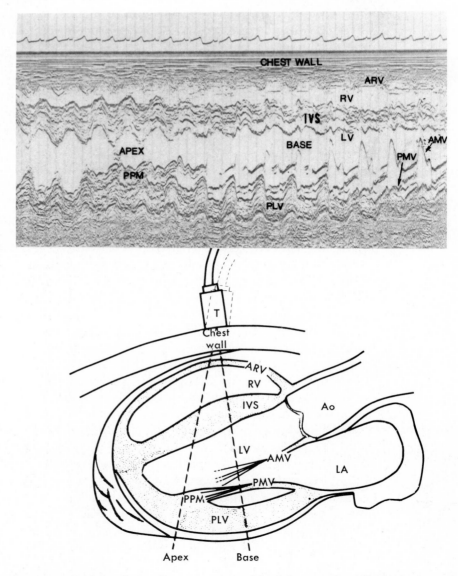

Fig. 5-6. Normal echocardiographic sector scan of the left ventricle and schematic presentation of the cardiac structures traversed by two echo beams. During ejection the left septal and posterior left ventricular wall echoes move toward the center of the left ventricular cavity. *AMV*, Anterior mitral valve leaflet; *AO*, aorta; *ARV*, anterior right ventricular wall; *IVS*, interventricular septum; *LA*, left atrium; *LV*, left ventricle; *PLV*, posterior left ventricular wall; *PMV*, posterior mitral valve leaflet; *RV*, right ventricle; *PPM*, posterior papillary muscle; *T*, transducer. (Reproduced with permission from Corya, B.C.: Applications of echocardiography in acute myocardial infarction, Cardiovasc. Clin. **2:**113, 1975.

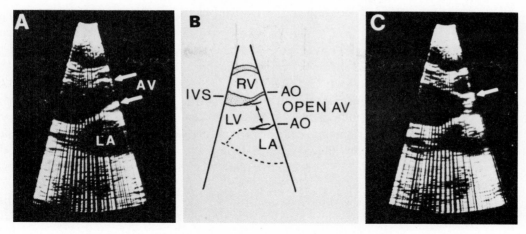

Fig. 5-7. Single frames of a long-axis, two-dimensional echogram of the aortic valve. **A** and **B,** Early systolic position of anterior aortic leaflet and posterior noncoronary aortic leaflet. **C,** Diastolic position of these leaflets. The leaflets curve inward toward the left ventricular outflow tract. Sound reflected from these curved surfaces produced multiple diastolic echoes. *AV,* aortic valve; *LA,* left atrium; *RV,* right ventricle, *LV,* left ventricle; *IVS,* interventricular septum; *Ao,* aorta; single *arrow* in **C,** closed and centrally positioned aortic leaflets. (From Chang, S.: Echocardiography: techniques and interpretations, ed. 2, Philadelphia, 1981, Lea & Febiger.)

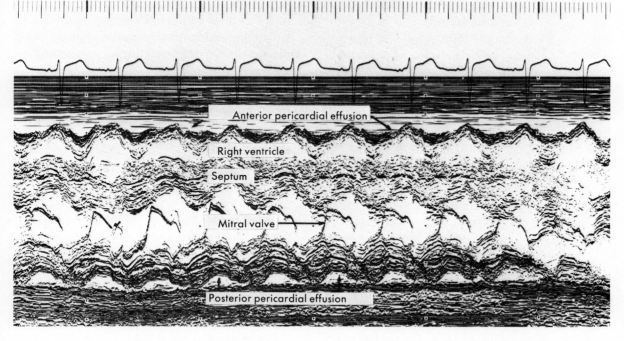

Fig. 5-8. M-mode echocardiogram in a patient with a pericardial effusion. Cardiac chambers (e.g., right ventricle) are depicted as echo-free spaces, whereas other cardiac structures (e.g., septum, mitral valve) are displayed with varying degrees of echo density. Anterior and posterior echo-free space (*arrows*) is consistent with a pericardial effusion.

tamponade.[15] For instance, an echocardiogram with a moderately sized pericardial effusion and a reduction in the size of the right ventricle or variations in the motion of the mitral valve suggests cardiac tamponade.[16]

Cardiac chamber size and function. The size of various cardiac chambers can be assessed with echocardiography. Accurate measurement of the diameter of the left ventricle, left atrium, and aortic root can be made. Measurements of the right ventricle are less reliable because of its irregular shape and variations in right ventricular size dependent on the patient's position. Two-dimensional echocardiography allows visualization of the cardiac apex and its motion during the cardiac cycle.[17] This is particularly useful in the identification of an apical thrombus.

Once the dimensions of the cardiac chambers are determined, the left ventricular shortening fraction can be determined. *Shortening fraction* is defined as:

$$\frac{\text{LV end-diastolic dimension} - \text{LV end-systolic dimension}}{\text{LV end-diastolic dimension}}$$

While the shortening fraction is an index of ventricular performance similar to the ejection fraction, it should be noted that this measurement is limited in the patient who has coronary artery disease, since the measurements obtained may be from a view in which regional wall motion abnormalities are not apparent.

Finally, information regarding the thickness of the left ventricular walls can be obtained. The existence and degree of left ventricualr hypertrophy may prove valuable in estimating the severity of other cardiac abnormalities. Also, changes in wall thickness during the cardiac cycle may help distinguish the ischemic myocardium from a myocardial scar in the patient who has ischemic heart disease.[18] Myocardial scar is more echo dense than viable myocardium and does not change in thickness, whereas a normal myocardium thickens during systole and an ischemic myocardium thins during systole.

Mitral valve function. Echocardiography can be used to evaluate the patient with mitral valve disease. The presence of a thickened, echo-dense mitral valve is highly suggestive of calcification of the mitral valve.[19] Furthermore, the extent of the opening of the mitral valve during diastole is decreased in a setting of mitral stenosis. This decrease in the mitral valve orifice size can be quantitated using two-dimensional echocardiography, in which the orifice size can actually be measured directly from the image.[20] Moreover, changes in chamber size, such as dilation of the left atrium, can further suggest the severity of the stenosis.

Mitral valve regurgitation, on the other hand, is not directly assessed with echocardiography, but its presence may be suggested by changes in left ventricular and left atrial size. In the patient with known mitral valve regurgitation, evidence of calcification of the mitral valve suggests the etiology of this lesion to be rheumatic.

Mitral valve prolapse is reliably assessed by echocardiography. The existence of a posterior displacement of the mitral valve in middle to late systole is indicative of mitral prolapse. Although this test is very specific, about 10% to 20% of patients with mitral valve prolapse fail to manifest this posterior displacement on echocardiographic examination.[21]

Finally, a flail mitral valve can be identified from the echocardiogram. The flailing leaflet may appear to displace posteriorly but to a much greater degree than in mitral valve prolapse.[22] Also, the motion of the mitral valve leaflets may be in an irregular pattern. With two-dimensional echocardiography the leaflet may be seen to prolapse entirely into the left atrium during systole.

Aortic valve function. The aortic valve, in the patient who has aortic stenosis, appears thickened and the opening appears to be narrowed, as with mitral stenosis.[23] Methods of measuring the opening are not very reliable, but the severity of the stenosis can be judged indirectly by the presence of left ventricular hypertrophy.

Aortic regurgitation is not easily assessed with echocardiography. In acute aortic regurgitation secondary to endocarditis, a vegetation on the valve leaflet itself may be seen. Furthermore, fine fluttering of the anterior mitral valve leaflet during diastole is suggestive of aortic regurgitation.[24] Other indirect evidence of aortic valve regurgitation includes left ventricular dilatation and early closure of the mitral valve.

Tricuspid and pulmonary valve function. Assessment of the tricuspid and pulmonary valves by echocardiography is less successful. Tricuspid valve stenosis is indicated by a decreased opening of the anterior leaflet. Tricuspid valve regurgitation manifests itself predominantly with signs of right ventricular overload.[25] Pulmonic valve stenosis appears as an early opening of the pulmonic valve caused by the right atrium contracting and ejecting blood into an overloaded right ventricle.[26]

Other applications. Echocardiography plays an important role in the assessment of congenital heart disease. The relative spatial arrangement of the cardiac structures as well as specific chamber abnormalities combine to provide useful information in the identification of various congenital lesions.[27]

Intracardiac masses such as tumors, vegetations, and thrombi are frequently identified through echocardiography. Although most masses can be identified through echocardiography, those in the left atrial appendage, such as thrombi, are not well visualized.[28]

Finally, idiopathic hypertrophic subaortic stenosis can be identified by the systolic anterior motion of the mitral valve, early closure of the aortic valve, and hypertrophy of the septum.[29] Differentiation of the patients with congestive cardiomyopathy and those with severe coronary artery disease is determined by the presence of diffuse hypokinesis of the ventricular wall as opposed to the regional wall motion abnormalities manifested in most patients who have coronary artery disease.[30]

In summary, echocardiography provides a sensitive, noninvasive means of assessing such cardiac conditions as valvular heart disease, pericardial disease, congenital heart disease, and coronary artery disease.

Long-term ECG recordings

Long-term ECG recording has widespread applications as a noninvasive tool. Lightweight, battery-powered recorders (Holter recorders) worn continuously for 24 hours or more collect 2-lead ECG data for subsequent analysis. Attached to a belt or shoulder strap, these recorders can be used in or out of the hospital. A clock on the recorder correlates ECG events with the patient's log of symptoms,

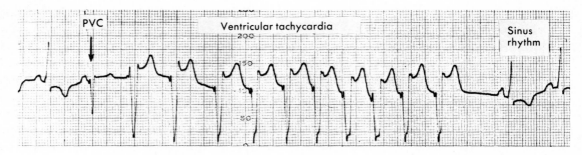

Fig. 5-9. Representative tracing of continuous ambulatory monitoring in a patient with a previous myocardial infarction. Preceded by a ventricular contraction, a run of ventricular tachycardia is seen with spontaneous resumption of normal sinus rhythm. The patient had no symptoms associated with this arrythmia.

activity, and medications. Some devices allow the patient to mark the tape to correspond with events entered in the log.

Computer-based systems scan and analyze the record with a technician's input for interpretation. Data are reported by mounting representative printout strips of abnormalities (Fig. 5-9), mounting strips corresponding with patient log entries, hourly analysis of the frequency of premature atrial and ventricular complexes, hourly heart rate, and any ST changes noted. The physician must correlate data from long-term ECG reports with the total patient picture, bearing in mind that it is not uncommon for 24-hour monitoring to show various abnormalities even in patients with normal cardiac function.[31]

Noncontinuous forms of ambulatory recording include recorders that can be intermittently activated by event (for example, bradycardia or tachycardia) or by patient and transtelephonic recording similar to that used for permanently implanted pacemaker follow-up. Limitations of these systems include lack of all ECG data, especially of arrhythmias that occurred but were not sensed and recorded by the device or the patient. Moreover, the transtelephonic device requires immediate access to a telephone and is of little value for transient arrhythmias or arrhythmias that markedly disable the patient. A new transtelephonic device that is patient activated records 30 seconds of the cardiac rhythm and then can be transmitted over the telephone at the patient's convenience. This may greatly improve the value of these devices in the detection of cardiac arrhythmias.

Indications for long-term ECG recording include the following: (1) documentation of a dysrhythmia or conduction disturbance as the cause of specific symptoms, (2) detection of significant ventricular arrhythmias that place patients at an increased risk of sudden death, (3) identification of the mechanism of a conduction disturbance, (4) determination of response to interventions such as antiarrhythmic drugs or permanent pacemaker implantation, and (5) recording and correlating ST-T changes with symptoms in the patient who has angina.

Symptoms of syncope, near syncope, dizziness, or palpitations may or may not arise from cardiac sources. However, ambulatory monitoring can document whether a significant arrhythmia is responsible for a specific symptom. This is most valuable when the activities that elicit symptoms are too sporadic or infrequent to be detected while the patient is under direct supervision. In addition, determining the onset and termination of an arrhythmia may reveal important information about its mechanism.

Complex ventricular arrhythmias (R on T, multifocal premature ventricular contractions [PVCs], ventricular bigeminy, ventricular coupling) in the presence of depressed left ventricular function are associated with a high incidence of sudden death in the first 12 months after myocardial infarction.[32] Documentation of these arrhythmias in the late hospital phase identifies this high-risk subgroup of patients as those who would most benefit from antiarrhythmic therapy, although there are no data to support that controlling these arrhythmias will decrease the risk of sudden death. In the patient who has known arrhythmias, long-term ECG recording can yield useful information regarding the electrophysiologic mechanisms of these conduction abnormalities.

Another indication for ambulatory monitoring comes from an assessment of the efficacy of antiarrhythmic drug therapy or other interventions such as permanent pacemaker implantation. Side effects, cost, and patient noncompliance in antiarrhythmic therapy must be weighed against its potential benefit. Pacemakers suspected of intermittent failure ca also be evaluated with continuous ambulatory monitoring. Finally, evaluation of ST-T changes on the ECG may provide insight about the etiology of chest pain.[33] This may be particularly useful in the patient who has angina at rest, such as Prinzmetal variant angina, or in patients who are unable to perform an adequate stress test.

Swan-Ganz catheterization

Right-sided heart catheterization with a Swan-Ganz thermodilution catheter involves passage of a balloon-tipped, flow-directed catheter through a vein to the right atrium. The balloon is inflated and the catheter is advanced through the right ventricle into the pulmonary artery until the balloon becomes wedged in a branch of it. There are two pressure lumens in the Swan-Ganz catheter. Once the catheter is in position, the proximal lumen opens into the right atrium and the distal lumen opens into the pulmonary artery at the tip of the catheter. A third lumen inflates the balloon on the tip of the catheter. Therefore, with the balloon deflated, pulmonary artery and right atrial pressures can be obtained. After inflation of the balloon, the branch of the pulmonary artery in which the catheter tip lies becomes occluded. The pressure recorded through the distal lumen then becomes the pressure that is reflected back to the catheter from the left atrium. The left atrial pressure thus obtained usually correlates quite well with the left ventricular end-diastolic pressure, provided that there is no obstruction between the pulmonary artery and left atrium, as in chronic obstructive lung disease.

Cardiac output can be easily assessed when the Swan-Ganz catheter is in position by using the thermodilution technique.[34] This involves the injection of a known volume of cold fluid into the right atrium. A thermistor located near the catheter tip detects the change in temperature as this cold fluid flows through the pulmonary artery. The change in temperature is inversely proportional to cardiac output; that is, the greater the temperature change, the lower the cardiac output.

Once the left atrial, right atrial, and pulmonary artery pressures, and cardiac output have been obtained, calculations of stroke volume (the amount of blood flow from a single heartbeat), left ventricular stroke work (the amount of work done by the ventricle in a single beat), and systemic and pulmonary vascular resistances (the forces the left and right ventricles respectively must overcome to produce blood flow) can be made. These measurements provide further information regarding the hemodynamic status of the patient.

Indications for use of the Swan-Ganz catheter include the following: (1) acute heart failure, (2) cardiac tamponade, (3) hypovolemia, and (4) intraoperative and postoperative management of high-risk surgical patients. In general, Swan-Ganz catheterization is indicated for any situation in which the obtained hemodynamic information substantially aids in choosing the best therapeutic modality for the patient.[35]

Cardiac catheterization and coronary angiography

Cardiac catheterization and angiography remain the definitive techniques for establishing the cause and severity of cardiac disease. These techniques provide physiologic data regarding cardiovascular hemodynamics; cardiac chambers and structures can be visualized on x-ray film by injection of radiopaque contrast media. This section concentrates on indications for these radiographic procedures in the patient who has coronary artery disease and on the methods of applying data obtained with these laboratory techniques to the diagnosis and management of ischemic heart disease.

Cardiac catherization involves passing a catheter through a vein or artery to the right or left cardiac chambers. With this technique, pressures and oxygen saturations within the chamber can be measured, and gradients across a cardiac valve, as in aortic stenosis, can be determined. In addition, radiopaque contrast media can be injected to visualize the cardiac chambers, great vessels, and coronary arteries with fluoroscopy and x-ray film. Through these laboratory techniques, for example, the presence of regional wall motion abnormalities such as a left ventricular aneurysm or the severity of mitral regurgitation due to myocardial infarction can be accurately assessed. Additional complications of myocardial infarction such as acquired ventricular septal defect with a left-to-right shunt can be detected and quantitated through measurements of oxygen saturations in the right cardiac chambers.

The most commonly performed angiographic procedure in the patient who has known or suspected coronary artery disease is coronary arteriography. With this technique, selective catheterization of the coronary arteries is performed by a brachial arteriotomy (Sones technique) or a percutaneous femoral puncture (Judkins technique). Coronary arteriography involves placing a specially designed catheter in the ostium of the left and right coronary arteries and injecting contrast media to visualize the coronary arterial circulation. A normal left coronary artery and its branches are shown in Fig. 5-10. Typically, several injections of both the left and right coronary arteries are performed in multiple x-ray projections to ensure adequate visualization of the proximal and distal portions of each vessel. A hemodynamically significant coronary artery stenosis is defined as a reduction in luminal diameter greater than or equal to 50% that of a normal segment of the same vessel (Fig. 5-11). In addition to atherosclerotic coronary artery lesions,

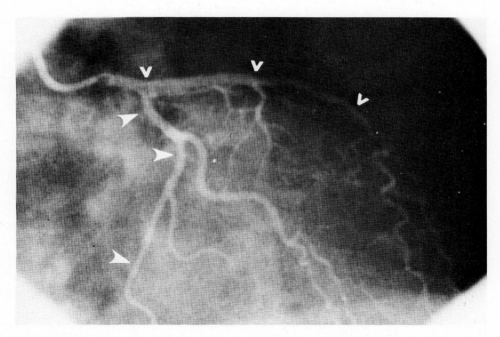

Fig. 5-10. Left coronary arteriogram in a patient with normal coronary arteries. Open arrows indicate the left anterior descending coronary artery, and closed arrows signify the circumflex coronary artery.

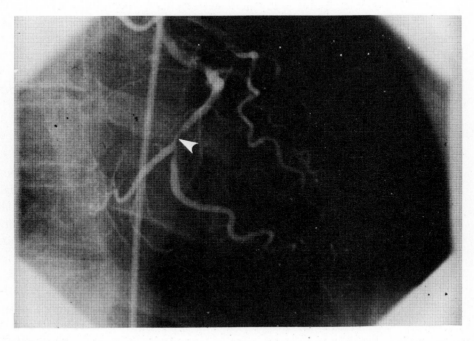

Fig. 5-11. Left coronary arteriogram in a patient with significant coronary artery disease. *Arrow* indicates a severe (90% to 95%) stenosis in the circumflex coronary artery. A hemodynamically significant coronary artery stenosis is defined as $\geq$50% reduction in luminal diameter as compared to normal segments of the same vessel.

conditions such as idiopathic hypertrophic subaortic stenosis or coronary artery spasm, which often mimic ischemic heart disease in their clinical presentation, can be diagnosed with cardiac catheterization and coronary arteriography. Serious complications occur in approximately 1 in every 1000 cardiac catheterizations and include death, stroke, myocardial infarction, loss of a peripheral pulse, and allergic reactions to contrast media.[36]

The indications for cardiac catheterization and coronary angiography vary somewhat among institutions. Moreover, the indications for these procedures have changed as data regarding the natural history of coronary artery and valvular heart disease and the effects of surgical therapy upon these lesions have become available. The measurement of valve areas or gradients and the assessment of indexes of left ventricular performance such as end-diastolic pressure or cardiac output are often required to determine the optimal timing for surgical intervention. A traditional use for coronary angiography in the patient who has classic angina unresponsive to standard medical therapy is to delineate the extent and anatomic sites of coronary artery lesions prior to considering aortocoronary bypass surgery. Even in the patient who has stable angina or myocardial infarction, coronary angiography is often performed to identify patients, such as those with left main coronary artery stenosis, in whom aortocoronary bypass surgery has been shown to improve long-term survival.[37] Coronary angiography may be indicated for the patient having atypical chest pain for whom noninvasive tests such as exercise with thallium imaging have been equivocal or nondiagnostic. For the patient who has chest pain following aortocoronary bypass surgery, coronary angiography may be required to assess graft patency or to determine if new coronary artery stenoses have developed in nonbypassed vessels. Variant, or Prinzmetal's, angina secondary to coronary artery spasm is best diagnosed through the use of angiography and provocation with agents such as ergonovine.[38] In summary, coronary angiography and cardiac catheterization are the techniques best able to assist in the precise evaluation of the etiology and severity of cardiac disease and in the determination of the prognosis and potential therapy for a given patient.

Serum enzymes in acute myocardial infarction

The diagnosis of acute myoardial infarction is typically confirmed by the patient's clinical history, electrocardiographic changes, and elevations of the serum enzymes released from the heart muscle after a myocardial injury. Necrosis or prolonged ischemia can result in increased permeability of cellular membranes, which allows these enzymes to leak into the bloodstream. There are three major enzymes that occur in abnormal levels in the serum following myocardial injury: creatine kinase, lactate dehydrogenase, and serum glutamic oxaloacetic transaminase. The relative rates at which each enzyme appears in the serum following infarction is shown in Fig. 5-12.

Creatine kinase (CK) is present in heart muscle, skeletal muscle, brain, and gastrointestinal tract. Abnormal elevations in serum CK begin to appear in the blood about 4 to 6 hours after the onset of acute myocardial infarction. Peak levels of this enzyme typically appear 16 to 30 hours after the onset of infarction and return to normal within 3 to 4 days. Elevations of serum CK, however, are

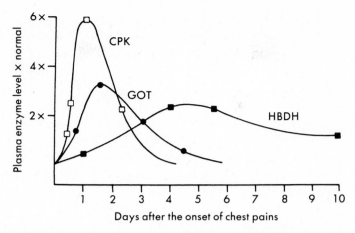

Fig. 5-12. Typical plasma profiles for creatine kinase (CPK), glutamic oxaloacetic transaminase (GOT), and lactate dehydrogenase (LDH) activities following the onset of acute myocardial infarction. (From Hearse, D.J.: Myocardial enzyme leakage, J. Mol. Med. **2:**185, 1977.)

nonspecific for cardiac injury. Thus in the patient with chest pain who may have received an intramuscular injection of analgesic, an elevation of serum CK may reflect either skeletal or cardiac muscle necrosis. To determine the precise source of the elevated serum CK, electrophoresis or radioimmunoassay can separate creatine kinase into three isoenzymes. The MM isoenzyme is found in skeletal muscle, and the BB isoenzyme appears to be uniquely present in brain tissue. The MB isoenzyme of creatine kinase is a fairly specific marker of cardiac muscle necrosis. This isoenzyme, like total serum CK, appears in the serum about 4 hours after the onset of the myocardial necrosis but has a shorter half-life than MM CK.

Creatine kinase levels in the serum have also been used to estimate the size of myocardial infarctions.[39] Canine studies have shown a correlation between serum CK levels drawn serially after myocardial infarction and the size of the infarction on postmortem studies. Although this technique appears to be less accurate in humans for a number of reasons, some studies still claim close correlations in human subjects.

Another enzyme that is released after myocardial infarction is lactate dehydrogenase (LDH). This enzyme appears in abnormal amounts in the peripheral blood about 24 to 48 hours after the onset of infarction. Peak levels occur in 3 to 6 days, and enzyme levels return to normal 10 to 12 days after infarction. LDH is widely distributed throughout such body organs as heart, kidney, skeletal muscle, lung, liver, and red blood cells. Like creatine kinase, LDH can be separated into five isoenzymes. Cardiac muscle is particularly rich in the isoenzyme LDH_1; therefore, after myocardial damage, the predominant isoenzyme found in the serum is LDH_1.

A third enzyme that appears in elevated levels in the serum is serum glutamic oxaloacetic transaminase (SGOT). Elevation of SGOT occurs about 12 to 18 hours after the onset of infarction, and peak levels occur about 24 to 48 hours after the onset of infarction. However, elevated levels of SGOT can occur in patients who have pulmonary embolism, myocarditis, pericarditis, or skeletal muscular disease. Since there are no specific isoenzymes of SGOT for myocardial tissue, this enzyme is not especially indicative of myocardial necrosis.

REFERENCES

1. Bruce, R.A.: Methods of exercise testing, Am. J. Cardiol. **33**:715, 1974.
2. Kattus, A.A.: Exercise electrocardiography: recognition of the ischemic response, false positive and negative patterns, Am. J. Cardiol. **33**:721, 1974.
3. DeBusk, R.F., and others: Serial ambulatory electrocardiography and treadmill exercise testing after uncomplicated myocardial infarction, Am. J. Cardiol.**45**:457, 1980.
4. Ellestad, M.H., Couke, B.M., Jr., and Greenberg, P.S.: Stress testing: clinical application and predictive capacity, Prog. Cardiovasc. Dis. **21**:431, 1979.
5. Rifkin, R.D. and Hood, W.B.: Bayesian analysis of electrocardiographic exercise stress testing, N. Engl. J. Med. **297**:681, 1977.
6. DiCola, V.C., and others: Pathophysiologic correlates of thallium 201 myocardial uptake in experimental infarction, Cardiovasc. Res. **11**:141, 1977.
7. Pohost, G.M., and others: Differentiation of transiently ischemic from infarcted myocardium by serial imaging after a single dose of thallium 201, Circulation **55**:294, 1977.
8. Beller, G.A. and Pohost, G.M.: Mechanism for thallium 201 redistribution after transient myocardial ischemia (abstract), Circulation **56**(3):141, 1977.
9. Okada, R.D., and others: Exercise radionuclide imaging approaches to coronary artery disease, Am. J. Cardiol. **46**:1188, 1980.
10. Buja, L.M., and others: Pathophysiology of thallium-201 scintigraphy of acute anterior myocardial infarcts in dogs, J. Clin. Invest. **57**:1508, 1976.
11. Holman, B.L., Tanaka, T.T., and Lesch, M.: Evaluation of radiopharmaceuticals for the detection of acute myocardial infarction in man, Radiology **121**:427, 1976.
12. Wackers, F.J.T., and others: Multiple-gated cardiac blood pool imaging for left ventricular ejection fraction: validation of the technique and assessment of variability, Am. J. Cardiol. **43**:1166, 1979.
13. Okada, R.D., and others: Observer variance in the qualitative evaluation of left ventricular wall motion and the quantitation of left ventricular ejection fraction using rest and exercise multigated blood pool imaging, Circulation **61**:128, 1980.
14. Borer, J.S., and others: Real-time radionuclide cineangiography in the noninvasive evaluation of global and regional left ventricular function and rest and during exercise in patients with coronary artery disease, N. Engl. J. Med. **296**:839, 1977.
15. Schiller, N.B., and Botvinick, E.H.: Right ventricular compression as a sign of cardiac tamponade: an analysis of echocardiographic ventricular dimensions and their clinical implications, Circulation **56**:744, 1977.
16. Setle, H.P., and others: Echocardiographic study of cardiac tamponade, Circulation **56**:951, 1977.
17. Hickman, H.O., and others: Cross-sectional echocardiography of the cardiac apex, abstract, Circulation **56**:111, 1977.
18. Corya, B.C. and others: Systolic thickening and thinning of the septum and posterior wall in patient with coronary artery disease, congestive cardiomyopathy, and atrial septal defect, Circulation **55**:109, 1977.
19. Joiner, C.R., Reid, J.M., and Bond, J.P.: Reflected ultrasound in the assessment of mitral valve disease, Circulation **27**:506, 1963.
20. Henry, W.L., and others: Measurement of mitral orifice area in patients with mitral valve disease by real-time, two-dimensional echocardiography, Circulation **51**:827, 1975.
21. DeMaria, A.N., and others: The variable spectrum of echocardiographic manifestations of the mitral valve prolapse syndrome, Circulation **50**:33, 1974.
22. Sweatman, T., and others: Echocardiographic diagnosis of mitral valve regurgitation due to ruptured chordae tendineae, Circulation **46**:580, 1972.
23. Gramiak, R., and Shah, P.M.: Echocardiography of the normal and diseased aortic valve, Radiology **96**:1, 1970.
24. Dillon, J.C., and others: Significance of mitral fluttering in patients with aortic insufficiency (abstract), Clin. Res. **18**:304, 1970.
25. Popp, R.L., and others: Estimation of the right and left ventricular size by ultrasound: a study of echoes from the interventricular septum, Am. J. Cardiol. **24**:253, 1969.
26. Weyman, A.E., and others: Echocardiographic patterns of pulmonic valve motion in pulmonic stenosis, Am. J. Cardiol. **34**:644, 1974.
27. Meyer, R.A., and others: Echocardiographic assessment of cardiac malposition, Am. J. Cardiol. **33**:896, 1974.
28. Spangler, R.D., and Okin, J.T.: Illustrative echocardiogram: echocardiographic demonstration of left atrial thrombus, Chest **67**:716, 1975.
29. Shah, P.M., and others: Role of echocardiography in diagnosis and hemodynamic assessment of hypertrophic subaortic stenosis, Circulation **44**:891, 1971.
30. Corya, B.C.: Echocardiographic feature of congestive cardiomyopathy compared with normal subjects and patients with coronary artery disease, Circulation **49**:1153, 1974.
31. Brodsky, M., and others: Arrhythmias documented by 24-hour continuous electrocardiographic monitoring in 50 male medical students without apparent heart disease, Am. J. Cardiol. **39**:390, 1977.
32. Schultze, R.A., Strauss, H.W., and Pitt, B.: Sudden

death in the year following myocardial infarction: relation to ventricular premature contractions in the late hospital phase and left ventricular ejection fraction, Am. J. Med. **62:**192, 1977.

33. Stern, S., and Tzivoni, D.: Early detection of silent ischaemic heart disease by 24-hour electrocardiographic monitoring of active subjects, Br. Heart J. **36:**481, 1974.

34. Forrester, J.S., and others: Thermodilution cardiac output determination with a single flow-directed catheter, Am. Heart J. **83:**306, 1972.

35. Swan, H.J.C.: the role of hemodynamic monitoring in the management of the critically ill, Crit. Care Med. **3:**83, 1975.

36. Grossman, W.: Complications of cardiac catheterization: incidence, causes and prevention. In Grossman, W., editor: Cardiac catheterization and angiography, ed. 2, Philadelphia, 1980, Lea & Febiger.

37. Zeft, J.H., Manley, J.C., and Huston, J.H.: Left main coronary artery stenosis: results of coronary bypass surgery, Circulation **49:**68, 1974.

38. Ricci, D.R. and others: Reduction of coronary blood flow during coronary artery spasm occurring spontaneously and after provocation by ergonovine maleate, Circulation **57:**137, 1978.

39. Shell, W.E., Kjekshus, J.K., and Sobel, B.E.: Quantitative assessment of the extent of myocardial infarction in the conscious dog by means of analysis of serial change in serum creatine phosphokinase activity, J. Clin. Invest. **50:**2614, 1971.

ADDITIONAL READINGS

Bailey, I.K., and others: Thallium 201 myocardial reperfusion imaging at rest and during exercise (comparative sensitivity to electrocardiography in coronary artery disease), Circulation **55:**79, 1977.

Berger, H.J., and others: Dual radionuclide study of acute myocardial infarction: comparison of thallium 201 and technetium 99m stannous pyrophosphate imaging in man, Ann. Intern. Med. **88:**145, 1978.

Berger, H.U., and others: First-pass radionuclide assessment of right and left ventricular performance in patients with cardiac and pulmonary disease, Semin. Nucl. Med. **9:**275, 1979.

Bodenheimer, M.M., and others: Nuclear cardiology. 1. Radionuclide angiographic assessment of left ventricular contraction: uses, limitations and future directions, Am. J. Cardiol. **45:**661, 1980.

Bruce, R.A., and others: Seattle Heart Watch: initial clinical, circulatory, and electrocardiographic responses to maximal exercise, Am. J. Cardiol. **33:**459, 1974.

DeBusk, R.F., and Haskell, W.: Symptom-limited vs heart rate-limited exercise testing soon after myocardial infarction, Circulation **61:**738, 1980.

Grossman, W.: Cardiac catheterization and angiography, Philadelphia, 1980, Lea and Febiger.

Morganroth, J., and Pohost, G.M.: Noninvasive approaches to cardiac imaging: comparisons and contrasts, Am. J. Cardiol. **46:**1093, 1980.

6

INTRODUCTION TO ELECTROCARDIOGRAPHY

Douglas P. Zipes
Kathleen Gainor Andreoli

This chapter explains some basic principles of electrocardiography, describes the use of the normal ECG, and introduces certain abnormalities commonly encountered in patients who have cardiac disease manifesting electrocardiographic changes. Additional electrocardiographic disorders are presented in Chapter 8.

Basic considerations

An ECG is a graphic tracing of the electrical forces produced by the heart. For patients who have heart disease this test is a frequently used and highly important diagnostic procedure. The ECG, however, has limitations, so it is important to evaluate the tracing in conjunction with a clinical examination of the patient. For example, electrocardiographic abnormalities may occur in healthy persons, and conversely, organic heart disease may occur in patients who have normal electrocardiographic patterns. Premature ventricular complexes found in the ECG of a young patient with no heart disease and complaints of palpitations raise different diagnostic considerations than do premature ventricular complexes found in the ECG of a middle-aged patient who has had a myocardial infarction and syncope. Thus the nature of the rhythm disturbance and the effect of the rhythm disturbance on the individual patient influence the clinical importance of the findings.

It is important to remember that the health care professional evaluates the patient who has an ECG abnormality, not the ECG in isolation. Some rhythm disturbances, for example, are hazardous to a patient regardless of the clinical setting, but others are hazardous only because of the clinical setting.

Numerous extrinsic factors not related to the heart per se such as drugs, metabolic changes, and electrolyte imbalances, may alter the final recording. Technical factors such as adequate skin preparation to reduce skin resistance, muscle tremor, 60-Hz cycle interference, and incorrectly applied electrodes also must be considered.

Standardization

The ECG comprises a series of horizontal and vertical lines that measure amplitude and duration of the various deflections, segments, and intervals. The

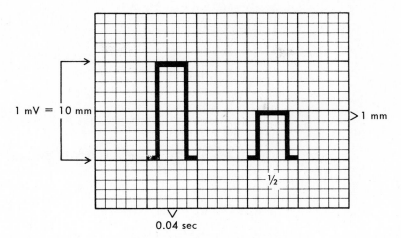

Fig. 6-1. Normal standardization of the ECG. One millivolt (mV) causes a deflection of 10 millimeters (mm). For large ECG deflections the standard must be halved so that 1 mV = 5 mm. For small ECG deflections the standard may be doubled so that 1 mV = 20 mm. Any changes in standardization must be noted on the ECG recording.

horizontal lines are 1 mm apart and are used to measure the *amplitude* of the ECG deflections. The vertical lines are also 1 mm apart and are used to measure the time or *duration* of the ECG events. Each fifth horizontal and vertical line is darker than the others, forming a large square that incorporates 25 smaller squares.

Conventionally, the ECG is *standardized* so that the amplitude of a 1 millivolt (mV) impulse causes a deflection of 10 mm that is two large squares (Fig. 6-1). Therefore each 1-mm deflection equals 0.1 mV. If the amplitude of the deflection recorded from the heart is too large for the ECG paper, the standardization must be halved so that 1 mV results in a deflection of 5 mm (one large square). If the standardization is halved, it must be noted on the ECG paper. The standardization may also be doubled so that 1 mV equals 20 mm.

The usual paper speed for recording is 25 mm/second, and therefore each vertical line separated by 1 mm equals 0.04 sec (40 msec). At twice the normal recording speed (50 mm/second), each small box equals 0.02 second (20 msec).

Deflections

Any wave or complex recorded in the ECG is inscribed as a *positive* (above the base line) or *negative* (below the base line) deflection. When a deflection is partly above the base line and partly below it, and the positive and negative components are approximately equal, the complex is called *diphasic* or *biphasic*. As previously mentioned, the amplitude of deflections is recorded in millimeters or millivolts. Measurement of positive deflections is made from the upper edge of the base line to the peak of the wave; negative deflections are measured from the lower edge of the base line to the lowest point of the wave. Deflections also have *duration*, recorded in seconds or milliseconds (msec).

The six major deflections of the normal ECG are designated by the letters P,

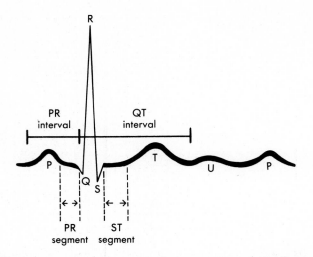

Fig. 6-2. The deflections in a normal ECG are the P wave (atrial depolarization), QRS complex (ventricular depolarization), and T wave (ventricular repolarization). The U wave is sometimes present and follows the T wave. The PR segment is the interval between the end of the P wave and the beginning of the QRS complex. The ST segment is the interval between the end of the QRS complex and the beginning of the T wave. Sometimes atrial repolarization, the Ta wave, can be recorded (see Fig. 6-5). The PR interval is from the onset of the P wave to the onset of the QRS complex. The QT interval is from the onset of the QRS complex to the end of the T wave.

Q, R, S, T, and U (Fig. 6-2). These waves are produced by the electrical energy caused by the movement of charged particles across the membranes of myocardial cells (depolarization and repolarization).

Electrophysiologic principles

The membrane surrounding a cell is a semipermeable two-layered lipid envelope that maintains inside the cell, a high concentration of potassium (K^+) and a low concentration of sodium (Na^+), and outside the cell, a high concentration of Na^+ and a low concentration of K^+. The voltage inside a resting (polarized) cardiac cell is negative with respect to the outside of the cell, in large part because of the cell membrane's relative permeability to K^+ and impermeability to Na^+ during diastole. The ratio of extracellular to intracellular potassium concentrations primarily determines the resting potential of the cell; when the cell becomes depolarized the cell membrane alters its permeability so that it becomes more permeable to Na^+ and less permeable to K^+. Na^+ rushes into the cell, making the voltage inside the cell positive with respect to the voltage outside the cell. These events occur in atrial and ventricular muscle and the His-Purkinje system. In the normal sinus and AV nodes, and possibly in other fibers if they become damaged, calcium appears to play a prominent role in the depolarization process. Calcium (and possibly sodium in some instances) enters the cell through the "slow channel," producing the slow response. It is called the *slow response* because the time to activate and inactivate the channel (in essence, turn it on and off) is slow, compared to the sodium or "fast channel," which is active in

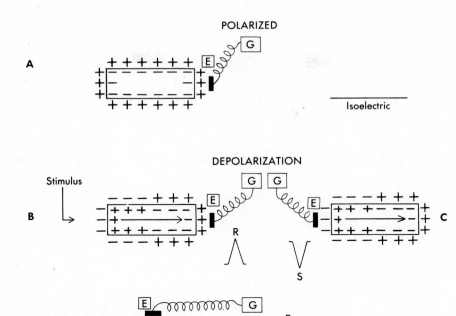

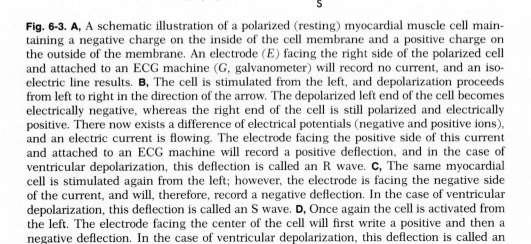

Fig. 6-3. A, A schematic illustration of a polarized (resting) myocardial muscle cell maintaining a negative charge on the inside of the cell membrane and a positive charge on the outside of the membrane. An electrode *(E)* facing the right side of the polarized cell and attached to an ECG machine *(G,* galvanometer) will record no current, and an isoelectric line results. **B,** The cell is stimulated from the left, and depolarization proceeds from left to right in the direction of the arrow. The depolarized left end of the cell becomes electrically negative, whereas the right end of the cell is still polarized and electrically positive. There now exists a difference of electrical potentials (negative and positive ions), and an electric current is flowing. The electrode facing the positive side of this current and attached to an ECG machine will record a positive deflection, and in the case of ventricular depolarization, this deflection is called an R wave. **C,** The same myocardial cell is stimulated again from the left; however, the electrode is facing the negative side of the current, and will, therefore, record a negative deflection. In the case of ventricular depolarization, this deflection is called an S wave. **D,** Once again the cell is activated from the left. The electrode facing the center of the cell will first write a positive and then a negative deflection. In the case of ventricular depolarization, this deflection is called an RS complex. *Continued.*

muscle and in His-Purkinje fibers. Understanding these ionic mechanisms is clinically important because of the development of drugs such as verapamil that *fairly* specifically block the slow channel. These drugs are often called "calcium entry blockers."

The cell in a resting, *polarized* state can be represented by negative and positive charges lining, respectively, the inside and outside of the cell membrane (Fig. 6-3, *A*). If an electrode of an ECG machine (galvanometer) were attached

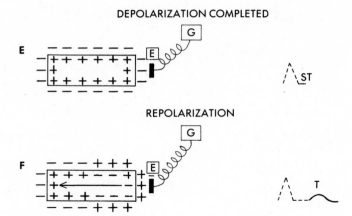

Fig. 6-3, cont'd. E, With the completion of depolarization, the outer surface of the myocardial cell becomes electrically negative; the flow of electric current ceases, and the R wave returns to the isoelectric line. The short period following complete ventricular depolarization is recorded as the ST segment. **F,** In the previous illustrations, the myocardial muscle cell was depolarized from left to right. Now the cell returns to the resting state, repolarization, in the opposite direction, from right to left. The right end of the cell becomes positive first and an electrode facing this site will inscribe a positive deflection. In the case of ventricular repolarization, this deflection is termed a T wave.

to this polarized cell, no electrical potential would be registered because no net change in ionic composition would occur. Hence, there would be no voltage shift and no deviation from the isoelectric base line (Fig. 6-3, *A*).

When a cell or, more likely, a group of cells is stimulated, and the change in membrane permeability permits sodium ions to migrate rapidly into the cell, making the inside positive with respect to the outside (*depolarization*), an electrical field is generated between the depolarized and polarized areas of myocardium. The *P wave* represents *atrial depolarization,* and the *QRS* complex represents *ventricular depolarization* (Fig. 6-3, *B,* to *D*).

A slower movement of ions across the membrane restoring the cell to the polarized state is termed *repolarization.* Movement of potassium ions out of myocardial cells primarily accounts for repolarization. In late diastole, after most of the repolarization has occurred, potassium and sodium reverse positions to restore ionic concentrations to the polarized state. The *Ta wave,* representing *atrial repolarization,* generally lies buried in the QRS complex and ST segment. The ST segment is an isoelectric line extending from the end of the QRS complex to the beginning of the T wave, during which early ventricular repolarization is beginning very slowly (Fig. 6-3, *E*). The *T wave* represents *ventricular repolarization* (Fig. 6-3, *F*).

Waves and complexes
P WAVE

As previously mentioned, the P wave represents atrial depolarization, and begins as soon as the impulse leaves the sinus node (sinoatrial, or SA, node) and

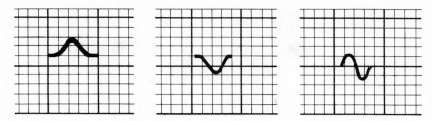

Fig. 6-4. The P wave is gently rounded in contour, may be normally positive, negative, or diphasic in different ECG leads, and should not exceed 2 or 3 mm.

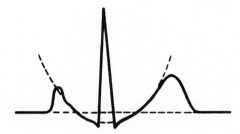

Fig. 6-5. Atrial repolarization as a cause of ST segment deviation. Note that the PQ (PR) and ST segments can be connected by a smooth curve, and that the direction of the deviation is opposite in direction to the P wave. (Adapted from Hurst, J.W. and others: The heart: arteries and veins, ed. 3, New York, 1974, McGraw-Hill Book Co.)

initiates atrial depolarization. Since the sinus node is situated in the right atrium, right atrial activation begins first and is followed shortly thereafter by left atrial activation. As left atrial activation begins, before the end of right atrial activation, the two processes overlap. This close overlap of the forces results in a gently rounded P wave. As will be discussed later in this chapter, the P wave normally may be positive, negative, or diphasic, depending on which lead of the ECG is recorded. Whatever the case, the amplitude of the P wave should not exceed 2 or 3 mm in any lead (Fig. 6-4).

Although usually not visible on the ECG, the Ta wave of atrial repolarization occurs in a direction opposite to that of the P wave and is recorded after the first portion of the P wave and continues through the PR interval. It is usually not identified unless the P wave occurs independently of the QRS, as in complete AV block (see Chapter 8). When the P wave is large, the Ta wave is also generally large and may be seen to extend beyond the QRS complex, resulting in a distortion of the initial portion of the ST segment. This may cause a depression of the ST segment that may be mistaken as having a pathologic significance. To make a correct interpretation in the setting of a depressed ST segment, one must (1) observe the configuration of the atrial repolarization wave (smooth curve with upward concavity), (2) recognize a similar deviation of the base line before the QRS is recorded, and (3) recognize a large P wave (Fig. 6-5).

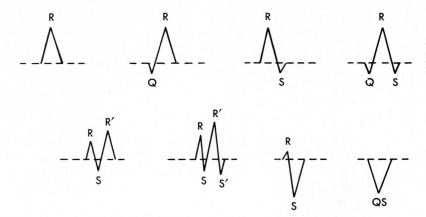

Fig. 6-6. Components of the QRS complex.

QRS COMPLEX

The QRS complex representing ventricular depolarization may have various components, depending on which lead of the ECG is recorded. These components are illustrated in Fig. 6-6 and described as follows:

R wave: The first positive deflection
Q wave: The initial negative deflection preceding an R wave
S wave: The negative deflection following an R wave
R′ wave: The second positive deflection
S′ wave: The negative deflection following the R′ wave
QS wave: The totally negative deflection

The QRS complexes should be examined for the following:
1. The *duration* of the complex (see Chapter 8 discussion of QRS interval)
2. The *amplitude* of the components
3. The general *configuration* of the complex, including the presence and location of any slurred component (see Chapter 8 discussion of bundle branch block and Wolff-Parkinson-White syndrome)
4. The presence of abnormal *Q waves* (discussed under myocardial infarction in this chapter)
5. The timing of the *intrinsicoid deflections* in precordial leads V_1 to V_6

Amplitude. The *amplitude* of the QRS complex has wide normal limits; however, it is generally agreed that if the total amplitude (above and below the base line) is 5 mm or less in all three standard leads, it is abnormally low. Such low voltage may be seen in patients who have cardiac failure, diffuse coronary disease, pericardial effusion, myxedema, primary amyloidosis, or any other conditions producing widespread myocardial damage. Furthermore, it may be found in patients who have emphysema, generalized edema, and obesity. The minimal normal QRS amplitude in precordial leads varies from right to left across the chest, being generally accepted as 5 mm in V_1 and V_6, 7 mm in V_2 and V_5 and 9 mm in V_3 and V_4.

Upper limits for normal QRS voltage (amplitude) have been difficult to set. Diagnostic evaluation is important when QRS amplitudes reach the following

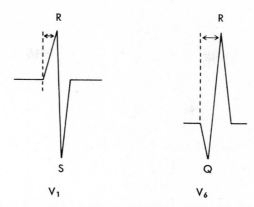

Fig. 6-7. The time of onset of the intrinsicoid deflection is measured from the beginning of the QRS complex to the peak of the R wave.

upper limits: V_1 an R wave of 5 mm; V_1, V_2 an S wave of 30 mm; V_5, V_6 an R wave of 30 mm; and in the limb leads an R or S wave of 20 mm.

Intrinsicoid deflection. Ventricular activation time is the interval between the beginning of the QRS complex and the onset of the intrinsicoid deflection. The time of onset of the intrinsicoid defelection is measured from the beginning of the QRS complex to the peak of the R wave, and it is measured in the precordial leads (Fig. 6-7). In right-sided precordial leads (V_1 or V_2) the time of onset for the intrinsicoid deflection is normally 0.03 second or less. In left-sided precordial leads (V_5 or V_6) the time of onset is normally 0.05 second or less in adults. If the time of onset for the intrinsicoid deflection exceeds 0.03 or 0.05 second, in right- and left-sided leads respectively, it is taken to indicate that the impulse arrived late at the epicardial surface of the ventricle under the electrode. Such delay may be caused by thickening or dilatation of the ventricular wall or a block in the conducting system to the ventricle involved (bundle branch block).

ST SEGMENT

The interval that occurs between the end of the QRS complex and the beginning of the T wave is called the ST segment. It represents the time during which the ventricles have been completely depolarized and are beginning ventricular repolarization. Usually, the ST segment is isoelectric (see Fig. 6-2), but it may normally deviate between -0.5 and $+1.0$ mm from the base line in the standard and unipolar leads (ECG leads are presented in the next section). In some instances, upward displacement of 2 or 3 mm may be normal, provided that the ST segment is concave upward and the succeeding T wave is tall and upright. This is called *early repolarization.* Downward displacement in excess of 0.5 mm generally is abnormal. In all situations, depression caused by a depressed PR segment must be considered. Maybe more important are ST segments, elevated or depressed, that vary temporarily (see discussions of myocardial infarction, pericarditis). Correlation with the clinical condition of the patient is often necessary to determine the significance of ST segment displacement.

Elevation of the ST segment is measured from the upper edge of the isoelectric

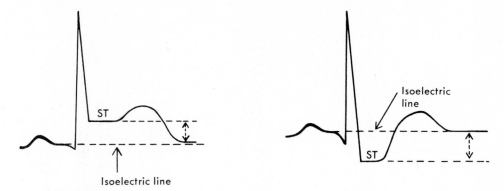

Fig. 6-8. Elevation of the ST segment is measured from the upper edge of the isoelectric line to the upper edge of the ST segment; depression is measured from the lower edge of the isoelectric line to the lower edge of the ST segment.

line to the upper edge of the ST segment; depression is measured from the lower edge of the isoelectric line to the lower edge of the ST segment (Fig. 6-8).

T WAVE

The T wave, normally slightly rounded and slightly asymmetric, represents the recovery period (repolarization) of the ventricles. Upright T waves are measured from the upper level of the base line to the summit of the T wave, whereas inverted T waves are measured from the lower level of the base line to the lowest point of the T wave. Diphasic T waves are measured by adding the amplitudes above and below the base line. T waves normally do not exceed 5 mm in any standard lead or 10 mm in any precordial lead. T wave contour is often very labile and, as with the ST segment, correlation with the clinical status of the patient, often in serially repeated ECGs, is necessary for correct interpretation.

U WAVE

The U wave is a small wave of low voltage sometimes observed following a T wave and in the same direction as its preceding T wave; that is, when the T wave is upright, the U wave normally will be upright. It is best observed in the chest leads, although it is present, but barely detectable, in the limb leads.

Relatively little is known about the U wave. Although the cause and clinical significance of the U wave are uncertain, the appearance of U waves or an increase in their magnitude is seen in certain disorders (see Chapter 8 discussion of hypokalemia). The U wave is generally upright in the precordial leads. A negative U wave may occur in patients who have left ventricular hypertrophy, hypertension, or coronary artery disease. An upright (positive) U wave that becomes inverted (negative) during an exercise stress test often indicates the presence of significant coronary artery obstruction in the main left or left anterior descending coronary artery.

Electrocardiogram leads

As previously mentioned, the deflections on the ECG are produced by the electrical energy owing to the movement of charged ions across the membranes of myocardial cells (depolarization and repolarization). This movement of charged particles results in a flow of electrical current. The pressure behind the flow of electrical current is called *electrical potential*, and it creates an electrical field. This electrical field extends to the body surface, where electrical potential can be measured by the ECG.

By convention there are 12 lead recordings in the ECG. Each lead has a positive and negative pole (electrode), and the location of these poles determines the *polarity* of the lead. A hypothetic line joining the poles of a lead is known as the *axis* of the lead. Moreover, every lead axis is oriented in a certain direction, depending on the location of the positive and negative electrodes.

Six of the twelve ECG leads measure cardiac forces in the *frontal plane* (I, II, III, aV_R, aV_L, and aV_F); the remaining six leads (V_1 to V_6) measure the cardiac forces in the *horizontal plane*. The frontal plane is measured by the standard limb leads and the augmented leads.

STANDARD (BIPOLAR) LIMB LEADS (I, II, III)

The standard limb leads, designated leads I, II, and III, were developed by Willem Einthoven (1860-1927), physiologist and inventor of the string galvanometer. Using the principle that the heart is situated in the center of the electrical field it generates, Einthoven placed the electrodes of the three standard leads as far away from the heart as possible, that is, on the extremities—the right arm, left arm, and left leg.* These three electrodes, therefore, are considered to be electrically equidistant from the heart. Consequently, the heart may be viewed as a point source in the center of an equilateral triangle, whose apices are the right arm, left arm, and left leg. This is called Einthoven's triangle (Fig. 6-9, *A*).

The standard biopolar limb leads measure the *difference* between two recording sites. The actual potential under either of the electrodes is not known, as it is for the unipolar leads. For lead I, the negative electrode is placed on the right arm and the positive electrode on the left arm. For lead II, the negative electrode is on the right arm and the positive electrode on the left leg. For lead III, the left arm electrode is negative, and the left leg electrode is positive (Fig. 6-9, *A*). This is summarized as follows:

Lead	Location
I	Right arm (−) to left arm (+)
II	Right arm (−) to left leg (+)
III	Left arm (−) to left leg (+)

Because of the established relationship of the standard limb leads to each other, at any given instant during the cardiac cycle the sum of the electrical potentials recorded in leads I and III equals the electrical potential recorded in lead II. This is *Einthoven's law,* and it applies to a triangle of any shape. The law stated mathematically is as follows:

$$Lead\ I + Lead\ III = Lead\ II$$

*The right leg serves as a ground electrode, thereby providing a pathway of least resistance for electrical interference in the body. Actually, the ground electrode can be placed at any location on the body.

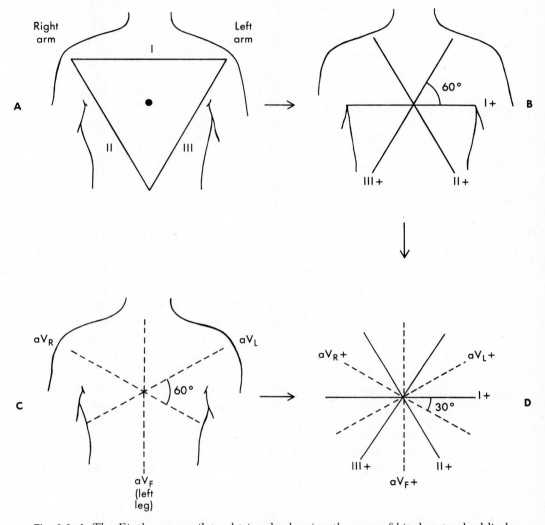

Fig. 6-9. A, The Einthoven equilateral triangle showing the axes of bipolar standard limb leads I, II, and III. The heart is at the center or zero point. **B,** The axes of the standard limb leads are shifted to the center of the triangle (zero point of the electrical field), forming a triaxial figure. **C,** The axes of the unipolar augmented leads. **D,** The axes of the standard and augmented limb leads are combined to form a hexaxial figure. Each lead is labeled at its positive pole.

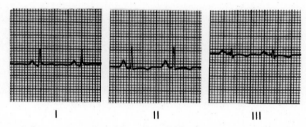

| I | II | III |

Fig. 6-10. Einthoven's law states: Lead I + Lead III = Lead II. The deflections in the ECG leads demonstrate this law.

Einthoven's law may be used to detect errors in electrode placement. Furthermore, it may clarify perplexing findings in one or another lead. If, for example, the deflections of lead II are obscured by muscular or electrical interference or by a wandering base line, the characteristics of the other two leads may be used to determine the presence of a Q wave or ST segment deviation in lead II. Einthoven's law also is helpful in evaluating serial tracings. For example, if in a given tracing the T wave in lead I appears to be more negative than in the previous tracing, changes must be present in the T waves of the other two limb leads as well, so that $T_1 + T_3 = T_2$ (Fig. 6-10).

To prevent confusion about polarities the ECG machine records a positive deflection in the bipolar leads when in lead I the left arm is in the positive portion of the electrical field, in lead II the left leg is in the positive portion of the electrical field, and in lead III the left leg is in the positive portion of the electrical field.

Triaxial reference figure. The three lead axes of the equilateral triangle can be shifted without changing their direction so that their midpoints intersect at the same point. Thus the *triaxial reference figure* is formed with each of the lead axes separated from one another by 60 degrees (Fig. 6-9, *B*).

AUGMENTED (UNIPOLAR) LEADS (aV$_R$, aV$_L$, aV$_F$)

All unipolar leads are called V leads and consist of extremity (limb) leads and precordial (chest) leads. The augmented leads aV$_R$, aV$_L$, and aV$_F$ use the same electrode locations as the standard limb leads. Therefore the positive electrode is attached to the right arm (aV$_R$), left arm (aV$_L$), or left leg (aV$_F$). The negative electrode, however, is formed by combining leads I, II, and III, whose algebraic sum is zero. Since the electrical center of the heart is at zero potential, the augmented leads measure the difference in potential between the limbs and the center of the heart.

The axis for each augmented lead is a line drawn from the extremity, where the positive electrode is placed, to the zero point of the electrical field of the heart, which is at the center of the equilateral triangle (Fig. 6-9, *C*). These three unipolar lead axes also form a triaxial reference system with the axes 60 degrees apart.

Hexaxial reference figure. When the triaxial figure of the standard leads and the triaxial figure of the augmented leads are combined, they form a *hexaxial reference figure* in which each augmented lead is perpendicular to a standard limb lead (Fig. 6-9, *D*). The hexaxial figure is a useful reference for plotting mean cardiac forces in the frontal plane.

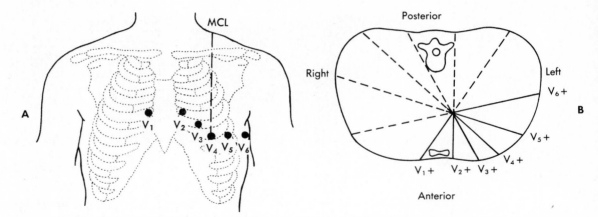

Fig. 6-11. A, Electrode positions of the precordial leads: V_1, fourth intercostal space at the right sternal border; V_2, fourth intercostal space at the left sternal border; V_3, halfway between V_2 and V_4; V_4, fifth intercostal space at the midclavicular line; V_5, anterior axillary line directly lateral to V_4; V_6, midaxillary line directly lateral to V_5. **B,** The precordial reference figure. Leads V_1 and V_2 are called right-sided precordial leads; leads V_3 and V_4, mid-precordial leads; and leads V_5 and V_6, left-sided precordial leads.

PRECORDIAL (UNIPOLAR) LEADS (V_1 TO V_6)

In the horizontal plane, precordial leads are utilized to determine how far anteriorly or posteriorly from the frontal plane the electrical forces of the heart are directed. The standard precordial ECG consists of six unipolar leads, V_1 through V_6. In Fig. 6-11, *A*, the V leads are shown with reference to their electrode positions on the anterior chest wall. These chest electrodes represent a positive pole (unipolar). Any electrical force traveling toward one of these leads will produce a positive deflection; traveling away from it will produce a negative deflection. For descriptive purposes, leads V_1 and V_2 are called right-sided precordial leads; leads V_3 and V_4, midprecordial leads; and leads V_5 and V_6, left-sided precordial leads.

Precordial reference figure. A transverse representation of the chest wall and the V leads results in the precordial reference figure (Fig. 6-11, *B*). This figure is a useful reference for plotting mean cardiac forces in the horizontal plane.

The vector approach to electrocardiography

The electrical potentials generated during the cardiac cycle can be described and measured. To adequately characterize such an electrical potential or force, both the magnitude and the direction of the force must be specified; this can be done by a *vector*. Briefly stated, a vector is a quantity of electrical force that has a known magnitude and direction. A vector may be illustrated graphically by an *arrow*, the length of the arrow representing the *magnitude* of the force and the direction of the arrow indicating the *direction* of the force. The *arrowhead* depicts the location of the positive field.

Representing electrical forces of the heart by vectors more easily explains the

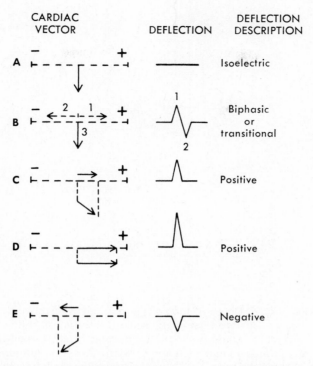

Fig. 6-12. Vectors and their electrocardiographic recordings. Each arrow represents the vector generated by an electrical force. This force produces an electrocardiographic deflection, shown on the right. **A,** Because the vector is perpendicular to the axis of the recording lead, no projection appears on that lead. The absence of a deflection establishes an uninterrupted isoelectric line. **B,** The mean vector (number 3) is perpendicular to the axis of the recording lead when the positive and negative forces are equal (the net area of the deflection is zero). A biphasic or transitional deflection is recorded because the initial forces moved rightward (vector 1) at the same distance that the later forces moved leftward (vector 2). The instantaneous vectors have equal magnitude but opposite direction. **C,** The vector projects on the positive side of the axis of the recording lead to inscribe a small positive deflection. **D,** When the vector is parallel with the lead axis, the projection onto the recording lead has its maximal magnitude. **E,** The vector projects on the negative side of the lead axis, and a small negative deflection is recorded.

relationship between the electrical activity generated by the heart and the recording of this electrical activity by a specific lead. When an electrical force (and therefore the vector that represents it) establishes a direction *parallel* to the lead that records it, this electrical force causes the *largest deflection* to be inscribed by that lead. An electrical force perpendicular to the recording lead produces no deflection in that lead. Forces in between these extremes generate deflections according to their directions: the more nearly parallel the force (and vector) to the recording lead, the larger the deflection produced in that lead; the more nearly perpendicular the force to the recording lead, the smaller the deflection. When the positive and negative forces on a lead are equal, the net area of the deflection is zero. This results in a biphasic or transitional deflection (Fig. 6-12).

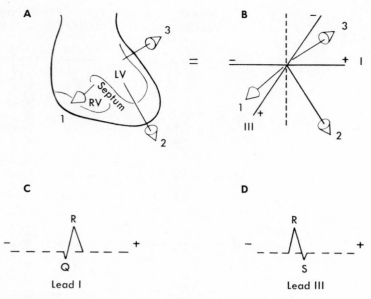

Fig. 6-13. A, Depolarization of the ventricles illustrated by instantaneous vectors. Arrow 1 depicts depolarization of the septum from left to right and is directed to the right and somewhat anteriorly. Arrow 2 illustrates depolarization of the apical region of the heart and is directed to the left and inferiorly. Arrow 3 represents depolarization of the posterior aspect of the left ventricle and is directed to the left and posteriorly. **B,** The instantaneous vectors representing ventricular depolarization are inscribed on lead I and lead III. **C** and **D,** Arrow 1 causes a small negative deflection in lead I, resulting in a Q wave, and a larger positive deflection in lead III, resulting in an R wave. Arrow 2 produces a small positive deflection (R wave) in lead I and an R wave in lead III. Arrow 3 causes a large R wave in lead I and S wave in lead III.

SEQUENCE OF ELECTRICAL EVENTS IN THE HEART

In the normal heart, depolarization of the ventricle is a seq
The process can be represented by *instantaneous vectors*, eac
responds to all the heart's electrical forces at a given momen
successive instantaneous vectors depicting ventricular depolari
in Fig. 6-13, *A*. Initial depolarization passes from left to right a
ventricular septum. During the second phase, depolarization of
muscle occurs near the apex. The last phase of depolarization oc
terior free wall of the left ventricle.

The deflection recorded by any given lead results from the p
cardiac vector generated during depolarization onto the axis of
arrow 1 (Fig. 6-13, *B*), depicting depolarization of the septum, u
small negative deflection in lead I, resulting in a Q wave and a
deflection in lead III, resulting in an R wave. Arrow 2, illustratin
of the apical region of the heart, usually produces a very small po
(R wave) in lead I because of its leftward orientation and an R w
Late depolarization of the heart, being from right to left in the po
of the left ventricle, causes a large positive deflection in lead I (th

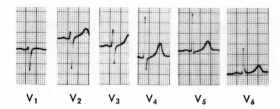

V₁	V₂	V₃	V₄	V₅	V₆

Fig. 6-14. Normal precordial lead ECG.

the R wave) and an S wave in lead III. Following the completion of depolarization of ventricles, the electrical wave returns to the base line. Therefore the three arrows have generated a small initial Q wave followed by a large R wave in lead I and an R wave followed by an S wave in lead III (Fig. 6-13, *C* and *D*).

As previously discussed, each ECG lead has a different orientation to the heart. Therefore the instantaneous vectors of ventricular depolarization will produce a different deflection in each lead. This is also true of ventricular repolarization and atrial depolarization.

In this chapter, detailed consideration is given to the vectors of the QRS complex. However, the positions of the P wave and T wave in the frontal plane are also important. Normally the P wave is upright in leads I and II and may be biphasic, flat, or inverted in lead III; inverted in lead aV_R; upright, biphasic, or inverted in lead aV_L; and upright in lead aV_F.

Normally the T wave is upright in leads I and II, flat, biphasic, or inverted in lead III, and inverted in lead aV_R. In lead aV_L, the T wave may be upright, flattened, or biphasic, according to the QRS pattern. It may also be inverted, provided that the T wave in lead aV_R is also inverted. In lead aV_F the T wave is usually upright; however, it can be normally flattened, biphasic, or inverted, provided that the T wave in lead aV_R is also inverted.

In the horizontal plane the P wave is normally upright in all precordial leads, but it may be inverted in V_1 and V_2 without being abnormal. The normal QRS complex is transitional at some point between V_3 and V_4. The precordial transition zone is characterized by the transition from the RS complexes recorded by the leads oriented to the right ventricle to the QR complexes recorded by the leads oriented to the left ventricle (Fig. 6-14). The normal T wave is upright in leads V_2 through V_6. The T wave may be flat or inverted in V_1 and still be normal.

THE MEAN CARDIAC VECTOR

The mean cardiac vector, which is the average of all the instantaneous vectors, can be expressed accurately on the hexaxial reference figure. Furthermore, since the hexaxial reference system divides the frontal plane into 30-degree intervals, the leads have been classified as follows: all degrees in the upper hemisphere of the hexaxial figure are labeled as negative degrees, and all degrees in the lower hemisphere are labeled as positive degrees. Accordingly, commencing at the positive end of the standard lead I axis (labeled 0 degrees and progressing counterclockwise), the leads are successively at -30, -60, -90, -120, -150, and

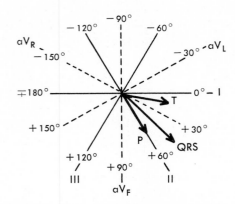

Fig. 6-15. The hexaxial reference system divides the frontal plane into 30-degree intervals. All degrees in the upper hemisphere are labeled as negative degrees, and all degrees in the lower hemisphere are labeled as positive degrees. The mean P vector normally lies along the +60-degree axis. The mean QRS vector normally lies anywhere between 0 and +90 degrees; in the figure the mean QRS vector lies on the +45-degree axis. The mean T vector normally lies between −10 and +75 degrees. In the figure the mean T vector lies on the +15-degree axis. The mean frontal plane QRS axis and T wave axis are usually similarly detected, and the angle between them normally does not exceed 60 degrees.

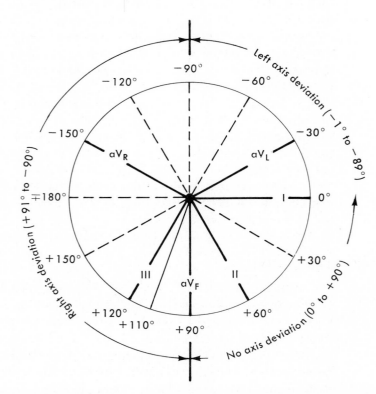

Fig. 6-16. Hexaxial reference figure indicating values for no axis deviation, left axis deviation, and right axis deviation.

−180 degrees. Progressing clockwise, the leads are successively at +30, +60, +90, +120, +150, and +180 degrees* (Fig. 6-15).

The position of the mean cardiac vector provides information about the electrical "position" of the heart, also expressed as the mean electrical axis, and is influenced by the anatomic position of the heart within the chest, the anatomy of the heart itself, and the pathway traveled by the depolarizing wave. If the P vector is projected on the hexaxial figure, the mean electrical axis of the P in the frontal plane lies approximately along the +60-degree axis (Fig. 6-15). The mean QRS vector lies normally between 0 and +90 degrees, whereas the mean electrical axis of the T wave lies between −10 and +75 degrees. The mean frontal plane QRS axis and T wave axis are usually similarly directed, and the angle between them normally does not exceed 60 degrees (Fig. 6-15).

MEAN QRS AXIS

The remainder of this section discusses the significance and determination of the mean QRS axis. The principles also may be applied to the mean P and T vectors.

Deviations in the mean electrical axis, even without other ECG abnormalities, may assist in the diagnosis of cardiac disease. As indicated in Fig. 6-16, the mean QRS vector normally lies between 0 and +90 degrees. Right axis deviation occurs when the mean QRS vector lies between +90 and −90 degrees. Right axis deviation with a mean QRS vector between +90 and +110 degrees may be abnormal, as in patients who have block in the posterior division of the left bundle branch (Chapter 8), but is frequently normal, as seen in young adults or asthenic individuals. This vector is illustrated in Fig. 6-17, A. *Abnormal right axis deviation* is present when the mean QRS vector lies between +110 and −90 degrees. This usually implies either delayed activation of the right ventricle as seen in right bundle branch block (Chapter 8) or right ventricular enlargement.

"Normal" left axis deviation is present when the mean QRS vector lies between 0 and −30 degrees. For example, this situation can occur in patients who have ascites or abdominal tumors, are pregnant, or are obese. *Abnormal left axis deviation,* however, is present when the mean QRS vector lies between −30 and −90 degrees. This vector is illustrated in Fig. 6-17, B. It may indicate delayed activation of the left ventricle as seen in left anterior hemiblock (Chapter 8) or left ventricular enlargement.

Occasionally the electrical position of the heart is described as horizontal, semihorizontal, intermediate, semivertical, or vertical. It has been convenient to refer to a heart with an axis in the range of 0 to −30 degrees as a *horizontal heart,* and to one with an axis between +60 and +90 degrees as a *vertical heart.* Semihorizontal and semivertical positions are halfway stations between the intermediate position and the horizontal and vertical extremes and are not very useful terms.

Determination of the frontal plane projection of the mean QRS vector. First, recall the following principles: an electrical force perpendicular to a lead axis will record

---

*The conventional labeling of the hexaxial reference figure as positive and negative units should not be confused with the positive and negative poles of the lead axes.

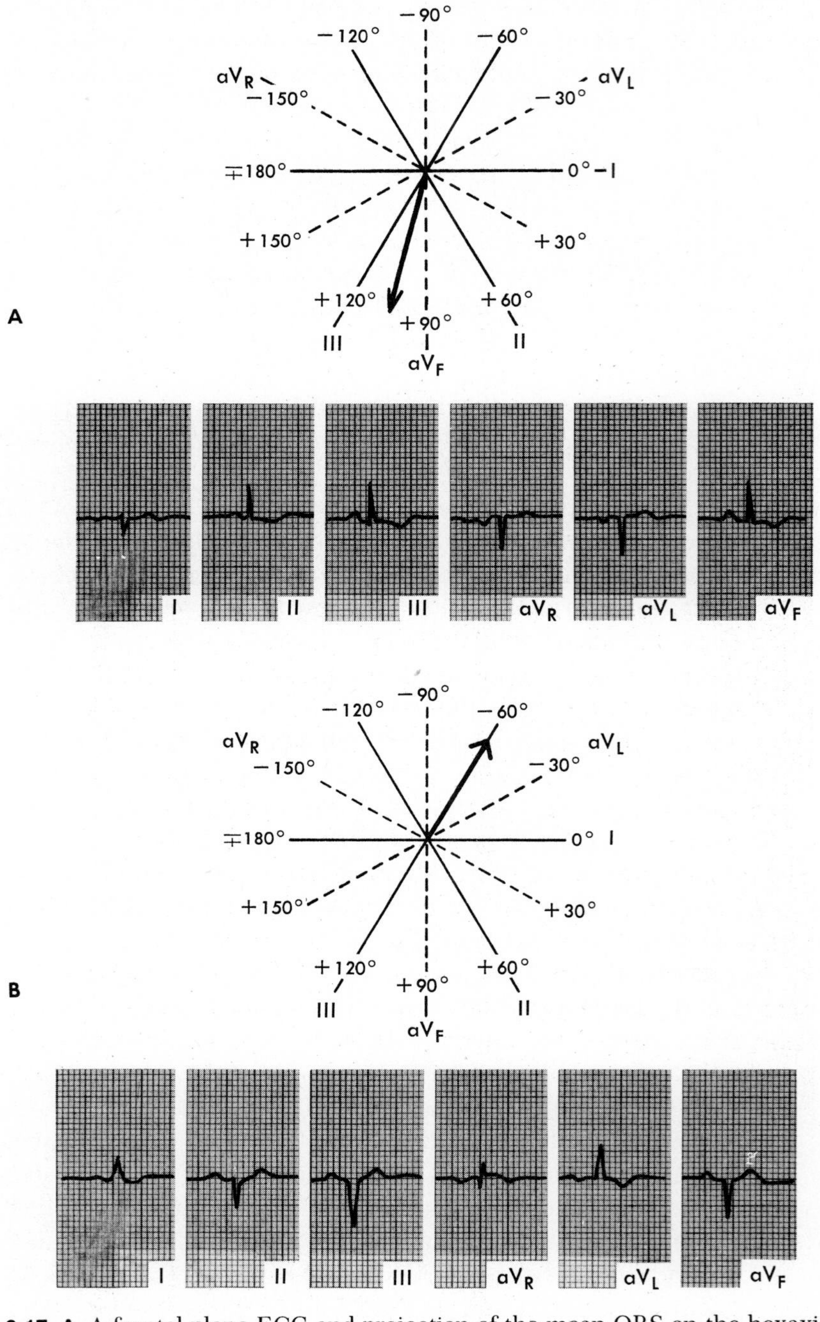

Fig. 6-17. A, A frontal plane ECG and projection of the mean QRS on the hexaxial figure. The mean QRS is located at +105 degrees and this is called right axis deviation. **B,** A frontal plane ECG and projection of the mean QRS on the hexaxial figure. The mean QRS is located at −60 degrees, and this is called left axis deviation.

a small or biphasic complex in the ECG lead. An electrical force parallel to a given lead axis will record its largest deflection in that ECG lead. With this in mind, follow the procedure below by referring to Fig. 6-17, *A*.

1. Examine the six frontal plane leads and identify the lead with the smallest or most diphasic deflection.
2. In Fig. 6-17, *A*, this is lead I.
3. The electrical axis must be near perpendicular to lead I, and it must run near parallel to the lead that intersects lead I at right angles. Perpendicular to lead I is aV_F.
4. The deflection in lead aV_F, therefore, must be largest in the frontal plane.
5. Since the deflection in lead aV_F is positive, the vector must be directed toward the positive pole of that lead.
6. Examine the six frontal plane leads to see if any other lead deflections are as large as lead aV_F. If the QRS complex is equal in amplitude in two leads, the mean QRS vector is directed halfway between the axes of these leads.
7. In this case the deflection in lead III is equal to that in lead aV_F.
8. The mean electrical axis of the QRS, therefore, lies between lead aV_F and lead III and is located at $+105$ degrees (right axis deviation).

In the example just given, if the deflection in lead aV_F had been greater than that in lead III, then the mean QRS vector would have been more parallel to lead aV_F, that is, at $+100$ or even $+95$ degrees, depending on how much larger the deflection in lead aV_F was compared with lead III.

Another example in which one can follow this procedure is shown in Fig. 6-17, *B*.

1. The smallest, or in this case the diphasic, deflection is seen in lead aV_R.
2. The mean QRS vector thus runs perpendicular to lead aV_R.
3. Since lead III runs perpendicular to lead aV_R, the deflection in lead III must be the largest.
4. The deflection in lead III is negative; therefore the mean axis is directed toward the negative pole of lead III.
5. The mean QRS vector in this figure is located at -60 degrees (left axis deviation).

Determination of the horizontal plane projection of the mean QRS vector

1. Identify the precordial lead with the transitional QRS deflection in Fig. 6-18, *A*.
2. Lead V_4 is transitional.
3. The QRS vector is perpendicular to the transitional lead (V_4).
4. The vector should be directed toward the positive sides of the leads with positive deflections, and on the negative sides of the leads with negative deflections, as shown in Fig. 6-18, *C*.
5. When the horizontal plane direction of the mean QRS is noted, an arrowhead may be placed on the mean QRS frontal plane vector to indicate the vector's anterior or posterior direction, as shown in Fig. 6-18, *B*.

It should be noted that the transitional QRS deflection may appear early, that is, between V_1 and V_2, or late, that is, between V_5 and V_6. One explanation for this is that the heart has rotated on its longitudinal axis. In describing the rotation about this axis, one must consider a view of the heart from under the diaphragm.

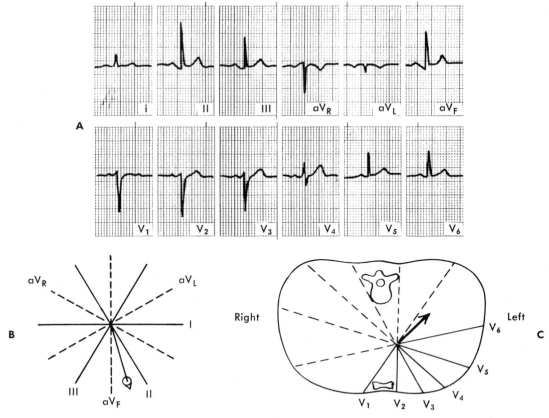

Fig. 6-18. Determination of the mean QRS vector in the frontal and horizontal planes. **A,** Twelve-lead ECG. **B,** The mean QRS vector in the frontal plane is located at + 70 degrees. The arrowhead indicates that the mean QRS vector points posteriorly in the horizontal plane. **C,** The horizontal plane projection of the mean QRS is drawn in a posterior direction on the precordial reference figure. This calculation gives information for the direction of the arrowhead in the frontal plane **(B).**

From this viewpoint, if the front of the heart rotates toward the left, this is called *clockwise rotation.* If the front of the heart rotates toward the right, this is called *counterclockwise rotation.* With a counterclockwise rotation the transitional zone will move toward the right (V_1, V_2). With a clockwise rotation the transitional zone will shift to the left (V_5, V_6). Such rotations may be normal or abnormal.

Left ventricular enlargement

It is not usually possible in the ECG to differentiate ventricular dilatation and hypertrophy. The term "hypertrophy" is commonly used; however, this presentation will use *enlargement,* since it includes both dilatation and hypertrophy.

Hypertension, aortic valvular disease, mitral insufficiency, coronary artery disease, and congenital heart disease (for example, patent ductus arteriosus and coarctation of the aorta) commonly produce left ventricular enlargement. Under these circumstances the wall of the left ventricle is thicker or more dilated than

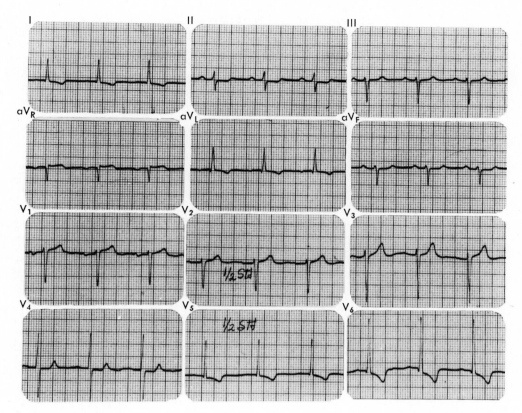

Fig. 6-19. Left ventricular enlargement. This tracing illustrates left ventricular hypertrophy using the Estes criteria: S wave in V_2 and R wave in V_5 and V_6 (note half standard in V_2 and V_5) exceed 30 mm (3 points); ST segment depression in the absence of digitalis (3 points); terminal negativity of P wave in V_1 (1 point). A score of 5 or more points is interpreted as indicating left ventricular hypertrophy. The "score" for this ECG is 7 points.

normal. Furthermore, this increase in muscle mass results in increased voltage of those QRS deflections that represent left ventricular potentials. Accordingly, the QRS interval may increase in duration to the upper limits of normal; the intrinsicoid deflection may be somewhat delayed over the left ventricle; and the voltage of the QRS complex will increase—producing deeper S waves over the right ventricle (leads V_1 and V_2) and taller R waves over the left ventricle (leads V_5, V_6, I, aV_L).

Leads oriented to the left ventricle may also demonstrate a *strain* pattern, that is, depressed ST segments and inverted T waves. "Strain" is a useful, non-committal term and its mechanism is not understood. It is known, however, to develop in patients who have long-standing left ventricular enlargement, and the pattern intensifies when dilatation and failure set in. Myocardial ischemia and slowing of intraventricular conduction are some of the important factors that probably contribute to the pattern.

In general, the voltage criteria proposed for the diagnosis of left ventricular enlargement are unreliable. However, the best approach so far is the Estes scoring system, which is as follows (compare with Fig. 6-19):

Points

1. R wave or S wave in limb lead = 20 mm or more; or
   S wave in V_1, V_2, or V_3 = 30 mm or more;   } 3
   or R wave in V_4, V_5, or V_6 = 30 mm or more
2. Any ST segment shift opposite to mean QRS vector (without digitalis)   3
   Typical "strain" ST segment, T wave (with digitalis)   1
3. Left axis deviation: −30 degrees or more   2
4. QRS interval: 0.09 second or more   1
   Intrinsicoid deflection in V_{5-6}: 0.05 second or more   1
5. Left atrial enlargement   3

Definite left ventricular enlargement is present with a *point score of 5 or more. Probable left ventricular enlargement* is present if the *point score is 4.*

It should be noted that left ventricular enlargement may be present without concomitant left axis deviation. Left axis deviation supports the diagnosis of left ventricular enlargement only when the voltage criteria are fulfilled. The voltage criteria just listed, however, include a small percentage of both false positive and false negative diagnoses. Therefore, in making an electrocardiographic diagnosis of left ventricular enlargement, it is wise to evaluate such factors as body build, the thickness of the chest wall, and the presence of complicating disease. Echocardiography has eliminated many uncertainties about the presence of ventricular enlargement.

Left atrial enlargement

Left atrial abnormality occurs frequently in left ventricular enlargement, but this is not always the case. For example, left atrial enlargement caused by mitral stenosis is not associated with left ventricular enlargement unless there is mitral insufficiency or concomitant aortic valvular disease.

The following criteria are used in the ECG diagnosis of left atrial enlargement (Fig. 6-20):

1. The duration of the P wave is often widened to 0.12 second or more. (Normal P wave duration is 0.11 second.)
2. The contour of the P wave is *notched* and slurred in leads I and II (*P mitrale*). (Notching per se is not abnormal unless the P wave shows increased voltage or duration or both, or the summits are more than 0.03 second apart.)
3. The right precordial leads (V_1, V_2) reflect diphasic P waves with a wide, deep, negative terminal component. The duration (in seconds) and amplitude (in millimeters) of the terminal component are measured and the algebraic product determined. A more negative value than −0.03 second is considered abnormal.
4. The mean electrical axis of the P wave may be shifted left, to between +45 and −30 degrees.

Right ventricular enlargement

Right ventricular enlargement is commonly seen with mitral stenosis, some forms of congenital heart disease, and chronic diffuse pulmonary disease such as pulmonary hypertension, emphysema, and bronchiectasis. For right ventricular

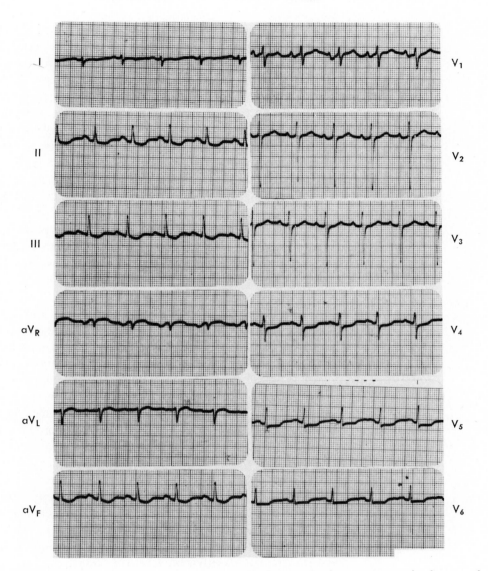

Fig. 6-20. Left atrial enlargement. In this example, left atrial enlargement may be diagnosed by the P terminal force abnormality seen in V_1. The negative portion of the diphasic P wave is approximately 0.04 second in duration and 1 mm in amplitude. The M-shaped broad contour seen prominently in leads I, II, III, and aV_F and the lateral precordial leads are also found in left atrial enlargement. In addition, right axis deviation of approximately +110 degrees exists in this patient with mitral stenosis.

enlargement in the adult to become evident electrocardiographically, however, the right ventricle must enlarge considerably, since the normal adult ECG reflects left ventricular predominance. This accounts for the relative frequency of a normal ECG in the presence of right ventricular enlargement.

Most of the criteria for diagnosing right ventricular enlargement focus on the QRS pattern in the right precordial leads. As the right ventricle enlarges, the height of the right precordial R waves increases, with a concomitant decrease in the depth of the S wave. When right ventricular enlargement becomes fully developed, the normal precordial pattern is completely reversed so that tall R waves (QR or RS) are recorded in V_1 with deep S waves (RS) in V_6.

Prolongation of the QRS interval does not develop unless an intraventricular conduction defect develops with the enlarged right ventricle. The time of onset of the intrinsicoid deflection, however, may be delayed in the right precordial leads because the vectors representing activation of the right ventricle usually occur later in the QRS interval than they do normally and are of increased magnitude.

Right axis deviation is the most common sign of right ventricular enlargement. The diagnosis of right ventricular enlargement, however, should not be made on this finding alone unless other causes for right axis deviation have been ruled out. Furthermore, right ventricular enlargement may occur without abnormal right axis deviation.

A right ventricular strain pattern is manifested in ST and T wave alterations, with T wave changes similar to those seen in left ventricular enlargement. The ST segment is depressed and the T wave is inverted in the right-sided precordial leads and often in leads II, III, and aV_F, as well. This is a nonspecific abnormality.

Right bundle branch block is seen in right ventricular enlargement, especially of the volume-overload variety. In the younger person, right ventricular enlargement is commonly associated with right bundle branch block, either complete or incomplete. In the older age group (40 years and up) coronary artery disease is the most common cause. The surface ECG is less useful than the vectorcardiogram in the assessment of the degree of right ventricular enlargement in cases of incomplete or complete right bundle branch block. Further elaboration on the vectorcardiogram is beyond the scope of this presentation; therefore the reader is encouraged to refer to other textbooks on this subject. See Chapter 8 for a discussion of right bundle branch block.

A summary of the features of right ventricular enlargement is given here; these should be compared with the example in Fig. 6-21.

1. Reversal of precordial lead pattern with tall R waves over the right precordium (V_1, V_2), and deep S waves over the left precordium (V_5, V_6); the R to S ratio in V_1 becomes greater than 1.0
2. Duration of QRS interval within normal limits (if no right bundle branch block)
3. Late intrinsicoid deflection in V_1, V_2
4. Right axis deviation
5. Typical strain ST segment T wave patterns in V_1, V_2, and in leads II, III, and aV_F

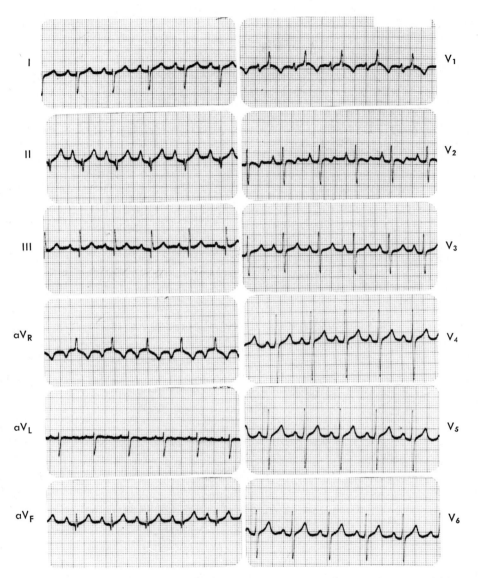

Fig. 6-21. Right ventricular enlargement. The presence of right axis deviation (approximately +160 degrees), an R wave in V_1 that exceeds 5 mm, and an R:S ratio in V_1 that exceeds 1.0 are all diagnostic of right ventricular hypertrophy. In addition, the totally upright R wave in V_1 suggests that the pressure in the right ventricle equals or almost equals the pressure in the left ventricle. The P waves suggest right atrial enlargement.

Right atrial enlargement

In the presence of right ventricular enlargement, it is not unusual to find an enlarged right atrium. Moreover, right atrial enlargement is often an indirect sign of right ventricular enlargement.

The following criteria are used in the ECG diagnosis of right atrial enlargement (Fig. 6-22):

1. The duration of the P wave is 0.11 second or less.
2. The contour of the P wave is tall, *peaked (P pulmonale)*, and measures 2.5 mm or more in amplitude in leads II, III, and aV_F.

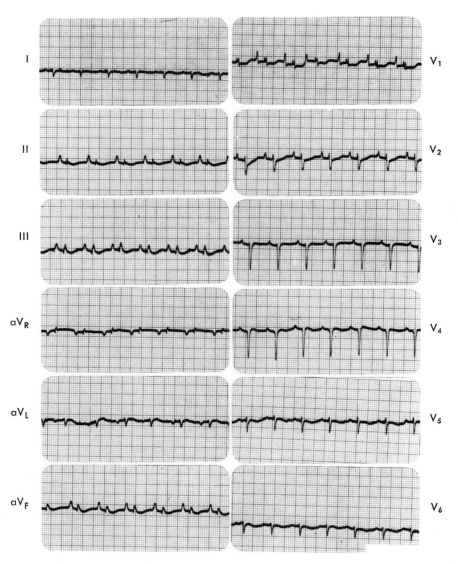

Fig. 6-22. Right atrial enlargement. The large peaked P waves in leads II, III, aV_F, and V_1, with an amplitude that exceeds 2.5 mm in leads II and III, characterize right atrial enlargement in this example. The mean P axis is more positive than +60 degrees, another criterion for right atrial enlargement. The patient has pulmonic stenosis.

3. The right precordial leads reflect diphasic P waves, often with increased voltage of the initial component.

4. The mean electrical axis of the P wave may be shifted right to +70 degrees or more.

It should be noted that abnormal P waves may occur in healthy patients. For example, acceleration of the heart rate alone may cause peaking and increased voltage of the P wave. Conversely, normal P waves may be identified in the presence of atrial disease.

Myocardial infarction

To diagnose myocardial infarction, the ECG should be used to confirm the clinical impression. Because the ECG may not be diagnostic in many instances, if a patient is suspected clinically of having experienced a myocardial infarction, he should be treated accordingly, regardless of what the ECG shows.

Only Q wave changes (necrosis) are diagnostic of infarction, but changes in the ST segments (injury) and T waves (ischemia) may be suspicious and provide presumptive evidence. These changes are illustrated in Fig. 6-23.

Q WAVE

The Q wave is one of the most important, and sometimes most difficult to interpret, assessors of myocardial infarction on the ECG. For example, with normal intraventricular conduction, small Q waves are present in leads V_5, V_6, aV_L, and I, particularly with a horizontal heart position or left axis deviation. Furthermore, with a vertical heart position or right axis deviation, small Q waves may be present in leads II, III, and aV_F. Finally, deep wide Q waves or QS complexes are normally present in aV_R and may be present in lead V_1.

Major importance is placed on the development of *new* Q waves in ECG leads where they previously were not present.

Accordingly, the *appearance* of abnormal Q waves must be considered in light

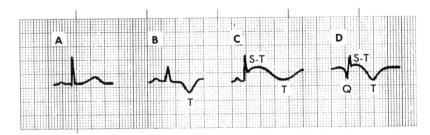

Fig. 6-23. ECG wave changes indicative of ischemia, injury, and necrosis of the myocardium. **A,** Normal left ventricular wave pattern. **B,** Ischemia indicated by inversion of the T wave. **C,** Ischemia and current of injury indicated by T wave inversion and ST segment elevation. The ST segment may be elevated above or depressed below the base line, depending on whether or not the tracing is from a lead facing toward or away from the infarcted area and depending on whether epicardial or endocardial injury occurs. Epicardial injury causes ST segment elevation in leads facing the epicardium. **D,** Ischemia, injury, and myocardial necrosis. The Q wave indicates necrosis of the myocardium.

of the overall picture, considering that pathologic Q waves have the following features:

1. Q waves are 0.04 second or longer in *duration*.
2. Q waves are usually greater than 4 mm in *depth*.
3. Q waves appear in *leads* that do not normally have deep, wide Q waves. V_1 and aV_R normally record Q waves. Pathologic Q waves are usually present in several leads that are oriented in similar directions (e.g., II, III, and aV_F; or I, aV_L.

VECTOR ABNORMALITIES

In acute myocardial infarction, electrical and anatomic death of the myocardium occurs in the region of the infarct; hence the initial forces of depolarization tend to point away from the infarcted area, producing Q waves in the ECG leads facing the involved site. The mean T vector also tends to point away from the site of infarction, presumably because of electrical ischemia in the tissues surrounding the infarct. The ST vector represents the effect of injury current. When

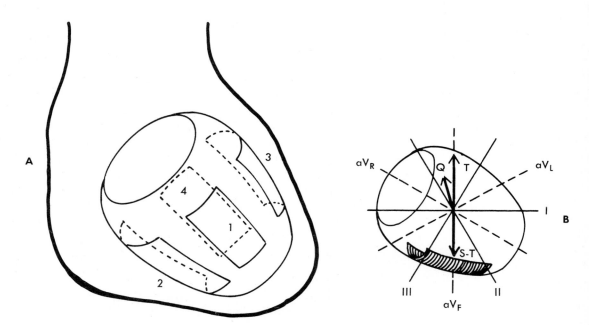

Fig. 6-24. A, Lie of the left ventricle in the chest as viewed frontally. The left ventricle has been divided into four topographic regions where infarctions may occur: (1) anterior, (2) diaphragmatic or inferior, (3) lateral, and (4) posterior (pure). **B,** Vectors of a diaphragmatic myocardial infarction. Hexaxial reference figure is superimposed on the left ventricle as viewed in **B.** The mean vector for the initial 0.04 second of the QRS complex points *away* from the infarcted area and indicates the dead zone. This produces Q waves in the leads "looking at" the infarction. The mean T vector indicates the ischemic zone surrounding the infarct and points *away* from the infarcted area. The ST vector indicates the injury zone and in the event of myocardial infarction, the ST vector points *toward* the injured area. In this example of a diaphragmatic myocardial infarction, leads II, III, and aV_F will exhibit the Q waves, ST segment elevation, and T wave inversion shown in Fig. 6-23, **D.**

the injury current is in the epicardial layers of the myocardium, as in myocardial infarction and pericarditis, the ST segment is elevated in leads facing the injury and the ST vector points toward the injured area. When the injury current is located in the subendocardial layers, as in angina pectoris, coronary insufficiency, and subendocardial infarction, the ST segment is depressed in leads facing the injury, and the ST vector points away from the site of injury (see Fig. 6-32). The ST displacement in subendocardial infarction persists longer than that of angina pectoris and coronary insufficiency.

Thus with an acute myocardial infarction the ST vector is opposite in direction to the Q vector and the mean T vector, resulting in ST segment elevation in those leads that have Q waves and inverted T waves. The relationship of these three vectors to one another is diagramed in Fig. 6-24, *B*.

LOCALIZATION OF INFARCTION

Localization of infarcts may be prognostically important. Localization is based on the principle that diagnostic signs of myocardial infarction (Fig. 6-23) occur in leads whose positive terminals face the damaged surface of the heart. To facilitate localization, the left ventricle has been divided into four topographic regions where infarctions may occur (Fig. 6-24, *A*). Although these locations represent electrical rather than anatomic sites of infarction, anatomic correlations occur with reasonable frequency, particularly for the first myocardial infarction.

An *anterior infarction* produces characteristic changes in leads V_1, V_2, and V_3; a *diaphragmatic* or *inferior infarction* affects leads II, III, and aV_F; a *lateral infarction* involves leads I, aV_L, V_5, and V_6. In strictly *posterior infarction*, there are no leads whose positive terminals are directly over the infarct. However, the changes of the electrical field produced by any infarction still apply; hence in purely posterior infarction the initial forces of the QRS complex and the T wave point anteriorly away from the site of the infarct, and the ST segment is directed posteriorly. This is recognized in the ECG as tall broad initial R waves, ST segment depression, and tall upright T waves in leads V_1 and V_2. In other words, a mirror image of the typical infarction pattern of an anterior myocardial infarction is recorded. Stated another way, infarction of the true posterior surface of the heart must be inferred from reciprocal (opposite) changes occurring in the anterior leads. These locations are summarized in Table 6-1.

It should be noted that although diagnostic signs of myocardial infarction appear in leads facing the infarcted heart surface, *reciprocal changes* occur con-

Table 6-1. Location of myocardial infarction

Area of infarction	Leads showing wave changes
Anterior	V_1, V_2, V_3
Diaphragmatic or inferior	II, III, aV_F
Lateral	I, aV_L, V_5, V_6
Posterior (pure)	V_1 and V_2: tall broad initial R wave, ST segment depression, and tall upright T wave

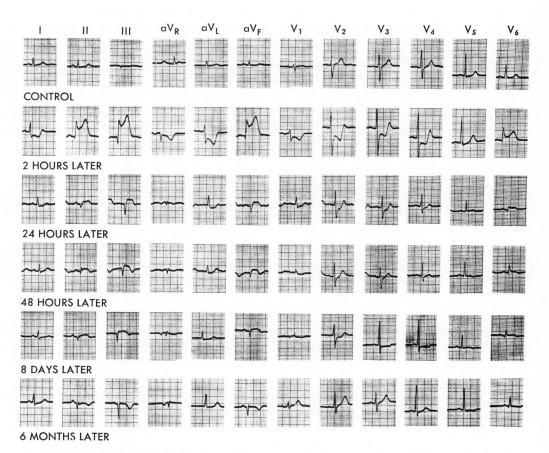

Fig. 6-25. Evolutionary changes in a posteroinferior myocardial infarction. *Control tracing* is normal. The tracing recorded 2 *hours* after onset of chest pain demonstrates development of early Q waves, marked ST segment elevation, and hyperacute T waves in leads II, III, and aV$_F$. In addition, a larger R wave, ST segment depression, and negative T waves have developed in leads V$_1$ to V$_2$. These are early changes indicating acute posteroinferior myocardial infarction. The *24-hour* tracing demonstrates evolutionary changes. In leads II, III, and aV$_F$ the Q wave is larger, the ST segments have almost returned to base line, and the T wave has begun to invert. In leads V$_1$ to V$_2$ the duration of the R wave now exceeds 0.04 second, the ST segment is depressed, and the T wave is upright. (In this classic example, ECG changes of true posterior involvement extend past V$_2$; ordinarily only V$_1$ and V$_2$ may be involved.) Only minor further changes occur through the *8-day* tracing. Finally, *6 months later* the ECG illustrates large Q waves, isoelectric ST segments, and inverted T waves in leads II, III, and aV$_F$, large R waves, isoelectric ST segment, and upright T waves in V$_1$ and V$_2$ indicative of an "old" posteroinferior myocardial infarction.

comitantly in leads facing the diametrically opposed surface of the heart. These changes include absence of a Q wave, some increase of the R wave, depressed ST segment, and upright tall T wave.

Reciprocal changes, therefore, in an anterior infarction will occur in leads II, III, and aV_F. In a diaphragmatic or inferior infarction, reciprocal changes occur in leads I, aV_L, and some of the precordial leads. In lateral wall infarction, lead V_1 may show reciprocal changes.

Frequently the localization of an infarction is not as strict as just described. If the anterior and lateral walls of the left ventricle are both involved in the process, it is called an *anterolateral infarction*. If the limb leads indicate an inferior infarction and diagnostic changes are also present in leads V_5 and V_6, then it is called an inferior infarction with lateral extension or an *inferolateral infarction,* and so on.

EVOLUTION OF A MYOCARDIAL INFARCTION

The evolution of a myocardial infarction is a sequential process, and it is important to record the time relationships in the diagnosis. Within the first few hours after an infarction, sometimes referred to as the hyperacute state, elevated ST segments and tall (hyperacute) upright T waves appear in those leads facing the infarction. Q waves may appear early or may not develop for several days. Within several days of the infarct the ST segment begins to return to base line, whereas the T waves develop progressively deeper inversion. After weeks or months the T waves become shallower and may finally return to normal. The Q waves are most likely to remain as a permanent record of the myocardial scar (Fig. 6-25). Persistent ST segment elevation (beyond 6 weeks) suggests the possibility of ventricular aneurysm (Table 6-2). The different locations of myocardial infarction in different stages of clinical evolution are shown in Figs. 6-26 to 6-32.

Table 6-2. Time relationships in the evolution and resolution of a myocardial infarction

ECG abnormality	Onset	Disappearance
ST segment elevation	Immediately	1 to 6 weeks
Q waves > 0.04 second	Immediately or in several days	Years to never
T wave inversion	6 to 24 hours	Months to years

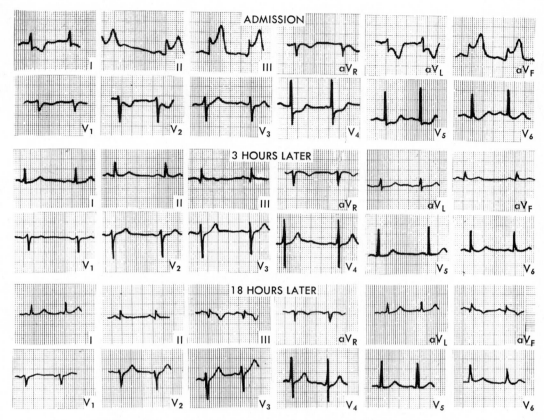

Fig. 6-26. These three 12-lead ECGs obtained at different time intervals from a patient who had an unequivocal myocardial infarction demonstrate that at one point during the electrocardiographic evolution of a myocardial infarction, the ECG may appear almost normal. Note the hyperacute T wave changes and unquestionable injury current portrayed in the admission ECG. Hyperacute T wave changes are normally upright; these enlarged T waves can occur very early after infarction, preceding the more characteristic T wave inversion. Three hours later, the ST segment has returned almost completely to the base line, significant Q waves have not yet appeared, and the T waves remain fairly normal. This ECG is at most "nonspecifically" abnormal. Eighteen hours after admission, classic changes in an acute diaphragmatic myocardial infarction have evolved. This illustration serves to deemphasize the value of a single ECG in diagnosing an acute myocardial infarction. The patient quite possibly would have been sent home if the determination for admission to the CCU had been based solely on a single ECG, that is, the second tracing.

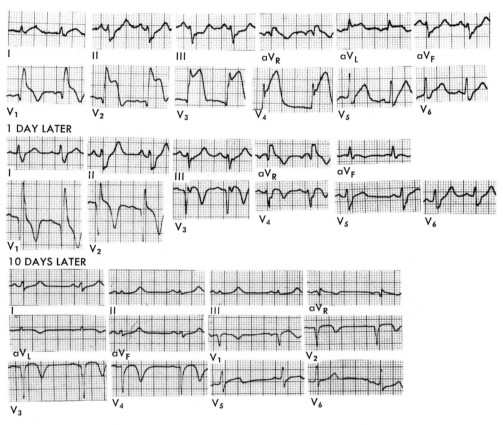

Fig. 6-27. Serial tracings on a patient with an acute anterior myocardial infarction. On admission patient's ECG showed left axis deviation (left anterior hemiblock) and right bundle branch block, thus supporting the presence of bifascicular block (see Chapter 8). Terminal T wave inversion in V_1 to V_2 and profound ST segment elevation are present in V_1 to V_5. These changes are not masked by the presence of the right bundle branch block. One day later the ST segments have returned toward the baseline, the Q waves in the anterior precordial leads have enlarged greatly, and there is now T wave inversion in these leads. Left anterior hemiblock and right bundle branch block are still present. In the tracing recorded 10 days later the right bundle branch block and left anterior hemiblock have disappeared, leaving the electrocardiographic changes of an anteroseptal myocardial infarction with Q waves in V_1 to V_3 and T wave inversion in V_1 to V_4.

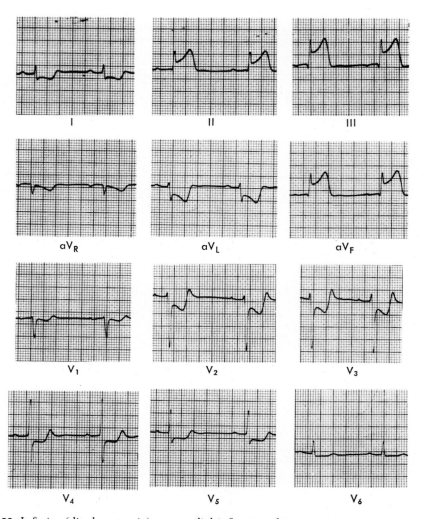

Fig. 6-28. Inferior (diaphragmatic) myocardial infarction, hyperacute stage. Note ST segment elevation in leads II, III, and aV$_F$, with reciprocal ST depression in the anterior precordial leads. The T waves in leads II, III, and aV$_F$ are still upright and pointed and indicate the hyperacute stage of myocardial infarction. Note the development of only very small Q waves in leads II, III, and aV$_F$. Subsequent evolution of this ECG will demonstrate the progressive development of significant (greater than 0.04 second) Q waves and T wave inversion in leads II, III, and aV$_F$; the ST segment will return to an isoelectric position.

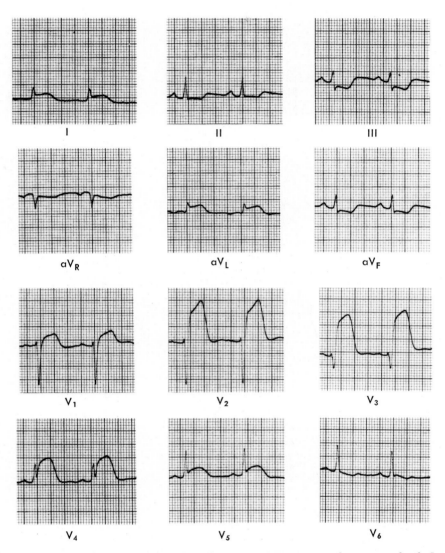

Fig. 6-29. Anterolateral myocardial infarction, acute. ST segment elevation in leads I, aV_L, and V_1 to V_5 indicate an acute anterolateral myocardial infarction. During the evolution of this tracing, one would expect the development of Q waves and T wave inversion in leads I and aV_L and the precordial leads, with the ST segment returning to baseline.

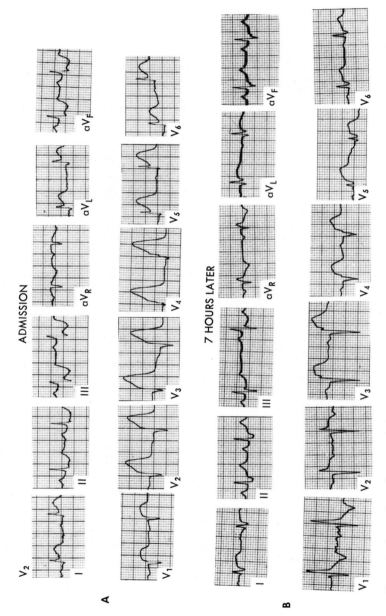

Fig. 6-30. Anterolateral myocardial infarction, acute. The 12-lead ECG on admission, **A,** demonstrates ST segment elevation in leads I, aV$_L$, and V$_1$ to V$_6$, indicating the anterolateral injury current of an acute anterolateral myocardial infarction. **B,** Seven hours later. The patient has developed right bundle branch block with abnormal Q waves in leads I, aV$_L$, and V$_2$ to V$_5$.

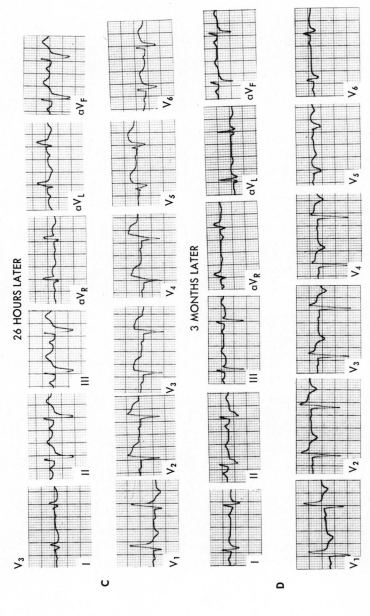

Fig. 6-30, cont'd. C, Twenty-six hours later. In addition to the right bundle branch block, the patient has now developed left anterior hemiblock. **D,** Three months later. The left anterior hemiblock and right bundle branch block are still present. The Q waves in leads I and aV_L are not as prominent as the Q waves in V_1 to V_5. Persistent ST segment elevation for a duration greater than 6 weeks after the myocardial infarction raises the possibility of a left ventricular aneurysm.

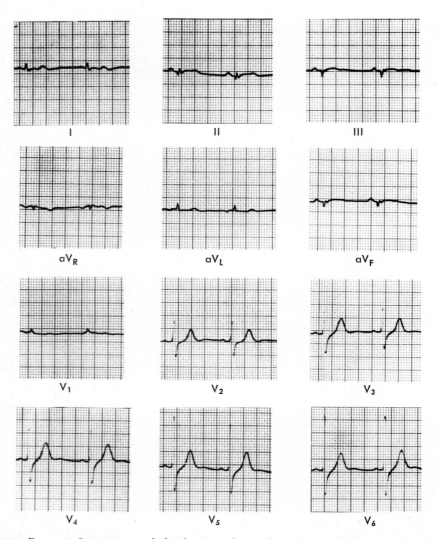

Fig. 6-31. Posteroinferior myocardial infarction, date indeterminant. Q waves in II, III, and aV$_F$ are consistent with an old inferior myocardial infarction. The large R wave in V$_1$ signifies true posterior infarction as well. Compare with Fig. 6-25 at 6 months.

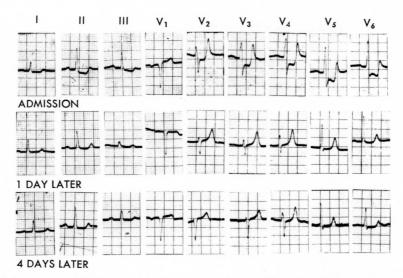

Fig. 6-32. Subendocardial myocardial infarction. Note slight ST segment depression in leads I, II, and III with marked ST segment depression in leads V$_2$ to V$_6$ on admission. One day later the ST segments have returned to normal and there is diminution of the height of the R wave in the precordial leads, but no other changes. The tracing 4 days later is essentially unchanged. Note failure to develop the classic Q waves of a transmural myocardial infarction. The patient died and at autopsy had an extensive subendocardial myocardial infarction.

SUGGESTED READINGS

Beckwith, J.R.: Grant's clinical electrocardiography; the spatial vector approach, New York, 1970, McGraw-Hill Book Co.

Burch, G.E., and Winsor, T.: A primer of electrocardiography, ed. 6, Philadelphia, 1971, Lea & Febiger.

Chung, E.K.: Electrocardiography: practical applications with vectorial principles, Hagerstown, Md., 1980, Harper & Row Publishers, Inc.

Friedman, H.D.: Diagnostic electrocardiography and vectorcardiography, ed. 2, New York, 1977, McGraw-Hill Book Co.

Hurst, J.W., and others, editors: The heart, ed. 5, New York, 1981, McGraw-Hill Book Co.

Lipman, B.S., Massie, E., and Kleiger, R.E.: Clinical scalar electrocardiography, ed. 6, Chicago, 1972, Year Book Medical Publishers, Inc.

Marriott, H.J.L.: Practical electrocardiography, ed. 6, Baltimore, 1977, The Williams & Wilkins Co.

Schamroth, L.: Diagnostic pointers in clinical electrocardiology, vol. 2, Bowie, Md., 1979, Charles Press.

7

COMPLICATIONS OF CORONARY ARTERY DISEASE

Paula Hindle
Andrew G. Wallace

To pump blood to all organs and tissues of the body, the heart muscle requires a substantial flow of blood (coronary perfusion) that can increase appropriately when cardiac demands increase with physical or emotional activity. A variety of functional disturbances in cardiac performance develop when disease of the coronary arteries compromises the supply of coronary blood flow.

During normal activity the heart extracts approximately 75% of the arterial oxygen supply. Other organs usually extract approximately 25% of this oxygen; thus the oxygen reserve available to the heart when it is stressed is very limited. Under these circumstances an increase in coronary blood flow is the only means by which increased myocardial needs are satisfied. If the coronary blood flow fails to meet the myocardial need for oxygen, ischemia results.[1]

The mean arterial blood pressure determines the rate of blood flow in most arteries throughout the body. Coronary blood flow, in contrast, is determined mainly by the diastolic arterial blood pressure. During ventricular systole the stress within the myocardial wall is high, and the heart muscle constricts the transmural coronary blood vessels. In diastole, wall stress drops precipitously, and coronary flow reaches its maximal velocity. Under any given set of conditions, a complex interaction between hydraulic factors (wall stress, arterial pressure, and heart rate) and local metabolic factors determines normal coronary blood flow. The activity of the autonomic nervous system, in turn, modulates these factors.

When these controls operate normally, the supply of coronary blood flow closely matches the metabolic requirements of heart muscle. When a hydraulically significant obstruction develops within a coronary artery, flow and the distribution of flow are compromised, and ischemia develops. The functional significance of any given coronary artery stenosis depends in part on the demands placed on the myocardium and in part on the extent of collateral vessels that provide an alternative source of perfusion to the muscle in the distribution area supplied by the stenosed vessel.

Clinical syndromes: an overview

Deficits in myocardial perfusion may result in or produce various clinical syndromes.

136

ANGINA PECTORIS

Pathophysiologically, this syndrome is a state of transient myocardial ischemia without clinically recognizable cell death. It is characterized by chest discomfort, which is usually precipitated by activities or events that increase the metabolic demand for oxygen. At the time of the first episode of anginal pain, the coronary artery obstruction is generally well developed. As the disease progresses, the anginal pain may change from its stable, predictable nature to "unstable" angina. In this state pain may be present even at rest, and despite aggressive medical therapy, relief of pain may be inconsistent.

MYOCARDIAL INFARCTION

This condition is defined as myocardial ischemia of sufficient intensity and duration to produce recognizable death (necrosis) of myocardial tissue. The most common symptom is severe, persistent chest pain, which may be accompanied by intense anxiety, nausea, vomiting, dyspnea, or diaphoresis. Ancillary clinical and laboratory tests show evidence of dead heart muscle. The patient may or may not be able to cite a precipitating factor, although approximately two-thirds of all such patients have premonitory symptoms. A myocardial infarction can be classified as subendocardial or transmural, depending on the extent of damage to the myocardial wall.

HEART FAILURE

In this state cardiac output fails to meet metabolic demands. Heart failure may involve either ventricle initially, but since they work in series, one ventricle does not fail for long before the other also becomes affected, leading to total cardiac decompensation. Pulmonary edema is a medical emergency caused by severe left-sided heart failure (Table 7-1). Cardiogenic shock, referred to as *pump failure*, is frequently caused by massive myocardial damage, which leaves the ventricle so disabled that it cannot generate an adequate cardiac output. Such profound failure is usually irreversible.

CARDIOMEGALY

Cardiomegaly is enlargement of the heart that may result from dilatation, hypertrophy, or both. Patients with long-standing angina or with recurrent infarctions demonstrate multiple scars and areas of replacement fibrosis in the heart. The heart appears to adapt to these changes by dilatation. In part because of dilatation and in part because the work load on the heart muscle shifts from areas of damage to residual health muscle, the remaining normal components undergo hypertrophy. As a result, the heart's size on x-ray examination, heart dimensions measured by angiography, and heart mass all increase.

ABNORMAL ELECTROCARDIOGRAM

Changes on the ECG may strongly indicate the presence of coronary insufficiency in an asymptomatic patient. On the other hand, the resting ECG may be normal in a patient with serious coronary artery disease. Therefore it is helpful to obtain an ECG during and after stress (exercise) to establish evidence of coronary insufficiency. The most significant change on the ECG is the devel-

Table 7-1. Treatment of acute pulmonary edema

Therapeutic goal	Therapy	Principle	Precaution
Improve gaseous exchange	Morphine sulfate, 8-15 mg IV	Morphine decreases anxiety, reduces venous return, and decreases musculoskeletal and respiratory activity	Monitor vital signs; hypoxic depression of respiratory system seriously aggravated by morphine; morphine antagonist nalorphine (Nalline) and respiratory stimulants should be available
	Intermittent positive pressure breathing (IPPB) apparatus delivering 100% O_2 via well-fitted nonrebreathing face mask, using airway pressure of 4-9 cm H_2O	IPPB decreases alveolar fluid, reduces ventilatory rate, increases arterial oxygen, facilitates uniformity of ventilation in all lung segments	Oxygen always administered with humidification to avoid airway drying and inspissation of bronchial secretions; antifoaming agents (20%-50% alcohol) may be used; remember that face mask is frightening to "suffocating" patient
	Aminophylline, IV at rate of about 20 mg/min, to total dose of 240-280 mg*	Aminophylline dilates bronchioles; also increases cardiac output, lowers venous pressure by relaxing smooth muscles of blood vessels	This drug injected slowly IV; otherwise headache, palpitation, dizziness, nausea, and fall in blood pressure occur; sedation required to relax anxious patient; cardiac arrhythmias may also occur
	Arterial line inserted for arterial blood gas determination	Normal blood gas values: pH: 7.38-7.42; Po_2: 90-100 mm Hg; Pco_2: 35-45 mm Hg; %O_2 saturation: 95%-100%	Keep arterial line open with heparin flush
Decrease intravascular volume	Diuretic therapy selecting one of the following: Furosemide (Lasix), 40-120 mg IV Ethacrynic acid (Edecrin), 50 mg IV	These rapidly acting diuretics given IV begin work within minutes; decrease in intravascular volume improves ability of lungs to exchange gases and decreases cardiac work	Monitor blood pressure and intake and output; given in excessive amounts these diuretics can lead to a profound diuresis with volume and electrolyte depletion; local infiltration of ethacrynic acid

*Aminophylline in suppository form has been used effectively for this stage of pulmonary edema and may be safer than IV administration.

†Rotating tourniquets are generally used only if other measures are unavailable or when all of the measures above have been tried without success.

Table 7-1. Treatment of acute pulmonary edema—cont'd

Therapeutic goal	Therapy	Principle	Precaution
	Phlebotomy of 300-500 ml	See preceding	If pulmonary edema has already precipitated circulatory collapse, phlebotomy will aggravate shock
Improve cardiac performance	All of the preceding	See preceding	See preceding
	Digitalis, IV administration of rapidly acting preparation (Appendix A)	Increase force of contraction and efficiency of heart	Monitor for arrhythmias; in presence of hypoxia in an acutely dilated heart, digitalis-induced arrhythmias likely to occur
Decrease venous return	Sitting (Fowler's) position	Sitting up increases lung volume and vital capacity, decreases venous return and work of breathing	In presence of hypotension, Fowler's position avoided or used cautiously
	IPPB	IPPB effectively reduces venous return by replacing normal negative intrathoracic pressure of spontaneous inspiration with positive pressure, varied as needed and impeding venous flow; reduces work of breathing to a degree	High-pressure settings avoided, since excessive reduction of peripheral venous return can cause circulatory collapse; also see preceding
	Tourniquets applied to three extremities with greater pressure than that of estimated venous pressure, but below arterial diastolic pressure; peripheral arterial pulses maintained at all times; tourniquets rotated so that each extremity is free, in sequence for 15 min†	Pooling of blood in the extremities retards venous return, reduces capillary-alveolar transudation, decreases cardiac work	Prolonged constriction of extremities causes pain and loss of function; resultant dramatic edema of extremities may be upsetting to patient; at conclusion of acute phase, tourniquets released one at a time, at 15-min intervals, to avoid flooding pulmonary circulation

opment of ST segment depression, seen most frequently in the lateral precordial leads (V_4, V_5, V_6), and less often in leads V_2, II, III, and aV_F. Frequently the ECG in a patient suffering an anginal attack also shows these changes. When the pain has subsided, the ST segments return to normal. Prinzmetal's angina, also called "atypical angina" or "variant angina," is characterized electrocardiographically by ST elevation, may occur unrelated to exertion, and is usually relieved by nitroglycerin. In most instances, transient coronary artery spasm is thought to play a role.

ARRHYTHMIAS

Disorders of impulse formation or abnormal conduction or both frequently signal the presence of coronary artery disease and may be caused by such factors as inadequate oxygenation, areas of scar formation, and acute infarction. The patient experiencing arrhythmias may complain of palpitations, dizziness, fatigue, or syncope.

SUDDEN DEATH

In this text sudden death is defined as unexpected death occurring within 1 hour of the onset of symptoms. In patients without apparent preexisting disease, sudden death is usually ascribed to ventricular fibrillation. Most sudden deaths occur before the patient reaches the hospital, and most patients who are resuscitated do not evolve an acute myocardial infarction.

MITRAL INSUFFICIENCY

The normal competence of the mitral valve depends on a structurally and functionally intact mitral valve apparatus. The components of this apparatus include the posterior left atrial wall, tne annulus, the leaflets, the chordae tendineae, and the papillary muscles and their base of support within the left ventricular wall. The most common cause of mitral insufficiency is probably coronary artery disease. Ischemic injury to the papillary muscle and its base of support or frank rupture of a papillary muscle or its chordae also may lead to mitral insufficiency. Murmurs caused by mitral insufficiency may develop during an angina attack or may be a stable consequence of the fibrotic changes that follow an old infarction. Mitral insufficiency may develop acutely in the setting of myocardial infarction and may contribute to or cause acute left-sided heart failure and pulmonary edema.

VENTRICULAR ANEURYSM

After transmural myocardial infarction the hydraulic stress on the necrotic portion of the ventricular wall may cause it to bulge during systole and to become extremely thin as the necrotic material is absorbed. If this occurs before a substantial scar has formed, the resulting scar may develop as an outward balloon or a bulge that communicates with the ventricular chamber through a narrow channel or "neck." If ventricular aneurysms develop, they usually do so during the early weeks that follow acute infarction. Their hemodynamic consequence can be related to their size, to the amount of residual normal muscle, and to their location, which sometimes involves the papillary muscles. For reasons that are not completely apparent, patients who have ventricular aneurysms are particularly prone to recurrent ventricular arrhythmias. Once a scar has developed, aneurysms seldom rupture. Hence they are detected either by x-ray examination, radionuclide studies, typical ECG changes, or during angiography.

VENTRICULAR RUPTURE

Just as hydraulic stress on necrotic myocardium may lead to aneurysm, it also may produce myocardial rupture.[2] When rupture of the heart occurs, it usually develops within 10 days after the onset of symptoms of infarction. The ventricle may rupture to the outside, producing acute cardiac tamponade, or, more often, the septum may rupture through necrotic muscle near its apical end. This rupture is called a *ventricular septal defect*. A holosystolic murmur at the apex and left sternal border that occurs in a patient who has acute myocardial infarction should always raise in the physician's mind the possibility that septal rupture exists. Heart failure usually develops or is worsened concurrently by this event. The diagnosis can be established by relatively simple, even bedside, catheter techniques. With the use of a balloon-tipped pulmonary artery catheter, blood samples from the superior vena cava, right atrium, right ventricle, and pulmonary artery are obtained. Normally the oxygen saturations of the blood samples are similar. However, a ventricular septal defect results in the flow of oxygenated blood from the left ventricle to the right ventricle. This flow increases the oxygen saturation in the right ventricle significantly, indicating the defect in the ventricular septal wall. Treatment consists of hemodynamic stabilization with drug therapy and intraaortic balloon counterpulsation and surgery to repair the ruptured septum.

Angina pectoris

The diagnosis of angina pectoris may be made from the characteristic history, since there are usually few abnormalities found on physical examination and the ECG may be normal at rest. It is important, then, to allow the patient to describe what he is feeling without influencing him by suggesting terms. Time and patience are necessary to explore all aspects of the patient's life-style, habits, and emotions, to obtain a clear picture of his chest discomfort.

Although the term *angina pectoris* is literally interpreted as "chest pain," it should perhaps be referred to as a discomfort, since some patients may deny chest "pain." They often refer to vague "sensations," "feelings," or "aches." This unpleasant feeling has been variously described as a sense of pressure, burning, squeezing, heaviness, smothering, and very frequently, as indigestion. Since the discomfort of angina is usually located in the retrosternal region, patients often illustrate the nature and location of their symptoms by placing a clenched fist against their sternum. Frequently the ache of angina pectoris is not confined to the chest but radiates to the neck, jaw, epigastrium, both shoulders, or arms. Most often it radiates to the left shoulder and left arm. Occasionally, angina pectoris may produce discomfort in an area of radiation without affecting the retrosternal region.

An elevation of blood pressure, heart rate, or both typically precedes attacks of angina. During the attack, pulse rate and blood pressure usually increase even further, presumably as a consequence of anxiety and as a physiologic response to pain. In some instances, however, blood pressure and pulse may fall dramatically because of vagally mediated reflexes analogous to vasopressor syncope or a faint. The patient may remain motionless; some patients experience a feeling of impending doom. The clenched fist over the sternum may graphically depict the constricting nature of the discomfort. Of more importance than the location is the duration of the pain and the circumstances under which it occurs. Angina pectoris usually lasts only a few minutes if the precipitating factor is relieved. Frequently attacks are induced by effort and tend to occur during rather than after the exertion. Exertion during cold weather or following meals is particularly likely to produce pain. Disturbing thoughts, smoking, stressful situations, worry, anger, hurry, and excitement are common precipitating factors. Patients have referred to the following situations as producing chest pain: running to catch a bus, driving in heavy traffic, nightmares, painful stimuli, sexual intercourse, and straining at stool.

Angina typically lasts from one to several minutes and usually no more than 3 to 5 minutes. It is relieved by rest, by nitroglycerin, or by any influence that reduces arterial pressure or heart rate and equalizes the supply of blood and nutrients with the demands.

Various types of anginal pain occur. During "walk-through" angina the patient is able to continue his activity until the pain gradually disappears. Angina decubitus is characterized by chest pain occurring at rest in the supine position. Nocturnal angina may awaken a patient from sleep (usually through dreams) with the same sensation he experiences during exertion.

Prinzmetal[3] (or "variant") angina produces symptoms similar to those of angina pectoris but is believed to be caused by coronary artery spasm. This chest pain frequently occurs at rest and can be difficult to induce by exercise testing. It is cyclical, frequently happening at the same time each day. ECG tracings show marked ST segment elevation that usually returns to baseline after relief of the pain (see Chapter 8). If the spasm is severe enough, however, the patient may subsequently suffer a myocardial infarction. To document the presence of variant angina, ergonovine maleate[4] can be injected into the coronary artery during cardiac catheterization to induce coronary artery spasm. Atherosclerotic lesions may or may not appear in the same vessel that exhibits spasm. Treatment for spasm[56] consists of rest, nitroglycerin, and longer acting nitrates. Recently calcium-blocking agents such as nifedipine, verapamil, and diltiazem have been found very effective.[38]

MEDICAL MANAGEMENT

The first principle in the medical management of angina pectoris is to reduce the discrepancy between the demand of the heart muscle for oxygen and the ability of the coronary circulation to meet this demand. Accordingly, the patient must learn to pace himself so that physical activity is kept below the threshold of discomfort. Moderate exercise performed below the angina threshold should be encouraged. Additional general measures include a diet designed to achieve the individual's ideal weight and cessation of smoking. Hypertension, if present, should be treated.

Pharmacologic treatment of angina has two objectives: first, relief of symptoms when they occur and second, prevention of angina. For the first objective, nitroglycerin taken sublingually is the preferred treatment. For prevention, beta-adrenergic blocking agents such as propranolol (Inderal), metoprolol tartrate (Lopressor), and nadolol (Corgard) are prescribed to slow the heart rate and attenuate the contractile response of the heart to physical or emotional activity. Long-acting nitrates such as isosorbide dinitrate (Isordil) and nitrol paste exert an action for 2 to 4 hours and are very effective. Recent reports[9] indicate that other vasodilators that act principally on the arterial system (for example, hydralazine or prazosin) may attenuate the hypertensive response to exertion and aid in preventing angina. Calcium-blocking agents[9-11] are another group of potent vasodilators for coronary and peripheral arteries. In addition, these drugs have an ability to decrease heart rate, afterload, and myocardial contractility. Thus coronary blood flow is enhanced.

Other general measures useful in treating angina include sedation, relief of anxiety, and supervised exercise programs designed to improve physical condition and thereby reduce the blood pressure and heart rate response to exercise.

Besides these more conventional methods of treatment, transluminal coronary angioplasty has recently been developed.[12] This procedure involves threading a balloon-tipped catheter into the coronary arteries, positioning it at the point of the atherosclerotic lesion, and inflating the balloon to compress the lesion into the arterial walls. The prime candidates for this procedure are patients who have recent onset of angina and who are candidates for coronary artery bypass surgery. The obstructive lesions must be located in the proximal portion of the artery; most attempts to date have been performed in patients who have single-vessel disease. Complications associated with this procedure are infrequent, but include artery occlusion, myocardial infarction, coronary artery dissection, and hematoma.

SURGICAL TREATMENT

In the past 10 years coronary artery surgery has become accepted as an effective treatment for angina pectoris caused by severe obstructive coronary artery disease. The saphenous vein or internal mammary artery is used as a graft to bypass the occlusion in one or more of the coronary arteries; thus dramatic relief from anginal pain is achieved in 80% to 90% of patients in the first year after surgery.[13,14] Bypass grafting is surgically feasible because of the pattern of disease in the coronary arteries. In most patients the occlusion principally involves the proximal one third to one half of the artery. Distal vessels are usually patent, thus allowing anastomosis. The bypass graft is illustrated in Fig. 7-1.

Coronary arteriograms verify the severity of the atherosclerotic occlusion in one or more arteries. A typical indication for surgery is a 75% or greater narrowing of the luminal diameter in one or more coronary arteries, coupled with the failure of aggressive medical treatment to successfully and consistently control the disabling pain. Usually operative risk is low, especially with new improvements in surgical techniques such as the use of cold potassium cardioplegia.[15] This solution, together with myocardial hypothermia during bypass surgery, provides metabolic protection for the ischemic heart, thus reducing operative risk. However, operative risk of death is increased if impaired cardiac contractility, cardiac

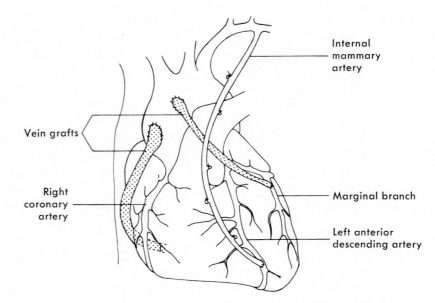

Fig. 7-1. Internal mammary artery attached as end-to-end anastomosis to anterior descending artery; vein grafts to distal right coronary and marginal branch of circumflex coronary arteries. (Adapted from Kirklin, J.W., editor: Advances in cardiovascular surgery, New York, 1973, Grune & Stratton, Inc., by permission.)

enlargement of heart failure exists. Another relative contraindication is occlusion of both the proximal and distal portions of the affected coronary artery. Significant distal disease greatly reduces the chances for long-term patency of the graft.

Since bypass grafting has been used aggressively for only 10 years, the efficacy of surgical treatment versus medical therapy for coronary artery disease remains controversial. The evidence to date indicates that after surgery most patients experience relief of symptoms. Two subsets of patients demonstrated an improvement in survival: patients who had stenosis of the left main coronary artery and patients who had lesions in three vessels.[16-18]

Acute myocardial infarction

Chest pain is the presenting symptom in a majority of patients with acute myocardial infarction. The pain is frequently severe, but there may be minimal discomfort and on occasion none. The pain is usually substernal in location and like angina may radiate to the epigastric region, jaw, shoulders, elbows, or forearms. The pain is usually described as a heaviness, tightness, or constriction but occasionally as indigestion or a burning sensation. It usually persists for 30 minutes or longer and often lasts until potent analgesics have been administered. In its classic presentation the symptoms of myocardial infarction differ in severity and duration from those of typical angina. On the other hand, the symptoms of myocardial infarction may be subtle, and very often severity and duration of pain do not help to distinguish prolonged angina from myocardial infarction.

In addition to chest pain, patients who have myocardial infarction may experience shortness of breath, sweating, weakness or extreme fatigue, nausea, vomiting, and severe anxiety. In a physical examination they may show evidence of overactivity of the sympathetic nerves, including tachycardia, sweating, and hypertension. Alternatively, evidence of vagal hyperactivity may predominate with bradycardia and hypotension. Many patients appear surprisingly normal. Hypotension with tachycardia and peripheral cyanosis suggests markedly reduced cardiac output and shock. In some patients normal blood pressure is maintained, but an S_3 gallop rhythm and pulmonary rales indicate acute left ventricular failure. Murmurs related to mitral insufficiency or a ruptured septum may develop, and a pericardial friction rub may be heard. The heart sounds are usually diminished in intensity, and, particularly with anterior infarction, a paradoxical precordial systolic lift inside the apex region can be felt.

The diagnosis of myocardial infarction is initially made on the basis of the patient's history and ECG tracings and finally by cardiac enzymes. Ancillary but nonspecific evidence of infarction includes low-grade fever, elevation of the white blood cell count, and elevation of the erythrocyte sedimentation rate. The ECG may show typical findings of infarction (see Chapter 8), or it may show nonspecific changes of the ST segment or T wave. Rarely if ever are *serial* ECGs normal in a patient with documented infarction.

With necrosis of heart muscle, enzymes that are normally confined within the cell leak out of the cell and eppear in peripheral blood; serum glutamic oxaloacetic transaminase (SGOT), lactic acid dehydrogenase (LDH), and creatine phosphokinase (CPK) are the enzymes measured most frequently. LDH and CPK appear in more forms than one, and these are referred to as isoenzymes. The isoenzymes of LDH and CPK are distributed differently in different tissues so that elevations of the "heart" isoenzymes are more specific evidence of heart muscle necrosis than elevation of the total CPK or LDH. Elevations of CPK-MB and of LDH_1 (the predominant heart isoenzymes) are typically observed in myocardial infarction.[19,20]

In the past 5 years two new imaging methods to establish the diagnosis of myocardial infarctions have received considerable attention. These methods are thallium 201 scintigraphy and technetium 99m pyrophosphate imaging.[21-24] Myocardial uptake of thallium 201 depends on blood flow; with decreased blood flow an area of diminished activity is visualized. However, one single study cannot differentiate ischemic and necrotic myocardium. This distinction is made by comparing images obtained immediately after injection of the isotope with those obtained 4 to 6 hours later to determine if the perfusion deficit is reversible or not. For optimal sensitivity the thallium 201 study should be done within 6 hours after the onset of symptoms. Thallium 201 scintigraphy in conjunction with other physical findings can be used to diagnose a myocardial infarction. In addition, this test can estimate the location and extent of decreased perfusion and necrosis.

The radionuclide imaging test using technetium 99m pyrophosphate is regarded as a sensitive technique to confirm myocardial damage. The isotope is taken up by necrotic cells within 12 to 18 hours after the onset of infarction; uptake persists for 4 or 5 days and then typically decays. Even small areas of infarction can be identified by appropriate scanning equipment from the "hot spot" produced on the scintigram. For optimal results the test should be done during the subacute phase, between 48 and 72 hours after the onset of infarction.

Thus the thallium 201 can supply diagnostic information during the acute phase while additional information from the technetium pyrophosphate is obtained during the subacute phase.

The mortality of patients with acute myocardial infarction is approximately 20% to 25%. About 50% of these deaths occur suddenly and prior to hospitalization. Mortality among patients who survive to reach the hospital is approximately 10% to 15%, and most of these deaths occur within the first 3 or 4 days. It is useful to distinguish between patients with complicated and uncomplicated acute myocardial infarction, since nearly all in-hospital deaths occur in the former group, whereas those in the latter group have an excellent prognosis and are candidates for early mobilization and discharge. These mortality figures are greatly determined by the patient's previous cardiac histories. If a patient has previously experienced a myocardial infarction or suffers from a congestive heart, cardiac reserve is reduced. Therefore another myocardial infarction continues to reduce cardiac function and is associated with a greater risk of death.

The site and extent of a myocardial infarction also influence mortality. The extent and site of the myocardial infarction indicate what changes occur in the normal anatomy and physiology. For example, a patient who has an anterior septal myocardial infarction has potentially more damage to the normal conduction pathways of the bundle branches than a patient who has an inferior myocardial infarction. Therefore the incidence of heart block and arrhythmias is greater in the patients who have the anterior wall damage.

The conditions that identify this complicated group include several factors.

1. *Persistent pain.* Pain that persists or recurs is frequently associated with unusually high enzyme elevations or secondary rises; it suggests that ischemia persists and infarction is in a process of evolution.

2. *Serious arrhythmia.* Nearly all patients with an acute infarction experience some transient alterations of rhythm. The alterations considered serious include ventricular fibrillation or ventricular tachycardia, second-degree or third-degree heart block, and atrial flutter or fibrillation, which develops in the setting of the acute infarction.[25] In addition, sinus tachycardia (>100 beats/minute) that persists for more than 24 to 48 hours in the absence of fever should alert those caring for the patient to heart failure.

3. *Pulmonary edema.* Pulmonary edema produces a sense of breathlessness, moist rales on examination, and typical changes on chest x-ray examination. It is nearly always accompanied by a significant rise in pulmonary artery and wedge pressure and indicates acute left ventricular failure.

4. *Persistent hypotension.* The arterial systolic blood pressure may drop below 90 mm Hg without accompanying signs of shock. Often this is an early and transient finding associated with bradycardia and other signs of vagal overactivity. Alternatively it may reflect an inadequate blood volume. When hypotension persists despite an adequate heart rate and left ventricular filling pressure, it usually signifies a markedly reduced cardiac output.

In a recent report patients with acute myocardial infarction were classified as complicated or uncomplicated on the basis of the presence or absence of complications during the first 4 days of hospitalization. Among the group of over 500 patients who were not free from complications through the fourth day, most patients either died subsequently in the hospital or suffered a serious late complication. Uncomplicated patients during the first 4 days appear to be candidates for early mobilization and early discharge. This possibility was tested by McNeer and co-workers. Among uncomplicated patients discharged on the seventh hospital day there were no serious complications or deaths at home during early follow-up.[26]

Patients who have acute myocardial infarction can be further categorized as those having nontransmural or transmural infarcts. In the past, nontransmural infarcts were classified as uncomplicated. Recent evidence suggests that patients who have nontransmural infarctions are at high risk for developing complications and sudden death after discharge from the hospital. The medical management of patients who have nontransmural infarctions is currently being reassessed.[27]

Methods of predicting which patients will experience complications prior to discharge are also utilized to predict further complications after discharge. Evidence indicates that patients with ST segment abnormalities, angina pectoris, or abnormal blood pressure responses during exercise testing are at higher risk of developing cardiac complications.[28,29]

MEDICAL MANAGEMENT

Pain, anxiety, and alterations of rhythm dominate the clinical picture in the early stages of acute myocardial infarction. After a route for intravenous therapy and ECG monitoring has been established, morphine should be given in doses of 2 to 3 mg intravenously; it eliminates or greatly reduces chest pain and relieves anxiety. Excessive bradycardia with a heart rate below 50 to 55 beats/minute (particularly if accompanied by hypotension and ectopic beats) should be treated with atropine, 0.4 to 1.0 mg intravenously.

The greatest threat to life in the early hours after myocardial infarction is ventricular fibrillation. In many patients episodes of fibrillation are preceded by ventricular premature beats. The high prevalence of premature beats and the fact that fibrillation is often not heralded by these changes have led in recent years to the use of prophylactic antiarrhythmic therapy. Lidocaine is given in an initial bolus (75 to 100 mg) followed by a rapid infusion of 150 mg over a period of 18 minutes and then by a continuous intravenous infusion at 2 to 3 mg/minute.[30] Conclusive studies[31] are currently available that indicate prophylactic lidocaine use is safe, and that the incidence of primary ventricular fibrillation is greatly reduced in patients treated prophylactically.

Oxygen is administered to all patients, since a decrease in arterial Po_2 caused by ventilation perfusion inequalities is common. Many physicians also advocate routine low-dose subcutaneous heparin administration during the initial stages of hospitalization to reduce the possibility of thromboembolic complications.[32-34] Once the patient ambulates, anticoagulation therapy is typically discontinued. However, the use of anticoagulant therapy for patients who have myocardial infarctions remains somewhat controversial; some physicians opt for full anticoagulation for 6 months after a myocardial infarction.

In patients who have persistent or recurrent chest pain despite therapy, efforts are made to balance the oxygen supply and demand and hence to diminish

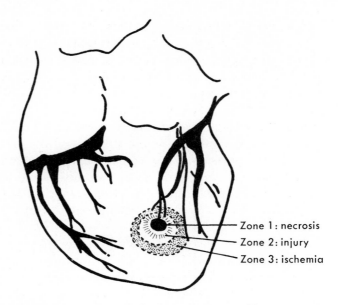

Zone 1: necrosis
Zone 2: injury
Zone 3: ischemia

Fig. 7-2. Tissue damage after myocardial infarction. *Zone 1*, Necrotic tissue; *zone 2*, injured tissue; *zone 3*, ischemic tissue.

ischemia. For example, if sinus tachycardia persists and signs of left ventricular failure are absent, propranolol in dosages of 0.05 to 0.10 mg/kg can be given to reduce heart rate. However, the hemodynamic response needs to be monitored closely.[35] In controlled studies this treatment has been shown to eliminate pain and reduce ST segment elevation. Other patients with persistent or recurrent pain have elevated arterial blood pressure. In these patients reducing blood pressure with propranolol or nitroprusside has a favorable effect. Finally, in patients with left ventricular failure and elevated pulmonary artery and wedge pressures, vasodilators such as nitroprusside or IV nitroglycerin reduce left ventricular end-diastolic pressure and often reduce pain and ST segment elevation.

Myocardial infarction is a dynamic process in which the ultimate fate of ischemic but still viable heart muscle is not determined until several hours or perhaps days after the onset of symptoms. Acute and late complications of infarction are determined at least in part by the ultimate size of the infarction. These considerations and the recognition that the balance between oxygen supply and demand can be altered have led to considerable efforts recently to protect ischemic muscle and to reduce infarct size (Fig. 7-2). These efforts have been hampered by the lack of a reliable and quantifiable index of the volume of ischemic muscle in patients; but despite this inability to quantitate ischemic muscle, favorable clinical results indicate directionally appropriate changes in the indexes of muscle death. Even a reduction in anticipated mortality has been reported with therapy directed toward reducing infarct size. Most of the interest in this area has focused on the use of hyaluronidase or solutions containing glucose-insulin-potassium, and propranolol or vasodilators.[36-39]

Under investigation is a technique to restore coronary blood flow to areas of myocardium that may be evolving from ischemia to infarction; it involves the use of thrombolytic agents such as streptokinase.[40-43] Some autopsy studies of patients with acute myocardial infarction have demonstrated a high prevalence of coronary artery thrombi within the infarct-related vessel.[44,45] Whether coronary thrombus is implicated as a primary event in the pathogenesis of myocardial infarction or results from stasis of coronary flow, lysis of thrombi with its ensuing restoration of coronary blood flow to ischemic myocardium is a logical means of reducing ischemic damage in an evolving myocardial infarction. Previous clinical trials employing the systemic administration of thrombolytic agents such as streptokinase and urokinase have produced conflicting results with few studies demonstrating a reduction in morbidity and mortality.[46-49]

A resurgence of interest in thrombolytic therapy has followed several recent reports of studies employing coronary angiography and direct intracoronary infusion of thrombolytic agents in patients who have an acute myocardial infarction.[41-43] This technique offers several advantages over systemic administration of thrombolytic agents. First, since coronary angiography is performed early in the course of infarction, the spectrum of coronary artery lesions responsible for acute myocardial infarction is now being accurately defined. Second, since thrombolytic agents are directly infused into the infarct-related coronary artery, the dosage can be greatly reduced, thus preventing the hemorrhagic complications frequently seen in systemic trials of thrombolytic agents. Intracoronary thrombolytic therapy in patients with acute myocardial infarction is typically performed as follows.

Cardiac catheterization and coronary angiography are performed within 4 to 6 hours after the onset of chest pain and following stabilization of the patient. Beyond 6 hours, necrosis from coronary artery occlusion is usually complete. A thrombus within a coronary artery typically appears as a total, abrupt occlusion of the coronary artery with little or no perfusion of the distal coronary artery. A catheter is threaded through the coronary artery to the site of the occlusion. The catheter is positioned within the artery. In some instances a guide wire is passed beyond the occlusion in the artery. Then thrombolytic agents, such as streptokinase or urokinase, are infused directly into the occluded coronary artery and continued until reperfusion of the distal vessel is achieved. Thrombi appear to be present in approximately 60% to 80% of totally occluded infarct-related coronary arteries. In the remainder of patients with acute myocardial infarction, myocardial necrosis appears to result from low coronary blood flow secondary to a high-grade atherosclerotic plaque, without evidence of total occlusion. Most studies have noted, following the lysis of an intracoronary thrombus, an atherosclerotic plaque at the site of previous total occlusion.[40-43] To prevent clot reformation, patients are anticoagulated with continuous intravenous heparin and warfarin for 3 to 6 months. Thus it is possible that in a high percentage of patients with acute myocardial infarction, ulceration or hemorrhage of an atherosclerotic plaque leads to platelet aggregation and formation of a thrombus within a coronary artery. Since many patients have coronary thrombi in the presence of atherosclerotic plaques, transluminal angioplasty may be an excellent adjunct to thrombolysis. However, this combination requires extensive clinical investigation.

A major problem in evaluating an intervention such as intracoronary thrombolytic therapy is how to measure its therapeutic impact in the patient with acute myocardial infarction. Previous techniques designed to measure infarct size, such as serial measurements of serum creatine kinase or ST segment elevation, have several practical and theoretical limitations. If restoration of coronary blood flow in evolving acute myocardial infarction saves potentially viable myocardium, left ventricular performance should be preserved or improved; this contrasts with patients in whom ischemic myocardium degenerates to complete necrosis. Thus changes in left ventricular performance following intracoronary thrombolytic therapy may provide a meaningful index of the functional impact of this intervention. Clinical studies of intracoronary thrombolytic therapy have demonstrated improved left ventricular performance in patients exhibiting coronary artery reperfusion compared with patients without coronary artery reperfusion.[50,51]

A pericardial rub is heard in about 25% of patients with transmural infarction, usually on the third to fifth day. Within 1 to 4 weeks after infarction, pericarditis with effusion and fever develops in about 2% to 5% of patients. This is referred to as Dressler's syndrome and is thought to result from an autoimmune response. Pericarditis, early or late, is generally treated symptomatically. Use of aspirin, indomethacin, or even steroids may be required; anticoagulation should be discontinued unless there is an overriding reason to continue its use, such as an overt pulmonary embolus.

Prolongation of the PR interval and Wenckebach cycles is common in patients who have posterior and inferior infarctions. The AV block usually regresses or can be treated with atropine. Third-degree AV block or conditions associated with a high incidence of progression to complete block, i.e., Mobitz type II second-degree block or new bifascicular bundle branch block, both of which are especially associated with PR prolongation, are regarded as indications for insertion of a temporary transvenous pacemaker. Use of the pacemaker is then determined primarily by the ventricular rate and the patient's hemodynamic response.

Heart failure

Heart failure may be defined as a state in which the cardiac output is insufficient to meet the metabolic needs of the body. This state can occur when the cardiac output is normal, increased, or decreased. However, in most cases patients with heart failure have a decreased cardiac output. Congestive failure indicates circulatory congestion resulting from heart failure and is manifested by retention of fluid and the formation of edema.[51] Low-output failure occurs when the heart as a pump is unable to supply the tissues with adequate perfusion. The basis for the inadequate perfusion lies in the inability of the failing heart to meet normal tissue demands. A number of cardiac disorders can result in low-output failure. For example, a myocardial infarction affecting a large area of the left ventricle, cardiomyopathy, or stenosis or insufficiency of the cardiac valves can impair the heart's ability to pump. Constrictive pericarditis or pericardial effusion can restrict the ability of the heart to fill and empty. Finally, heart block, because of the excessively slow ventricular rate, may lead to heart failure.

Less commonly, heart failure occurs when peripheral demands exceed the capacity of even a normal heart to adequately perfuse the tissues. This is called high-output failure and can occur in severe anemia, thyrotoxicosis, and in patients who have arteriovenous fistulas.

The basic defect in heart failure is a decrease in the pumping capacity of the heart. Patients who have early or mild heart disease may show no significant abnormalities when they are at rest, since the reserve in cardiac function provides compensation. Despite a normal cardiac output in these patients at rest, their cardiac output with exercise is subnormal, and they demonstrate decreased tolerance for exercise.

PATHOPHYSIOLOGY OF HEART FAILURE

As the heart begins to fail, many compensatory mechanisms are activated to maintain cardiac output at a level that is adequate to meet the metabolic needs of the body. Most of these adaptations employ the same mechanisms as those utilized by normal persons during exercise or during periods of increased stress. The principal initial adjustments are a reflex increase in sympathetic nerve discharge and a decrease in parasympathetic activity. These autonomic alterations, affecting the heart, arteries, and veins, maintain arterial pressure despite a possible decrease in stroke volume. Venous tone increases, which in turn increases venous pressure and helps to maintain venous return. The resulting increase in end-diastolic volume helps to maintain stroke volume. Normally some blood remains in the ventricles after contraction. The volume of blood ejected during each ventricular contraction is the difference between the volume of blood contained in the ventricle at the end of diastole (end-diastolic volume) and the volume remaining at the end of systole (end-systolic volume). The fraction ejected (ejection fraction) equals the end-diastolic volume minus the end-systolic volume, divided by the end-diastolic volume; it is an important measurement of cardiac performance. An increase in end-diastolic volume helps maintain stroke volume because cardiac muscle increases its strength of contraction when it is stretched. Starling's law of the heart states that a direct proportion exists between the diastolic volume of the heart—that is, the length of cardiac muscle fibers during diastole—and the force of contraction of the following systole. Increased fiber length immediately prior to contraction increases the strength of that contraction. Consequently, the distended heart *(within certain limits)* contracts forcefully enough to maintain arterial perfusion. Furthermore, the contraction is not only more powerful but occurs more frequently as well (i.e., heart rate increases).

An increase in heart rate (tachycardia) by itself may increase cardiac output when mechanisms to improve stroke volume are exhausted. Above a certain rate, however, cardiac output may actually begin to decrease. This rate is about 170 to 180 beats/minute for most normal young individuals. In trained athletes the rate may be 200 to 220, whereas in patients with myocardial disease the rate limit may be 120 to 140. This decrease in cardiac output above a certain heart rate is due to shortening of diastole, which limits the time for adequate filling of the ventricles and for coronary blood flow. Slow heart rates allow more complete diastolic filling. When the rates decrease below 40 to 50 beats/minute, however, no further increase of stroke volume occurs, and cardiac output drops.

When cardiac output falls, from whatever cause, the kidneys retain salt and water as an early compensatory mechanism. This is due in part to sympathetic stimulation, which produces renal vasoconstriction and reduces renal blood flow. Sympathetically mediated activation of the renin-angiotensin system triggers al-

Table 7-2. Edema formation

Organ	Edema	Description
Skin	Dependent edema, pitting type	Increased venous pressure forces fluid through capillary walls into subcutaneous tissues; in ambulatory patients edema localized in dependent parts of body (hands and feet); patients in bed may lose edema of legs and feet, have it only in presacral region
Liver	Hepatomegaly	Increased pressure in hepatic veins causes accumulation of fluid in liver, which becomes enlarged and tender
Pleural cavity	Pleural effusion; hydrothorax	Venous congestion forces fluid into pleural cavity
Pericardial cavity	Pericardial effusion	Fluid accumulation in pericardial cavity

dosterone release and further promotes sodium retention. Expansion of the intravascular blood volume brings about increases in the end-diastolic volume and pressure that, when elevated, result in transudation of fluid from the vascular bed to edema formation (Table 7-2).

A major long-term hemodynamic adjustment to heart failure is ventricular hypertrophy. This is presumably caused by a chronic increase in the systolic force or tension developed by the myocardium. The hypertrophied myocardium may maintain compensation because the total mass of myocardium is increased. If the pumping capacity of the ventricle is restored by hypertrophy, tachycardia and edema may no longer be present.

LEFT-SIDED HEART FAILURE

The heart is really comprised of two pumps in series, the right ventricle and the left ventricle. Certain events may alter the function of one of these pumps without significantly impairing function of the other at first. In acute myocardial infarction, for example, the primary insult is usually to the performance of the left ventricle. When the ability of the left ventricle to pump blood is compromised without compromising the right ventricle, a temporary imbalance in the output between the two sides of the heart results. The right side of the heart continues to pump blood into the lungs. At the same time the left side of the heart is unable to pump the blood adequately into the systemic circulation. This results in an accumulation of blood in the lungs and increases the pressures in all the pulmonary vessels. Consequently, one of the cardinal symptoms associatd with acute left ventricular failure is dyspnea. If dyspnea occurs when the patient is recumbent, it is called orthopnea and is usually relieved by the patient sitting up. When the patient is lying down, there is decreased vital capacity because the volume of blood in the pulmonary vessels is increased in the recumbent patient.

Paroxysmal nocturnal dyspnea is an almost specific sign of left ventricular failure. The patient awakens suddenly at night, extremely breathless, and seeks relief by sitting up or running to an open window for fresh air. The mechanism for this type of dyspnea is uncertain, but it represents a form of acute pulmonary edema. When the patient goes to sleep the metabolic needs of the body may decrease. As a result the cardiac output, which had previously been inadequate, may be adequate to supply the body needs. Fluid that had been pocketed away may be mobilized into the vascular system, thus increasing the blood volume. This action in turn may increase the hydrostatic pressure in the lungs and lead to nocturnal pulmonary congestion. The second and more plausible mechanism is redistribution of fluids to the lungs in a recumbent patient.

As the heart's compensatory mechanisms fail, the already elevated diastolic filling pressure continues to increase; stroke volume does not, so left atrial pressure necessarily increases. To maintain flow, the pressure in the pulmonary veins and capillaries exceeds the intravascular oncotic pressure (approximately 30 mm Hg), and fluid rapidly leaks into the interstitial regions of the lung tissue. Pulmonary edema greatly reduces the amount of lung tissue available to exchange gases and consequently results in a dramatic clinical presentation characterized by extreme dyspnea, cyanosis, and severe anxiety. This is called acute pulmonary edema.

In the early stages of pulmonary edema the patient appears anxious, restless, or vaguely uneasy. Wheezing, orthopnea, and pallor appear as left-sided heart failure progresses. A third heart sound (S_3) may be heard as the distensibility of the ventricle decreases. Tachycardia and increased systemic arterial pressure are common during the attempt of neural reflexes to correct the imbalance. If these physiologic compensations fail, hypotension occurs, respirations become bubbling (rales), and copious, blood-tinged, frothy sputum is expectorated. As pulmonary interstitial and intraalveolar fluids accumulate, arterial hypoxemia and cyanosis occur in varying degrees. This deterioration in pulmonary function is reflected in the patient's mental status. Anxiety progresses to mental confusion and eventually to stupor and coma. The patient is literally drowning in his own secretions. The situation is critical and demands immediate emergency action.

RIGHT-SIDED HEART FAILURE

Usually right-sided heart failure follows left-sided heart failure. Right-sided heart failure without left-sided heart failure may be caused by pulmonary hypertension (secondary to lung disease) or recurrent pulmonary emboli and is referred to as *cor pulmonale*. Pressure increases in the pulmonary vasculature during right-sided heart failure and prompts a rise of pressure in the right side of the heart. This impedes venous return, and, consequently, organs become congested. This is manifested in two ways: (1) distention of the neck veins and (2) development of body edema (Table 7-2). When the accumulation of fluid becomes extensive and generalized, with edema of the tissues throughout the body, the patient is said to have *anasarca*.

TREATMENT OF HEART FAILURE

Treatment of patients with heart failure requires an understanding of the condition(s) that led to this clinical state and of the mechanisms that produce heart failure and congestion regardless of the primary cardiac problem.

When heart failure results from certain specific mechanical problems—such as aortic or mitral valve stenosis or insufficiency, persistent uncontrolled arrhythmias, severe anemia, hypertension, or a congenital cardiac lesion—therapy is directed at correcting the cause. It is important to recognize that, regardless of cause, infections, arrhythmias, anemia, thryotoxicosis, and pregnancy may all place an added burden onto the heart sufficient to precipitate heart failure. Thus appropriate treatment of these conditions may convert a patient with heart disease from a decompensated to a compensated state.

We have previously defined heart failure as a condition in which the cardiac output is not sufficient to meet the metabolic demands of the body. Essentially all of the situations that aggravate heart failure do so by placing metabolic demands on a heart that is not capable of responding with an adequate output. A favorable response in patients with heart failure often can be observed with rest. Indeed, bed rest is the first principle of treating heart failure, since it reduces metabolic demands of the body. Defining the level of physical activity that a patient can tolerate without precipitating failure is a major objective of subsequent follow-up and treatment.

In addition to prescribing rest and defining the level of physical activity a patient can tolerate, therapy is directed at improving cardiac performance and cardiac output. Obviously, if tight aortic stenosis or another structural defect is present, surgery is indicated. On the other hand, digitalis, which increases the contractility of heart muscle, has a favorable effect on cardiac performance and output. It is used routinely in most instances of heart failure, with beneficial results. In acute myocardial infarction, particularly in the early phases, the evidence of benefit from digitalis is minimal, and because of an increased sensitivity to toxic manifestations of digitalis excess, its use in this situation is still controversial. In patients with severely decompensated congestive hearts, the renin-angiotensin system is activated, resulting in the maintenance of elevated systemic vascular resistance. A drug that inhibits the angiotensin-converting enzyme, captopril, reduces afterload and results in the clinical improvement of congestive heart failure.[52,53] Vasodilator agents are a recent and important addition to the treatment of heart failure. This class of agents includes IV nitroglycerin, nitroprusside, hydralazine, minoxidil, and prazosin.[54-59] Some of these agents may be given intravenously and some orally. Some act predominantly on the arterial system, and others exert significant actions on veins as well. The use of these agents is aimed at reducing arterial resistance, which is accompanied by an increase in cardiac output, a reduction in left atrial and pulmonary venous pressure, and a decrease in left ventricular end-diastolic volume and pressure. These agents have proved very useful in the treatment of heart failure that is caused by a variety of disorders such as myocardial infarction, mitral insufficiency, or cardiomyopathy. The benefits of vasodilator therapy are greatest when left atrial and pulmonary artery pressures are elevated. Vasodilators are useless for and may even be detrimental to patients who have a normal or reduced left ventricular filling pressure because they decrease peripheral resistance and may result in a mild or significant drop in the arterial blood pressure. Vasodilators can be used with digitalis to produce additive effects.

In the discussion of vasdilator therapy the principles of cardiac function are important to remember. As previously discussed, Starling's law states that as cardiac output increases proportionally, within certain limits, to increases in ventricular filling pressure, there results an increase in ventricular diastolic length. Cardiac output is the product of heart rate and stroke volume (the difference between left ventricular end-diastolic volume and left ventricular end-systolic volume). At any moment, cardiac output is dependent on myocardial oxygen consumption. The determinants of this oxygen consumption include heart rate, contractility, preload, and afterload. *Preload* is the venous filling pressure, that is, the pressure exerted by the blood volume and venous return to the heart. *Afterload* is the resistance the heart pumps against, that is, arterial blood pressure. Therefore, in patients with congestive heart failure, drugs that modulate the heart rate, contractility, preload, and afterload are used to improve cardiac function. For example, vasodilators are effective in the reduction of afterload, and diuretic therapy reduces preload. Drugs such as dopamine exert a positive inotropic effect on the heart; that is, they increase myocardial contractility.

The third aim in the treatment of patients with heart failure is directed toward achieving and maintaining an appropriate blood volume. As noted before, several compensatory mechanisms, invoked when cardiac output is insufficient, affect sodium and water balance by the kidneys. The net effects of these influences are sodium (and water) retention and a diminished ability to excrete a sodium load. A normal sodium intake of 5 to 8 g/day cannot be tolerated by patients with heart failure and should be reduced to 2 g or even less. Diuretics promote the excretion of sodium and hence water by the kidneys through one or more of several specific actions. Thiazide diruetics inhibit sodium transport primarily in the distal or cortical segment of the nephron. Loop diuretics such as ethacrynic acid and furosemide are very potent and act on both the cortical and medullary segments of the nephron. Spironolactone is a diuretic that specifically antagonizes the effect of aldosterone on the collecting duct. Triamterene has an action on sodium transport identical to that of spironolactone, but its action is not dependent on blocking aldosterone. In general, thiazides and loop diuretics also cause potassium loss, whereas spironolactone and triamterene do not. These agents vary in potency but with appropriate selection and dosage can promote a diuresis in patients with edema caused by heart failure and with chronic use can diminish the tendency of patients with heart failure to retain salt and water.

Mild to moderate heart failure in patients who have acute myocardial infarction is usually managed successfully with bed rest, morphine, careful attention to fluid balance, and the use of vasodilators and diuretics when indicated. The pulmonary artery wedge pressure is a helpful indicator of the patient's fluid balance. For example, if a patient is receiving intravenous fluid at a rate of 150 ml/hour and the wedge pressure measure exceeds 18 mm Hg, fluid overload is indicated.

Cardiogenic shock

When oxygen and other nutrients become unavailable to the cells of the body, shock may occur. Shock is a descriptive term, denoting a clinical picture that develops in the presence of inadequate tissue perfusion. It occurs in about 15% of patients hospitalized with an acute myocardial infarction. The clinical picture is characterized by a systolic blood pressure of less than 90 mm Hg or at least 30 mm Hg lower than the prior basal level, and signs of impaired tissue perfusion such as pallor, cyanosis of varying degrees, cool clammy skin, mental confusion or obtundation, and a urine output of less than 20 ml/hour. Shock may be caused by a variety of conditions unrelated to myocardial infarction such as, severe dehydration, hyperinsulinism that produces severe hypoglycemia, severe trauma, massive hemorrhage, and overwhelming infection. Before treating shock, it is essential that its cause be determined.

For the purposes of this discussion, cardiogenic shock is present when the aforementioned clinical characteristics occur in a patient with acute myocardial infarction. Patients who have hypotension related to pain or vasovagal reactions responsive to atropine are specifically excluded from the group defined as having cardiogenic shock. Although cardiac arrhythmias such as excessive tachycardia or bradycardia can cause the symptoms of shock, the following remarks are intended to describe abnormalities noted in patients in whom these rhythm disturbances either are not present or have been corrected and the symptoms of shock persist.

HEMODYNAMIC ASSESSMENT

In recent years a technique has been developed that permits bedside hemodynamic assessment of the patient without significant risk or discomfort. With the aid of fluoroscopy or a pressure recorder or both, a balloon-tipped, flow-directed catheter[60,61] is inserted into the brachial vein and directed into the right ventricle and pulmonary artery (Fig. 7-3, *A* and *B*). This catheter provides a guide for more precise management of heart failure and especially cardiogenic shock by furnishing a means to measure the pulmonary artery end-diastolic pressure (PAEDP) and pulmonary capillary wedge pressure (PCWP). Since there is a direct relationship between the PAEDP, the PCWP, and the pressure in the left ventricle immediately before systole (the left ventricular end-diastolic pressure [LVEDP],

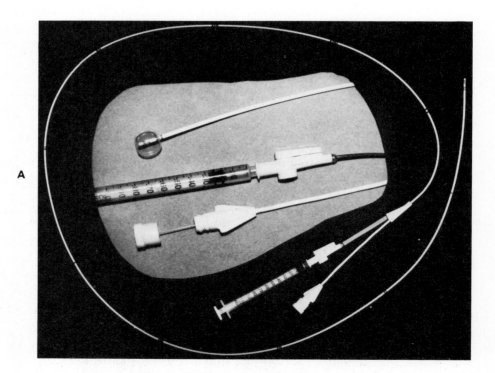

Fig. 7-3. A, The Swan-Ganz flow-directed catheter.

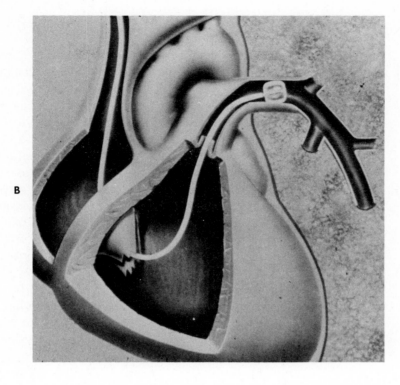

B

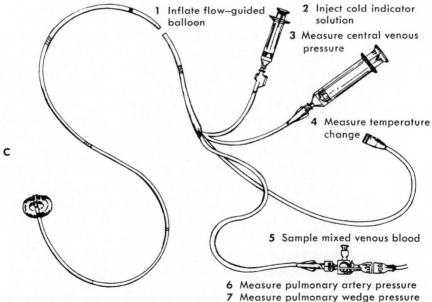

1 Inflate flow–guided balloon

2 Inject cold indicator solution

3 Measure central venous pressure

4 Measure temperature change

C

5 Sample mixed venous blood

6 Measure pulmonary artery pressure
7 Measure pulmonary wedge pressure

Fig. 7-3, cont'd. B, The Swan-Ganz flow-directed catheter with *partially inflated* balloon is passed through the superior vena cava and into the right atrium, where the balloon is then inflated to its maximum recommended capacity. Continued catheter advancement propels the balloon-tipped catheter into the right ventricle, pulmonary artery, and finally into the wedged position that is evidenced by a characteristic change in pressure waveform. **C,** The Swan-Ganz flow-directed thermodilution catheter (**A** and **C** with permission of Edwards Laboratories, Division of American Hospital Supply Corp., Santa Ana, Calif.)

an elevated PAEDP or PCWP reflects the elevated LVEDP that occurs when left ventricular contractility is impaired sufficiently to prevent normal emptying. A PAEDP or PCWP valve exceeding 12 mm Hg is considered abnormal. This balloon-tipped catheter, furthermore, may aid in establishing the cause of heart failure or shock, as well as in evaluating the effectiveness of the therapy. For example, in a state of hypotension caused by hypovolemia, infusing normal saline, whole blood, or low–molecular weight dextran elevates the systemic pressure. In this case the PAEDP and PCWP, initially low, return to normal when the blood volume has been restored. If the PAEDP is elevated because of congestive heart failure that has caused pulmonary edema, for example, effective therapy should be to reduce the pressure readings that were initially elevated.[60-62]

The use of the central venous pressure (CVP) to measure right atrial pressure (RAP) is no longer considered sufficiently accurate because the relationship between the RAP and LVEDP is inconsistent. Therefore PAEDP and PCWP, rather than CVP, should be accepted as major guides in the treatment of heart failure and shock.

As the clinical features of heart failure worsen, they may be paralleled by an elevation of the PAEDP and PCWP, a decrease in cardiac output, a decrease in arterial and right atrial oxygen tension, and a widening of the oxygen difference (in volume percent) between arterial and venous blood samples, commonly referred to as the *AV oxygen difference.*

To complement the picture of pump failure, a fall in arterial oxygen tension (a sign of abnormal lung function) occurs and is thought to result, at least in part, from elevation of left atrial pressure. The changes in pulmonary function include (1) abnormalities of diffusion, particularly of oxygen, (2) a redistribution of pulmonary blood flow into the less well-ventilated upper lobes, and (3) right-to-left shunting, that is, not all blood circulates through ventilated areas of the lungs. Not only is the arterial oxygen tension reduced in patients with acute infarction and shock, but it also fails to increase to expected values with the administration of oxygen until pulmonary congestion has cleared.[63]

When the right atrial oxygen saturation is reduced, a wider AV oxygen difference and a lower cardiac output can be suspected. If arterial oxygen saturation remains constant, reduced right atrial oxygen saturation reflects increased tissue extraction of oxygen during the passage of blood from the arterial to the venous circulation. This observation implies that the determination of right atrial oxygen saturation can be a useful index of circulatory failure in patients with acute infarction. If the AV oxygen difference is known, the product of it and the AV oxygen difference can determine systemic oxygen consumption. *Systemic oxygen consumption* indicates the amount of oxygen used by the body each minute and is an indication of the metabolic state of the patient. In addition to the bedside techniques for measuring pulmonary artery and pulmonary capillary wedge pressure and left ventricular end-diastolic pressure, the simple test of determining whether the right atrial oxygen saturation is above or below 65% is a useful guide to therapy. The use of this variable is based on the Fick equation for measuring cardiac output:

$$\text{Cardiac output} = \frac{\text{Oxygen consumption}}{\text{AV oxygen difference}}$$

A specially designed cardiac catheter with a thermistor (temperature) electrode has been used to measure cardiac output by using the principle of thermodilution. The procedure involves injecting a cold solution into the right atrium or superior vena cava. The temperature change is registered by the thermistor electrode in the pulmonary artery. Cardiac output is inversely proportional to the temperature change, that is, the greater the cardiac output the less the temperature change. The use of such a catheter facilitates measurement of the cardiac output and eliminates the need for a systemic arterial blood sample to determine cardiac output (Fig. 7-3, C).

The cardiac output varies inversely with the AV oxygen difference, since oxygen consumption under basal conditions is stable. Right atrial oxygen saturation may be reduced by (1) hypoventilation, (2) ventilation perfusion abnormalities, (3) diffusion abnormalities, or (4) intrapulmonary shunting. Hypoventilation occurs when alveolar ventilation is low in relation to the uptake of O_2 and CO_2 output; it results in hypoxia and hypercapnia. Ventilation perfusion abnormalities are seen in all generalized lung diseases (e.g., chronic bronchitis, emphysema, asthma) and result in an inequality of ventilation and blood flow. Diffusion abnormalities occur with pulmonary diseases in which there is marked thickening of the alveolar wall, such as sarcoidosis. This thickening limits the diffusion of gases. In intrapulmonary shunting, blood from the right side of the heart enters the left side of the heart without exchange with alveolar gas. Then oxygenated blood from the lungs mixes with the unoxygenated blood, resulting in a decreased oxygen content. Giving 100% oxygen will correct the effects of the first three abnormalities. (Normal cardiac chamber oxygen values are found in Fig. 7-4.)

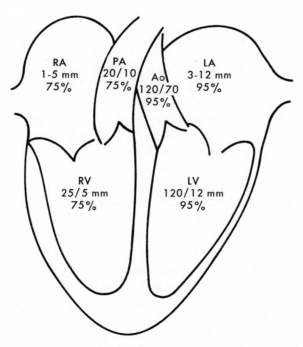

Fig. 7-4. Normal average cardiac pressures (mm Hg) and normal oxygen content (%) in each chamber.

TREATMENT OF SHOCK

The current term to describe the problem of patients who develop cardiogenic shock with or without congestive heart failure is *pump failure*. Most studies indicate a mortality of at least 80% among those visited with cardiogenic shock during the course of acute myocardial infarction; unfortunately, current therapeutic measures have not reduced this figure.

The primary therapeutic goals are to increase cardiac output and to maintain renal blood flow, but there is no clear-cut regimen for the treatment of cardiogenic shock that can be applied to all patients, since therapy depends on the specific findings in the individual patients. Therefore, for the physician to direct treatment intelligently, as much clinical and hemodynamic information as possible should be available. Therapy, as well as the natural evolution of the shock state, may change these values, so measurements should be repeated as often as necessary. Clinical management of the patient in cardiogenic shock is divided into general and specific measures as follows.

A. General therapeutic measures
   1. Have patients assume a supine position with a pillow. Trendelenburg's position is not recommended for treating cardiogenic shock.
   2. Relieve pain with just enough IV morphine to be effective (5 to 10 mg initially). Large doses of morphine sulfate should be avoided if possible. Observe for lowering of arterial pressure.
   3. Insert a Foley catheter to measure hourly urine output as an index of renal function. Maintain urine output at a minimum of 20 ml/hour to prevent renal failure.
   4. Insert an intraarterial needle or catheter to monitor arterial blood pressure, blood gases, pH, cardiac output, AV oxygen difference, and peripheral resistance.
   5. Insert a balloon-tipped, flow-directed catheter[61] to monitor PAEDP and PCWP as a reflection of left ventricular performance.

B. Specific therapeutic goals
   1. Correct arrhythmias and establish appropriate heart rate. If the heart rate is above normal but not in the abnormal tachycardia range (90 to 100 beats/minute), no special therapy is necessary. If the rate is abnormally slow, atropine administration in patients with myocardial infarction may be considered. For the symptomatic (premature ventricular complexes, hypotension, and so forth) patient who has sinus bradycardia, atropine is clearly indicated. Also isoproterenol in a continuous infusion at 2 to 4 μg/minute may be indicated to increase heart rate. However, isoproterenol may increase myocardial oxygen consumption and also may further decrease arterial blood pressure. For the asymptomatic patient with sinus bradycardia, it would appear best not to administer atropine, but to monitor closely. When atropine is indicated, the initial dose should be in the range of 0.4 to 0.6 mg IV, with another dose of 0.2 to 0.4 mg if the initial dose does not produce the desired effect. If atropine does not raise the heart rate sufficiently to eliminate the symptoms accompanying the slower rate, or if the cause of the low heart rate is complete heart block, then electrical pacing should be considered.

The other common rhythm disturbance is premature ventricular beats. Ventricular ectopic beats may be seen singularly, in a pattern (bigeminy, trigeminy), or consecutively. If the patient is symptomatic from the premature ventricular beats, prompt treatment is required, and lidocaine is indicated. As previously discussed, the patient is given a bolus of 75 to 100 mg lidocaine followed by a rapid infusion of 150 mg over a period of 18 minutes and then a continuous drip of 2 to 4 mg/minute. If the patient continues to experience premature ventricular beats, procainamide is the next antiarrhythmic of choice. Initially, the patient is given 100 mg IV over 3 to 5 minutes until 500 mg to 1 g is given. Then a continuous infusion of procainamide is added at a rate of 2 to 4 mg/minute. Bretylium tosylate is a useful drug in the treatment of ventricular tachycardia and ventricular fibrillation. It is initiated with intravenous administration of 5 mg/kg followed by a continuous infusion at a rate of 2 to 4 mg/minute or intramuscular injections of 5 mg/kg of body weight every 6 hours. An adverse effect of bretylium is severe hypotension; thus the patient's blood pressure must be monitored daily. If the patient experiences symptomatic ventricular tachycardia or ventricular fibrillation, electrical cardioversion or defibrillation is indicated to terminate the arrhythmia.

2. Correct hypovolemia. Elderly patients who have myocardial infarction are prime candidates for the development of relative hypovolemia, especially if they have been receiving diuretics or are on a low-sodium diet. The acute stages of myocardial infarction are associated with a reduced fluid intake (because of pain), analgesic therapy, nausea, and vomiting. Further routes of fluid loss are profuse sweating, diarrhea secondary to medication, vigorous treatment with diuretics, and phlebotomy. Consequently, patients showing evidence of low cardiac output syndrome with hypotension and oliguria may be given a trial of fluid loading, particularly if PAEDP and PCWP are low.

   Patients with evidence of severe pulmonary congestion are not suitable for this therapy. With low PAEDP and PCWP values, normal saline (e.g., blood products) or low–molecular weight dextran may be infused until the PCWP reaches 15 to 18 mm Hg.

   Current experience indicates that PCWP should be kept slightly elevated in patients who have cardiogenic shock.

3. Correct hypoxemia. Hypoxia with Po_2 values below 70 to 75 mm Hg in the patient who is receiving nasal oxygen indicates that additional oxygen support is necessary. If a 100% oxygen mask fails to increase the Po_2 values, intubation and positive pressure or volume and 100% oxygen are indicated.

4. Correct acidosis. When circulatory impairment exists, the metabolic activity of the perfused cells of the body changes, and lactic acid and other metabolic products are released into the vascular system and ineffectively metabolized. Consequently, systemic acidosis develops. This state is indicated by the blood pH and contributes to poor tissue perfusion. The complication is treated with intravenous sodium bicarbonate, taking precautions not to produce sodium overload.

5. Improve cardiac contractility. Use of digitalis in the management of cardiogenic shock is not well supported by existing data. Recent experimental studies show that the positive inotropic effect of digitalis preparations improves contractility but significantly increases myocardial oxygen demand.[64,65] Other agents that enhance the state of cardiac contractility have been employed in cardiogenic shock. In patients with adequate filling pressures and normal or increased peripheral resistance, dopamine hydrochloride or dobutamine can cause a significant increase in cardiac output. Dopamine has a strong inotropic effect. In a low dose (1 to 10 mg/kg/minute) dopamine increases myocardial contractility, increases heart rate, and results in mesenteric and renal vasodilatation. At higher doses dopamine causes vasoconstriction, thus increasing impedance to ventricular ejection. Also, at high doses, the patient's heart rate increases and arrhythmias may occur.

   Dobutamine is a relatively new positive inotropic agent. It increases myocardial contractility and cardiac output with minimal changes in the heart rate and blood pressure. Also, fewer arrhythmias are seen with dobutamine therapy than with dopamine. In left ventricular failure, dobutamine decreases preload and afterload, thus improving cardiac output. This drug is administered by intravenous infusion at a rate of 2.5 to 10.0 mg/kg/minute.[66-68]

6. Improve circulation. Clinical estimates of the degree of increased peripheral resistance usually present in the shock syndrome can be made by considering the degree of increased venous pressure, the amount of decrease in pulse pressure, the decrease in cutaneous blood flow with cold and cyanotic extremities, the poorly palpable peripheral pulses in spite of bounding carotid pulsations, reduced urine flow, and the clinical appearance of the patient. If these findings persist, a dangerously inappropriate prolonged period of peripheral vasoconstriction may exist. If the patient exhibits signs of the shock syndrome with a low or normal calculated peripheral resistance, an infusion of a drug with combined alpha- and beta-adrenergic properties may be considered. Norepinephrine [levarterenol (Levophed)] is used to increase arterial blood pressure and improve perfusion of ischemic areas of myocardium that are functionally depressed. The elevated pressure may open existing or latent coronary collateral channels, which require a relatively high pressure to maintain blood flow through them, and bypass concomitant areas of arterial atherosclerosis. Consequently, this drug improves myocardial function and increases cardiac output. However, at the same time, it increases cardiac afterload (resistance against which the ventricle pumps) and thus myocardial oxygen consumption. Therefore the use of this agent should be aimed at producing a balance between coronary perfusion and ventricular afterloading. Norepinephrine is used less frequently because of its vasoconstrictive effects and increased demands for myocardial oxygen. Dopamine and dobutamine are the preferred drugs.

Several groups of investigators are evaluating agents that produce vasodilatation and decrease peripheral resistance, thereby increasing cardiac output in patients who exhibit clinical signs of shock with an increased peripheral resistance. Such agents include nitroprusside and intravenous nitroglycerin. Current studies show the promise of these drugs in patients who have an increased pulmonary capillary wedge pressure and signs of left-sided heart failure. They should not be used if arterial pressure is below 90 mm Hg unless they are used in conjunction with dopamine to maintain an adequate blood pressure.

A technique currently receiving evaluation in the management of cardiogenic shock is mechanical circulatory assistance in the form of intraaortic balloon counterpulsation. The balloon is inserted percutaneously into the femoral artery and connected to a console that controls the inflation of the balloon with helium. Timing for inflation and deflation of the balloon is correlated with the ECG. The intraaortic balloon is deflated during ventricular systole and thus partially empties the aorta. The effect is to potentiate forward stroke volume, reduce developed ventricular pressure caused by reduced afterload, and enhance myocardial oxygen consumption. In diastole the balloon is inflated, restoring arterial pressure and coronary perfusion. In patients, counterpulsation improves cardiac output, reduces evidence of myocardial ischemia, and frequently relieves pain and reduces ST segment elevation. Patients with shock usually demonstrate a favorable hemodynamic and systemic metabolic response to balloon pumping. A minority of patients can be weaned from the pump. Most revert to the symptoms of shock when pumping is stopped. Thus balloon pumping per se has a minimal effect on mortality associated with shock, despite its temporary utility. However, several groups have reported that of patients in shock who receive balloon counterpulsation and then in 12 to 24 hours undergo cardiac catheterization to define surgical candidates, significant numbers can be saved.[69-72] A recent report by Resnekov describes 35 patients who were pumped and studied by catheterization. Of these, 28 were felt to be surgical candidates (80%), and of these, 21 were discharged alive after surgery (55%). Others have reported survival with balloon pumping and surgery in patients who have cardiogenic shock ranging from 40% to 50%. This should be compared with a mortality of 80% to 90% in comparable patients treated only medically. So, balloon pumping as a support device, if diagnostic and subsequent surgical therapy are contemplated, has a much more favorable outcome than pumping alone. Based on these data, counterpulsation probably is indicated for the treatment of shock at institutions where an experienced pump team, catheterization laboratory, and coronary surgery program are established.

Other indications for intraaortic balloon counterpulsation include severe congestive heart failure, medically refractory ischemia, ventricular septal defects, and left main coronary stenosis in patients who have shock. In most instances the intraaortic balloon pump provides additional protection for the myocardium until surgery can be done.

Hagemeijer and co-workers studied the effectiveness of intraaortic balloon pumping in patients who had severe congestive heart failure associated with a recent myocardial infarction and did not undergo subsequent surgery. Of 25 patients, 20 were successfully weaned from the pump. Thirteen of these patients lived for more than 1 year; 12 patients improved their functional class and returned to work.[74]

Intraaortic balloon counterpulsation is not without risk. The most common serious complication associated with it is limb ischemia, which occurs in approximately 14% of patients. Other less common complications include dissection of the aorta, septicemia, localized groin sepsis, and thrombocytopenia. The least serious common complication is catheter injury of the atherosclerotic aortic wall. Subsequent thrombectomies are required.[73,75]

Besides the intraaortic balloon, another mechanical device has received recognition in recent years. This device is a paracorporeal left ventricular assist device (LVAD). This device is used postoperatively in subjects of open-heart surgery who have developed cardiogenic shock unresponsive to adjunctive drug therapy, pacing, and intraaortic counterpulsation. Many of these patients are unable to be disconnected from cardiopulmonary bypass. A variety of devices have been developed to unload the left ventricle and pump an adequate volume for systemic blood flow. The LVAD actually takes over the pumping action for the left ventricle, thus decreasing the workload and myocardial oxygen consumption. The LVAD has had only limited success to date, and its use is restricted by protocols. The LVAD is still experimental and will require more clinical investigation before it receives widespread acceptance in the treatment of postoperative cardiogenic shock.[76-80]

Acknowledgement is extended to Gregory C. Freund, Brenda Lewis, R.N., and Lawrence Reduto, M.D., for the discussion of coronary artery reperfusion in evolving acute myocardial infarction.

REFERENCES

1. Harrison, T.R., and Reeves, T.J.: Principles and problems of ischemic heart disease, Chicago, 1968, Year Book Medical Publishers, Inc.
2. Matsui, K., and others: Ventricular septal rupture secondary to myocardial infarction: clinical approach and surgical results, J.A.M.A. **245**:1537, 1981.
3. Prinzmetal, M., and others: Angina pectoris. I. A variant form of angina pectoris: a preliminary report, Am. J. Med. **27**:35, 1959.
4. Schroeder, J.S., and others: Provocation of coronary spasm with ergonovine maleate: new test results with 57 patients undergoing coronary arteriography, Am. J. Cardiol. **40**:487, 1977.
5. Schroeder, J.S., and others: Medical therapy of Prinzmetal's variant angina, Chest (suppl.) **78**:231, 1980.
6. Bertrand, M.E., and others: Treatment of Prinzmetal's variant angina: role of medical treatment with nifedipine and coronary revascularization combined with plexectomy, Am. J. Cardiol. **47**:174, 1981.
7. Nevins, M.A., Lyon, L.S., and Pantazapaulous, J.: Pharmacotherapy of variant angina, Cardiovascu. Med. **3**:445, 1978.
8. Muller, J.E., and Gunther, S.S.: Nefedipine therapy for Prinzmetal's angina, Circulation **57**:137, 1978.
9. Turner, G.G.: Reassessment of vasodilator therapy in angina: effects of oral isosorbide dinitrate and hydralazine on exercise tolerance in patients receiving Inderal, Am. J. Cardiol. **47**:910, 1981.
10. Hindman, M.C., and others: Rest and exercise hemodynamic effects of oral hydralazine in patients with coronary artery disease and left ventricular dysfunction, Circulation **61**:751, 1980.
11. Stone, P.H., and others: Calcium channel blocking agents in the treatment of cardiovascular disorders. II. Hemodynamic effects and clinical applications, Ann. Intern. Med. **93**:886, 1980.
12. Check, W.: Calcium antagonists: long awaited new therapy for heart disease, J.A.M.A. **245**:807, 1981.
13. Pepine, C.J., and others: Transluminal coronary angioplasty, J.A.M.A. **244**:1966, 1980.
14. Tyras, D.H., and others: Left main equivalent: results of medicine and surgical and surgical therapy, Circulation **64**(suppl. 2):7, 1981.
15. O'Donoghue, M.J., Engelman, R.M., and Auvil, J.: Multidose cardioplegia for myocardial preservation during prolonged ischemic arrest, Surg. Forum **19**:274, 1978.
16. Loop, F.D., and others: The efficacy of coronary artery surgery, Am. Heart J. **101**:86, 1981.
17. Peter, R.H., and others: A new approach to clinical decision making in coronary artery disease: observations on subsets within Duke University data bank, Adv. Cardiol. **27**:199, 1980.
18. Conti, C.R., and Curry, R.C.: Unstable angina: results of medical and surgical treatment: status report, Adv. Cardiol. **27**:94, 1980.
19. Romhilt, D.W., and Fowler, N.O.: Physical signs in acute myocardial infarction, Heart Lung **2**:74, 1973.
20. Harvey, W.P.: Some pertinent physical findings in the clinical evaluation of acute myocardial infarction, Circulation **39**(suppl. 4):175, 1969.

21. Pitt, B.: Clinical application of myocardial imaging with radioisotopes in the evaluation and management of patients with coronary artery disease, Adv. Cardiol. **26**:30, 1980.

22. Wackers, F.J.T.: Current status of radionuclide imaging in the management and evaluation of patients with cardiovascular disease, Adv. Cardiol. **27**:40, 1980.

23. Wackers, F.J.T.: Radionuclide evaluation of patients in the CCU, Adv. Cardiol. **27**:105, 1980.

24. Willerson, J.T., and others: Radionuclide imaging in acute myocardial infarction, Cardiovasc. Med. **3**:69, 1978.

25. Waugh, R.A.: Immediate and remote prognostic implications of fascicular block during acute myocardial infarction, Circulation **47**:765, 1973.

26. McNeer, J.F., and others: Hospital discharge the week after acute myocardial infarction, N. Engl. J. Med. **298**:229, 1978.

27. Cannon, D.S., and others: The short- and long-term prognosis of patients with transmural and nontransmural infarction, Am. J. Med. **61**:452, 1976.

28. Haskell, W.L., and DeBusk, R.: Cardiovascular responses to repeated treadmill exercise testing soon after myocardial infarction, Circulation **60**:1247, 1979.

29. Starling, M.R., and others: Exercise testing early myocardial infarction: predictive value for subsequent unstable angina and death, Am. J. Cardiol. **46**:909, 1980.

30. Stargel, W.W., and others: Clinical comparison of rapid infusion and multiple injection methods for lidocaine loading, Am. Heart J. **102**:872, 1981.

31. Lie, K.L., Wellens, H.J., and Durrer, D.: Characteristics and predictability of primary ventricular fibrillation, Eur. J. Cardiol. **1**:379, 1974.

32. Rackley, E., and others: Modern approach to myocardial infarction: determination of prognosis and therapy, Am. Heart J. **101**:75, 1981.

33. Resnekov, L.: Management of acute myocardial infarction, Cardiovasc. Med. **2**:949, 1977.

34. Ewy, G.A.: Anticoagulation in patients with acute myocardial infarction, Pract. Cardiol. **4**:25, 1978.

35. Mueller, H., and Ayers, S.: Propranolol in the treatment of acute myocardial infarction, Circulation **49**:1078, 1974.

36. Bodenheimer, M.M., and others: Effect of progressive pressure reduction with nitroprusside on acute myocardial infarction in humans: determination of optimal afterload, Ann. Intern. Med. **94**:435, 1981.

37. Braunwald, E., and Maroko, P.R.: The reduction of infarct size: an idea whose time (for testing) has come, Circulation **50**:206, 1974.

38. Maroko, P.R., and others: Infarct size reduction: a critical review, Adv. Cardiol. **27**:127, 1980.

39. Rogers, W.J., and others: Reduction of hospital mortality rate of acute myocardial infarction with glucose-insulin-potassium infusion, Am. Heart J. **92**:441, 1976.

40. McEwan, M.P., and others: Effect of intravenous and intracoronary nitroglycerin in left ventricular wall motion and perfusion in patients with coronary artery disease, Am. J. Cardiol. **47**:102, 1981.

41. Ganz, W., and others: Intracoronary thrombolyses in evolving myocardial infarction, Am. Heart J. **101**:4, 1981.

42. Rentrop, P., and others: Acute myocardial infarction: intracoronary application of nitroglycerin and streptokinase in combination with transluminal recanalization, Clin. Cardiol. **2**:354, 1979.

43. Rentrop, P., and others: Selective intracoronary thrombolysis in acute myocardial infarction and unstable angina pectoris, Circulation **63**:307, 1981.

44. Reduto, L.A., and others: Intracoronary infusion of streptokinase in patients with acute myocardial infarction: effects of reperfusion of left ventricular performance, Am. J. Cardiol. **48**:403, 1981.

45. Brosius, F.C., and Roberts, W.C.: Significance of coronary arterial thrombus in transmural acute myocardial infarction: a study of 54 necropsy patients, Circulation **63**:810, 1981.

46. Chandler, A.B., and others: Coronary thrombosis in myocardial infarction: report of a workshop on the role of coronary thrombosis in the pathogenesis of acute myocardial infarction, Am. J. Cardiol. **34**:823, 1974.

47. Aber, C.P., and others: Streptokinase in acute myocardial infarction: a controlled multicentre study in the United Kingdom, Br. Med. J. **2**:1100, 1976.

48. European Working Party: Streptokinase in recent myocardial infarction: a controlled multicentre trial, Br. Med. J. **3**:325, 1971.

49. European Collaborative Study: A controlled trial of urokinase in myocardial infarction, Lancet **2**:624, 1975.

50. European Cooperative Study Group for Streptokinase Treatment in Acute Myocardial Infarction: Streptokinase in acute myocardial infarction, N. Engl. J. Med. **301**:797, 1979.

51. Markis, J.E., and others: Myocardial salvage after intracoronary thromboly with streptokinase in acute myocardial infarction, N. Engl. J. Med. **1**:305, 1981.

52. Muller, J.E., and others: Sounding boards: let's not let the genie escape from the bottle again, N. Engl. J. Med. **304**:1294, 1981.

53. Harlan, W.R., and others: Chronic congestive heart failure in coronary artery disease: clinical criteria, Ann. Intern. Med. **87**:133, 1977.

54. Dzau, V.J., and others: Relation of renin-angiotensin-aldosterone system to clinical state in congestive heart failure, Circulation **63**:645, 1981.

55. Dzau, V.J., and others: Sustained effectiveness of converting enzyme inhibition in patients with severe congestive heart failure, N. Engl. J. Med. **302**:1371, 1980.

56. Chatterjee, J., and Parmley, W.W.: The role of vasodilator therapy in heart failure, Prog. Cardiovasc. Dis. **19**:301, 1977.

57. Cohn, J.N.: Choice and rationale for vasodilators in treatment of hypertension or relief of heart failure, Cardiovasc. Rev. **1**:686, 1980.

58. Mason, D.T., and others: Treatment of acute and

chronic congestive heart failure by vasodilator after-load reduction, Arch. Intern. Med. **140:**1577, 1980.

59. Massie, B., and others: Long-term vasodilator therapy for heart failure: clinical response and its relationship to hemodynamic measurements, Circulation **63:**269, 1981.

60. Franciosa, J.A., and others: Hemodynamic improvement after oral hydralazine in left ventricular failure, Ann. Intern. Med. **86:**388, 1977.

61. Franciosa, J.A., and Cohn, J.N.: Effects of minoxidil on hemodynamics with congestive heart failure, Circulation **63:**652, 1980.

62. The Path finder family of Swan-Ganz flow-directed right heart catheters, Edwards Laboratories, Division of American Hospital Supply Corp., Santa Ana, Calif., 1973.

63. Walinsky, P.: Acute hemodynamic monitoring, Heart Lung **6**(suppl. 5):838, 1977.

64. Ratshin, R.A., and others: Hemodynamic elevation of left ventricular function in shock complicating myocardial infarction, Circulation **45:**127, 1972.

65. Rotman, M., and others: Pulmonary artery diastolic pressure in acute myocardial infarction, Am. J. Cardiol. **33:**357, 1974.

66. Shubin, H., and Weil, M.H.: Practical considerations in the management of shock complicating acute myocardial infarction: a summary of current practice, Am. J. Cardiol. **26:**603, 1970.

67. Loeb, H.S., and Gunnau, R.M.: Treatment of pump failure in acute myocardial infarction, J.A.M.A. **245:**2093, 1981.

68. Holzer, J., and others: Effectiveness of dopamine in patients with cardiogenic shock, Am. J. Cardiol. **32:**79, 1973.

69. Loeb, H.S., and others: Acute hemodynamic effects of dopamine in patients with shock, Circulation **44:**163, 1971.

70. Keung, E.C.H., and others: Dobutamine therapy in myocardial infarction, J.A.M.A. **245:**13, 1971.

71. Lamberti, J., and others: Mechanical circulatory assistance for the treatment of complications of coronary artery disease, Surg. Clin. North Am. **56:**83, 1976.

72. Ehrich, D.A., and others: The hemodynamic response to intraaortic balloon counterpulsation in patients with cardiogenic shock complicating acute myocardial infarction, Am. Heart J. **93:**274, 1977.

73. Mueller, H., and Ayers, S.: The effects of intraaortic balloon counterpulsation on cardiac performance and metabolism in shock associated with acute myocardial infarction, J. Clin. Invest. **50:**1885, 1971.

74. Hagemeijer, F., and others: Effectiveness of intraaortic balloon pumping without cardiac surgery for patients with severe heart failure secondary to a recent myocardial infarction, Am. J. Cardiol. **40:**951, 1977.

75. Berger, R.L., and others: Applications of intraaortic balloon counterpulsation, Isr. J. Med. Sci. **11:**231, 1975.

76. Beckman, C.B., and others: Results and complications of intraaortic balloon counterpulsation, Ann. Thorac. Surg. **24:**550, 1977.

77. McCabe, J.C., and others: Complications of intraaortic balloon insertion and counterpulsation, Circulation **57:**769, 1978.

78. McGee, M.G., and others: Retrospective analyses of the need for mechanical support (IABP/ALVAD or partial artificial heart) after cardiopulmonary bypass, Am. J. Cardiol. **46:**135, 1980.

79. Barnhard, W.F., and others: A new method for temporary left ventricular bypass, J. Thorac. Cardiovasc. Surg. **70:**880, 1975.

80. Berger, R.L., and others: Successful use of a left ventricular assist device in cardiogenic shock from massive postoperative myocardial infarction, J. Thorac. Cardiovasc. Surg. **78:**626, 1979.

8
ARRHYTHMIAS

Douglas P. Zipes

Normal cardiac cycle

Before discussing electrocardiographic interpretation of cardiac arrhythmias, a review of the normal electrical events that occur during a cardiac cycle, as well as a discussion of basic electrophysiologic principles is necessary. During sinus rhythm the cardiac impulse originates in the sinus node and then travels to right and left atria. Sinus node discharge and conduction from the sinus node to the atria are not recorded from the body surface and therefore these events are not present in the ECG. In response to the sinus node impulse, the atria depolarize and generate the P wave; atrial repolarization (Ta wave) is generally obscured by the QRS complex and is therefore not usually seen. Atrial conduction probably proceeds through both atria in a more or less radial fashion (like spreading ripples caused by a rock thrown into still water), eventually reaching the AV node and His bundle. Some data suggest that conduction through the atria travels preferentially through loosely connected bundles of atrial muscle called the anterior, middle, and posterior internodal pathways, which, it is argued, provide specialized pathways of conduction from the sinus node to the left atrium (via Bachmann's bundle, a division of the anterior internodal pathway) and to the AV node. However, the functional importance of these pathways in providing specialized tracts for conduction is unsettled. The speed at which the impulse travels (conduction velocity) becomes reduced as the impulse traverses the AV node but once again accelerates through the His bundle, bundle branches, and Purkinje fibers. These fibers distribute the impulse rapidly and uniformly over the ventricular endocardium, finally depolarizing the ventricular myocardium (Fig. 8-1). It is important to remember that the surface ECG records only ventricular muscle depolarization (QRS) and repolarization (T wave), atrial depolarization (P wave), and sometimes repolarization (Ta wave). Activity from the SA and AV nodes, His bundle, bundle branches, and Purkinje fibers is not recorded in the ECG. Special intracardiac electrodes can be employed to record activity from some of these structures and is discussed briefly later in this chapter.

It has been postulated that the bundle branches are really composed of three divisions, called fascicles, that are formed by the right bundle branch and two divisions of the left bundle branch, the anterosuperior division, and the postero-inferior division. The term "hemiblock" has been used to describe block in one of these fascicles.[1] A more accurate term is *fascicular block*. Although a number of careful anatomic and pathologic studies of human hearts have failed to substantiate the anatomic separation of the left bundle branch into two distinct and specific divisions, the fascicular block concept has been useful to explain observed electrocardiographic and clinical entities (see discussion of bundle branch block).

The electrical activity of the heart is recorded by an ECG machine onto ECG paper. This graph paper is divided into a series of vertical lines measuring time and horizontal lines measuring voltage (Fig. 8-2). The electrical pattern of a typical cardiac cycle is displayed in Fig. 8-3 and is discussed in Table 8-1. (See also Chapter 6.)

The atrial rate in beats per minute may be determined by dividing the *time* interval between regularly occurring consecutive P waves (PP interval) into 60. A similar procedure performed for the interval between ventricular beats (RR interval) determines the ventricular rate (Fig. 8-4). The rate can be more rapidly determined by dividing the *number* of large (0.2-second) divisions between two consecutive complexes into 300 or *small* squares into 1500. For irregular rhythms, the rate must be averaged over a longer interval; for example, the number of large divisions separating four QRS complexes (three complete cardiac cycles) may be divided into 900. Table 8-2 can be used to calculate the rate of a regular rhythm.

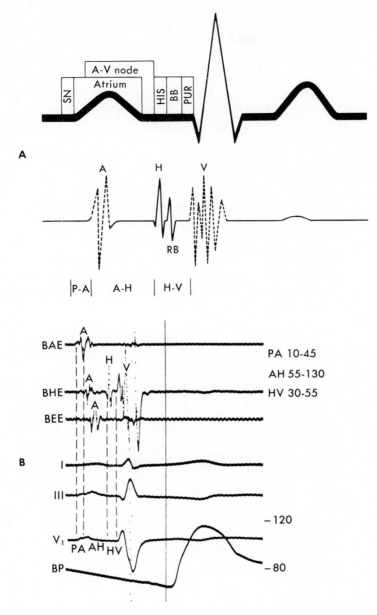

Fig. 8-1. A, Schematic illustration of a cardiac cycle, demonstrating the normal ECG (top) and a His bundle recording (bottom). The diagram illustrates the approximate time of activation of various structures in the specialized conduction system. It is important to emphasize that conduction has already reached the Purkinje fibers just prior to the onset of the QRS complex. *SN,* Sinus node; *HIS,* bundle of His; *BB,* bundle branches; *PUR,* Purkinje fibers; *A,* low right atrial deflection; *H,* His bundle deflection; *RB,* right bundle branch deflection; *V,* ventricular septal muscle depolarization; *P-A,* interval from the onset of the P wave in the surface tracing to the onset of the low right atrial deflection, serving as a measure of intraatrial conduction; *A-H,* measurement of conduction across the AV node; *H-V,* measurement of conduction through the His bundle distal to the recording electrode, the bundle branches, and the Purkinje system up to the point of ventricular activation. (Top panel modified from Hoffman, B.F., and Singer, D.H.: Prog. Cardiovasc. Dis. **7**:226, 1964.) **B,** Electrophysiologic and blood pressure recordings during one cardiac cycle. *BAE,* Bipolar high right atrial electrogram; *BHE,* bipolar His electrogram; *BEE,* bipolar esophageal electrogram. Normal intervals in milliseconds to the right.

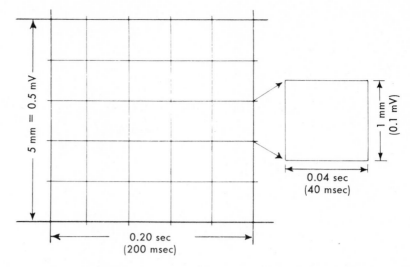

Fig. 8-2. Time and voltage lines of the ECG. The interval between two heavy vertical lines is 0.20 second (200 msec) and between each light line 0.04 second (40 msec). The voltage between each heavy horizontal line is 0.5 mV.

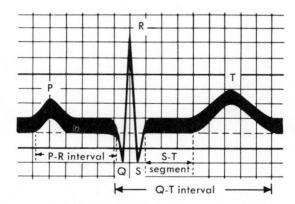

Fig. 8-3. Electrical pattern of cardiac cycle. (Refer to Table 8-1.)

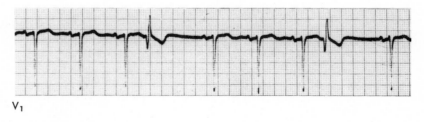

Fig. 8-4. Calculation of the atrial and ventricular rates. The heart rate is 75 beats/minute, determined by dividing 60 seconds by 0.80 second, the time interval between consecutive P waves and/or consecutive R waves or by dividing four large squares into 300 or 20 small squares into 1500. Two premature ventricular extrasystoles are present. See Table 8-2.

Table 8-1. Definition and significance of ECG intervals*

Description	Duration	Significance of disturbance
PR interval: from beginning of P wave to beginning of QRS complex; represents time taken for impulse to spread through the atria, AV node and His bundle, the bundle branches and Purkinje fibers, to a point immediately preceding ventricular activation	0.12 to 0.20 second	Disturbance in conduction usually in AV node, His bundle, or bundle branches but can be in atria as well
QRS interval: from beginning to end of QRS complex; represents time taken for depolarization of both ventricles	0.06 to 0.10 second	Disturbance in conduction in bundle branches and/or in ventricles
QT interval: from beginning of QRS to end of T wave; represents time taken for entire electrical depolarization and repolarization of the ventricles	0.36 to 0.44 second	Disturbances usually affecting repolarization more than depolarization such as drug effects, electrolyte disturbances, and rate changes

*Heart rate influences the duration of these intervals, especially that of the PR and QT intervals.

Table 8-2. Determination of heart rate from the ECG

Time (second)	No. of small squares	Rate (beats per minute)	Time (second)	No. of small squares	Rate (beats per minute)
0.10	2.5	600	0.60	15.00	100
0.12	3.0	500	0.64	16.00	94
0.15	3.75	400	0.70	17.50	86
0.16	4.0	375	0.72	18.00	83
0.20	5.0	300	0.76	19.00	79
0.24	6.0	250	0.80	20.00	75
0.26	6.5	230	0.84	21.00	71
0.28	7.0	214	0.88	22.00	68
0.30	7.5	200	0.92	23.00	65
0.32	8.0	188	0.96	24.00	63
0.34	8.5	176	1.00	25.00	60
0.36	9.0	167	1.08	27.00	56
0.38	9.5	158	1.14	28.50	53
0.40	10.0	150	1.20	30.00	50
0.42	10.5	143	1.40	35.00	43
0.44	11.0	136	1.50	37.50	40
0.46	11.5	130	1.60	40.00	38
0.48	12.0	125	1.80	45.00	33
0.50	12.5	120	2.00	50.00	30
0.52	13.0	115	2.50	62.50	25
0.56	14.0	107	3.00	75.00	20

Electrophysiologic principles

Certain specialized cells, such as those in the sinus node, some parts of the atria, AV node, and His-Purkinje system, are able to discharge spontaneously; they do not require an external or propagated stimulus to fire. This property, known as *automaticity* (also called diastolic depolarization), creates the potential for these cells to depolarize the rest of the heart. Normally the sinus node rules as the pacemaker, since it spontaneously discharges faster than these other latent pacemakers.

Should a latent pacemaker possessing the property of automaticity discharge more rapidly than the sinus node, it may depolarize atria, ventricles, or both. This may occur in two ways. If the SA node discharges more slowly than the discharge rate of the latent pacemaker (Fig. 8-12), or if the sinus impulse is blocked before reaching the latent pacemaker site (Fig. 8-59), the latent pacemaker may passively *escape* sinus domination and discharge automatically at its own intrinsic rate. Such escape beats are slower than normal, since the AV junction and bundle branch–Purkinje system (two probable escape focus sites) generally beat at 40 to 60 times/minute and 30 to 40 times/minute, respectively. However, should a latent pacemaker abnormally accelerate its discharge rate and actively *usurp* control of the heartbeat from the sinus node, a premature beat results. This may happen in the atria, ventricles, or AV junction. A series of these premature beats in a row produces a tachycardia. A shift in the normal manner of atrial or ventricular activation, such as might be produced by a shift in pacemaker focus, is reflected by a change in P or QRS contour.

Automatic discharge of a pacemaker focus is not sufficient to depolarize a cardiac chamber; the impulse must also be conducted from its site of origin to surrounding myocardium. The heart possesses the property of *excitability*, which is a characteristic enabling it to be depolarized by a stimulus; this is an integral part of the propagation or conduction of the impulse from one fiber to the next. Many factors may influence the level of excitability but the most important, in the normal state, is how long after depolarization the heart is restimulated. Cardiac tissue requires a recovery period following depolarization. If a stimulus occurs too early, the heart has had insufficient time to recover, and it will not respond to the stimulus no matter how intense it is (absolute refractory period, excitability zero). A slightly later stimulus allows more time for recovery (relative refractory period, excitability improving), and a still later stimulus finds the heart completely recovered (no longer refractory, full excitability).

If conduction becomes unevenly depressed, with block in some areas and not in others, some regions of the myocardium (unblocked areas) must necessarily be activated (and recover) earlier than others. Under appropriate circumstances, when the block is in only one direction (unidirectional), this uneven conduction may allow the initial impulse to *reenter* areas previously inexcitable but that have now recovered. Should the reentering impulse then be able to depolarize the entire atria and/or ventricles, a corresponding premature extrasystole results; maintenance of the *reentrant excitation* establishes a tachycardia. A special form of reentry may produce echo or reciprocal beats (Fig. 8-41, *D*).

Thus disorders of impulse *formation* (automaticity) or *conduction* (unidirectional block and reentry) or, at times, combinations of both may initiate arrhythmias.

Only indirect evidence exists to enable a clinical classification of arrhythmias according to electrophysiologic mechanisms. In addition, an arrhythmia may be initiated and perpetuated by different mechanisms. For example, spontaneous diastolic depolarization (automaticity) may trigger a premature atrial or ventricular systole that initiates an arrhythmia caused by reentry. Also, the work of Moe and Jalife on parasystole,[2] a type of automaticity, and reflection,[3] a form of reentry, is causing us to rethink many of our clinical definitions. Thus the clinical classification of arrhythmias according to mechanism remains speculative. Antiarrhythmic agents specifically indicated to treat one mechanism or the other do not yet exist[4] (Table 8-3).

Depolarization of cells in the atria, ventricles, and His-Purkinje system depends on a rapid movement of sodium into the cell. Such an event is called the *fast response*. In the sinus and AV nodes depolarization depends primarily on intracellular movement of calcium and is called the *slow response*.[5] The slow response may play a role in the genesis of certain cardiac arrhythmias and is affected by a specific class of drugs called calcium entry blockers and typified by verapamil.

Table 8-3. Probable electrophysiologic mechanism responsible for various cardiac arrhythmias

Automaticity	Reentry	Automaticity or reentry
Escape beats—atrial, junctional, or ventricular	Paroxysmal supraventricular tachycardia	Premature systoles—atrial, junctional, or ventricular
Atrial rhythm	Reciprocating tachycardia using an accessory (WPW) pathway	Flutter and fibrillation
Atrial tachycardia with or without AV block	Atrial flutter	Ventricular tachycardia
Junctional rhythm	Atrial fibrillation	
Nonparoxysmal AV junctional tachycardia	Ventricular tachycardia	
Accelerated idioventricular rhythm	Ventricular flutter	
Parasystole	Ventricular fibrillation	

Arrhythmia analysis (Table 8-4)

For proper analysis, each arrhythmia must be approached in a systematic manner. A suggested guide follows:

1. What is the rate? Is it too fast or too slow? Are P waves present? Are atrial and ventricular rates the same?
2. Are the PP and RR intervals regular or irregular? If irregular, is it a consistent, repeating irregularity?
3. Is there a P wave (and therefore atrial activity) related to each ventricular complex? Does the P wave precede or follow the QRS complex? Is the PR or RP interval constant?
4. Are all P waves and QRS complexes identical and normal in contour? To determine the significance of changes in P or QRS contour or amplitude, one must know the lead being recorded.
5. Are the PR, QRS and QT intervals normal?
6. Considering the clinical setting, what is the significance of the arrhythmia?
7. How should the arrhythmia be treated?

Table 8-4. Classification of normal and abnormal cardiac rhythms

Rhythms originating in the sinus node
  Sinus rhythm
  Sinus tachycardia
  Sinus bradycardia
  Sinus arrhythmia
  Sinus arrest
  Sinus exit block
  Sinus nodal reentry
Rhythms originating in the atria
  Wandering pacemaker between sinus node
    and atrium or AV junction
  Premature atrial systole (or complex)
  Intraatrial reentry
  Atrial flutter
  Atrial fibrillation
  Atrial tachycardia with block
  Multifocal atrial tachycardia
Rhythms originating in the AV junction (AV
  node–His bundle)
  Premature AV junctional systole (or complex)
  AV junctional escape beats
  AV junctional rhythm
  AV nodal reentry
  Reciprocating tachycardia using an accessory
    (WPW) pathway

Rhythms originating in the ventricles
  Ventricular escape beats
  Premature ventricular systole (or complex)
  Ventricular tachycardia
  Idioventricular tachycardia (accelerated idio-
    ventricular rhythm)
  Ventricular flutter
  Ventricular fibrillation
AV block
  First-degree
  Second-degree
    Type I (Wenckebach)
    Type II
  Third-degree (complete)
Bundle branch block
  Right
  Left
  Fascicular blocks (hemiblocks)
Parasystole
  Atrial
  Junctional
  Ventricular

Therapy of arrhythmias (Table 8-5)
GENERAL THERAPEUTIC CONCEPTS[8]

Initial assessment. The therapeutic approach to a patient who has a cardiac arrhythmia begins with an accurate electrocardiographic *interpretation* of the arrhythmia and continues with determination of the *cause* of the arrhythmia (if possible), the nature of the underlying *heart disease* (if any), and the *consequences* of the arrhythmia for the individual patient. Thus one cannot treat arrhythmias as isolated events without having knowledge of the clinical situation; *patients* who have arrhythmias, not arrhythmias themselves, are treated.

Electrophysiologic and hemodynamic consequences. The ventricular rate and duration of an arrhythmia, its site of origin, and the cardiovascular status of the patient primarily determine the electrophysiologic and hemodynamic consequences of a particular rhythm disturbance. Electrophysiologic consequences, often influenced by the presence of underlying heart disease such as acute myocardial infarction, include the development of serious arrhythmias as a result of rapid (and slow) rates, initiation of sustained arrhythmias by premature systoles, or the degeneration of rhythms like ventricular tachycardia into ventricular fibrillation. Hemodynamic performance of the heart and circulation may be altered by extremes of heart rate or by loss of atrial contribution to ventricular filling. Rapid rates greatly shorten the diastolic filling time, and, particularly in diseased hearts, the increased heart rate may fail to compensate for the reduced stroke output; blood pressure, along with cardiac output, declines. Arrhythmias that prevent sequential AV contraction mitigate the hemodynamic benefits of the atrial booster pump, whereas atrial fibrillation causes complete loss of atrial contraction and may reduce cardiac output.

Slowing the ventricular rate. When a patient develops a tachyarrhythmia, slowing the ventricular rate is the initial and frequently the most important therapeutic maneuver. Since medical therapy frequently involves a time-consuming and potentially dangerous biologic titration of drugs such as digitalis or quinidine, electrical direct current (DC) cardioversion may be preferable, depending on the clinical situation. Therapy may differ radically for the very same arrhythmia in two different patients because the consequences of the tachycardia on the individual patients differ. For example, a supraventricular tachycardia at 200 beats/minute may produce little or no symptoms in a healthy young adult and therefore require little or no therapy; the very same arrhythmia may precipitate pulmonary edema in a patient with mitral stenosis, syncope in a patient with aortic stenosis, shock in a patient with an acute myocardial infarction, or hemiparesis in a patient with cerebrovascular disease. In these situations the tachycardia requires prompt electrical conversion.

Etiology. The etiology of the arrhythmia may influence therapy markedly. Electrolyte imbalance (potassium, magnesium, calcium), acidosis or alkalosis, hypoxemia, and many drugs may produce arrhythmias. Because heart failure may cause arrhythmias, digitalis may effectively suppress arrhythmias during heart failure when all other agents are unsuccessful or prevent more severe arrhythmias by reversing early congestive heart failure. Similarly, an arrhythmia secondary to hypotension may respond to leg elevation or vasopressor therapy. Mild sedation or reassurance may be successful in treating some arrhythmias related to emotional stress. Precipitating or contributing disease states such as infection, hypovolemia, anemia, and thyroid disorders should be sought and treated. Aggressive management of premature atrial or ventricular systoles that often presage or precipitate the occurrence of sustained tachyarrhythmias may prevent later occurrence of more serious tachyarrhythmias.

Table 8-5. Cardiac arrhythmias*

Type of arrhythmia	P waves			QRS complexes		
	Rate	Rhythm	Contour	Rate	Rhythm	Contour
Sinus rhythm	60 to 100	Regular†	Normal	60 to 100	Regular	Normal
Sinus bradycardia	<60	Regular	Normal	<60	Regular	Normal
Sinus tachycardia	100 to 180	Regular	May be peaked	100 to 180	Regular	Normal
Paroxysmal supraventricular tachycardia	150 to 250	Very regular except at onset and termination	Retrograde; difficult to see; lost in QRS complex	150 to 250	Very regular except at onset and termination	Normal
Atrial flutter	250 to 350	Regular	Sawtooth	75 to 175	Generally regular in absence of drugs or disease	Normal
Atrial fibrillation	400 to 600	Grossly irregular	Base line undulations; no P waves	100 to 160	Grossly irregular	Normal

*In an effort to summarize these arrhythmias in a tabular form, generalizations have to be made, particularly under therapy. Particularly, acute therapy to terminate a tachycardia may be different from chronic therapy to prevent a recurrence. Some of the exceptions are indicated by the footnotes, but the reader is referred to the text for a complete discussion.
†P waves initiated by sinus node discharge may not be precisely regular because of sinus arrhythmia.
‡Often, carotid sinus massage fails to slow a sinus tachycardia.

Risks of therapy. Since therapy always involves some risk, one must decide, particularly as the therapeutic regimen escalates, if the risks of not treating the arrhythmia continue to outweigh the risks of the therapy. The antiarrhythmic agents[11] lidocaine, procainamide, quinidine, propranolol, disopyramide, and phenytoin exert negative inotropic effects on the myocardium, and when given parenterally, they may produce hypotension. Antiarrhythmic agents may slow conduction velocity, depress the activity of normal (sinus) as well as abnormal (ectopic) pacemaker sites, and cause arrhythmias. It should be remembered that doses of all drugs may need to be adjusted according to the size of the patient, routes of excretion or degradation, presence of impaired organ function (heart, liver, kidney), degree of absorption (if given orally), adverse side effects, interaction with other drugs, electrolyte imbalance, hypoxemia, and the like.

The remainder of this chapter will be devoted to a discussion of cardiac arrhythmias (see Tables 8-4 and 8-5). An analysis similar to that presented in the discussion of arrhythmia analysis will be employed.

Ventricular response to carotid sinus massage	Physical examination			Treatment
	Intensity of S_1	Splitting of S_2	A waves	
Gradual slowing and return to former rate	Constant	Normal	Normal	None
Gradual slowing and return to former rate	Constant	Normal	Normal	None, unless symptomatic; atropine
Gradual slowing‡ and return to former rate	Constant	Normal	Normal	None, unless symptomatic; treat underlying disease
Abrupt slowing caused by termination of tachycardia, or no effect	Constant	Normal	Constant cannon A waves	Vagal stimulation, verapamil, digitalis, propranolol, DC shock, pacing
Abrupt slowing and return to former rate; flutter remains	Constant; variable if AV block changing	Normal	Flutter waves	DC shock, digitalis, quinidine, propranolol, verapamil
Slowing; gross irregularity remains	Variable	Normal	No A waves	Digitalis, quinidine, DC shock, verapamil

§Any independent atrial arrhythmia may exist or the atria may be captured retrogradely.
‖Constant if atria captured retrogradely.
¶Atrial rhythm and rate may vary, depending on whether sinus bradycardia or tachycardia, atrial tachycardia, or something else is the atrial mechanism.
**Regular or constant if block is unchanging.   *Continued.*

Table 8-5. Cardiac arrhythmias—cont'd

Type of arrhythmia	P waves			QRS complexes		
	Rate	Rhythm	Contour	Rate	Rhythm	Contour
Atrial tachycardia with block	150 to 250	Regular; may be irregular	Abnormal	75 to 200	Generally regular in absence of drugs or disease	Normal
AV junctional rhythm	400 to 100§	Regular	Normal	40 to 60	Fairly regular	Normal; may be abnormal but <0.12 second
Reciprocating tachycardia using an accessory (WPW) pathway	150 to 250	Very regular except at onset and termination	Retrograde; difficult to see; follows the QRS complex	150 to 250	Very regular except at onset and termination	Normal
Nonparoxysmal AV junctional tachycardia	60 to 100§	Regular	Normal	70 to 130	Fairly regular	Normal; may be abnormal but <0.12 second
Ventricular tachycardia	60 to 100§	Regular	Normal	110 to 250	Fairly regular; may be irregular	Abnormal, >0.12 second
Accelerated idioventricular rhythm	60 to 100§	Regular	Normal	50 to 110	Fairly regular; may be irregular	Abnormal, >0.12 second
Ventricular flutter	60 to 100§	Regular	Normal; difficult to see	150 to 300	Regular	Sine wave
Ventricular fibrillation	60 to 100§	Regular	Normal; difficult to see	400 to 600	Grossly irregular	Base line undulations; no QRS complexes
First-degree AV block	60 to 100¶	Regular	Normal	60 to 100	Regular	Normal
Type I second-degree AV block	60 to 100¶	Regular	Normal	30 to 100	Irregular**	Normal
Type II-second-degree AV block	60 to 100¶	Regular	Normal	30 to 100	Irregular**	Abnormal, >0.12 second
Complete AV block	60 to 100§	Regular	Normal	<40	Fairly regular	Abnormal, >0.12 second
Right bundle branch block	60 to 100	Regular	Normal	60 to 100	Regular	Abnormal, >0.12 second
Left bundle branch block	60 to 100	Regular	Normal	60 to 100	Regular	Abnormal, >0.12 second

Ventricular response to carotid sinus massage	Physical examination			Treatment
	Intensity of S_1	Splitting of S_2	A waves	
Abrupt slowing and return to former rate; tachycardia remains	Constant; variable if AV block changing	Normal	More A waves than CV waves	Stop digitalis if toxic; digitalis, if not toxic; possibly verapamil
None; may be slight slowing	Variable‖	Normal	Intermittent cannon waves‖	None, unless symptomatic; atropine
Abrupt slowing caused by termination of tachycardia, or no effect	Constant but decreased	Normal	Constant cannon waves	See paroxysmal supraventricular tachycardia above
None; may be slight slowing	Variable‖	Normal	Intermittent cannon waves‖	None, unless symptomatic; stop digitalis if toxic
None	Variable‖	Abnormal	Intermittent cannon waves‖	Lidocaine, procainamide, DC shock, quinidine
None	Variable‖	Abnormal	Intermittent cannon waves‖	None, unless symptomatic; lidocaine, atropine
None	None	None	Cannon waves	DC shock
None	None	None	Cannon waves	DC shock
Gradual slowing caused by sinus slowing	Constant, diminished	Normal	Normal	None
Slowing caused by sinus slowing and an increase in AV block	Cyclic decrease and then increase after pause	Normal	Normal; increasing AC interval; A waves without C waves	None, unless symptomatic; atropine
Gradual slowing caused by sinus slowing	Constant	Abnormal	Normal; constant AC interval; A waves without C waves	Pacemaker
None	Variable‖	Abnormal	Intermittent cannon waves‖	Pacemaker
Gradual slowing and return to former rate	Constant	Wide	Normal	None
Gradual slowing and return to former rate	Constant	Paradoxical	Normal	None

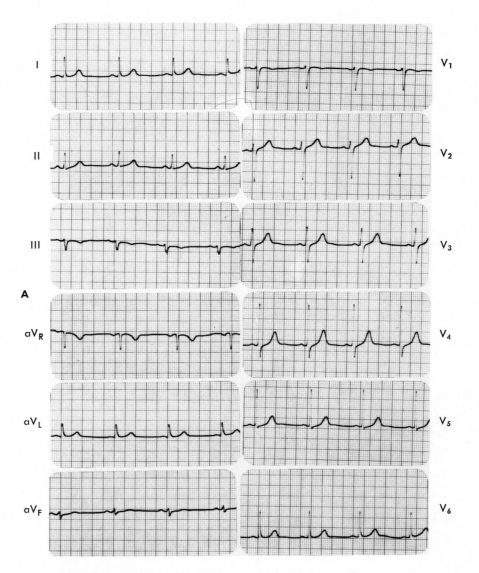

Fig. 8-5. A, Normal sinus rhythm. The ECG is normal. Schematic illustration in **B.**

Rate: 60 to 65 beats/minute.

Rhythm: Fairly regular.

P waves: Precede each QRS with normal, unchanging contour. Note P wave contour in each of the 12 leads.

PR interval: 0.14 second.

QRS: 0.08 second.

Significance and treatment: For significance and treatment of this and the following arrhythmias, see discussion under each arrhythmia.

NORMAL SINUS RHYTHM (Fig. 8-5, *A* and *B*)

Normal sinus rhythm is arbitrarily limited to rates of 60 to 100 beats/min. The P wave is upright in leads I and II and negative in lead aV_R with a vector in the frontal plane between 0 and +90 degrees. In the horizontal plane the P vector is directed anteriorly and slightly leftward and may therefore be negative in V_1 and V_2 but is positive in V_3. The PP interval characteristically varies slightly but by less than 0.16 second. The PR interval is greater than 0.12 second and may vary slightly with rate. The sinus node responds readily to autonomic stimuli; parasympathetic (cholinergic) stimuli slow and sympathetic (adrenergic) stimuli speed the rate of discharge. The resulting rate depends on the net effect of these two opposing forces.

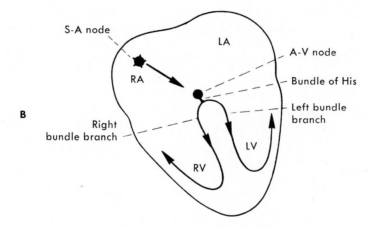

Fig. 8-5, cont'd. For legend see opposite page.

SINUS TACHYCARDIA (Figs. 8-6 and 8-7)

Sinus tachycardia, because of enhanced discharge of the sinus node from vagal inhibition or sympathetic stimulation, maintains a rate between 100 to 180 beats/min but may be higher with extreme exertion and in infants. It has a gradual onset and termination, and the PP interval may vary slightly from cycle to cycle. P waves have a normal contour, but may develop a larger amplitude and become peaked. Carotid sinus massage and Valsalva or other vagal maneuvers gradually slow a sinus tachycardia, which then accelerates to its previous rate. More rapid sinus rates may fail to slow in response to a vagal maneuver.

Significance. Sinus tachycardia is the normal reaction to a variety of physiologic stresses such as fever, hypotension, thyrotoxicosis, anemia, anxiety, exertion, hypovolemia, pulmonary emboli, myocardial ischemia, congestive heart failure, or shock. Inflammation such as pericarditis may produce sinus tachycardia. Sinus tachycardia is usually of no physiologic significance; however, in patients with organic myocardial disease, reduced cardiac output, congestive heart failure, or arrhythmias may result. Since heart rate is a major determinant of oxygen requirements, angina or perhaps an increase in the size of an infarction may accompany persistent sinus tachycardia in patients with coronary artery disease.

Treatment. Therapy should be directed toward correcting the underlying disease state that caused the sinus tachycardia. Elimination of tobacco, alcohol, coffee, tea, or other stimulants (for example, vasoconstrictors in nose drops) may be helpful. If sinus tachycardia is not secondary to a correctable physiologic stress, treatment with sedatives, reserpine, or clonidine is occasionally useful. The only currently available medication that consistently slows a sinus tachycardia directly is propranolol, administered orally, 10 to 60 mg, four times daily. Drugs that block the slow inward current (see Chapter 10), such as verapamil, may also slow the rate of sinus node discharge but at present are available for oral use in the United States only as an investigational drug.

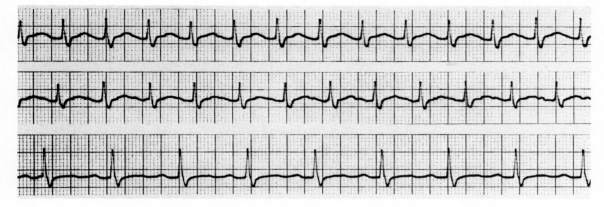

Fig. 8-6. Sinus tachycardia. Sinus tachycardia gradually slows to reveal clearer P waves in the bottom tracing. Monitor lead.

Rate: Top, 125 beats/minute; middle, 122 beats/minute; bottom, 82 beats/minute.
Rhythm: Regular.
P waves: Difficult to see in top strip. Precede each QRS complex at a regular interval with unchanging contour in middle and bottom strip.
PR interval: Top, cannot measure; middle, 0.20 second; bottom, 0.24 second.
QRS: 0.09 second.

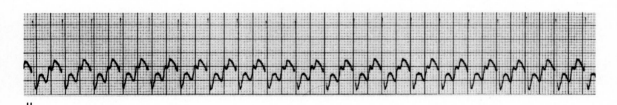

II

Fig. 8-7. Sinus tachycardia. Patient complained of chest pain and was noted to have a sinus tachycardia with ST segment depression, consistent with an anginal episode. Lead II.

Rate: 150 beats/minute.
Rhythm: Regular.
P waves: Normal, precede each QRS complex with regular contour at fixed interval.
PR interval: 0.12 second.
QRS: Normal, 0.09 second. ST segments are depressed.

SINUS BRADYCARDIA (Figs. 8-8 and 8-9)

Sinus bradycardia exists in the adult when the sinus node discharges at a rate less than 60 beats/minute. P waves have a normal contour and occur before each QRS complex with a constant PR interval exceeding 0.12 second. Sinus arrhythmia is frequently present.

Significance. Sinus bradycardia results from excessive vagal or decreased sympathetic tone. Eye surgery, meningitis, intracranial tumors, cervical and mediastinal tumors, and certain disease states such as myocardial infarction, myxedema, obstructive jaundice, and cardiac fibrosis may produce sinus bradycardia. In most instances, sinus bradycardia is a benign arrhythmia and may actually be beneficial by producing a longer period of diastole and increased ventricular filling. It occurs commonly during sleep, vomiting, or vasovagal syncope and may be produced by carotid sinus stimulation or by the administration of parasympathomimetic drugs. Sinus bradycardia occurring in patients who have myocardial infarction, more commonly diaphragmatic or posterior, may compromise optimal myocardial function and predispose to premature systoles and sustained tachyarrhythmias. More recent data suggest sinus bradycardia actually is beneficial in some patients who have acute myocardial infarction because it reduces oxygen demands, may help to minimize the size of the infarction, and may lessen the frequency of some arrhythmias. Patients with acute myocardial infarction who have sinus bradycardia generally have lower mortality than patients who have sinus tachycardia.

Treatment. Treatment of sinus bradycardia per se usually is not needed. If the patient with an acute myocardial infarction is asymptomatic, it is probably best not to try to speed the sinus rate. If the cardiac output is inadequate, or if arrhythmias are associated with the slow rate, atropine (0.5 mg IV as an initial dose, repeated if necessary) or isoproterenol (1 or 2 μg/minute IV) is usually effective. These drugs should be used cautiously, with care taken not to produce too rapid a rate. In patients who experience congestive failure as a result of chronic sinus bradycardia, electrical pacing may be needed. Atrial pacing is preferable to ventricular pacing, to preserve sequential AV contraction (see Chapter 11).

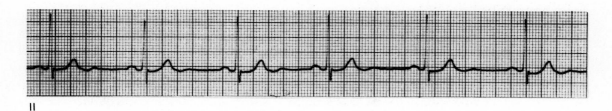

II

Fig. 8-8. Sinus bradycardia. Sinus bradycardia is present in this patient because of administration of propranolol. Lead II.

Rate: 46 beats/minute.
Rhythm: Regular.
P waves: Precede each QRS with a normal contour.
PR interval: 0.19 second.
QRS: 0.09 second.

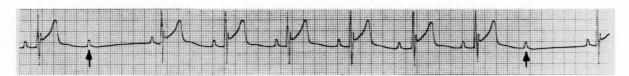

Fig. 8-9. Sinus bradycardia in a young patient. Type I (Wenckebach) AV block is also present and probably represents excessive vagal tone that may be normal in young individuals. Monitor lead. ST elevation is early repolarization.

Rate: Atrial, 55 beats/minute.
Rhythm: Atrial, regular; ventricular, irregular because of nonconducted P waves *(arrows)*.
PR interval: Increasing slightly from 0.18 second to 2.2 seconds.
QRS: 0.09 second.

SINUS ARRHYTHMIA (Figs. 8-10 to 8-12)

Sinus arrhythmia is characterized by a phasic variation in cycle length of greater than 0.16 second during sinus rhythm. It is the most frequent form of arrhythmia and occurs as a normal phenomenon. The P waves do not vary in morphology, and the PR interval is greater than 0.12 second and remains unchanged, since the focus of discharge is fixed within the sinus node. Occasionally the pacemaker focus may wander within the sinus node, producing P waves of slightly different contour (but not retrograde) and a changing PR interval (but not less than 0.12 second). Sinus arrhythmia commonly occurs in the young or aged, especially with slower heart rates or following enhanced vagal tone from digitalis or morphine administration. Sinus arrhythmia appears in two basic forms. In the respiratory form the PP interval cyclically shortens during inspiration as a result of reflex inhibition of vagal tone or enhancement of sympathetic tone or both. Breath holding eliminates the cycle length variation. Nonrespiratory sinus arrhythmia is characterized by a phasic variation unrelated to the respiratory cycle.

Significance. Symptoms produced by sinus arrhythmias are rare, but on occasion, if the pauses between beats are excessively long, palpitations or dizziness may be experienced. Marked sinus arrhythmia can produce a sinus pause sufficiently prolonged to induce syncope if not accompanied by an escape rhythm.

Treatment. Treatment is usually not necessary. Increasing the heart rate by exercise or drugs will abolish sinus arrhythmia. Symptomatic individuals may experience relief from feelings of palpitations through the use of sedatives, tranquilizers, atropine, ephedrine, or isoproterenol administration, as in the treatment of sinus bradycardia.

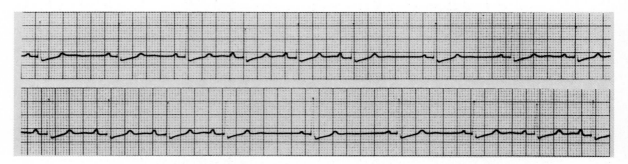

Fig. 8-10. Respiratory sinus arrhythmia. The phasic variation in heart rate corresponds to a respiratory rate of approximately 12 beats/minute. Monitor lead.

Rate: Sinus rate increases with inspiration and decreases with expiration at a rate of 53 to 80 beats/minute.

Rhythm: Irregular with repetitive phase variation in cycle length according to respiratory cycles. Cycle lengths vary by more than 0.16 second. Breath-holding eliminates the rate variations (not shown).

P waves: Precede each QRS complex with a normal, fairly constant contour.

PR interval: Normal, constant, 0.18 second.

QRS: Normal, 0.18 second.

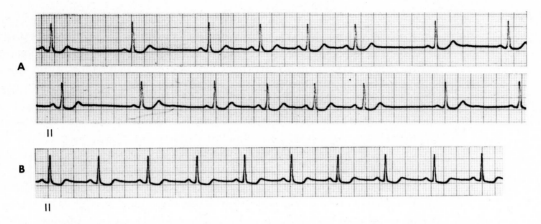

Fig. 8-11. Nonrespiratory sinus arrhythmia. In this instance it was caused by digitalis toxicity **(A)**. One week following discontinuation of digitalis the nonrespiratory sinus arrhythmia disappeared **(B)**.

Rate: Rate increases and decreases independently of respiration in **A** (47 to 80 beats/minute). Rate constant (78 beats/minute) in **B**.
Rhythm: **A,** Irregular with a repetitive phasic variation in cycle length which continues during breath-holding. **B,** Regular.
P waves: Precede each QRS with a normal, fairly constant contour.
PR interval: 0.12 second.
QRS: Normal, 0.06 second.

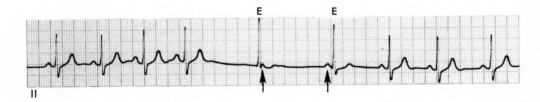

Fig. 8-12. Respiratory sinus arrhythmia. The first four P waves are fairly regular; the PR interval is 0.16 second and constant. Then the sinus node slows and the next two P waves occur much later (*arrows*). The marked sinus slowing allows a latent pacemaker—possibly located in the His bundle or high in the fascicles—to escape sinus domination, depolarize automatically, and discharge the ventricles (*E,* junctional escapes). A slight change in QRS contour is apparent in these beats. The sinus node then speeds up to resume control. This slightly complex arrhythmia is completely normal in an otherwise healthy person.

Rate: Rate increases with inspiration and decreases with expiration (55 to 80 beats/minute).
Rhythm: Irregular with a repetitive phasic variation in cycle length.
P waves: Normal, fairly constant contour.
PR interval: 0.16 second during sinus-conducted beats.
QRS: Normal, 0.08 second during sinus-conducted beats.

SINUS ARREST (Figs. 8-13 and 8-14)

Failure of sinus node discharge results in absence of atrial depolarization and periods of ventricular asystole if escape beats produced by latent pacemakers do not discharge. Sinus arrest may be produced by involvement of the sinus node or the sinus node artery by acute myocardial infarction, digitalis toxicity, excessive vagal tone, or degenerative forms of fibrosis.

Significance. Transient sinus arrest may have no clinical significance by itself if latent pacemakers promptly escape to prevent ventricular asystole (Fig. 8-13). Prolonged ventricular asystole results should the latent pacemakers fail to escape. Other arrhythmias may be precipitated by the slow rates (Fig. 8-14).

Treatment. Atropine (0.5 mg IV initially, repeated if necessary) or isoproterenol (1 or 2 μg/minute IV) may be tried as the first therapeutic approach. If these drugs are unsuccessful, atrial or ventricular pacing may be required. In patients who have a chronic form of sinus node disease characterized by marked sinus bradycardia or sinus arrest (sick sinus syndrome), permanent pacing is often necessary. Some of these patients experience sinus bradycardia alternating with periods of supraventricular tachycardia (bradycardia-tachycardia syndrome). These patients are best treated by a combination of drugs (to slow the ventricular rate during the supraventricular tachycardia) and implantation of a permanent demand pacemaker (to prevent the slow rate when the tachycardia terminates).

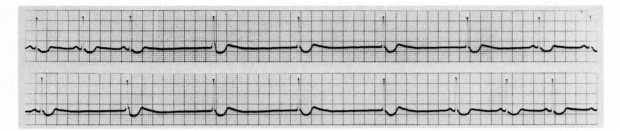

Fig. 8-13. Sinus arrest. After three sinus beats in the top strip, sinus arrest occurs followed by junctional escape beats. The sinus rhythm returns at the end of the strip and once again restores sinus rhythm for the last two beats. A similar event happens in the lower recording. Monitor lead.

Rate: Varying: junctional escape rate, 38 beats/minute; sinus rate, 70 beats/minute.
Rhythm: Irregular.
P waves: Normal contour, intermittently precede QRS complexes.
PR interval: Constant when P waves precede QRS contours, 0.18 second.
QRS: Normal, 0.09 second.

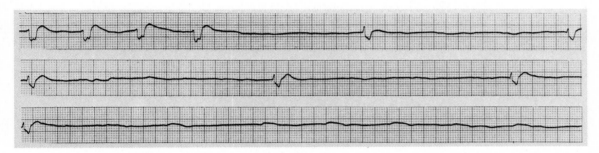

Fig. 8-14. Sinus arrest with asystole. These monitor lead tracings were recorded during a resuscitation procedure in a patient with recurrent syncope. No atrial activity is apparent, and the slight undulations in the base line represent chest compression during resuscitation. The patient has intermittent junctional or most probably ventricular escapes and then develops complete atrial and ventricular asystole.

Rate: Varying.
Rhythm: Irregular.
P waves: Not seen.
PR interval: Not measurable.
QRS: 0.16 second.

SINOATRIAL EXIT BLOCK (Figs. 8-15 and 8-16)

Sinoatrial (SA) block is a conduction disturbance during which an impulse formed within the SA node is blocked from depolarizing the atria. SA exit block is indicated on the ECG by the absence of the normally expected P wave(s). The length of the pause between P waves is a multiple of the basic PP interval, approximately two, less commonly three or four times the normal PP interval (type II exit block). Type I (Wenckebach) SA exit block may also occur, in which case the PP interval progressively shortens prior to the pause, and the duration of the pause is less than two PP cycles.

Significance. SA exit block may be caused by excessive vagal stimulation, by acute infections such as diphtheria or rheumatic carditis, by atherosclerosis involving the SA nodal artery, or by fibrosis involving the atrium. Occlusion of the SA nodal artery owing to acute myocardial infarction may result in an atrial infarction and produce SA exit block. Medications such as quinidine, procainamide, and digitalis may lead to SA exit block. SA block is usually transient and often of no clinical importance except to prompt a search for the underlying cause. Syncope may result if the SA block is prolonged and unaccompanied by an AV junctional or ventricular escape rhythm. Digitalis produces type II SA exit block (but not type I AV block).

Treatment. Therapy for symptomatic SA exit block is directed toward increasing sympathetic tone and decreasing parasympathetic tone. Thus atropine and isoproterenol are useful, as described under sinus bradycardia. If the clinical situation demands therapy and pharmacologic measures are not effective, atrial or ventricular pacing may be indicated.

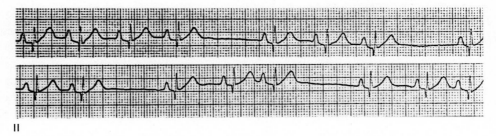

II

Fig. 8-15. Sinoatrial (SA) exit block (type II). The longer PP intervals are approximately twice the shorter PP intervals, indicating an intermittent 2:1 sinus exit block of the type II variety.

Rate: Varying, slow (43 to 68 beats/minute).
Rhythm: Irregular; pauses are twice as long as the shorter intervals.
P waves: Contour normal, precede each QRS complex; intermittent loss of P wave.
PR interval: 0.16 second.
QRS: Normal, 0.08 second.

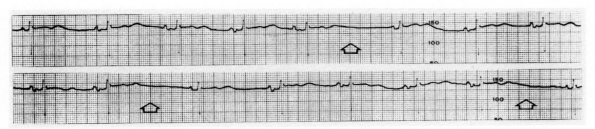

Fig. 8-16. Sinoatrial (SA) exit block, type I (Wenckebach block). The following characteristics of this tracing suggest the diagnosis of a Wenckebach exit block from a sinus node. *1,* The PP intervals progressively shorten until (*2*) a pause in atrial activity occurs. *3,* The duration of the pause is less than twice the shortest PP interval. *4,* The PP interval after the pause exceeds the PP interval preceding the pause, which is the shortest PP interval. Monitor lead.

Rate: Varying from 33 to 50 beats/minute.
Rhythm: The four features mentioned above.
P waves: Biphasic, but fairly constant contour; intermittent loss of P wave, producing a pause *(arrows)*.
PR interval: 0.24 second.
QRS: 0.07 second.

WANDERING PACEMAKER (Figs. 8-17 and 8-18)

Wandering pacemaker, a variant of sinus arrhythmia, involves the passive transfer of the dominant pacemaker focus from the sinus node to latent pacemakers with the next highest degree of automaticity, in other atrial sites or in the AV junctional tissue. Thus only one pacemaker is operative at a time. As with other forms of sinus arrhythmia, the change occurs in a gradual fashion over the duration of several beats. The ECG displays a cyclic increase of the RR interval, a PR interval that gradually shortens and may become less than 0.12 second, and a change in P wave configuration until it becomes negative in lead I or II or becomes buried in the QRS complex. A slight change in QRS configuration may occur owing to aberrant conduction. Generally these changes occur in reverse as the pacemaker shifts back to the sinus node. Rarely a wandering pacemaker may appear without changes in rate.

Significance. Wandering pacemaker is a normal phenomenon that is often seen in the very young or in the aged, and particularly in athletes. Persistence of an AV junctional rhythm for long periods of time, however, usually indicates underlying heart disease.

Treatment. Treatment of a wandering pacemaker usually is not indicated. Sympathomimetic agents such as ephedrine or isoproterenol or parasympatholytic agents such as atropine can be used if necessary (see discussion of sinus bradycardia).

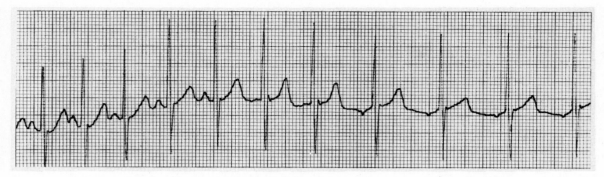

Fig. 8-17. Wandering atrial pacemaker. When the heart rate is fast, the P wave is upright and gradually becomes inverted as the heart rate slows and P wave activation changes. Monitor lead.

Rate: Varying, 80 to 135 beats/minute.
Rhythm: Irregular with a repetitive phasic variation in cycle length, as in sinus arrhythmia.
P waves: Varying contour, indicating shift in pacemaker site or change in activation sequence.
PR interval: Constant, 0.13 second.
QRS: 0.10 second.

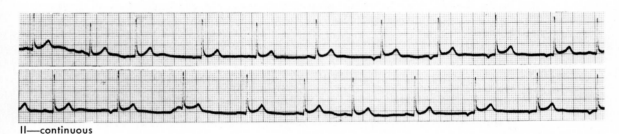

II—continuous

Fig. 8-18. Wandering atrial pacemaker. As the heart rate slows, the P waves become inverted and then gradually revert toward normal as the heart rate speeds. The PR interval shortens to 0.14 second with the inverted P wave and is 0.16 second with the upright P wave.

Rate: Varying, slow (52 to 72 beats/minute).
Rhythm: Irregular with a repetitive phasic variation in cycle length as in sinus arrhythmia.
P waves: Varying contour, indicating shift in pacemaker site. Become negative in lead II.
PR interval: Varies, 0.14, 0.16 second.
QRS: Normal, 0.08 second.

PREMATURE ATRIAL SYSTOLES (Figs. 8-19 to 8-22)

Premature systoles are the most common cause of an intermittent pulse. They may originate in any area of the heart, most frequently in the ventricles, less often in the atria and the AV junctional region, and rarely in the sinus node. Although premature systoles arise in normal hearts, they are more often associated with organic disease, particularly in older patients.

The diagnosis of premature atrial systoles is indicated by a premature P wave and a PR interval greater than 0.12 second. Although the contour of the premature P wave may resemble the normal sinus P wave, it generally is different. Variations in the basic sinus rate at times may make the diagnosis of prematurity difficult, but differences in the contour of the P wave are usually quite apparent and indicate a different focus of origin. When a premature atrial systole occurs early in diastole, conduction may not be completely normal. The AV junction may still be refractory from the preceding beat and will prevent propagation of the impulse (blocked premature atrial systole) or cause conduction to be slowed (prolonged PR interval). As a general rule, a short RP interval produced by an early premature atrial systole close to the preceding QRS complex is followed by a long PR interval. On occasion, when the AV junction has sufficiently repolarized to conduct normally, the supraventricular QRS complex may be aberrant in configuration because the ventricle has not completely repolarized (see discussion of supraventricular arrhythmias with abnormal QRS complexes, Figs. 8-21 and 8-22).

The length of the pause following any premature beat or series of premature beats is determined by the interaction of several factors. If the premature atrial systole occurs when the sinus node is not refractory, the impulse may conduct to the sinus node, discharge it prematurely, and cause the next sinus cycle to begin from that point. The interval between the two normal beats flanking a premature atrial systole that has reset the timing of the basic sinus rhythm is less than twice the normal cycle, and the pause after the premature atrial systole is said to be "noncompensatory." The interval following the premature atrial systole is generally longer than one sinus cycle, however. Less commonly the premature atrial systole may find the sinus node refractory, in which case the timing of the basic sinus rhythm is not altered, and the interval between the two normal beats flanking the premature atrial systole is twice the normal PP cycle. The interval following this premature atrial discharge is therefore said to be a "full compensatory pause." A *compensatory pause* is one of sufficient duration to make the interval between the two normal beats on each side of the premature beat equal to twice the basic cycle length. However, sinus arrhythmia may lengthen or shorten this pause.

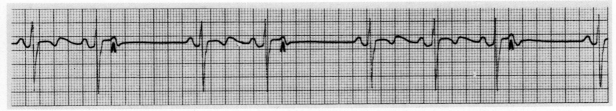

Fig. 8-19. Premature atrial systoles, blocked and hidden in the T wave. The deformed T waves (*arrows*) indicate a nonconducted premature atrial systole that blocks within the AV node or His bundle. The premature atrial complex discharges the sinus node and delays its return so that the PP interval from the premature atrial complex to the next sinus P wave exceeds the normal sinus PP interval. Monitor lead.

Rate: 67 beats/minute during sinus rhythm.
Rhythm: Varying due to premature atrial systoles.
P waves: Premature atrial systoles are hidden within and deform the T waves.
PR interval: Of normal sinus beats, 0.18 second.
QRS: 0.10 second; monitor lead.

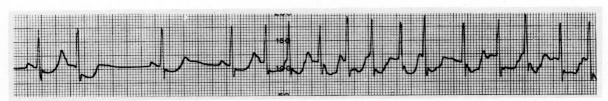

Fig. 8-20. Premature atrial systole precipitating atrial flutter-fibrillation. A premature atrial complex is hidden within the T wave of the first QRS complex and occurs again in the T wave of the fourth QRS complex. This premature atrial complex precipitates atrial flutter-fibrillation. Monitor lead.

Rate: Varying.
Rhythm: Varying due to premature atrial complexes and atrial flutter-fibrillation.
P waves: Premature atrial complexes hidden in the T waves.
PR interval: Of normally conducted beats, 0.14 second.
QRS: 0.08 second.

Significance. Premature atrial systoles may occur in a variety of situations: for example, during infection, inflammation, or myocardial ischemia, or they may be provoked by a variety of medications, by tension states, or by tobacco and caffeine. Premature atrial systoles may precipitate or presage the occurrence of a sustained supraventricular tachycardia.

Treatment. In the absence of organic heart disease, treatment may not be necessary, unless the patient complains of symptoms such as palpitations or has recurrent tachycardias or an excessive number of atrial extrasystoles. If treatment is indicated, for example, in a patient with acute myocardial infarction, initial therapy should probably be with digitalis, combined with quinidine or procainamide if digitalis alone is not successful. Sedation and/or omission of alcohol, caffeine, or smoking may be helpful in some patients.

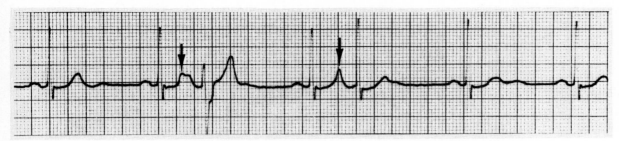

Fig. 8-21. Premature atrial systoles with and without aberrancy. The first premature atrial systole *(arrow)* occurs at a shorter RP interval than does the second premature atrial systole *(arrow)* and conducts with a bundle branch block contour (probably right bundle branch block in this monitor lead). The first premature atrial systole conducts with aberrancy while the second does not because the first reaches the bundle branch system before complete recovery of repolarization.

Rate: 50 beats/minute during the normally conducted beats.

Rhythm: Irregular because of the premature atrial systoles.

P waves: Normal for the normally conducted sinus beats. Premature atrial systoles deform the T waves.

PR interval: Of premature atrial systoles, prolonged because the AV node and/or His bundle has incompletely recovered. PR interval of first premature atrial asystole is approximately 0.26 second and that of the second premature atrial systole approximately 0.22 second. The PR interval of normally conducted sinus beats is 0.19 second.

QRS: Of normally conducted beats, 0.07 second; of aberrantly conducted QRS complex, 0.12 second.

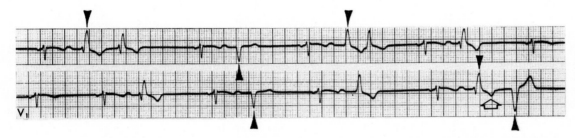

Fig. 8-22. Premature atrial systoles that produce functional right and functional left bundle branch block. Upright arrowheads point to QRS complexes that conduct with complete or incomplete functional left bundle branch block while inverted arrowheads point to some of the QRS complexes that conduct with functional right bundle branch block. Note that the latter have both a monophasic and triphasic contour. The deformed T waves *(open arrow* at end of the last strip) indicate a premature atrial complex. They occur singly and in pairs.

Rate: Varying due to premature atrial systoles.

Rhythm: Irregular because of premature atrial systoles.

P waves: During sinus rhythm, normal; P waves of premature atrial systoles are hard to discern because they occur in the preceding T wave.

PR interval: Of normal sinus beats, 0.12 second; of premature atrial complexes, prolonged and of differing durations because of differences in RP intervals.

Paroxysmal supraventricular tachycardia (Figs. 8-23 to 8-25)

The tachycardias formerly called paroxysmal atrial (PAT) and junctional (PJT) tachycardias, are caused most commonly by AV nodal reentry or reentry over an accessory pathway and are often called, nonspecifically, paroxysmal supraventricular tachycardia (PSVT) when the mechanism responsible for the tachycardia cannot be determined with certainty. In this section AV nodal reentry is examined. Reentry over an accessory pathway is dealt with in the section on Wolff-Parkinson-White syndrome.

AV NODAL REENTRY

AV nodal reentry is characterized by a rapid, regular tachycardia of sudden onset and termination, occurring at rates generally between 150 and 250 beats/minute. Uncommonly the rate may be as low as 110 beats/minute and occasionally, especially in children, the rate may exceed 250 beats/minute. Unless aberrant ventricular conduction exists, the QRS complex is normal in contour and duration. The retrograde P wave is usually lost within the QRS complex.

AV nodal reentry recorded at the onset begins abruptly, usually following a premature atrial systole that conducts with a prolonged PR interval; the abrupt termination is sometimes followed by a brief period of asystole. The RR interval may shorten during the course of the first few beats at the onset or lengthen during the course of the last few beats preceding termination of the tachycardia. Variation in cycle length is usually caused by variation in AV nodal conduction time. The mechanism of the tachycardia is reentry within the AV node (see Fig. 8-82).

Significance. AV nodal reentry may occur at any age and is often unassociated with underlying heart disease. The arrhythmia may be related to specific inciting causes such as overexertion, emotional stimuli, and coffee and smoking, although this is often difficult to prove; it may follow a specific pattern, or its onset may be unrelated to any particular event.

Symptoms frequently accompany the attack and range from feelings of palpitations, nervousness, or anxiety to angina, frank heart failure, or shock, depending on the duration and rate of the PSVT and the presence of organic heart disease. The PSVT may cause syncope because of the rapid ventricular rate, reduced cardiac output, and cerebral circulation or because of asystole when the PSVT terminates, owing to tachycardia-induced depression of sinus node automaticity. The prognosis for patients without heart disease is usually quite good.

Treatment. Treatment of the acute attack depends on the clinical situation, how well the PSVT is tolerated, the natural history of the attacks in the individual patient, and the presence of associated disease. For some patients, rest, reassurance, and sedation may be all that are required to abort an attack.

1. Vagal maneuvers, including carotid sinus massage, Valsalva, and gagging, serve as the first line of therapy and either terminate PSVT or leave it unaffected (actually, slight slowing may occur during vagal stimulation). These maneuvers should be retried after *each* pharmacologic approach.
2. Cholinergic drugs, particularly edrophonium chloride (Tensilon), a short-

acting cholinesterase inhibitor, may terminate PSVT when administered initially at a dose of 3 to 5 mg IV and, if unsuccessful, repeated at a dose of 10 mg IV. Its action is rapid in onset and short in duration, with minimal side effects. Edrophonium chloride should be used cautiously or not at all in patients who are hypotensive or who have lung disease, especially asthmatics.

3. Verapamil, one of the new, so-called calcium antagonists, at a dose of 5 to 10 mg IV, terminates PSVT successfully in about 2 minutes in over 90% of instances. It has become the preferred treatment if the simple vagal maneuvers fail.[12]

4. Pressor drugs may terminate PSVT by inducing reflex vagal stimulation mediated via baroreceptors in the carotid sinus and aorta when the systolic blood pressure is acutely elevated to levels of about 180 mm Hg. One of the following drugs, diluted in 5 to 10 ml of 5% dextrose and water, may be given over a period of 1 to 3 minutes; phenylephrine hydrochloride (Neo-Synephrine), 0.5 to 1.0 mg; methoxamine hydrochloride (Vasoxyl), 3 to 5 mg; or metaraminol (Aramine), 0.5 to 2.0 mg. Pressor drugs should be used cautiously or not at all in the elderly or in patients with organic heart disease, significant hypertension, hyperthyroidism, or acute myocardial infarction. This potentially dangerous and almost always uncomfortable procedure is rarely needed any longer, unless the patient is also hypotensive. Other, safer procedures are preferred.

5. If these approaches are unsuccessful, IV digitalis administration may be attempted next, using one of the following short-acting digitalis preparations: ouabain, 0.25 to 0.50 mg IV, followed by 0.1 mg every 30 to 60 minutes if needed, keeping the total dose less than 1.0 mg within a 24-hour period; digoxin (Lanoxin), 0.5 to 1.0 mg IV, followed by 0.25 mg every 2 to 4 hours, with a total dose less than 1.5 mg within a 24-hour period; or deslanoside (Cedilanid-D), 0.8 mg IV, followed by 0.4 mg every 2 to 4 hours, restricting the total dose to less than 2.0 mg within a 24-hour period. Oral digitalis administration to terminate an acute attack is generally not indicated. Vagal maneuvers, previously ineffective, may terminate PSVT following digitalis administration and therefore should be repeated.

6. Propranolol (Inderal) given IV at a rate of 0.5 to 1 mg/minute for a total dose of 0.5 to 3 mg may be tried if digitalis administration is unsuccessful. Propranolol must be used cautiously, if at all, in patients who have heart failure or chronic lung disease because its adrenergic beta-receptor blocking action depresses myocardial contractility and may produce bronchospasm.

Prior to administering digitalis or propranolol, it is advisable to reassess the clinical status of the patient and consider whether DC cardioversion may be advisable at this stage. DC shock, administered to patients who have received excessive amounts of digitalis, may be dangerous and result in serious postshock ventricular arrhythmias (see Chapter 12 for discussion).

7. Particularly if signs or symptoms of cardiac decompensation occur, DC electrical shock should be attempted next. DC shock, synchronized to the QRS complex to avoid precipitating ventricular fibrillation, successfully terminates PSVT with energies in the range of 10 to 50 watt-seconds; higher energies may be required in some instances. Short-acting barbiturates like sodium methohexital (Brevital), 50 to 120 mg given IV at a rate of 50 mg/30 seconds, may be used to provide anesthesia, or diazepam (Valium), 5 to 15 mg given IV at a rate of 5 mg/minute, may be used to provide sedation and amnesia. Doses must be individualized and in general should be reduced for patients who have heart failure, hypotension, or liver disease. During DC cardioversion a physician skilled in airway management should be in attendance, an IV route established, and all equipment and drugs necessary for emergency resuscitation immediately accessible. One hundred percent oxygen is administered throughout the procedure, employing manually assisted ventilation if necessary.

    If DC shock becomes necessary in patients who have received large amounts of digitalis, one should begin with 1 to 5 watt-seconds and gradually increase the energy level in increments of approximately 25 to 50 watt-seconds as long as premature ventricular systoles do not result. If premature ventricular systoles occur but can be suppressed with lidocaine or phenytoin, the next higher energy level may be tried.

8. In the event that digitalis has been given in large doses and DC shock is contraindicated, right atrial pacing may restore sinus rhythm, presumably by prematurely depolarizing one of the pathways required for continued reentry (Fig. 8-25).[14] In some patients, right atrial pacing may precipitate atrial fibrillation; however, because the latter is generally accompanied by a slower ventricular rate, the patient's clinical status improves.

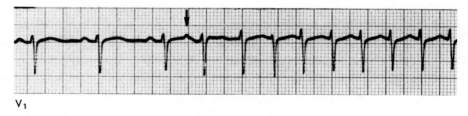

V₁

Fig. 8-23. Paroxysmal supraventricular tachycardia. Three sinus beats are interrupted by a premature atrial systole *(arrow)*, which conducts with PR prolongation and initiates the supraventricular tachycardia.

Rate: Sinus rhythm, 83 beats/minute; paroxysmal supraventricular tachycardia, 190 beats/minute.
Rhythm: Regular during sinus rhythm and during paroxysmal supraventricular tachycardia.
P waves: Seen in first four beats but not afterward.
PR interval: Normal during sinus beats, 0.16 second; slightly prolonged (0.20 second) during premature atrial systole.
QRS: Normal, 0.08 second.
Arrhythmia: Sudden initiation of paroxysmal supraventricular tachycardia by a premature atrial systole that conducts with PR prolongation.

9. Procainamide (Pronestyl), quinidine, disopyramide (Norpace), or phenytoin (Dilantin) may be required to terminate PSVT in some patients. Unless contraindicated, DC cardioversion should be employed prior to using these agents, which are more often administered to prevent recurrences.

Prevention of recurrences is often more difficult than terminating the acute episode. Smoking, alcohol, or excessive fatigue, if identified as precipitating factors, should be avoided. Initially, one must decide whether the frequency and severity of the attacks warrant drug prophylaxis. For example, an attempt should probably not be made to suppress PSVT occurring twice yearly in an otherwise healthy patient.

1. If drug prophylaxis is indicated, digitalis is the initial drug of choice. The speed at which digitalization is achieved is determined by the clinical situation. Using digoxin, rapid oral digitalization can be accomplished in 24 to 36 hours with an initial dose of 1.0 to 1.5 mg, followed by 0.25 to 0.5 mg every 6 hours for a total dose of 2.0 to 3.0 mg. A less rapid oral regimen digitalizes in 2 to 3 days with an initial dose of 0.75 to 1.0 mg, followed by 0.25 to 0.5 mg every 12 hours for a total dose of 2.0 to 3.0 mg.

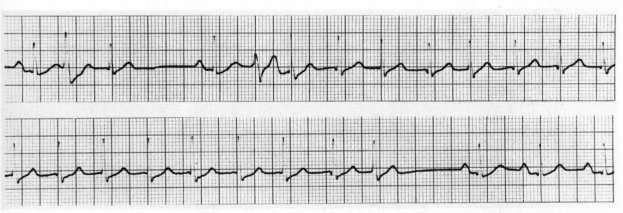

Fig. 8-24. Initiation of paroxysmal supraventricular tachycardia (PSVT) following a premature ventricular complex and spontaneous termination of PSVT. In the top panel, PSVT begins following the fifth QRS complex, which is a premature ventricular complex. Two interpretations are possible. The first possibility is that the normally conducted sinus complex occurs in the T wave of the premature ventricular complex (PVC) and conducts with a prolonged PR interval (i.e., the PVC is interpolated) and initiates PSVT. The second possibility is that the PVC conducts retrogradely to the atrium and initiates the PSVT in that manner. In the bottom strip, the PSVT terminates spontaneously with a slight pause. Monitor lead.

Rate: During PSVT, 120 beats/minute.
Rhythm: Fairly regular during PSVT.
P waves: Cannot be seen during PSVT.
PR interval: Cannot determine during PSVT.
QRS: Normal, 0.07 second.

Alternatively, digoxin administered as a maintenance dose of 0.125 to 0.5 mg achieves digitalization in about 1 week. Because of its shorter half-life, digoxin may provide more effective control when administered twice daily. Digitoxin, which has a longer duration of action, may be used instead of digoxin. Oral digitalization with digitoxin may be accomplished in 24 to 36 hours with an initial dose of 0.5 to 0.8 mg, followed by 0.2 mg every 6 to 8 hours until reaching a total dose of 1.2 mg. A slower approach involves administering 0.2 mg three times daily for 2 to 3 days. Complete digitalization can also be accomplished in about 1 month by simply giving a maintenance dose of 0.05 to 0.2 mg daily.

2. If digitalis alone is unsuccessful, one can then add quinidine, 200 to 400 mg every 6 hours, or propranolol (Inderal), 10 to 40 mg every 6 hours. Verapamil (80 to 120 mg every 6 to 8 hours) combined with digitalis may be very effective treatment. Oral verapamil is still an investigational drug at the time of this writing.[13]

3. If a combination of digitalis and quinidine or digitalis and propranolol is unsuccessful, concomitant administration of all three drugs, that is, digitalis, quinidine, and propranolol, may be tried. If this regimen also fails, empiric trials with other antiarrhythmic agents such as procainamide, disopyramide, or phenytoin may be warranted.

4. For many patients, pacemaker implantation is an acceptable treatment. Rapid atrial pacing promptly terminates PSVT, restoring sinus rhythm immediately or sometimes after a transient episode of atrial fibrillation. Some pacemaker units need to be activated by the patient when PSVT occurs; other units discharge automatically when they detect the onset of PSVT. Such pacing devices can be combined with drug therapy (see Chapter 11).

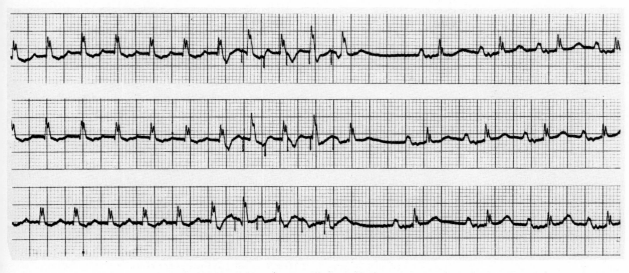

Fig. 8-25. Pacing-induced termination of PSVT. The patient had recurrent episodes of PSVT that were easily terminated by rapid atrial pacing. Pacing stimuli can be seen prior to the onset of sinus rhythm in the midportion of each monitor lead tracing.

Rate: During PSVT, 150 beats/minute.
Rhythm: During PSVT, regular.
P waves: Not seen during PSVT. P waves during sinus rhythm were abnormal with a low-amplitude biphasic component following an initial positive component.
PR interval: During sinus rhythm, 0.24 second; during PSVT, cannot be discerned.
QRS: 0.08 second.

ATRIAL FLUTTER (Figs. 8-26 to 8-29)

The atrial rate during atrial flutter is usually 250 to 350 beats/minute; antiarrhythmic drugs such as quinidine or procainamide may reduce the rate to 200 beats/minute. In patients who have untreated atrial flutter the ventricular rate is usually half the atrial rate, that is, 150 beats/minute. A significantly slower ventricular rate (in the absence of drugs) suggests abnormal AV conduction. Atrial flutter in children, in patients who have the preexcitation syndrome or hyperthyroidism, and occasionally in otherwise normal adults may conduct to the ventricle in a 1:1 fashion, producing a ventricular rate of 300 beats/minute. In patients whose atrial flutter rate has been slowed by drugs, 1:1 conduction to the ventricle may also occur.

The ECG reveals identically recurring, regular, sawtooth-shaped flutter waves and evidence of continual electrical activity (lack of an isoelectric interval between flutter waves), often best visualized in leads II, III, aV_F, or V_1. Commonly the flutter waves appear inverted in these leads. Less commonly the flutter waves are upright (positive) in these leads. If the AV conduction ratio remains constant, the ventricular rhythm will be regular; if the ratio of conducted beats varies (usually the result of a Wenckebach AV block), the ventricular rhythm will be irregular. Impure flutter (flutter-fibrillation), occurring at a faster rate than pure flutter, shows variability in the contour and spacing of the flutter waves and may represent dissimilar atrial rhythms, that is, fibrillation in one atrium or part of the atrium and a slower, more regular rhythm in the opposite atrium.

Significance. Atrial flutter is a less common tachyarrhythmia than is atrial fibrillation. Although paroxysmal atrial flutter usually indicates the presence of cardiac disease, it may occur in normal hearts. Chronic (persistent) atrial flutter

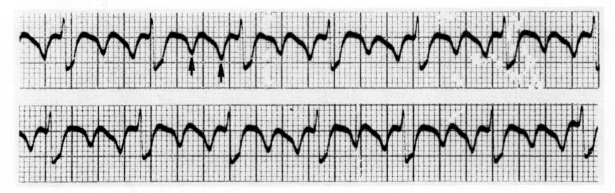

Fig. 8-26. Atrial flutter. Flutter waves indicated by arrows. The conduction ratio is 3:1, that is, three flutter waves to one QRS complex and is a less common conduction ratio. Monitor lead.

Rate: Atrial, 270 beats/minute; ventricular, 90 beats/minute.
Rhythm: Atrial, regular; ventricular, regular.
P waves: Flutter waves with regular oscillations resembling a sawtooth pattern are apparent.
PR interval: Flutter-R interval is constant. Assuming that the flutter wave immediately preceding the QRS complex conducts to the ventricle, the flutter-R interval is approximately 0.18 second.
QRS: 0.12 second.

rarely occurs in the absence of underlying heart disease. Atrial flutter usually responds to carotid sinus massage with a decrease in ventricular rate in stepwise multiples, reversing to the former ventricular rate at the termination of carotid massage. The ratio of conducted atrial impulses to ventricular responses is most often an even number, for example, 2:1 or 4:1. Very rarely will sinus rhythm follow carotid sinus massage. Exercise, by enhancing sympathetic tone, lessening parasympathetic tone, or both, may reduce the AV conduction delay and produce an increase in the ventricular rate.

Treatment. Treatment for atrial flutter is as follows:

1. Synchronous DC cardioversion is commonly the preferred initial treatment for atrial flutter, since it promptly and effectively restores sinus rhythm with energies less than 50 watt-seconds. If DC shock results in atrial fibrillation, a second shock with a higher energy level may be used to restore sinus rhythm, or, depending on the clinical circumstance, the atrial fibrillation may be left untreated. The untreated fibrillation will usually revert to atrial flutter or sinus rhythm.

2. If the patient cannot be cardioverted or the DC cardioversion is contraindicated (for example, after administering large amounts of digitalis) rapid atrial pacing can effectively terminate atrial flutter in many patients.

3. If the patient cannot be cardioverted or if the atrial flutter recurs at frequent intervals, therapy with a short-acting digitalis preparation, such as digoxin or deslanoside, should be prescribed. The dose of digitalis necessary to slow the ventricular response varies and at times may result in toxic levels because it is often difficult to slow the ventricular rate during atrial flutter. Frequently, atrial fibrillation develops after digitalization and may revert to normal sinus rhythm on withdrawal of digitalis; occasionally, normal sinus rhythm may occur without intervening atrial fibrillation.

4. Verapamil, in an initial bolus of 5 to 10 mg IV followed by a constant infusion at a rate of 0.005 mg/kg/minute, may be used to slow the ventricular response. Verapamil less commonly restores sinus rhythm in patients who have atrial flutter.[12]

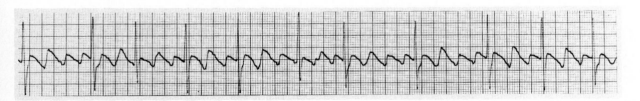

Fig. 8-27. Atrial flutter slowed by an antiarrhythmic agent. The atrial flutter in this patient had a rate of 300 beats/minute prior to therapy but was slowed by an experimental antiarrhythmic agent, amiodarone. Monitor lead.

Rate: Atrial, 200 beats/minute; ventricular, 52 to 86 beats/minute.
Rhythm: Atrial, regular; ventricular, irregular.
P waves: Flutter waves are apparent.
PR interval: The flutter-R interval varies as the conduction ratio varies.
QRS: Normal, 0.08 second.

5. If the atrial flutter persists after digitalization, quinidine, 200 to 400 mg orally every 6 hours, is used to restore sinus rhythm. Large doses of quinidine, formerly used to terminate atrial flutter prior to the development of DC cardioversion, are no longer warranted. If atrial flutter persists after

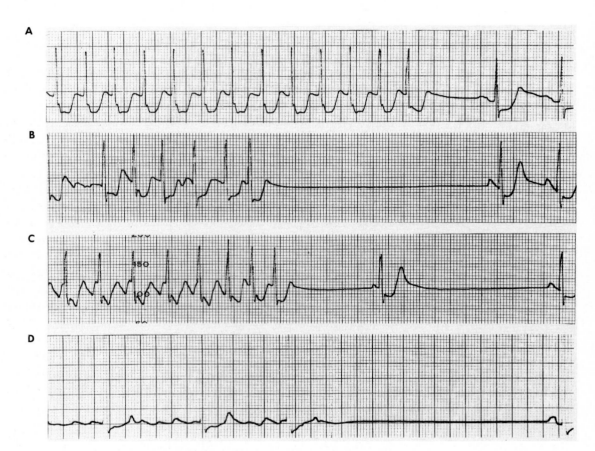

Fig. 8-28. Termination of multiple supraventricular tachycardias. In panel **A**, paroxysmal supraventricular tachycardia abruptly terminates with only a short pause before restoration of sinus rhythm. In panels **B** and **C**, atrial flutter-fibrillation and pure atrial flutter, respectively, terminate on separate occasions in the same patient. In panel **B**, a fairly long period of asystole results before restoration of the first sinus beat while the lengthy pause is interrupted by an escape beat in panel **C**. In panel **D**, termination of atrial flutter-fibrillation in another patient results in a long period of asystole before the first sinus beat occurs. The long pauses in **B, C,** and **D** are consistent with sick sinus syndrome and episodes of bradycardia-tachycardia. Monitor leads.

Rate: 158 beats/minute in panel **A**; varying ventricular rate, approximately 150 beats/minute in panel **B**; 136 beats/minute in panel **C**; 48 beats/minute in panel **D**.

Rhythm: Atrial and ventricular rhythm regular in panel **A**; atrial and ventricular rhythm irregular in panel **B**; atrial rhythm regular and ventricular rhythm irregular in panel **C**; atrial rhythm and ventricular rhythm irregular in panel **D**.

PR interval: Not measurable.

QRS: Normal in all panels.

digitalis and quinidine administration, termination may be attempted with DC cardioversion and the patient maintained on both digitalis and quinidine following reversion to sinus rhythm. Sometimes, treatment of the specific, underlying disorder, for example, thyrotoxicosis, is necessary to effect conversion to sinus rhythm.

6. In certain instances atrial flutter may continue, and if the ventricular rate can be controlled with digitalis, conversion may not be indicated. Quinidine maintenance therapy should be discontinued if flutter remains. It is important to remember that quinidine and procainamide should *not* be used unless the patient is fully digitalized. Both drugs have a vagolytic action and also directly slow the atrial rate. These two effects may facilitate AV conduction sufficiently to result in a 1:1 ventricular response to the atrial flutter, unless digitalis has been administered previously.

7. Propranolol effectively diminishes the ventricular response to atrial flutter and may be used together with digitalis in patients in whom the ventricular rate is not decreased after digitalization. Propranolol does not appear to affect the atrial rate during atrial flutter.

8. Uncommonly, atrial flutter may be resistant to cardioversion as well as to the AV blocking effects of digitalis. Rapid atrial pacing, on a temporary or permanent basis, may be used to convert flutter to fibrillation with a decrease in the ventricular rate.

9. Rarely, neostigmine (Prostigmin), 0.25 to 0.5 mg subcutaneously, or edrophonium (Tensilon), 0.25 to 2.0 mg/minute in an IV solution, may be administered over a few days to control the ventricular rate.

Prevention of recurrent atrial flutter is often difficult to achieve but should be approached as outlined for the prevention of PSVT caused by AV nodal reentry. If recurrences cannot be prevented, the aim of therapy is directed toward a controlled ventricular rate when the flutter does recur, with digitalis alone or combined with propranolol, or with oral verapamil. (At the time of this writing, oral verapamil is still an investigational drug, whereas IV verapamil is approved.)

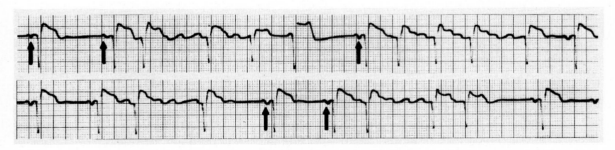

Fig. 8-29. Intermittent atrial flutter. Atrial flutter starts and stops intermittently throughout this continuous recording. Monitor lead.

Rate and rhythm: Both atrial and ventricular rate and rhythm vary.

P waves: Precede some QRS complexes. Atrial flutter waves precede other QRS complexes. Several P waves indicated by arrows.

PR interval: 0.14 second when it can be measured.

QRS: 0.08 second.

ATRIAL FIBRILLATION (Figs. 8-30 and 8-31)

Atrial fibrillation is characterized by a total disorganization of atrial activity without effective atrial contraction. The ECG reveals small deflections appearing for the most part as irregular base-line undulations of variable amplitude and contour at a rate of 305 to 600 per minute. The ventricular response is totally irregular, and if the patient is untreated, the rate is usually between 100 and 160 beats/minute. Carotid sinus massage slows the ventricular rate, but the rhythm remains completely irregular. The conversion of atrial flutter to atrial fibrillation is usually accompanied by a *slowing* of the ventricular rate because more atrial impulses become blocked at the AV node. As a result, it is generally easier to slow the ventricular rate with digitalis during atrial fibrillation than during atrial flutter. When the ventricular rhythm becomes regular in patients with atrial fibrillation, four explanations are possible: conversion to sinus rhythm, conversion to atrial flutter, development of atrial tachycardia, or development of an independent junctional or ventricular rhythm (or tachycardia) controlling the ventricles and giving rise to AV dissociation. In the last two instances, digitalis intoxication must be suspected. If after a period of regularization the ventricular rhythm becomes irregular again in a patient who has been given an excessive amount of digitalis, it may be due to an exit block, generally of the Wenckebach type (see p. 243), from the junctional or ventricular focus.

Significance. Similar to other tachyarrhythmias, atrial fibrillation may be chronic or paroxysmal; the former is almost always associated with underlying heart disease, whereas the latter may occur in clinically normal patients. Underlying heart disease is more frequent in patients who have atrial fibrillation than in patients who have atrial flutter. The arrhythmia is commonly seen in patients who have rheumatic mitral stenosis, thyrotoxicosis, cardiomyopathy, hypertensive heart disease, pericarditis, and coronary heart disease.

Approximately 30% of all patients who have atrial fibrillation experience systemic or pulmonary emboli. Such a catastrophe is most common in patients who have rheumatic mitral valvular disease. Of the emboli that occur in patients with mitral stenosis, 90% occur in patients who have atrial fibrillation.

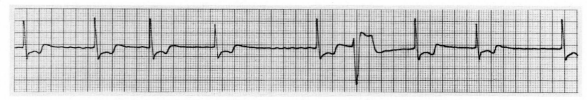

Fig. 8-30. Atrial fibrillation. Atrial activity is present as the undulating wavy base line seen in the midportion of the ECG strip. Note that the premature ventricular complex follows the longest RR cycle. This conforms to a phenomenon known as the "rule of bigeminy," that is, ventricular ectopy during atrial fibrillation more commonly follows the long RR cycles. The premature ventricular complex would have to be differentiated from aberrant supraventricular conduction. Monitor lead.

Rate: Atrial, cannot be determined accurately; ventricular, 36 to 105 beats/minute.
Rhythm: Atrial and ventricular are both irregularly irregular.
P waves: Only the fibrillatory (*F*) waves of atrial fibrillation can be seen.
PR interval: Not measurable.
QRS: 0.08 second.

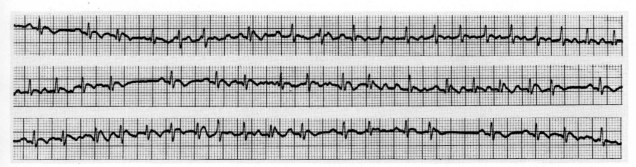

Fig. 8-31. Intermittent, "coarse" atrial flutter-fibrillation. Throughout this recording, sinus beats are interrupted by premature atrial complexes that initiate episodes of atrial flutter-fibrillation. The fibrillatory waves appear more coarse than usual, and the flutter waves are irregularly spaced and of varying amplitude. Such atrial rhythms are often called *coarse atrial flutter* and are probably due to portions of the atria that are fibrillating and other portions that are fluttering. A more appropriate term might be *flitter*. Monitor lead.

Rate: Atrial, varying; ventricular, 69 to 150 beats/minute.
P waves: Appear before the sinus beats; otherwise the undulating base line indicates flutter-fibrillation.
PR interval: 0.16 second for the sinus beats.
QRS: 0.08 second.

Treatment. It is of paramount importance in treating the patient who has atrial fibrillation for the first time to search for a precipitating cause. Thyrotoxicosis, mitral stenosis, acute myocardial infarction, pericarditis, and other known associated causes should be considered.

1. Initial therapy is determined by the patient's clinical status. The primary therapeutic objective is to slow the ventricular rate and, secondarily, to restore atrial systole. DC cardioversion may accomplish both of these objectives. If the sudden onset of atrial fibrillation with a rapid ventricular rate results in acute cardiovascular decompensation, DC cardioversion is the preferred treatment, beginning with 50 to 100 watt-seconds.

2. In the absence of decompensation the patient may be given digitalis to maintain a resting apical rate of 60 to 80 beats/minute, which does not exceed 100 beats/minute after slight exercise. The speed, route, dosage, and type of digitalis preparation administered are determined by the degree of cardiovascular compensation (see the discussion of the treatment of PSVT, AV nodal reentry). The ventricular rate cannot be slowed sufficiently by digitalis administration in some patients, and digitalis toxicity may result before slowing the ventricular rate. In such cases, complicating factors such as pulmonary emboli, atelectasis, myocarditis, infection, congestive heart failure, and hyperthyroidism should be ruled out and treated if found. In some instances[11] verapamil may be useful (see atrial flutter).[12]

3. The combined use of digitalis and propranolol or digitalis and verapamil may be used to slow the ventricular rate when digitalis alone fails. Occasionally, conversion of atrial fibrillation to normal sinus rhythm may result from this combination or following the administration of digitalis alone.

4. Most often the use of quinidine together with digitalis administration is necessary to convert the rhythm to a sinus mechanism. Because of the availability and safety of the electric cardioverter, it is preferable not to administer the large doses of quinidine that were used formerly to produce drug reversion to normal sinus rhythm. Rather, maintenance doses in the range of 1.2 to 2.4 g/day should be administered for a few days prior to the planned DC cardioversion. During this time, 10% to 15% of patients establish a normal sinus rhythm. If sinus rhythm does not occur, digitalis is withheld for 1 or 2 days (while continuing quinidine), and DC cardioversion is carried out. Recent experience suggests that digitalis may not have to be discontinued prior to cardioversion if the patient has not received an excessive amount of digitalis. Pretreatment with quinidine establishes an effective tissue concentration, determines whether the drug will be tolerated, improves chances of maintaining normal sinus rhythm after

cardioversion, and reduces the number of shocks and level of energy required to restore normal sinus rhythm. Successful establishment of normal sinus rhythm by electrical DC cardioversion occurs in over 90% of patients; with maintenance quinidine therapy approximately 30% to 50% remain in normal sinus rhythm for 12 months. In patients who do not tolerate quinidine, disopyramide or procainamide may be tried.

Certain patients should not be considered for cardioversion. These include patients who have (1) known sensitivity or intolerance to quinidine or other antiarrhythmic agents (according to some studies, the recurrence rate of atrial fibrillation is higher in the absence of prophylactic quinidine administration), (2) repetitive paroxysmal atrial fibrillation that cannot be prevented by quinidine, (3) digitalis intoxication, (4) numerous conversion procedures without clinical improvement or preservation of sinus rhythm, (5) difficult-to-control atrial tachyarrhythmias that finally eventuate into atrial fibrillation, (6) cardiac surgery planned in the near future, (7) a high degree of partial or complete AV block and thus a slow ventricular response, and (8) sick sinus syndrome (Fig. 8-28).

Many elderly patients in the last two groups tolerate the atrial fibrillation well because the ventricular rate is slow, and they often do not require treatment with digitalis, unless the ventricular rate increases or congestive heart failure develops. These patients may demonstrate serious supraventricular and ventricular arrhythmias after cardioversion because concomitant sinus node disease becomes manifest after cardioversion. A related group of patients may have supraventricular tachycardias that alternate with bradycardias, and represent a subgroup of the sick sinus syndrome called "bradycardia-tachycardia syndrome." Usually, these patients are best treated with a ventricular pacemaker (to correct the slow rates) and digitalis (to control the ventricular rates during the supraventricular tachycardia).

In general, all other patients in whom improved circulatory hemodynamics are desirable may be considered candidates for electrical cardioversion. Failure to maintain normal sinus rhythm after electrical reversion is related to the duration of atrial fibrillation, the functional classification of the patient, and the cause of the underlying heart disease. The likelihood of establishing and maintaining sinus rhythm should be weighed against the risks of cardioversion or other forms of therapy. The presence of multiple factors that adversely affect maintenance of sinus rhythm militates against cardioversion attempts.

Anticoagulation before cardioversion is indicated in patients with a high risk of emboli, that is, those who have mitral stenosis, recent onset of atrial fibrillation, recent or recurrent emboli, or enlarged heart. The incidence of embolization during conversion to normal sinus rhythm is 1% to 3%.

ATRIAL TACHYCARDIA WITH AV BLOCK (Figs. 8-32 and 8-33)

The atrial rate is usually between 150 and 200 beats/minute, with a range, similar to PSVT caused by AV nodal reentry, of 150 to 250 beats/minute. When caused by digitalis excess, the atrial rate is generally less than 200 beats/minute and may be noted to gradually increase as the digitalis is continued. The PR interval also may gradually lengthen until Wenckebach second-degree AV block develops. On occasion the degree of AV block may be more advanced. Frequently other manifestations of digitalis excess, such as premature ventricular systoles, coexist. In nearly 50% of cases of atrial tachycardia with block the atrial rate is irregular, whereas in PSVT caused by AV nodal reentry the atrial rate is generally exceedingly regular. Characteristic isoelectric intervals between P waves, in contrast to atrial flutter, are usually present in all leads. However, at rapid atrial rates the distinction between atrial tachycardia with block and atrial flutter may be quite difficult. As in atrial flutter, carotid sinus massage slows the ventricular rate by increasing the degree of AV block, but does not terminate the tachycardia.

Significance. Atrial tachycardia with block occurs most commonly in patients who have significant organic heart disease such as coronary artery disease or cor pulmonale. It is associated with digitalis excess in 50% to 75% of such patients.

A different type of atrial tachycardia, multifocal atrial tachycardia, is characterized by atrial rates of 100 to 250 beats/minute and marked variation in P wave morphology and in the PP interval, is associated with a high mortality, and is rarely produced by digitalis.

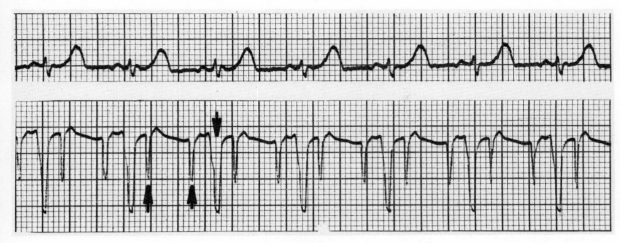

Fig. 8-32. Atrial tachycardia with 2:1 block. In the top tracing (lead II) alternate P waves cannot be seen because they are lost within the ST segment, and the ECG appears to be sinus rhythm at a rate of 95 beats/minute. The extra deflection in the terminal portion of the T wave suggests the presence of a second P wave which is revealed in the esophageal recording (*bottom* tracing). The atrial rate actually is 190 beats with 2:1 conduction to the ventricle. Upright arrows indicate P waves, inverted arrow indicates QRS complex. Monitor lead.

Rate: Atrial, 190 beats/minute; ventricular, 95 beats/minute.
Rhythm: Atrial and ventricular, regular.
P waves: Seen with clarity in the esophageal recording.
PR interval: 0.14 second for the conducted beats.
QRS: 0.07 second.

Treatment. If the ventricular rate is in a normal range and the patient is asymptomatic, often no therapy at all may be necessary.

1. Very slow ventricular rates may respond to atropine (0.5-mg increments IV) or, rarely, require ventricular pacing.
2. Atrial tachycardia with block in a patient who is not taking digitalis may be treated with digitalis to slow the ventricular rate.
3. If atrial tachycardia with block remains after digitalization, oral quinidine, disopyramide, or procainamide may be added.
4. The rhythm in some patients may resist termination by pharmacologic means, and, if digitalis excess is not the cause, DC cardioversion may be tried.
5. If atrial tachycardia with block appears in a patient receiving digitalis, it should be assumed initially that the digitalis is responsible for the arrhythmia, especially if the patient recently has received diuretics, the serum potassium level is low, the digitalis dose has been increased, quinidine has been added to the therapeutic regimen, or multiple premature ventricular systoles are also present. In such patients, initial therapy includes omission of digitalis and potassium-depleting diuretics (discontinuation of quinidine if it has been started recently) and the administration of potassium chloride, orally (30 to 45 mEq initially, repeated if necessary in 1 hour) or intravenously (0.5 mEq/minute in 5% dextrose and water during constant electrocardiographic monitoring, for a total of 30 to 60 mEq initially). A gradual slowing of the atrial rate with a decrease in AV block usually occurs if the arrhythmia is caused by digitalis. In the presence of advanced AV block, potassium, as well as other antiarrhythmic agents, must be given with great caution and under constant electrocardiographic monitoring. It should be remembered that renal dysfunction, acidosis, and excess digitalis predispose to the development of hyperkalemia, and therefore potassium must be administered cautiously, along with frequent ECG, serum potassium, and blood urea nitrogen (BUN) checks.
6. Propranolol, 0.5 to 1 mg/min IV for a total dose of 0.5 to 3 mg, or phenytoin, 50 to 100 mg IV every 5 minutes until the tachycardia terminates, the patient develops signs of toxicity such as nystagmus, vertigo, or nausea, or a total dose of 1 g is given, may be quite useful for digitalis-induced arrhythmias, including atrial tachycardia with block. The latter agent, since it does not appear to slow AV conduction, may be particularly useful.
7. If these agents are not effective, further short-acting digitalis preparations may be given cautiously, assuming that the development of atrial tachycardia with block was not caused by digitalis.

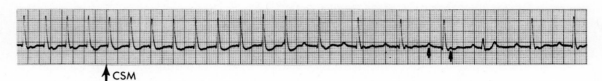

↑CSM

Fig. 8-33. Atrial tachycardia with 1:1 conduction becoming 2:1 conduction during carotid sinus massage. At the left portion of the ECG, P waves can be seen to conduct to each QRS complex. Carotid sinus massage, performed at the large arrow, precipitates 2:1 conduction, and clear atrial activity can be seen (*arrows*) as 2:1 conduction occurs. Monitor lead.

Rate: Atrial, 150 beats/minute; ventricular, 150 beats/minute in left portion and 75 beats/minute in right portion.

Rhythm: Atrial, regular; ventricular, regular.

P waves: Can be seen in the ST segment in the left portion of the tracing and are quite clear in the right portion of the tracing.

PR interval: Difficult to measure in the left portion of the tracing, but P waves conduct with a PR interval of 0.25 second in the right portion of the tracing.

QRS: 0.09 second.

PREMATURE AV JUNCTIONAL SYSTOLES (Fig. 8-34)

Rhythms formerly called nodal, coronary nodal, and coronary sinus are now termed *AV junctional*. This term, which includes the AV nodal–His bundle area, is preferred to terms that imply a more exact site of impulse origin because the exact location at which the impulse originates often cannot be determined from the surface ECG. A premature AV junctional systole arises in the AV junction and spreads in an anterograde and retrograde fashion. If unimpeded in its course, the impulse discharges the atrium to produce a premature retrograde P wave and a QRS complex with a supraventricular contour. Retrograde atrial activation generally results in a negative P wave in leads II, III, aV_F, and V_6, with positive P waves in leads I, aV_L, aV_R, and V_1. The retrograde P wave may occur before, be buried in, or (less commonly) follow the QRS complex. The site at which the impulse originates, as well as the relative speeds of anterograde and retrograde conduction, determines the relationship of the P wave to the QRS complex. A compensatory pause commonly follows a premature AV junctional systole, but if the atrium and sinus node are discharged retrogradely, a noncompensatory pause results.

Significance and treatment. The significance of premature AV junctional systoles is discussed under premature ventricular systoles.

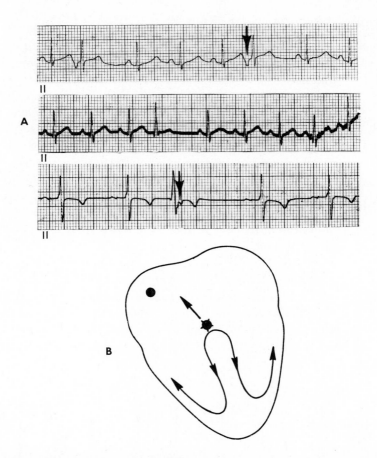

Fig. 8-34. A, Premature AV junctional systoles. Premature junctional systoles seen in the top, middle, and bottom tracings were formerly called upper, middle, and lower nodal premature systoles, respectively, because the retrograde P wave was inscribed before, during, and after the QRS complex. Since not only the site of origin, but also the relative speeds of anterograde and retrograde conduction determine the P-QRS complex relationships during a premature AV junctional systole, it is best to use the nonspecific term "premature AV junctional systole" for all three types. Note that the QRS complex maintains an almost identical contour to the normally conducted beats. Slight QRS aberration occurs in the middle recording. Monitor lead from three different patients; arrows indicate P waves. In **B** schematic illustration is presented.

Rate: Determined by basic rate and number of premature systoles.
Rhythm: Irregular because of premature systoles; may be a regular irregularity, as in bigeminy or trigeminy.
P waves: Atria discharged in a retrograde direction, producing negative (inverted) P waves in lead II. P waves occur before (top), during (middle), and after (bottom) the QRS complex, depending on the site of origin of the premature systole and the status of anterograde and retrograde conduction.
PR interval: Less than 0.12 second.
RP interval: If P wave follows QRS, less than 0.20 second.
QRS: Normal 0.08 second, reflecting normal anterograde conduction to the ventricles. Contour may differ slightly from normal.

AV JUNCTIONAL RHYTHMS (Figs. 8-35 to 8-37)

An AV junctional escape beat occurs when the rate of impulse formation of the primary pacemaker (usually sinus node) becomes less than that of the AV junctional pacemaker, or when impulses from the primary pacemaker do not penetrate to the region of the escape focus (AV block). The interval from the last normally conducted beat to the escape beat therefore exceeds the normal RR interval and is a measure of the initial rate of discharge of the AV junctional focus. The inherent discharge rate of the AV junctional escape focus (usually 40 to 60 per minute) determines when the junctional escape beat occurs. A continued series of AV junctional escape beats is called an AV junctional rhythm. An AV junctional escape rhythm is usually fairly regular. Intervals between subsequent escape beats after the initial escape beat may gradually shorten as the rate of discharge of the escape focus increases (rhythm of development). The configuration of the QRS complex may differ from the normal sinus-initiated QRS complex; usually, it maintains the same contour as the normally conducted QRS.

The atria may be under retrograde control of the AV junctional pacemaker, or the atria may discharge independently (see discussion of AV dissociation).

Significance. An AV junctional escape beat(s) or rhythm may be a normal phenomenon owing to the effects of vagal tone on higher pacemakers, or it may occur during pathologic slow sinus discharge and heart block. The escape beat

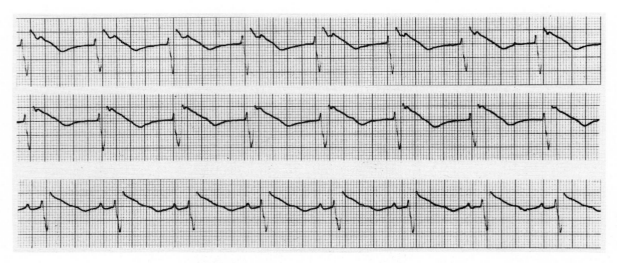

Fig. 8-35. AV junctional rhythm. The top two tracings are a continuous recording, whereas the bottom tracing is recorded some time later. In the top two tracings, isorhythmic AV dissociation is present. P waves are in the ST segment and gradually move into the QRS complex (compare the QRS-P relationship in the first complex in the top strip with the last complex in the second strip). In the top strip, sinus slowing initially allowed the escape of the junctional rhythm (not shown). Monitor lead.

Rate: Top two strips, atrial is 60 beats/minute and ventricular is 58 beats/minute; bottom strip, atrial and ventricular rate 57 beats/minute.
Rhythm: Atrial, regular; ventricular, regular.
P waves: Normal.
PR interval: Varying in the top two strips; regular (0.22 second) in the bottom strip.
QRS: 0.10 second (appears prolonged in this monitor lead but was normal by 12-lead ECG).

or rhythm serves as a safety mechanism that assumes control of the cardiac rhythm owing to *default* of the primary pacemaker, so as to prevent the occurrence of complete ventricular asystole.

Treatment. Treatment, if indicated, lies in increasing the discharge rate of higher pacemakers or improving conduction with atropine or isoproterenol. Rarely, pacing may be needed.

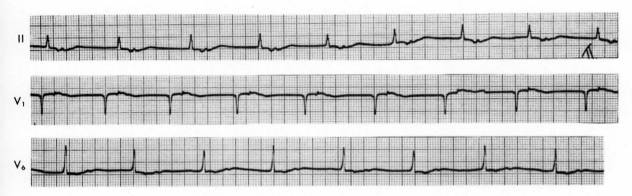

Fig. 8-36. AV junctional rhythm. The patient has an AV junctional rhythm with 1:1 retrograde capture. Thus AV dissociation is not present.

Rate: Atrial and ventricular, 55 beats/minute.
Rhythm: Regular.
P waves: Retrograde.
RP interval: 0.18 second.
QRS: 0.06 second.

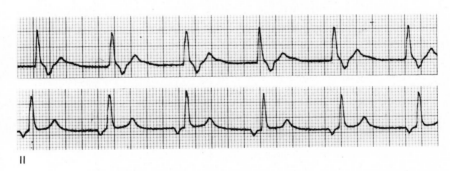

II

Fig. 8-37. AV junctional rhythm with a changing P-QRS relationship. In the top tracing, retrograde atrial activity follows the QRS complex. In the bottom tracing, retrograde atrial activity precedes the QRS complex. Thus, with the same AV junctional rhythm in the same patient, atrial activity first followed and then preceded the QRS complex.

Rate: Atrial, 65 beats/minute; ventricular, 65 beats/minute.
Rhythm: Regular.
P waves: Inverted; follow QRS in top tracing; precede QRS in bottom tracing.
PR interval: 0.12 second, bottom.
RP interval: 0.12 second, top.
QRS: Generally normal, 0.08 second.

NONPAROXYSMAL AV JUNCTIONAL TACHYCARDIA (Figs. 8-38 and 8-39)

Accepted terminology confers the label of tachycardia to rhythms that exceed 100 beats/min. However, since rates greater than 60 to 70 beats/min represent, in effect, a tachycardia for the AV junctional tissue, the term *nonparoxysmal AV junctional tachycardia* (NPJT), although not entirely correct, has been generally accepted when the rate of junctional discharge exceeds 60 to 70 beats/min.[15] NPJT usually has a more gradual onset and termination than does PSVT caused by AV nodal reentry, with a ventricular rate commonly between 70 and 130 beats/min. The rate sometimes may be slowed by vagal maneuvers, as in sinus tachycardia, and the rhythm may not always be entirely regular. Although retrograde atrial activation may occur, more commonly the atria are controlled by an independent sinus or atrial focus resulting in AV dissociation.

Significance. The distinction between NPJT and PSVT caused by AV nodal reentry is etiologically and therapeutically quite important. NPJT occurs most commonly in patients who have underlying heart disease, such as inferior wall infarction, and acute rheumatic myocarditis, and following open-heart surgery. Probably the most important cause is excessive digitalis, which only rarely produces PSVT caused by AV nodal reentry. It is especially important to recognize slowing and regularization of the ventricular rhythm caused by NPJT as an early sign of digitalis intoxication in a patient who has atrial fibrillation.

Treatment. The treatment for NPJT is as follows:

1. If the ventricular rate is rapid, the cardiovascular status compromised, and the patient is not taking digitalis, digitalization should be the first measure.
2. Uncommonly in an emergency situation or if the arrhythmia does not respond to digitalization and is *clearly not induced by digitalis,* electrical DC cardioversion may be employed.
3. However, if the patient tolerates the arrhythmia well, careful monitoring and attention to the underlying heart disease is usually all that is needed. The arrhythmia will usually abate spontaneously.
4. If digitalis toxicity is the causative factor, the drug must be immediately stopped. Potassium may be given (see the discussion of treatment of atrial tachycardia with block). The ECG should be monitored, since the blocking effects of potassium administration and digitalis are additive in the AV junctional tissue, and advanced AV heart block may result. The rate of potassium administration is important, since a rapid infusion of the potassium, especially in a potassium-depleted patient, may result in transient cardiac arrest or depression of AV conduction.
5. Lidocaine, propranolol, or phenytoin also may be tried.

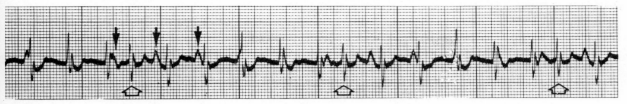

Lead II

Fig. 8-38. Nonparoxysmal AV junctional tachycardia. Atrial activity (inverted dark arrows) intermittently capture the ventricles (upright arrow outlines) to produce incomplete AV dissociation. The junctional tachycardia fails to capture the atria retrogradely, but the sinus tachycardia intermittently captures the ventricles. Unidirectional block (i.e., retrograde) is present. Incomplete AV dissociation occurs because of the accelerated AV junctional discharge.

Rate: Atrial, 111 beats/minute; ventricular, 125 beats/minute.
Rhythm: Atrial, regular; ventricular, fairly regular with intermittent speeding due to sinus captures.
P waves: Normal and can be "marched out." P waves are not influenced by ventricular activity.
PR interval: Difficult to measure but prolonged before the captures.
QRS: 0.06 second.

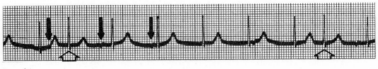

Lead I

Fig. 8-39. Nonparoxysmal AV junctional tachycardia. Atrial activity (inverted dark arrows) can be seen as small inverted P waves that occur regularly throughout the QRS complex, uninfluenced by ventricular activity. The ventricular rhythm is regular except for intermittent atrial captures indicated by the unfilled upright arrows. The rhythm is explained as in Fig. 8-38 except that an ectopic pacemaker, rather than a sinus pacemaker, controls the atria. This ectopic pacemaker could be an atrial focus or an upper junctional focus. Incomplete AV dissociation is present with unidirectional conduction from atria to ventricles but retrograde block (the ventricular rhythm does not capture the atria retrogradely).

Rate: Atrial, 72 beats/minute; ventricular, 79 beats/minute.
Rhythm: Atrial, regular; ventricular, irregular due to intermittent atrial captures.
P waves: Abnormal.
PR interval: Prolonged during ventricular captures.
QRS: 0.06 second.

VENTRICULAR ESCAPE BEATS (Fig. 8-40)

A ventricular escape beat results when the rate of impulse formation of supraventricular pacemakers (sinus node and AV junctional) becomes less than that of potential ventricular pacemakers or when supraventricular impulses do not penetrate to the region of the escape focus because of SA or AV block. The inherent rate of discharge of ventricular escape pacemakers is usually 20 to 40 per minute. A continued series of ventricular escape beats is called a ventricular escape rhythm. The ventricular rhythm is usually fairly regular, although the rhythm may accelerate for a few complexes shortly after its onset (rhythm of development). The duration of the QRS complexes is prolonged to greater than 0.12 second because the origin of ventricular discharge is located in the ventricles. Sometimes the escape focus may shift from one to another portion of ventricle and may generate QRS complexes with a different contour and rate.

Significance. The presence of ventricular escape beats indicates significant slowing of supraventricular pacemakers or a fairly high degree of SA or AV block, and would therefore generally be considered abnormal.

Treatment. Depending on the cause, atropine, isoproterenol, or pacing generally would represent the therapeutic approach.

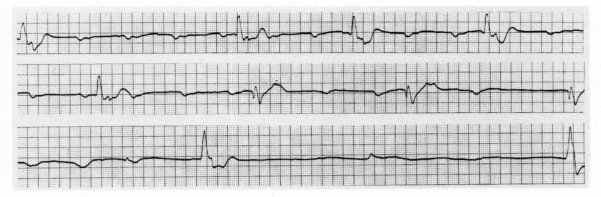

Fig. 8-40. Ventricular escape beats occurring in a dying patient. Ventricular escape beats occur with changing contour and at irregular intervals in this ECG from a dying patient. AV block is also present, since the P waves do not appear to conduct to the ventricles. The changing QRS contour may be caused by shifting pacemakers or changing activation sequence. Continuous recording from a monitor lead.

Rate: Varying.
Rhythm: Atrial and ventricular rhythms are varying.
P waves: Can be seen in the top strip and then more intermittently in the second and third strips.
PR interval: Varying.
QRS: Varying but approximately 0.16 second.

PREMATURE VENTRICULAR SYSTOLES (Figs. 8-41 to 8-43, 8-48)

A premature ventricular systole is characterized by the premature occurrence of a QRS complex, initiated in the ventricle, that has a contour different from the normal supraventricular complex and a duration usually greater than 0.12 second. The T wave is generally large and opposite in direction to the major deflection of the QRS. The QRS complex generally is not preceded by a premature P wave but may be preceded by a sinus P wave occurring at its expected time. One must remember, however, that these criteria may be met by a supraventricular beat or rhythm that conducts aberrantly through the ventricle; in fact, aberrant supraventricular conduction may mimic all the manifestations of ventricular arrhythmia except ventricular fibrillation (see p. 266).

Retrograde transmission to the atria from premature ventricular systoles occurs more frequently than has often been affirmed but still probably does not occur commonly. The retrograde P wave produced in this fashion is often obscured by the distorted QRS complex. Usually a fully compensatory pause follows a premature ventricular systole. If the retrograde impulse discharges the sinus node prematurely and resets the basic timing, it may produce a pause that is not fully compensatory. A compensatory pause results when the premature systole does not alter the discharge rate or rhythm of the sinus node, so that a P wave occurs at its normal time. The P wave does not reach the ventricle, since the AV node is refractory because of (concealed) retrograde penetration into the AV node by the premature junctional or ventricular systole. Therefore the RR interval produced by the two QRS complexes on either side of the premature complex equals twice the normally conducted RR interval. A compensatory pause occurs more commonly with ventricular and AV junctional premature systoles, but the presence of a compensatory pause is not invariably diagnostic of the site of origin of the premature complex.

The normal sinus P wave following a premature ventricular systole may conduct to the ventricles with a long PR interval, in which case a pause does not follow the premature ventricular systole, and the premature ventricular systole is said to be *interpolated*. A *ventricular fusion beat* (the simultaneous activation of one chamber by two foci) represents a blend of the characteristics of the normally conducted beat and the beat originating in the ventricles, indicating that the ventricle has been depolarized from both atrial and ventricular directions. *Atrial fusion beats* may occur during ectopic atrial discharge and represent a blend of the characteristics of the sinus-initiated and ectopic atrial P waves. Whether a compensatory or noncompensatory pause, a retrograde atrial excitation, an interpolated systole, a fusion systole, or an echo beat (see Fig. 8-41) occurs is merely a function of how well the AV junction conducts and the timing of the events taking place. The term *bigeminy* refers to pairs of beats or two complexes and may be used to indicate couplets of normal and ectopic ventricular systoles. Premature ventricular systoles may have differing contours and often are called multifocal. More properly they should be called multiform, since it is not known that there are multiple foci discharging.

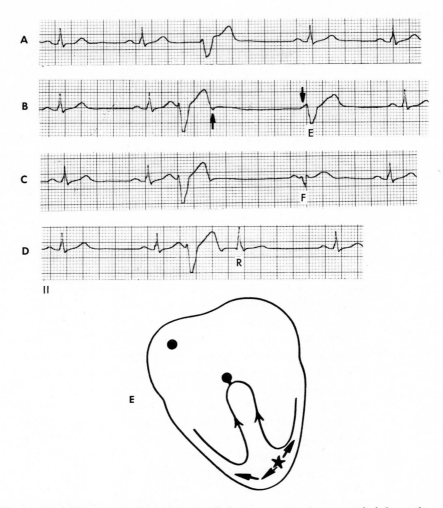

Fig. 8-41. Premature ventricular systoles. All four tracings were recorded from the same patient. In **A** a relatively late premature ventricular systole is followed by a full compensatory pause. Sinus slowing makes the pause after the ventricular systole minimally greater than compensatory, but its characteristics are essentially the same, that is, the interval between the two normal QRS complexes flanking the premature ventricular systole is twice the basic RR interval. In **B** an earlier premature ventricular systole in the same patient retrogradely discharges the atria (↑). This resets the sinus node and a ventricular escape beat (*E*) escapes before the next P wave (↓) can conduct to the ventricles. In strip **C** the sequence is the same as in **B,** except that the atrial rate is faster. This permits the P wave, following the premature ventricular systole and retrograde P wave, to partially depolarize the ventricles at the same time the ventricular escape beat occurs, resulting in a fusion beat (*F*). In **D,** the sequence is the same as in **C,** except that after the impulse from the ventricle retrogradely discharges the atria, it returns to the ventricles to produce a ventricular echo, or reciprocal beat (*R*). In **E,** a schematic illustration is presented.

Rate: Determined by basic rate and number of ventricular systoles.
Rhythm: Irregular because of premature systoles.
P waves: Generally normal; may be captured retrogradely; often lost in QRS or T wave of premature ventricular systole.
PR interval: Determined by whether P wave is blocked, conducted with a prolonged PR interval, or retrogradely activated.
QRS: 0.14 second.

Significance. The frequency of premature ventricular systoles increases with age. In individuals without organic heart disease the presence of premature systoles may be manifested by the symptoms of palpitations or discomfort in the chest or neck; this is caused by the greater than normal contractile force of the postectopic beats or the feeling that the heart has stopped during the long pause after the premature systoles. Long runs of premature systoles in patients who have heart disease may produce angina or hypotension. Frequent interpolated premature systoles actually represent a doubling of the heart rate and may compromise the patient's hemodynamic status. In the absence of underlying heart disease the presence of premature systoles may have no significance and not require suppression. Premature ventricular systoles and complex ventricular arrhythmias occurring in asymptomatic middle-aged men are associated with the presence of coronary heart disease and with a greater risk of subsequent death from coronary heart disease. However, it has not been demonstrated that the premature ventricular systoles or complex ventricular arrhythmias play a *precipitating* role in the genesis of sudden death; they may be simply a marker of heart disease. Nor has it been shown unequivocally that antiarrhythmic therapy given to suppress the premature ventricular systoles or complex ventricular arrhythmias reduces the incidence of sudden death in these patients.

Most of the drugs used to suppress premature systoles also may produce them on certain occasions. This is especially true of the digitalis preparations. On the other hand, digitalis often is effective in controlling premature atrial and ventricular systoles, especially those related to the presence of congestive heart failure. In patients suffering from acute myocardial infarction, it has been commonly held that so-called warning arrhythmias (premature ventricular systoles occurring close to the preceding T wave, greater than five or six per minute, bigeminal, multiform, or occurring in salvos of two, three, or more) may presage or precipitate ventricular tachycardia or fibrillation. However, it has been demonstrated that about half of the patients who develop ventricular fibrillation have no warning arrhythmias, and half of those who do have warning arrhythmias do not develop ventricular fibrillation.[16]

Treatment. In the patient who has an acute myocardial infarction, extremes of heart rate, both fast and slow, may provoke the development of premature ventricular systoles. Frequently, premature systoles accompanying the slow ventricular rates caused by sinus bradycardia or AV block may be abolished by increasing the basic rate with atropine or isoproterenol or by pacing at a faster rate with an artifical pacemaker. If the patient with sinus bradycardia has no hypotension, heart failure, or premature ventricular systoles and can be monitored closely, it appears best not to increase the heart rate. Faster rates increase the oxygen needs of the heart and may increase the degree of ischemia and precipitate ventricular arrhythmias.

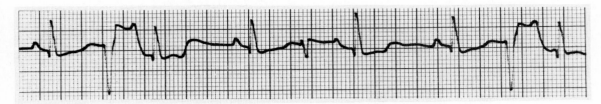

Fig. 8-42. Interpolated premature ventricular systoles. The second, fifth, and eighth QRS complexes are premature ventricular systoles. The sinus P wave that follows those premature ventricular complexes conducts to the ventricle with a long PR interval. Thus the normally expected compensatory pause is not present. The premature ventricular systole does not replace a normally conducted complex (see Fig. 8-41, *A*) but occurs in addition to the normally conducted complex. The PR interval following the premature ventricular systole is prolonged due to incomplete recovery of the AV node because of partial retrograde penetration by the interpolated premature ventricular systole. Monitor lead.

Rate and rhythm: Varying because of the premature ventricular systoles.
P waves: Normal.
PR interval: 0.16 second for the normally conducted beats and 0.20 to 0.25 second after the interpolated premature ventricular complexes.
QRS: 0.09 second for the normal beats and 0.12 second for the premature ventricular complexes.

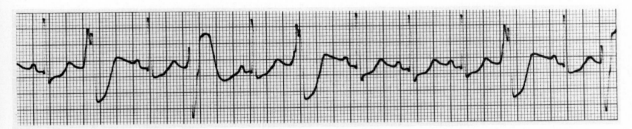

Fig. 8-43. Multiform premature ventricular systoles. Each sinus beat is followed by premature ventricular complexes that have two contours, one predominantly upright and the other predominantly negative. These premature ventricular complexes of different contours are more properly called multiform rather than multifocal, since one cannot be certain that more than one focus is active rather than simply different activation sequences emerging from the same focus. Monitor lead.

Rate: 100 beats/minute but varying.
Rhythm: Varying due to premature ventricular complexes.
P waves: Normal preceding the normally conducted beats.
PR interval: 0.14 second preceding the normally conducted beats.
QRS: 0.09 second for the normally conducted beats and 0.16 second for the premature ventricular complexes.

1. In the hospitalized patient, lidocaine, 1 to 2 mg/kg (50 to 100 mg) given as an IV bolus followed by an IV drip in a dosage of 1 to 4 mg/minute, is the initial treatment of choice. A second or third IV injection using half the initial dose may be given at approximately 20- to 60-minute intervals after the first dose if necessary, but care should be taken not to exceed 400 to 500 mg/hour. A loading dose may also be given by rapid infusion, with an effective serum concentration maintained by constant infusion. In some instances, lidocaine may be given intramuscularly in a dose of 250 to 300 mg. The onset of action of lidocaine given IV is 45 to 90 seconds and the duration of action is 10 to 20 minutes. Lidocaine produces less hypotension and negative inotropic effects than procainamide or quinidine in doses having equivalent antiarrhythmic effects. It is ideal for use in patients who have renal disease, since less than 10% is excreted unaltered in the kidney and the rest is metabolized by the liver. In patients exhibiting allergic reactions to quinidine or procainamide, lidocaine is useful, since there appears to be no cross-sensitivity.[17]

2. If maximum doses of lidocaine are unsuccessful, then procainamide, administered IV (50 to 100 mg/1 to 3 minutes until suppression of the premature ventricular systoles occurs, toxic effects such as QRS widening or hypotension result, or 750 to 1000 mg is administered) may be tried. If successful, procainamide may then be given as a continuous IV infusion (2 to 6 mg/min).

3. Oral maintenance therapy can be achieved with procainamide, 375 to 500 mg every 3 to 4 hours to produce therapeutic blood levels of 4 to 8 mg/L, or with quinidine sulfate, 200 to 400 mg every 6 hours to produce serum levels of 3 to 6 mg/L. A long-acting procainamide preparation is now available (see Chapter 10).

4. Disopyramide (Norpace), 100 to 250 mg every 6 hours, may be useful at serum concentrations of 2 to 5 mg/ml.

5. Propranolol or phenytoin may be tried if lidocaine, quinidine, procainamide, and disopyramide fail (see discussion of treatment of ventricular tachycardia).

VENTRICULAR TACHYCARDIA (Figs. 8-44 to 8-46)

Ventricular tachycardia is usually an ominous finding, indicating the presence of significant underlying cardiac disease. In many instances the responsible electrophysiologic mechanism is probably reentry.[18] Although ventricular tachycardia occurs most commonly in patients who have acute myocardial infarction and coronary artery disease, this arrhythmia also occurs in patients who have a variety of cardiac diseases, including cardiomyopathy, mitral valve prolapse, prolonged QT syndrome, and other problems. It has been reported in patients who have no evidence of structural heart disease.

The electrocardiographic diagnosis of ventricular tachycardia is suggested when a series of three or more bizarre, premature ventricular systoles occur that have a duration exceeding 0.12 second, with the ST-T vector pointing opposite to the major QRS deflection. The ventricular rate is between 110 and 250 beats/minute, and the RR interval may be exceedingly regular, or it may vary. Atrial activity may be independent of ventricular activity (AV dissociation) or the atria may be depolarized by the ventricles in a retrograde fashion (in which case AV dissociation is *not* present). Ventricular tachycardia may be sustained or nonsustained, and the patient's prognosis as well as the electrophysiologic mechanism may differ for the two forms. One type of nonsustained ventricular tachycardia is characterized by bursts of premature ventricular systoles separated by a series of sinus beats. Another type is called *torsade de pointes* and is characterized by a QRS contour that gradually changes its polarity from negative to positive or vice versa over a series of beats. It often occurs in a setting of QT prolongation.

The distinction between supraventricular and ventricular tachycardia may be difficult to tell at times because the features of both arrhythmias frequently overlap, and under certain circumstances a supraventricular tachycardia can mimic the criteria established for ventricular tachycardia. Ventricular complexes with abnormal configurations indicate only that conduction through the ventricle is not normal; they do not necessarily indicate the origin of impulse formation or the reason for the abnormal conduction (see discussion of supraventricular arrhythmia with abnormal QRS complex, p. 266).

The presence of *fusion* and *capture* beats provides evidence in favor of ventricular tachycardia. Fusion beats indicate simultaneous activation of the ventricles by two separate impulses (suggesting that one of the impulses arose in the ventricles), whereas the capture beats signal supraventricular control of the ventricles, generally at a rate faster than the ventricular tachycardia. This proves that normal ventricular conduction can occur at cycle lengths equal to or shorter than the tachycardia in question, again implying that the origin of the wide QRS complexes lies in the ventricles rather than in aberrant supraventricular conduction.

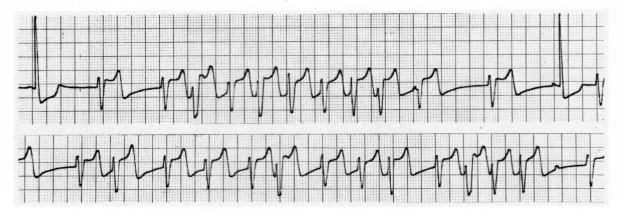

Fig. 8-44. Ventricular tachycardia. Ventricular tachycardia may be irregular at times, as exemplified in this ECG. The origin of the ventricular tachycardia was documented by His bundle electrocardiography. The interectopic intervals do not conveniently fit a diagnosis of exit block. Monitor lead.

Rate: Atrial, cannot be determined; ventricular, varying.

Rhythm: Atrial, cannot be determined; ventricular, irregular.

P waves: Can be seen occasionally and precede the first and next to last QRS complexes in the top strip, which are the only normally conducted QRS complexes. The nonconducted P wave at the terminal portion of the bottom strip is probably due to incomplete AV nodal recovery of refractoriness caused by retrograde penetration from the last beat in the ventricular tachycardia.

PR interval: 0.12 second for the normally conducted beats.

QRS: 0.08 second for the normally conducted beat and 0.11 second for the ventricular tachycardia.

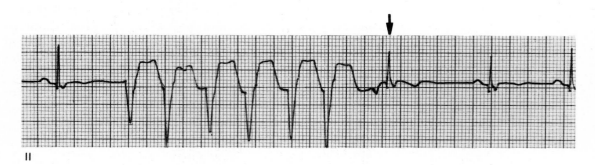

II

Fig. 8-45. Ventricular tachycardia ending with a ventricular echo. Six beats of ventricular tachycardia occur following the first sinus beat. The last ventricular tachycardia beat conducts retrogradely to the atrium (note the small negative P wave in lead II), which then returns to reexcite the ventricle (ventricular echo, *arrow*).

Rate: Atrial, 55 to 75 beats/minute; ventricular, approximately 150 beats/minute.

Rhythm: Atrial, cannot be determined during ventricular tachycardia; regular during sinus rhythm. Ventricular, slightly irregular during ventricular tachycardia.

P waves: Normal during sinus-conducted beats; retrograde P wave following the last ventricular tachycardia beat.

PR interval: 0.16 second during sinus rhythm. RP interval following the last ventricular tachycardia beat, 0.52 second.

QRS: 0.08 second during sinus rhythm and 0.10 second during ventricular tachycardia.

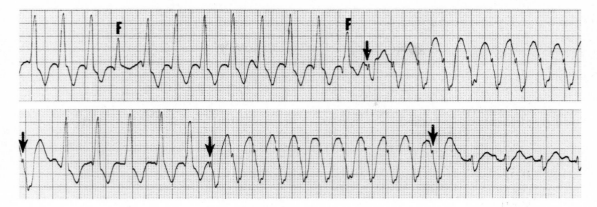

Fig. 8-46. Termination of ventricular tachycardia by rapid ventricular pacing. Intermittent fusion beats *(F)* in the top strip support the diagnosis of ventricular tachycardia. Between the first and second arrows, competitive ventricular pacing is performed at a rate of 166 beats/minute, but the ventricular tachycardia continues. Between the third and fourth arrows, competitive ventricular pacing is performed at a rate of 176 beats/minute, and following cessation of pacing, sinus rhythm occurs. Monitor lead, continuous recording.

Rate: Atrial, cannot be determined; ventricular, 136 beats/minute.
Rhythm: Atrial, cannot be determined; ventricular, fairly regular.
P waves: Cannot be seen.
PR interval: Cannot be determined.
QRS: 0.13 second.

Significance. Symptoms occurring during ventricular tachycardia depend on the ventricular rate, the duration of the tachyarrhythmia, and the severity of the underlying heart disease. The location of impulse formation and therefore the way in which the depolarization wave spreads across the myocardium also may be important because it influences the ventricle's contraction. The immediate significance of ventricular tachycardia to the patient relates to the hemodynamic dysfunction it produces and the possible development of ventricular fibrillation.

A premature ventricular (rarely, atrial) complex can initiate ventricular tachycardia or ventricular fibrillation when the premature systole occurs during the vulnerable period of the antecedent T wave. The vulnerable period represents an interval of 20 to 40 msec located near the apex of the T wave during which the heart, when stimulated, is prone to develop ventricular tachycardia or fibrillation (see discussion of ventricular fibrillation). The stimulus may be from an intrinsic source such as a spontaneous premature systole or from an extrinsic source such as a pacemaker or DC shock. During the interval of the vulnerable period, maximal electrical nonuniformity in the ventricular muscle is present; that is, ventricular muscle fibers are at varying stages of recovery of excitability. Some fibers may have completely repolarized, others may have only partially repolarized, and still others may be completely refractory. Therefore stimulation during this period establishes nonuniform conduction with some areas of slowed conduction or actual block and sets the stage for repetitive ventricular discharge possibly due to reentrant excitation. Equally important, however, is that ventricular tachycardia or fibrillation may begin without preexisting or precipitating premature ventricular systoles or may be ushered in by a *late* premature ventricular systole.

Treatment. The treatment for ventricular tachycardia is as follows:

1. Ventricular tachycardia that does not cause any hemodynamic decompensation may be treated medically, to achieve acute termination, by administering lidocaine IV in an initial bolus of 1 to 2 mg/kg body weight. A second or third IV injection of one half the initial dose may be given at approximately 20- to 40-minute intervals if necessary, but care should be taken not to exceed 400 to 500 mg/hour. The dosage should be reduced in patients who have liver disease, heart failure, or shock. If lidocaine abolishes the ventricular tachycardia, then a continuous IV infusion of about 40 mg/kg/minute or 1 to 4 mg/minute can be given to the patient. Other infusion schedules also are effective.[17]

2. If maximum doses of lidocaine are unsuccessful, procainamide administered IV (up to 100 mg/1 to 3 minutes until termination of the tachycardia occurs, toxic effects such as QRS widening or significant hypotension result, or 750 to 1000 mg is administered) may be tried. If successful, procainamide may then be given as a continuous IV infusion (2 to 6 mg/minute).

3. Recently intravenous bretylium has been approved for use in treating ventricular tachycardia or ventricular fibrillation when first-line antiarrhythmic agents such as lidocaine or procainamide have failed. A dose of 5 mg/kg is given over several minutes and may be increased to 10 mg/kg 15 to 30 minutes later. Doses may be repeated at 15- to 30-minute intervals, not to exceed a total of 30 mg/kg.

4. If the arrhythmia does not respond to medical therapy, electrical DC cardioversion may be used. Ventricular tachycardia that precipitates hypotension, shock, angina, or congestive heart failure should be treated *promptly* with DC cardioversion. Very low energies may terminate ventricular tachycardia; we generally begin with a synchronized shock of 10 to 50 watt-seconds (see discussion of treatment of ventricular fibrillation). Digitalis-induced ventricular tachycardia is best treated medically. After reversion of the arrhythmia to a normal rhythm, it is essential to institute measures to prevent a recurrence (see Chapter 8 for discussion of cardioversion).

5. Striking the patient's chest, sometimes called *"thumpversion,"* may terminate ventricular tachycardia by mechanically inducing a premature ventricular systole that presumably interrupts the reentrant pathway necessary to support the ventricular tachycardia. Stimulation at the time of the vulnerable period during ventricular tachycardia may provoke ventricular fibrillation.

6. In patients who have recurrent ventricular tachycardia a pacing catheter can be inserted into the right ventricle, and single, double, or multiple stimuli can be introduced competitively to terminate the ventricular tachycardia (Fig. 8-46). This procedure incurs the risk of accelerating the ventricular tachycardia to ventricular flutter or ventricular fibrillation. A new catheter electrode has been recently developed through which synchronized cardioversion can be performed. In the awake, conscious patient shocks of 0.25 watt-seconds that successfully terminate ventricular tachycardia can be delivered through this catheter electrode.[19]

7. A search for reversible conditions contributing to the initiation and maintenance of ventricular tachyarrhythmias should be made and the conditions corrected if possible. For example, ventricular arrhythmia related to hypotension or hypokalemia at times may be terminated by vasopressors or potassium, respectively. Slow ventricular rates that are caused by sinus bradycardia or AV block may permit the occurrence of premature ventricular systoles and ventricular tachyarrhythmias that can be corrected by administering atropine, 0.5 to 2.0 mg IV, temporary isoproterenol administration (1 to 2 μg/minute in an IV drip), or temporary transvenous pacing.

8. Intermittent ventricular tachycardia, interrupted by one or more supraventricular beats, generally is best treated medically. Lidocaine or procainamide should be tried. If they prove unsuccessful, then quinidine (200 to 400 mg orally or intramuscularly every 6 hours), disopyramide (100 to 250 mg q6 hours IV; IV administration is approved for investigational use only), propranolol (0.5 to 3 mg IV, 10 to 60 mg orally every 6 hours), or phenytoin IV (50 to 100 mg IV every 5 minutes until the tachycardia terminates, 1000 mg is given, or toxic symptoms such as nausea, ataxia, or vertigo result) or orally (250 mg every 6 hours the first day, followed by 100 mg every 6 to 8 hours thereafter) may be tried. Maintenance oral therapy with a long-acting procainamide preparation (500 to 1000 mg every 6 hours) may be useful.

Prevention of recurrences may be difficult at times.

1. Initial preventive drug therapy for recurrent ventricular arrhythmias in the ambulatory patient should be with quinidine, procainamide, or disopyramide. Procainamide is given as a loading dose of 0.5 to 1 g orally, followed by 375 to 500 mg three to six times daily. Because procainamide has a shorter duration of action than quinidine, giving procainamide at 6-hour intervals may fail to provide therapeutic blood levels for the entire 6-hour period. If the arrhythmia fails to respond, procainamide should be administered at 3-hour intervals to ensure adequate therapeutic serum levels in the range of 4 to 8 mg/L at all times. Hard-to-control arrhythmias may reflect poor absorption of the drug or nontherapeutic blood levels between too widely spaced doses. A long-acting procainamide preparation, as indicated (see also Chapter 10), is now available and can be given every 6 hours.

2. Alternatively, quinidine may be tried, administered at a dose of 200 to 400 mg four times daily, to achieve therapeutic blood levels of 3 to 6 mg/L.

3. If quinidine is unsuccessful, disopyramide, 100 to 250 mg every 6 hours, may be tried.

4. Following an initial approach with procainamide or quinidine, phenytoin or propranolol may be tried. However, these latter two drugs are often not very effective in preventing recurrences of ventricular tachyarrhythmias.

5. Combinations of drugs with different mechanisms of action may be successful and allow one to use low doses of both agents rather than high or toxic doses of one drug. For example, propranolol, 40 mg daily, combined with average doses of quinidine or procainamide may be efficacious. Similarly, procainamide or quinidine might be effectively combined with phenytoin.

6. Administration of potassium to maintain serum potassium levels in the 5+ range, in addition to antiarrhythmic agents, may be helpful on occasion.

7. A trial of ventricular or atrial pacing, combined with antiarrhythmic agents if necessary, may be tried empirically; if successful, permanent pacing may be instituted. Generally, unless the initiation of the ventricular tachycardia is related to significant bradycardia, such as ventricular rates in the 30s caused by complete AV block, attempts at rapid "overdrive" pacing are often ineffective long term.[14]

8. Surgery[20] may be used in selected patients to treat ventricular tachycardia. A ventriculotomy in patients who have ventricular tachycardia related to right ventricular dysplasia, encircling endocardial ventriculotomy, or endocardial resection (directed by electrophysiologic mapping techniques in patients who have ventricular tachycardia related to coronary artery disease) may eliminate recurrences or may make previously ineffective drug regimens efficacious. Coronary bypass surgery alone, without electrophysiologic mapping and myocardial resection, in patients who do not have ventricular tachycardia definitely associated with ischemia, for example, ventricular tachycardia induced by stress testing, has not been very successful.

9. A number of new antiarrhythmic agents (see Chapter 10) offer promise to control recurrent, life-threatening ventricular tachyarrhythmias.[13]

Evaluation of therapy. Evaluating adequate drug therapy in patients who have widely spaced episodes of ventricular tachycardia is a difficult problem because there exists no adequate end point to judge therapy until the patient has another spontaneous recurrence. Because of this, many groups have taken a more aggressive approach. The patient undergoes a control electrophysiologic study, during which the ventricular tachycardia is initiated and a variety of electrophysiologic and hemodynamic parameters are assessed. Then the patient is treated with a drug and the electrophysiologic study is repeated. If the drug prevents reinduction of the ventricular tachycardia, there is a high likelihood that the drug will also prevent spontaneous recurrences. If the drug fails to prevent reinitiation of the tachycardia, in many instances the drug may slow the rate of the ventricular tachycardia, convert a sustained form to a nonsustained episode, and still be useful clinically.[21] See Chapter 10 for a more detailed discussion.

ACCELERATED IDIOVENTRICULAR RHYTHM (Figs. 8-47 and 8-48)

The ventricular rate, commonly between 50 and 110 beats/minute, usually hovers within 10 beats of the sinus rate so that control of the cardiac rhythm may be passed back and forth between these two competing pacemaker sites. Consequently, long runs of fusion beats often appear at the onset and termination of the arrhythmia as the pacemakers vie for control of ventricular discharge. Because of the slow rates, capture beats are common. The onset of this arrhythmia is generally gradual (nonparoxysmal) and occurs when the rate of ectopic ventricular discharge exceeds the sinus rate because of sinus slowing, or SA or AV block. The ectopic mechanism may also begin following a premature ventricular complex or the ectopic ventricular rate may simply accelerate sufficiently to overtake the sinus focus. The slow rate and nonparoxysmal onset usually avoid the problems initiated by excitation during the vulnerable period, and consequently, precipitation of more rapid ventricular arrhythmias is rarely seen. Termination of the rhythm generally occurs gradually as the dominant sinus rhythm accelerates or the ectopic ventricular rhythm decelerates. Occasionally, an accelerated idioventricular rhythm may be present in a patient who also has a more rapid ventricular tachycardia at other times.

Significance. The arrhythmia occurs as a rule in patients with heart disease such as in a setting of acute myocardial infarction or as an expression of digitalis toxicity. It is transient and intermittent, with episodes lasting a few seconds to a minute, and does not appear to seriously affect the course or prognosis of the disease. Suppressive therapy is usually unnecessary because the ventricular rate is generally less than 100 beats/minute. Basically, five conditions exist during which therapy may be considered: (1) when AV dissociation results in loss of sequential AV contraction and, with it, the hemodynamic benefits of atrial contraction; (2) when accelerated idioventricular rhythm occurs together with more rapid forms of ventricular tachycardia; (3) when accelerated idioventricular rhythm begins with a premature ventricular complex that has a short coupling interval and causes discharge in the vulnerable period; (4) when the ventricular rate is too rapid and produces symptoms; and (5) if ventricular fibrillation develops. The latter appears only rarely.

Treatment. Treatment for accelerated idioventricular rhythm is as follows:

1. The best initial therapeutic approach would appear to be close observation, rhythm monitoring, and care for the underlying heart disease.
2. Digitalis administration should be discontinued if the drug is implicated in the genesis of the arrhythmia.
3. Atropine, 0.5 mg IV initially, repeated if necessary, may be used to speed the sinus rate and capture the ventricles. Rarely, pacing may be considered to speed the basic heart rate and suppress the accelerated idioventricular rhythm.
4. Lidocaine or other antiarrhythmic drugs may be given to suppress the ectopic ventricular focus.

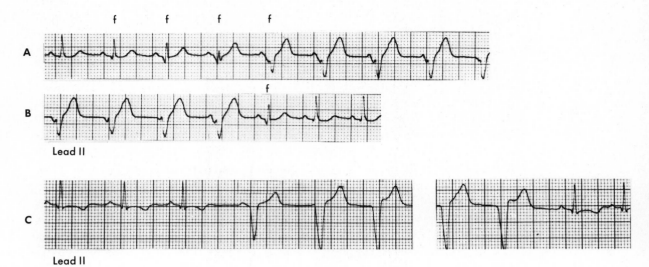

Fig. 8-47. Accelerated idioventricular rhythm. In panel **A** the sinus rate slows slightly and allows the escape of an idioventricular rhythm. A series of fusion beats (*F*) result. In panel **B** the sinus rate speeds slightly and once again regains control of the ventricular rhythm. A similar sequence occurs in panel **C**.

Rate: In panels **A** and **B** the atrial rate is 94 beats/minute but slows and speeds; ventricular is 90 beats/minute. In panel **C** the atrial rate is 75 beats/minute but slows and speeds; ventricular rate is 75 beats/minute but speeds to 86 beats/minute.

Rhythm: Fairly regular.

P waves: Normal P waves preceding each normally conducted QRS complex.

PR interval: 0.14 second for the normally conducted beats.

QRS: 0.06 second for the normally conducted beats and 0.14 second for the accelerated idioventricular beats.

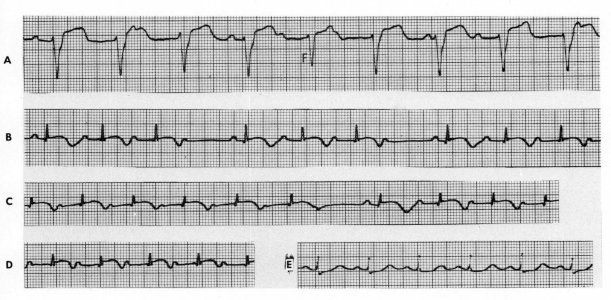

Fig. 8-48. Accelerated idioventricular rhythm and second-degree AV block. This series of trac-ings was recorded over a period of several days in a patient who had an acute inferior myocardial infarction. In panel **A** an accelerated idioventricular rhythm occurs at a rate of 70 beats/minute. Note the fusion QRS complex (*F*) in the midportion of the strip preceded by a long PR interval. The long PR interval suggests the presence of an AV conduction disturbance, but its exact degree cannot be determined from this ECG. Thus incomplete AV dissociation is present, caused by a combination of accelerated idioventric-ular rhythm and AV block. In panel **B** the accelerated idioventricular rhythm has stopped, but Wenckebach second-degree AV block is present with a conduction ratio of 4:3. In panel **C** the Wenckebach second-degree AV block is still present, but the conduction ratio has increased significantly. On the following day **(D)** the second-degree AV block has disappeared and is now replaced by first-degree AV block. Finally, after several days the first-degree AV block is barely present **(E). A,** Monitor lead. **B-E,** Lead II.

Rate: Panel **A:** atrial, 88 beats/minute; ventricular, 70 beats/minute. Panel **B:** atrial, 87 beats/minute; ventricular, varying. Panel **C:** atrial, 86 beats/minute; ventricular, varying. Panel **D:** atrial and ventricular, 88 beats/minute. Panel **E:** atrial and ventricular, 88 beats/minute.

Rhythm: Panel **A:** atrial and ventricular, regular. Panel **B:** atrial, regular; ventricular, irregular. Panel **C:** atrial, regular; ventricular, irregular. Panel **D:** atrial and ventricular, regular. Panel **E:** atrial and ventricular, regular.

P waves: Normal in all traces.

PR interval: Not measurable in panel **A,** progressively increasing in panels **B** and **C,** regular at 0.3 second in panel **D,** and regular at 0.20 second in panel **E.**

QRS: 0.12 second in panel **A** and 0.06 second in panels **B** to **E.**

VENTRICULAR FLUTTER AND VENTRICULAR FIBRILLATION (Figs. 8-49 to 8-51)

Ventricular flutter and ventricular fibrillation represent severe derangements of the heartbeat that usually terminate fatally within 3 to 5 minutes unless they are promptly stopped. Ventricular flutter resembles a sine wave in appearance, with regular, large oscillations occurring at a rate between 150 and 300 beats/minute, usually about 200 beats/minute. Ventricular fibrillation is recognized by the presence of irregular undulations of varying contour and amplitude. Distinct QRS complexes, ST segment, and T waves are absent. The difference between rapid ventricular tachycardia and ventricular flutter may be difficult and is usually of academic interest only.

Significance. Ventricular fibrillation occurs in a variety of clinical situations but is most commonly associated with coronary heart disease, acute myocardial infarction, and advanced forms of heart block. The arrhythmia occurs frequently as the terminal event in a variety of diseases. It also may be seen during cardiac pacing, cardiac catheterization, operation, anesthesia, drug toxicity (for example, digitalis, quinidine, procainamide), and hypoxia. It may occur after electric shock administered during cardioversion or accidentally by improperly grounded equipment. Premature stimulation during the vulnerable period (R-on-T phenomenon; see discussion of ventricular tachycardia) may precipitate ventricular tachycardia, flutter, or fibrillation, particularly when the electrical stability of the heart has been altered by the ischemia of an acute myocardial infarction, for example. In many patients, sustained ventricular tachycardia may precede ventricular fibrillation.[22] However, ventricular fibrillation may occur without antecedent or precipitating ventricular tachycardia or premature ventricular complexes. Experimentally, it may occur when a previously occluded coronary artery undergoes sudden restoration of flow. Clinically, this condition may be replicated by streptokinase infusion that restores flow to an occluded coronary artery, or possibly when coronary spasm relaxes. Conceivably, the latter event could result in ventricular fibrillation without myocardial infarction.

Ventricular flutter or fibrillation results in faintness followed by loss of consciousness, seizures, apnea, and, if the rhythm continues untreated, death. The blood pressure is unobtainable, and heart sounds are usually absent. The atria may continue to beat at an independent rhythm or be retrogradely captured for a time. Eventually, electrical activity of the heart is completely absent.

Many patients who suffer ventricular fibrillation out of hospital have been resuscitated. It is interesting that only a small percentage of them evolve a myocardial infarction, and that they have a 2% to 3% recurrence rate of ventricular fibrillation in the first year. However, those patients who are resuscitated from out-of-hospital ventricular fibrillation but do not evolve a myocardial infarction have a 1-year recurrence rate of almost 25% (see Chapter 9).[23]

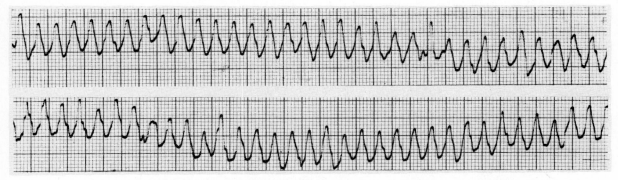

Fig. 8-49. Ventricular flutter. During ventricular flutter, ventricular depolarization and re-polarization appear as a sine wave with regular oscillations. The QRS complex cannot be distinguished from the ST segment or T wave. Monitor lead is continuous recording.

Rate: Ventricular, 300 beats/minute.
Rhythm: P waves cannot be seen; ventricular, fairly regular.
PR interval: Not measurable.
QRS: 0.18 second.

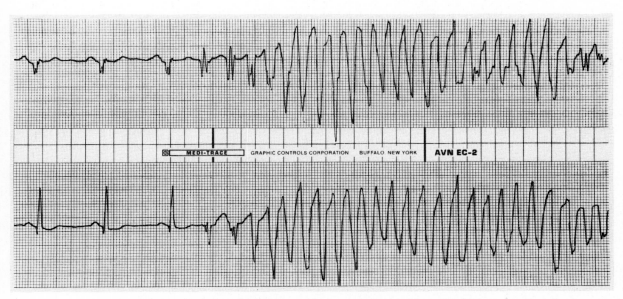

Fig. 8-50. Ventricular fibrillation. During a 24-hour ambulatory ECG recording the patient experienced sudden death. The ECG demonstrated the development of a rapid ventricular tachycardia that progressed promptly to ventricular fibrillation. Ventricular fibrillation at its onset may appear fairly regular. Dual tracing records simultaneously.

Rate: During sinus rhythm, 65 beats/minute; ventricular rate during the rapid ventricular tachycardia is approximately 300 beats/minute.
Rhythm: During sinus rhythm, regular; during rapid ventricular tachycardia, grossly irregular.
P waves: Normal during sinus rhythm. Cannot be seen during ventricular tachycardia-fibrillation.
PR interval: 0.16 second during sinus rhythm.
QRS: 0.08 second during sinus rhythm. Cannot be measured accurately during the ventricular tachycardia-fibrillation.

Treatment. Ventricular flutter and ventricular fibrillation are totally unphysiologic life-threatening arrhythmias for which immediate electrical (nonsynchronized) DC cardioversion, using 200 to 400 watt-seconds, is the only reliable treatment. When ventricular tachycardia produces the same hemodynamic response as ventricular flutter or fibrillation, it also must be immediately terminated by DC shock. A sharp blow to the chest may terminate some forms of ventricular tachyarrhythmias ("thumpversion"), but time should not be wasted on this procedure if one or two sharp blows fail.

Termination of ventricular flutter or fibrillation within 30 to 60 seconds prevents the biochemical derangements accompanying ventricular fibrillation, eliminates the need for endotracheal intubation, and significantly increases the success rate of such procedures. If necessary, artificial ventilation by means of mouth-to-mouth resuscitation or a well-fitting rubber face mask and an Ambu bag is quite satisfactory and eliminates the delay attending intubation by inexperienced personnel. Chest compression to achieve cardiac massage may be instituted, but *there must be no delay in administering the DC shock.* If the patient is not monitored and it cannot be established whether asystole or ventricular fibrillation has caused the cardiovascular collapse, the electric shock should be administered *without* wasting precious seconds attempting to record the ECG. The DC shock may cause the asystolic heart to begin discharging, as well as terminate ventricular fibrillation if the latter is present. Following a successful cardioversion, measures must be taken to prevent a second episode of ventricular fibrillation, including monitoring of the cardiac rhythm, administration of lidocaine, procainamide, and bretylium, and so forth.

Ventricular fibrillation is quickly followed by severe metabolic acidosis, and sodium bicarbonate, 1 to 3 ampules containing 44 mEq of sodium bicarbonate per ampule, may be used initially. The exact amount necessary depends on the pH, which in turn is related to the duration of the ventricular fibrillation. An additional ampule is given every 5 to 8 minutes until adequate cardiorespiratory function is achieved. Blood gases and pH should be obtained as soon as possible and further bicarbonate administration adjusted accordingly.

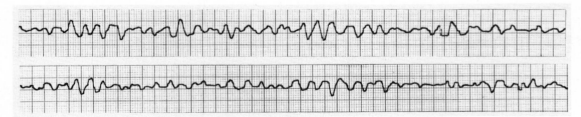

Fig. 8-51. Ventricular fibrillation. In this monitor lead the irregular, undulating base line without any electrical evidence of organized ventricular activity is characteristic of ventricular fibrillation. The rhythm in Fig. 8-50 proceeds to resemble the rhythm in 8-51.

Rate: Cannot be determined.
Rhythm: Grossly irregular.
P waves: Cannot be seen.
PR interval: Cannot be determined.
QRS: Cannot be measured.

FIRST-DEGREE AV BLOCK (Figs. 8-52 and 8-53)

During first-degree heart block AV conduction is abnormally prolonged, manifested by a PR interval exceeding 0.20 second in the adult. PR intervals as long as 1.0 second have been recorded. Every atrial impulse is conducted to the ventricles, producing a regular ventricular rhythm.

Atropine, isoproterenol, and exercise normally shorten the PR interval as the atrial rate increases; when the atrial rate is increased by atrial pacing, the PR interval lengthens. Steroids and thyroid hormones tend to improve AV conduction, which may lengthen during adrenal insufficiency or myxedema. Myocarditis or myocardial ischemia can cause transient AV conduction abnormalities.

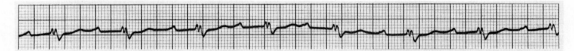

Fig. 8-52. First-degree heart block. In this monitor lead one cannot be certain of the type of intraventricular conduction delay. The prolonged AV conduction time may be due to conduction delay within the AV node and/or His-Purkinje system (see His bundle section).

Rate: 60 to 70 beats/minute.
Rhythm: Regular.
P waves: Normal contour and precede each QRS complex.
PR interval: Prolonged 0.36 to 0.40 second.

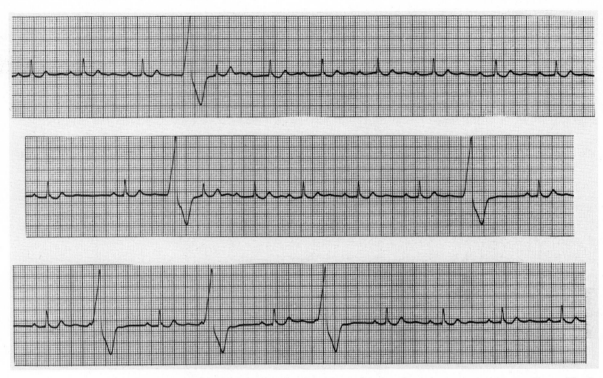

Fig. 8-53. First-degree AV block. In the selected strips from a continuous recording of lead I, premature ventricular systoles occur and are either interpolated (PVC in the first strip and first PVC in the second strip) or result in a compensatory pause. The PR interval of the QRS complexes preceding the PVC is slightly prolonged. However, following the interpolated PVC the PR interval prolongs further and remains prolonged for a series of beats, finally returning to the resting PR interval duration. When the premature ventricular complex produces a compensatory pause, additional PR prolongation does not occur. Monitor lead.

Rate: 63 beats/minute.
Rhythm: Regular for the most part; irregularities caused by premature ventricular complexes.
P waves: Normal.
PR interval: 0.22 to 0.24 second prior to the interpolated premature ventricular complexes, lengthening to 0.4 second immediately following the interpolated premature ventricular complex.
QRS: 0.07 second for the normally conducted beats and 0.16 second for the PVC.

SECOND-DEGREE AV BLOCK[24] (Figs. 8-54 to 8-58)

Failure of some atrial impulses to conduct to the ventricles at a time when physiologic interference would not be expected constitutes second-degree AV block. The nonconducted P wave may be intermittent, frequent, or infrequent, occur at regular or irregular intervals, and may be preceded by fixed or lengthening PR intervals. A distinguishing feature is that conducted P waves relate to a QRS complex with recurring PR intervals, that is, the association of P with QRS is not random. The two types of second-degree AV block can be distinguished with an acceptable degree of accuracy by analysis of the PR intervals. In a classic type I (Wenckebach) second-degree AV block a gradual lengthening of the PR interval occurs because of lengthening AV conduction time, until an atrial impulse is nonconducted. Then the sequence begins again. The ratio of atrial impulses to ventricular responses is frequently 5:4, 4:3, 3:2, or 3:1. Because the increment in conduction time is greatest in the second beat of the Wenckebach group and then *decreases* progressively over succeeding cycles, the interval between successive RR cycles prior to the nonconducted P wave progressively *decreases*, the duration of the pause produced by the nonconducted P wave is less than twice the shortest cycle, and the duration of the RR cycle following the pause exceeds the RR cycle preceding the pause. In atypical Wenckebach (which occurs commonly) the increment in AV conduction time may increase in the last beat so

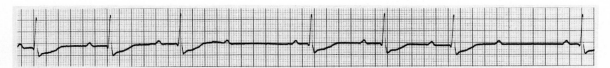

Fig. 8-54. Second-degree AV heart block (type I, Wenckebach). In this monitor lead classic AV Wenckebach heart block is characterized by four features in the surface electrocardiogram: (1) progressive PR prolongation preceding the nonconducted P wave; (2) progressive shortening of the RR interval because the increment in PR interval decreases in succeeding cycles; (3) the duration of the pause (generated by the blocked P wave) being less than twice the duration of the shortest cycle, which is the cycle that precedes the nonconducted P wave; and (4) the duration of the RR cycle following the pause exceeding the duration of the RR cycle preceding the pause. The increment in PR interval is greatest in the second cycle following the pause. Wenckebach AV block commonly may be "atypical" during which the increment in PR interval does not decrease but rather increases, so that the last RR interval preceding the nonconducted P wave lengthens rather than shortens. In the setting of a normal QRS complex, Wenckebach almost always occurs at the level of the AV node.

Rate: Atrial, 54 beats/minute; ventricular, varying.

Rhythm: Atrial, regular; ventricular, varying.

P waves: More numerous than QRS complexes but are related to ventricular beats in a consistent repetitive fashion.

PR interval: Progressive PR prolongation preceding the nonconducted P wave. Finally, one P wave is blocked, and the cycle then repeats.

QRS: Prolonged, 0.14 second. Therefore in this tracing one cannot be certain that the level of block is at the AV node but indeed could occur distal to the His bundle recording site (see His bundle section).

that the last RR cycle preceding the blocked P wave lengthens rather than shortens. The duration of the QRS complex may be normal or prolonged. Type I AV block occurs most commonly in the AV node but can occur in the His-Purkinje system as well.

In type II second-degree AV block a P wave is blocked without progressive antecedent PR prolongation and occurs almost always in a setting of bundle branch block. The PR interval of the conducted atrial impulses may be prolonged or normal but usually remains fairly constant. The pause caused by the nonconducted P wave is equal to or may be slightly less than twice the normal RR interval. Sinus arrhythmia, premature beats, AV junctional escape beats, or changes in neurogenic influences may disturb the timing of the expected pauses. Type II AV block almost always occurs in the His-Purkinje system.

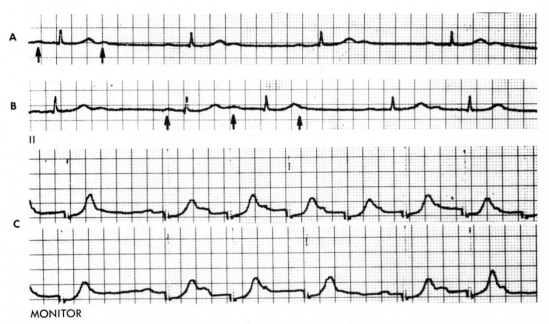

MONITOR

Fig. 8-55. Second-degree AV heart block (type I Wenckebach). In **A,** 2:1 conduction occurs (arrows indicate P waves). Since 2:1 conduction can occur with either type I or type II second-degree heart block, one sometimes cannot readily differentiate the two. The presence of a normal QRS complex is certainly in favor of this being type I second-degree AV heart block, however. In **B** the 2:1 AV heart block becomes 3:2 and PR prolongation for the second conducted P wave (second arrow) establishes the diagnosis of type I second-degree AV heart block. **C** (continuous recording) illustrates the response of Wenckebach AV block to intravenous atropine. Both the atrial rate and the conduction ratio increase.

Rate: Atrial: in **A** and **B,** 72 beats/minute; in **C,** 79 beats/minute; ventricular: in **A,** 36 beats/minute; in **B,** varying; in **C,** varying but increased.
Rhythm: Atrial, regular; ventricular, varying, depending on the degree of AV block.
P waves: Normal.
PR interval: Progressive increase in PR interval until one P wave fails to conduct.
QRS: Normal, 0.07 second.

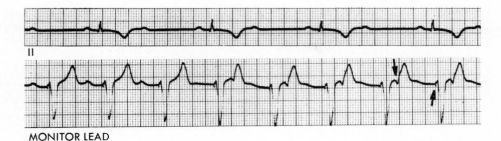

MONITOR LEAD

Fig. 8-56. 2:1 anterograde AV block and 1:1 retrograde VA conduction. In the top tracing alternate P waves conduct to the ventricles. In the lower tracing (same patient) ventricular pacing (upright arrow indicates pacemaker artifact) establishes 1:1 retrograde atrial conduction beginning with the fourth paced QRS complex. Inverted arrow indicates retrograde atrial activation.

Rate: Atrial: top tracing, 68 beats/minute; bottom tracing, 70 beats/minute; ventricular: top tracing, 34 beats/minute; bottom tracing, 70 beats/minute.
Rhythm: Atrial, regular; ventricular, regular.
P waves: Top tracing, normal; bottom tracing, normal and retrograde.
PR interval: Top tracing, 0.20 second; conduction of alternate P waves.
RP interval: Bottom tracing, 0.16 second.
QRS: Top tracing, 0.08 second; bottom tracing, 0.14 second.

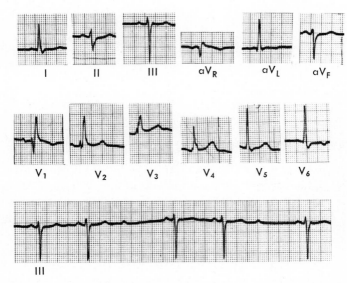

Fig. 8-57. Second-degree AV heart block, type II. The 12-lead ECG indicates the presence of left anterior fascicular block and right bundle branch block. In the rhythm recording (lead III) sudden failure of AV conduction results without antecedent PR prolongation.

Rate: 62 beats/minute.
Rhythm: Atrial, regular; ventricular, varying, depending on the degree of AV block.
P waves: Normal.
PR interval: Normal, constant (0.14 second) or may be prolonged, constant; sudden failure of conduction.
QRS: Prolonged, 0.12 second.

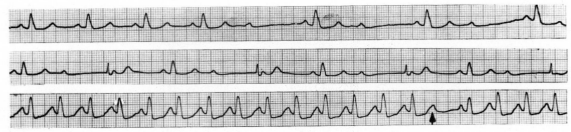

Isoproterenol

Fig. 8-58. Second-degree AV heart block, type II. Left bundle branch block is present in this recording of lead I. Sudden failure of AV conduction results, without antecedent PR prolongation. In the second strip the escape beats interrupt the pause produced by the blocked P wave. In the bottom strip isoproterenol infusion has increased the atrial rate and also increased the conduction ratio significantly. Only one nonconducted P wave occurs (*arrow*).

Rate: Atrial, 62 beats/minute in the top strip, 71 beats/minute in the middle strip, and 122 beats/minute in the bottom strip; ventricular, varying.
Rhythm: Atrial, regular; ventricular, varying depending on the degree of AV block.
P waves: Normal.
PR interval: Normal and constant at 0.19 second in the top and middle strips and difficult to measure in the bottom strip.
QRS: Prolonged to 0.12 second with a left bundle branch block contour.

COMPLETE AV BLOCK (Figs. 8-59 to 8-61)

Complete AV block occurs when no P waves are conducted to the ventricles. The atria and ventricles are controlled by independent pacemakers, and, as such, complete AV block constitutes one form of complete AV dissociation. The atrial pacemaker may be of sinus or ectopic atrial origin (tachycardia, flutter, or fibrillation). The ventricular focus may be above or below the His bundle bifurcation, depending on the site of the block. In congenital complete AV block, the block is usually at the level of the AV node, proximal to the His bundle. The escape focus is supraventricular and, as such, is more stable and faster than that which occurs with distal His block. The rhythm, usually regular, may vary because of premature ventricular beats, a shift in pacemaker site, or an irregularly discharging pacemaker focus. The QRS is normal, and Adams-Stokes syncope occurs less often. In acquired complete AV block, the ventricular rate is 30 to 40 beats/minute because the site of block is distal to the His bundle and consequently the escape focus is in the bundle branch–Purkinje system (Fig. 8-59). Less commonly, block within the bundle of His may occur (Fig. 8-61).

Significance. In the adult, drug toxicity (predominantly digitalis, but other drugs as well) and degenerative heart disease are the most common causes of acquired AV heart block. The degenerative process produces partial or complete anatomic or electrical disruption within the AV nodal region, the His bundle, or both bundle branches. Multiple factors may contribute to this degenerative process. They include fibrosclerosis of the cardiac skeleton, fibrosis of the conduction system, coronary artery disease, myocarditis, and cardiomyopathies. Cardiac surgery has become an infrequent but still important cause of heart block. Less commonly, electrolyte disturbances, endocarditis, tumors, Chagas' disease, syphilitic gummas, rheumatoid nodules, myxedema, infiltrative processes such as amyloidosis, sarcoidosis, or scleroderma, and other systemic illnesses may lead to AV heart block. Calcium deposition in the region of the aortic and mitral valves may extend to involve the conduction pathways. Digitalis excess produces type I, not type II, second-degree AV block.

AV heart block occurring during a myocardial infarction may be divided into two groups: that which occurs during an anterior or anteroseptal infarction and that which occurs during a diaphragmatic (inferior) infarction. When an anterior wall infarction produces AV block, it is usually the result of extensive necrosis of the summit of the interventricular septum, which spares the AV node and His bundle but inflicts severe damage to the bundle branches. Consequently, the block is apt to be distal to the His bundle (type II) and associated with right bundle branch block and a form of fascicular block. Complete AV block may develop, during which the ventricular rate is less than 40 beats/minute, asystole and syncope occur more commonly, and mortality is 75% or higher. Death results from pump failure or shock, owing to the large size of the infarction.

When AV block results from diaphragmatic infarction, the block, type I, usually occurs in the region of the AV node, owing to inflammation or edema that results from ischemia or infarction of neighboring myocardium. The ventricular pacemaker is faster and more stable, located in the region of the AV node or His bundle, and the block is usually transient, without residua. Advanced block and syncope are uncommon, and the mortality in patients without associated heart failure does not appear to be increased. Some overlap occurs between these two divisions.

Symptoms during second-degree AV block are infrequent unless long periods of AV block occur. The slow ventricular rate during complete heart block may not maintain circulation effectively and may result in angina, congestive heart failure, or syncope. Ventricular asystole may occur or the slow rate may initiate premature ventricular systoles or tachyarrhythmias.

Treatment

First-degree AV block. Generally no therapy is required. If digitalis, quinidine, or procainamide is implicated, the offending drug must be stopped or its dosage reduced.

Second-degree AV block

TYPE I. Generally no therapy is required. Treatment may be necessary for patients who are symptomatic with very slow ventricualr rates. Atropine, in 0.5-mg increments IV, or isoproterenol, 1 or 2 µg/minute, may be tried initially, with

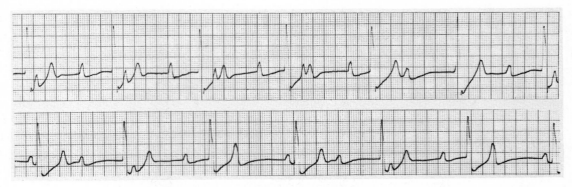

Fig. 8-59. Third-degree (complete) AV heart block. Complete AV dissociation is present due to complete AV heart block. Atria and ventricles are under control of separate pacemakers, the sinus node and an idioventricular escape rhythm, respectively. Monitor lead.

Rate: Atrial, slightly irregular but in the range of 75 beats/minute; ventricular, 39 beats/minute.
Rhythm: Atrial, slightly irregular. At times the PP interval surrounding the QRS complex is shorter than the PP interval without a QRS complex in between; this is called ventriculophasic sinus arrhythmia. Ventricular, regular.
P waves: Appear large but the standardization is not given.
PR interval: Completely variable.
QRS: Prolonged, 0.16 second.

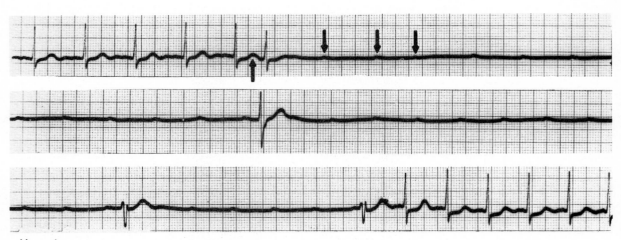

V₄ continuous

Fig. 8-60. Paroxysmal AV block. Periods of complete AV block interrupted only by an occasional escape beat occurred in this patient who had recurrent syncope. Each episode of AV block was always introduced by a premature atrial complex (*upright arrow*) which then resulted in a series of successive nonconducted P waves (*inverted arrows*). Finally, an escape beat occurred and restored conduction (bottom strip of this continuous recording of V₄). Electrophysiologic mechanism responsible for this form of paroxysmal AV block is not clear.

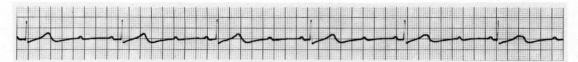

Fig. 8-61. Third-degree (complete) AV heart block. This tracing was recorded from an 80-year-old man who had recurrent syncope caused by an acquired complete AV block. The ECG is uncommon, since the QRS complexes are normal in this monitor lead and suggest that the site of block is AV nodal or, more likely, intra-Hisian. Congenital complete AV block has this appearance, although with a faster ventricular rate. His bundle recording would be necessary to establish site of block.

Rate: Atrial, 107 beats/minute; ventricular, 36 beats/minute.
Rhythm: Atrial, regular; ventricular, regular.
P waves: Normal.
PR interval: Totally variable.
QRS: Normal, 0.6 second.

care taken not to produce a sinus tachycardia in patients who have an acute myocardial infarction. If there is no response or if the block remains for prolonged periods, pacemaker therapy may be used. Digitalis, if implicated, must be stopped.

TYPE II. If type II block develops in the setting of an acute myocardial infarction, temporary transvenous pacing is necessary because this form of block often presages the occurrence of sudden complete AV block with ventricular asystole and Adams-Stokes syncope. Prior to pacemaker insertion, isoproterenol may be used temporarily. Atropine, by increasing the atrial rate without decreasing the AV block, may cause more P waves to block and reduce the ventricular rate. Symptomatic (for instance, with syncope, or presyncope) patients who do not have an acute myocardial infarction should receive a permanent pacemaker. For asymptomatic patients, many physicians recommend permanent pacemaker implantation prophylactically, since the natural history of type II AV block is to progress to complete AV block.

Third-degree (complete) AV block. If third-degree (complete) AV block develops in a setting of an acute myocardial infarction, temporary transvenous pacing is necessary; isoproterenol may be used initially if required. Asymptomatic patients with chronic stable complete AV block may need no specific therapy, although many physicians recommend prophylactic pacemaker implantation for them, to prevent an Adams-Stokes attack. For those patients with symptoms of congestive heart failure or Adams-Stokes syncope, caused by ventricular asystole, severe ventricular bradycardia, or ventricualr tachyarrhythmias occurring as a result of the AV block, long-term drug therapy is generally unreliable, and permanent pacemaker implantation is indicated. It has been suggested that patients who develop transient high-degree AV block during myocardial infarction and survive should receive prophylactic permanent pacemaker implantation even though the block resolves.[25] This conclusion needs to be supported by other studies.

BUNDLE BRANCH BLOCK[26] (Figs. 8-62 and 8-63)

Anatomic or functional discontinuity in one of the bundle branches may prevent or slow conduction so that the ventricle on the affected side becomes activated late, because this ventricle, normally supplied by the blocked bundle branch, must be activated by impulses traveling through the ventricular wall and interventricular septum from the unaffected side. Conduction along this circuitous route proceeds more slowly, and therefore the QRS complex becomes widened to 0.10 to 0.12 second (incomplete) or more than 0.12 second (complete right or left bundle branch block). Transient bundle branch block may occur as a result of tachycardia, bradycardia, pulmonary embolism, anemia, infection, myocardial ischemia or infarction, congestive heart failure, metabolic derangements, hypoxia, and other causes.

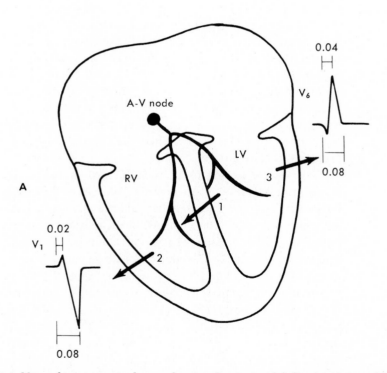

Fig. 8-62. A, Normal intraventricular conduction. Intrinsicoid deflection (interval from onset of QRS complex to peak of R wave, upper brackets) is usually about 0.02 second in right precordial leads and 0.03 to 0.04 second in left precordial leads. The intrinsicoid deflection prolongs during bundle branch block.

LEFT BUNDLE BRANCH BLOCK (Fig. 8-62)

In complete left bundle branch block (LBBB) the QRS complex becomes prolonged more than 0.12 second, with the major slowing occurring in the middle and terminal forces. The initial forces are deformed and prevent the development of the normal septal Q wave in I or V_6. Initial R waves in V_1 to V_3 are small or absent, followed by deep, large, slurred S waves, and large, prolonged R waves in V_5 and V_6. Significant mean axis deviation is usually absent. The ST segment and T wave shift are characteristically 180 degrees opposite the major QRS deflection.

Significance. LBBB is often associated with serious heart disease such as coronary artery disease, valvular heart disease, and hypertension. Although both RBBB and LBBB can occur in patients without apparent heart disease, LBBB correlates significantly with cardiomegaly and suggests a more serious prognosis. The conduction defect caused by LBBB alters the initial QRS vector, often obscuring the normal ECG signs of an acute myocardial infarction.

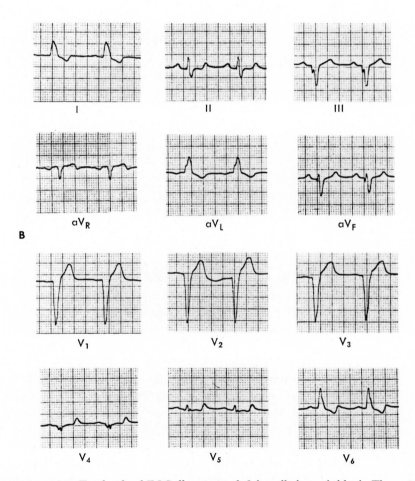

Fig. 8-62, cont'd. B, Twelve-lead ECG illustrating left bundle branch block. The axis is −30 degrees. *Continued.*

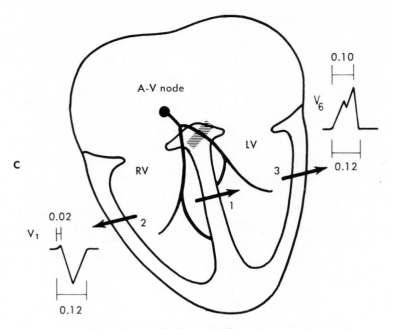

Fig. 8-62, cont'd. C, Schematic illustration is presented.

RIGHT BUNDLE BRANCH BLOCK (Fig. 8-63)

In uncomplicated complete right bundle branch block (RBBB) the QRS complex is 0.11 second or wider. The initial and middle forces of the vector loop are in a normal direction, and the terminal force is directed to the right and anteriorly. These changes produce large S waves in I, II, V_5, and V_6, often a terminal R wave in III, and R′ in V_1 and V_2. Incomplete RBBB is associated with the same electrocardiographic pattern, but the QRS complex is 0.10 second or less.

Significance. In a young individual, right ventricular hypertrophy may produce RBBB; in an older patient, coronary artery disease is a more likely cause. Early supraventricular complexes that are conducted aberrantly through the ventricle are more likely to develop an RBBB than LBBB, presumably because the right bundle branch takes longer to repolarize than does the left bundle branch. The initial forces in RBBB are not altered, and therefore the ECG signs of myocardial infarction are not obscured.

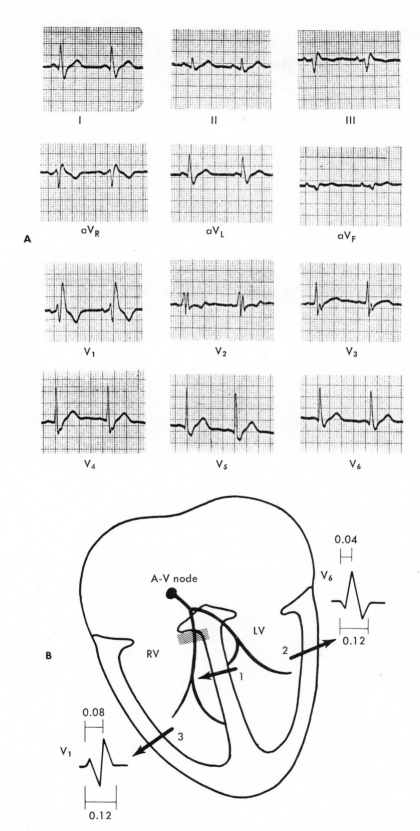

Fig. 8-63. A, Twelve-lead ECG illustrating right bundle branch block. **B,** Schematic illustration is presented.

FASCICULAR BLOCKS (Figs. 8-64 and 8-65)

According to electrocardiographic concepts, the left bundle branch divides into anterior and posterior divisions or fascicles.[1] Block may occur in one or the other division (hemiblock) and give rise primarily to a shift in the frontal plane QRS axis without significant QRS prolongation. *Left anterior fascicular block* results in a QRS angle in the frontal plane of about -60 degrees, an initial Q wave in lead I, a terminal S wave in lead III, and a normal or slightly prolonged QRS duration. *Left posterior fascicular block* produces a QRS angle in the frontal plane of about $+120$ degrees, an initial Q wave in lead III, and a terminal S wave in lead I; forces of the first half of the QRS complex are also directed toward $+120$ degrees. Right ventricular hypertrophy and a vertical heart must be excluded. Fascicular blocks may combine with RBBB, thus representing examples of bilateral bundle branch block.

Significance. Fascicular blocks may result from coronary artery disease, particularly in the setting of an acute anteroseptal myocardial infarction that simultaneously involves the right bundle branch and one of the divisions of the left bundle branch. Two large groups of patients develop ventricular conduction disorders owing to a sclerodegenerative process limited to the conduction system (Lenegre's disease) or to fibrosclerosis of structures adjacent to the conduction system (Lev's disease). Patients with Lenegre's disease appear to be younger than those with Lev's disease and more prone to developing AV block.

If left anterior or left posterior fascicular block is present with RBBB, it must be remembered that the unblocked fascicle may constitute the only conduction pathway from the His bundle to the ventricle. The posterior division of the left bundle branch seems to be the least vulnerable segment of the specialized ventricular conduction system and, therefore, left posterior fascicular block, with or without RBBB, occurs least often. When lesions are sufficiently extensive to involve the posterior fascicle, they often involve the anterior fascicle and right bundle branch as well. Left posterior fascicular block carries a worse prognosis than does left anterior fascicular block, with increased likelihood to progress to more advanced stages of AV block.

Treatment. In the presence of an acute myocardial infarction, the development of RBBB with left anterior or posterior fascicular block generally requires prophylactic temporary transvenous pacemaker insertion because more advanced AV block may follow. Pacemaker implantation usually is not necessary for the asymptomatic patient without acute myocardial infarction who develops one of the chronic forms of unilateral or bilateral bundle branch block as a result of degenerative cardiac changes, since their rate of progression to forms of symptomatic AV block is fairly slow. Also, these patients do not require temporary prophylactic pacing prior to undergoing surgical procedures.

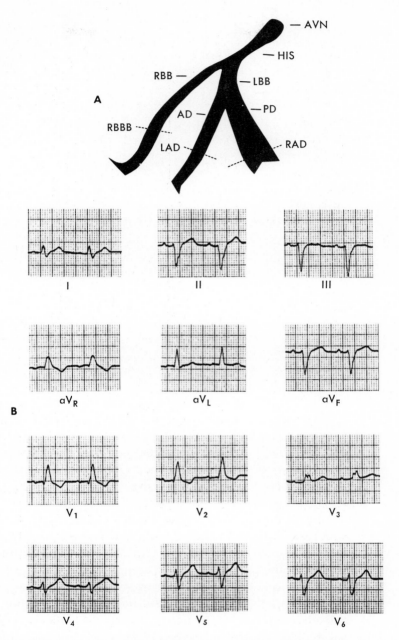

Fig. 8-64. A, Schematic illustration of the trifascicular nature of ventricular conduction. *AVN,* Atrioventricular node; *HIS,* bundle of His; *RBB,* right bundle branch; *LBB,* main portion of left bundle branch; *AD,* anterior division (fascicle) of left bundle branch; *PD,* posterior division (fascicle) of left bundle branch. Interrupted lines indicate block or delay in conduction, with resultant right bundle branch block *(RBBB),* left axis deviation *(LAD),* right axis deviation *(RAD).* LAD and RAD, in this context, are called left anterior fascicular and left posterior fascicular block, respectively. **B,** Twelve-lead ECG illustrating right bundle branch block and left anterior fascicular block. See also Fig. 8-57.

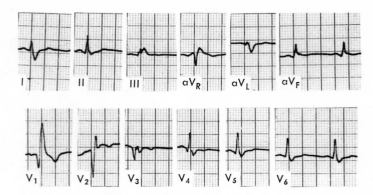

Fig. 8-65. Twelve-lead ECG illustrating right bundle branch block and left posterior fascicular block. The abnormal Q waves in leads V_1 to V_4 indicate the presence of an anteroseptal myocardial infarction. See also Fig. 5-7.

PARASYSTOLE (Fig. 8-66)[2]

Premature systoles that lack a fixed relationship to the preceding complex (varying coupling intervals) may result from parasystole. As classically defined, a parasystolic focus is a protected pacemaker focus that discharges at a fixed rate. Parasystolic discharge becomes manifest when the area in which the parasystolic focus originates has recovered excitability. The parasystolic focus then may depolarize the atrium or ventricle to produce a premature systole. The resulting P wave or QRS complex has a configuration different from that of the dominant rhythm, depending on the site of origin. Although the dominant rhythm may be discharged by the parasystolic focus, the dominant rhythm does not depolarize the parasystolic focus because the latter is protected by unidirectional entrance block; that is, impulses may exit from the parasystolic focus to discharge the surrounding myocardium, but no impulse may enter the parasystolic focus and discharge it. For learning purposes, it can be thought of as a fixed-rate pacemaker that does not sense spontaneous complexes and is not reset by them. The manifest parasystolic rate may be much less than the actual rate because of exit block from the parasystolic focus. That is, the parasystolic focus discharges at more rapid rates than are apparent in the ECG because many of the discharges fail to exit and depolarize the surrounding myocardium. Exit block from the parasystolic focus may produce irregular spacing of the interectopic intervals. However, since the rate of discharge of the parasystolic focus is constant, the interectopic intervals between parasystolic impulses reduce to a common denominator. Premature systoles that are caused by a parasystolic focus ordinarily have no fixed relationship to the basic rhythm and often result in the production of fusion beats.

Recent experimental and preliminary clinical data suggest that these comments about parasystole are too restrictive, and that the dominant cardiac rhythm can and does modulate the discharge rate and rhythm of the parasystolic focus.[2] Further discussion of this concept is beyond the scope of this chapter.

Significance. Atrial and junctional parasystole may occur in patients without clinical evidence of heart disease. Ventricular parasystole generally manifests in patients with heart disease; it is rarely, if ever, caused by digitalis excess.

Treatment. The therapeutic approach is basically the same as that discussed for premature atrial, junctional, and ventricular systoles.

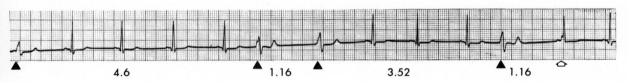

Fig. 8-66. Ventricular parasystole. The parasystolic ventricular beats are indicated by the solid triangles and the open arrow. The interval between parasystolic ventricular complexes is 1.16 seconds. The intervals of 4.6 and 3.52 seconds are four times and three times, respectively, the interectopic interval of 1.16 seconds. Note that the coupling interval varies and that a fusion beat (next to last QRS complex, indicated by open arrow) is also present. Ventricular refractoriness prevents emergence of the parasystolic ventricular rhythm during the long intervals in which it is absent. This tracing was recorded from an otherwise healthy 15-year-old boy.

Rate: 65 beats/minute, with some variation; parasystolic rate, 63 beats/minute.
Rhythm: Atrial and ventricular rhythms during normally conducted beats, regular; parasystolic ventricular interval, regular.
P waves: Normal.
PR interval: 0.11 second during the normally conducted beats.
QRS: Of normally conducted beats, 0.09 second; of parasystolic ventricular beats, 0.12 second.

PREEXCITATION (WOLFF-PARKINSON-WHITE) SYNDROME (Figs. 8-67 to 8-72)

Preexcitation[27] exists when the atrial impulse activates the whole or some part of ventricular muscle earlier than would be expected if the atrial impulse reached the ventricles by way of the normal specialized conduction system only. Four basic features typify the usual ECG of a patient with the preexcitation syndrome: (1) PR interval less than 0.12 second during sinus rhythm, (2) QRS complex duration greater than 0.12 second with a slurred, slow-rising onset of the R wave upstroke in some leads (delta wave) and usually normal terminal QRS portion, (3) secondary ST-T wave changes that are usually directed opposite the major delta and QRS vectors, and (4) paroxysmal tachyarrhythmias in 4% to 80% of patients. The explanation for those findings is the presence of a rapidly conductive accessory pathway that bypasses the AV node by communicating directly from atrium to ventricle. Other patients may possess variants of the preexcitation syndrome that are explained by the presence of bypass tracts between the AV node and ventricle (nodoventricular) or between the fascicles and ventricle (fasciculoventricular). The group of patients who have a short PR interval (less than 0.12 second) and a normal QRS complex with supraventricular tachycardias may not have a bypass tract from atrium to His bundle. These patients may simply possess an AV node that conducts rapidly, and also have episodes of supraventricular tachycardia.

Patients with the Wolff-Parkinson-White (WPW) variety of preexcitation syndrome may be divided into two broad types, depending on the form of QRS in the leads recorded from the right precordium, particularly V_1 and V_2. In type A the R wave is the sole or largest deflection in V_1 and V_2, and the accessory pathway is located between the left atrium and the left ventricle. In type B the S or QS deflection is largest in V_1 and V_2, and the accessory pathway is located between the right atrium and the right ventricle. Actually, the accessory pathway may be located at many different sites around the circumference of the AV groove, including septal areas. Each location results in a different QRS contour and delta wave,[28] and the classification into types A and B represents an oversimplification but is useful for our purposes.

Significance. The reported incidence of the preexcitation syndrome averages about 1.5 in 1000 persons, although the actual incidence is unknown. It occurs in all age groups and more often (60% to 70%) in males. Two thirds of patients with the short PR interval and normal QRS complex are female. Patients may seek help because of recurrent supraventricular tachycardia, atrial fibrillation with a rapid ventricular response, heart failure, syncope, or symptoms related to associated cardiac anomalies; or the symptoms may be discovered during examination for noncardiac-related reasons. Of adults with preexcitation syndrome, 60% to 70% have normal hearts; a higher proportion of children have heart disease. A variety of acquired and congenital cardiac defects have been reported in patients with the preexcitation syndrome, including Ebstein's anomaly, cardiomyopathies, and mitral valve prolapse.

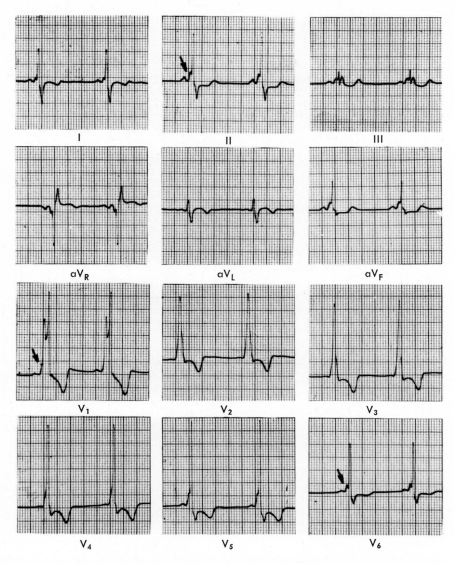

Fig. 8-67. Twelve-lead ECG illustrating preexcitation (Wolff-Parkinson-White) syndrome, type A indicated by positive delta wave and QRS complex in V_1 and V_6. Arrows indicate delta waves. The short PR interval is apparent.

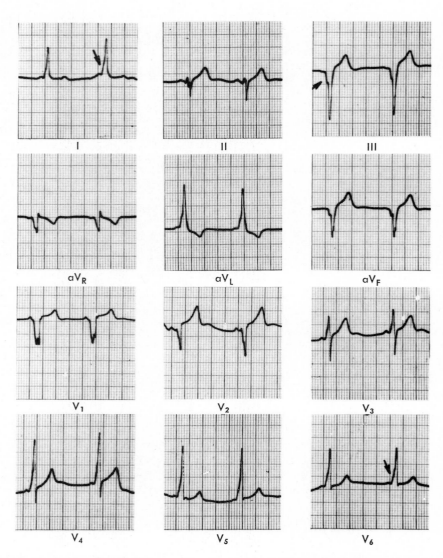

Fig. 8-68. Twelve-lead ECG illustrating preexcitation (Wolff-Parkinson-White) syndrome, type B indicated by negative delta wave and QRS complex in V_1 and positive delta wave and QRS complex in V_6. Arrows indicate delta waves. The short PR interval is apparent.

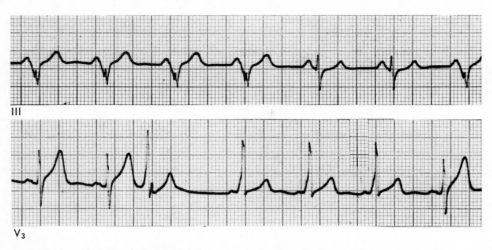

III

V₃

Fig. 8-69. Preexcitation (Wolff-Parkinson-White) syndrome, type B. Spontaneous onset and termination of preexcitation conduction account for the variable QRS conduction in lead III and V₃. The fifth and sixth QRS complexes in III and the first, second, and last QRS complexes in V₃ are normally conducted. In lead V₃ the onset of anomalous conduction follows a premature atrial systole (third QRS) with a Wolff-Parkinson-White pattern. This patient was erroneously admitted to the coronary care unit because of the Q waves in lead III, which were misinterpreted as indicating an inferior myocardial infarction.

Rate: 78 beats/minute.
Rhythm: Regular.
P waves: Normal.
PR interval: Varies between 0.10 and 0.13 second.
QRS: Normal (0.08 second) during conduction over the AV node with a normal PR interval; abnormal (0.12 second) during conduction over the bypass tract with a short PR interval.

Of patients with the preexcitation syndrome, 4% to 80% experience recurrent tachyarrhythmias; paroxysmal supraventricular (reciprocating) tachycardia occurs most often (80%), followed by atrial fibrillation (15% to 30%) and atrial flutter (5%). Ventricular tachycardia rarely occurs, and most reports have misdiagnosed as ventricular tachycardia the aberrant QRS complexes caused by anomalous conduction. Recognition of the preexcitation syndrome is clinically important, since the tachyarrhythmias at times do not respond to conventional therapy and may be associated with very rapid ventricular rates. For example, digitalis may accelerate the ventricular rate in some patients who have atrial fibrillation and the WPW syndrome. The anomalous complexes may mask or mimic myocardial infarction, bundle branch block, or ventricular hypertrophy, and the presence of the preexcitation syndrome may call attention to an associated cardiac defect.

The prognosis is excellent in patients without tachycardia or associated cardiac anomaly. In most patients with recurrent tachycardia the prognosis is good, but sudden unexpected death can occur, especially when the ventricular rate during tachycardia is rapid or associated congenital defects are present. Ventricular fibrillation has been documented in human and dogs and is probably caused by extremely rapid ventricular rates, permitted by the bypass during atrial flutter or fibrillation, that exceed the ability of the ventricle to follow in an organized fashion. Consequently, fragmented, disorganized ventricular activation results and leads to fibrillation. Alternatively, supraventricular discharge, bypassing the AV nodal delay, may activate the ventricle during the vulnerable period of the antecedent T wave and precipitate fibrillation.

Treatment. The tachycardia in patients who have the WPW syndrome may not respond to conventional therapy and may be associated with very rapid ventricular rates. Many patients with the preexcitation syndrome have rare or infrequent bouts of tachycardia that are not incapacitating and subside spontaneously or with vagal maneuvers. Some patients are moderately or severely incapacitated by recurrent tachyarrhythmias that require suppressive therapy. In this category are patients with frequent attacks of tachycardia, patients with very fast heart rates during attacks, and patients experiencing severe hypotension, heart failure, or syncope during attacks. In addition, prophylactic suppressive therapy may be considered in those patients whose accessory pathway has a short refractory period (established by electrophysiologic techniques) and who therefore might develop a very rapid ventricular reponse to atrial flutter or fibrillation.

A paroxysmal supraventricular tachycardia (PSVT) that exhibits normal QRS complexes can be approached as an ordinary PSVT, as if it were not associated with the preexcitation syndrome. The reason for this is that the cardiac impulse in this type of reciprocating tachycardia usually travels anterogradely to the ventricle over the normal AV node–His bundle route and retrogradely to the atrium over the accessory pathway (Fig. 8-70). Therefore, agents that slow AV nodal

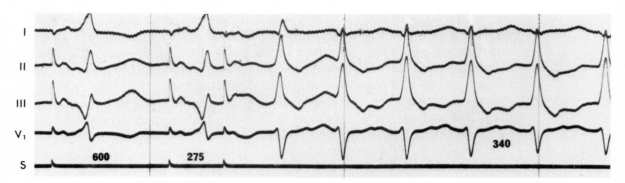

Fig. 8-70. Onset of reciprocating tachycardia in a patient with preexcitation (WPW) syndrome. The first two beats are paced from the right atrium (cycle length 600 msec) and conduct over the accessory pathway. The third beat is premature (275 msec) and conducts over the normal AV node–His bundle (note loss of delta wave). Following this a reciprocating tachycardia occurs at a cycle length of 340 msec. This is a typical example of the tachycardia in a patient with WPW syndrome. *S*, Stimulus.

conduction and prolong AV nodal refractory period, such as cholinergic drugs, verapamil, digitalis, reflex-induced vagal stimulation, propranolol, or any other agent that depresses AV nodal conductivity, may terminate the PSVT; digitalis, verapamil, quinidine, and propranolol may be used prophylactically (see discussion of therapy for PSVT). When PSVT is characterized by widened QRS complexes of WPW contour, digitalis alone may be contraindicated, and quinidine or other drugs that depress conduction in the accessory pathway, such as procainamide or disopyramide, may be required.

For atrial flutter or fibrillation, atrial impulses are not obliged to travel the normal AV node–His bundle route but can reach the ventricles via the bypass. Drugs possessing a vagal action (such as digitalis) may actually *speed* the ventricular rate, since they may improve conduction and shorten the refractory period in the accessory pathway in some patients. Quinidine, procainamide, and disopyramide prolong the refractory period of the accessory pathway and are useful in treating atrial flutter and fibrillation. Frequently the combination of digitalis and quinidine may be effective in slowing conduction in both the normal and the accessory pathways. Some patients who have PSVT may also intermittently develop atrial fibrillation. In these patients digitalis should not be used alone but can be combined, with quinidine, for example. If one is concerned about the effects of digitalis on the accessory pathway, then quinidine can be combined with propranolol or verapamil and digitalis not given at all.

If the ventricular rate is exceedingly rapid, in the range of 250 beats/minute, the development of ventricular fibrillation is possible, and DC shock should be considered the initial preferred treatment (Fig. 8-71).

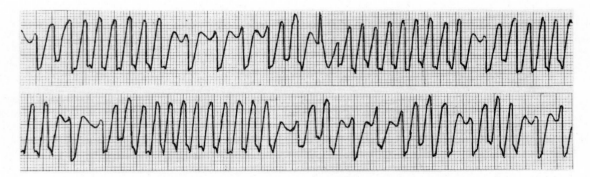

Fig. 8-71. Atrial fibrillation with an extremely rapid ventricular response in a patient who has the preexcitation (Wolff-Parkinson-White) syndrome. In this monitor lead the extremely rapid ventricular rates and gross irregularity of the RR intervals (remember, ventricular tachycardia can be irregular also; see Fig. 8-44) suggest the diagnosis of atrial fibrillation in a patient who has the Wolff-Parkinson-White syndrome. The atrial fibrillatory impulses conduct to the ventricle over the accessory pathway, bypassing the AV node.

Rate: Atrial, indeterminant; ventricular, 150 to 350 beats/minute.
Rhythm: Irregular.
P waves: Cannot be seen.
PR interval: Cannot be determined.
QRS: Difficult to determine, but approximately 0.12 to 0.14 second.

For patients who are symptomatic owing to drug-refractory, recurrent tachycardia, surgery to interrupt the accessory pathway has been extremely useful.[28]

It is now known that some patients who have PSVT without any overt evidence of WPW may have an accessory pathway that only conducts retrogradely (concealed WPW).[29] The surface ECG during PSVT may provide some clues as to the presence of a concealed accessory pathway by demonstrating the retrograde P wave to be in the ST segment (rather than simultaneous with the QRS, as in AV nodal reentry) and, if the accessory pathway is left sided, a negative P wave in lead I. Naturally, the short PR interval, delta wave, and prolonged QRS duration during sinus rhythm are not present.

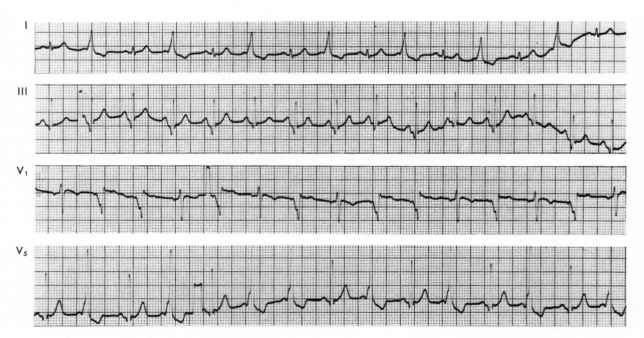

Fig. 8-72. Alternating conduction over the accessory pathway in type B preexcitation (Wolff-Parkinson-White) syndrome. Almost throughout the entire recording, the QRS complexes alternate between conduction over the accessory pathway and conduction over the normal pathway. Occasionally two consecutive beats conduct over the accessory pathway. Conduction over the accessory pathway is characterized by a short PR interval, delta wave, prolonged QRS duration, and secondary T wave changes. Such intermittent conduction over an accessory pathway suggests that its refractory period is prolonged and implies that extremely rapid rates during atrial flutter or atrial fibrillation, as seen in Fig. 8-71, would not occur.

Rate: 105 beats/minute.
Rhythm: Regular.
P waves: Normal.
PR interval: Alternating between 0.08 and 0.12 second.
QRS: Normal, 0.06 second during conduction over the AV node and abnormal, 0.12 second, during conduction over the accessory pathway.

AV DISSOCIATION[30]

As the words imply, AV dissociation means that atria and ventricles are dissociated; they are controlled by separate pacemakers for one or more beats. The term used generically tells nothing regarding the nature of atrial or ventricular activity, except that these chambers are beating independently for a period of time. It is as if the term described a "symptom" without indicating what caused it. The atria may be fibrillating, fluttering, or responding to an ectopic tachycardia or sinus impulses; the ventricles may be controlled by AV junctional or ectopic ventricular beating. The only fact conveyed is that whatever controls one chamber does not also control the other during the period of AV dissociation.

AV dissociation is *never* a primary disturbance of rhythm but rather a consequence of a more basic disorder; for the term to be used properly, the cause(s) producing AV dissociation must also be described. Examples can be found throughout this chapter; some of them are as follows:

1. Slowing of the primary pacemaker to allow the escape of a subsidiary (latent) focus. In Fig. 8-12, sinus slowing allows two ventricular beats to escape under the control of a separate focus while the sinus node still controls the atria. During these two beats, AV dissociation exists.

2. Accelerated discharge of subsidiary focus. In Fig. 8-38, accelerated AV junctional discharge results in a nonparoxysmal AV junctional tachycardia without retrograde atrial capture. Since the atria remain under sinus domination, separate pacemakers control atria and ventricles, resulting in AV dissociation. Fig. 8-136 presents a similar example, called "isorhythmic" AV dissociation because atria and ventricles maintain similar rates and rhythms. AV dissociation may also occur during ventricular tachycardia if retrograde atrial capture does not ensue (see Figs. 8-44 to 8-47).

3. AV block. In Fig. 8-58, AV block reduces the number of effective (conducted) atrial impulses; this allows the escape of a subsidiary focus to produce AV dissociation. When AV block results in AV dissociation, the atrial rate generally exceeds the ventricular rate (see Fig. 8-59).

4. Combinations of 1, 2, or 3 may initiate AV dissociation, as, for example, when digitalis causes both first-degree (or Wenckebach) AV block and NPJT, or when acute myocardial infarction produces AV block and an accelerated idioventricular rhythm (Fig. 8-48).

In all these examples, but for diverse reasons, the ventricular rate either exceeds or becomes equal or nearly equal to the effective (conducted) atrial rate. It is this fact that allows AV dissociation to occur.

The preceding discussion makes it apparent that the presence or absence of AV dissociation depends on the rate and temporal relationships of the two pacemakers and the intactness of AV and VA conduction. Should the atrial pacemaker capture control of the ventricle, or vice versa, AV dissociation would be terminated during that period of capture (incomplete AV dissociation).

SUPRAVENTRICULAR ARRHYTHMIA WITH ABNORMAL QRS COMPLEXES (Figs. 8-73 to 8-76)

Wide, bizarre QRS complexes may occur during isolated supraventricular beats or sustained supraventricular rhythms. The term *aberrant ventricular conduction* is commonly applied to such complexes. Thus QRS contours that display prolonged abnormal configuration indicate that conduction through the ventricle is abnormal; they do not necessarily mean that the impulse *originated* in the ventricles. The presence of fusion and capture complexes strongly supports the diagnosis of ventricular tachycardia or accelerated ventricular rhythm. However, the electrocardiographic manifestations of ventricular tachycardia, including the presence or absence of AV dissociation, and complexes that appear to represent capture or fusion beats, may be mimicked, under certain circumstances, by supraventricular arrhythmias.

Intraventricular conduction defects, bundle branch blocks, and anomalous pathway conduction all may initiate abnormal ventricular depolarization with widened QRS complexes. Also, premature supraventricular stimulation may conduct to the ventricles before ventricular repolarization has been completed, causing the impulse to conduct aberrantly. The resulting widened QRS complex may display characteristic features that distinguish it from those beats arising in the ventricles during a true ventricular tachycardia. The following analysis may be helpful in distinguishing aberrant ventricular conduction initiated by a supraventricular impulse from ventricular tachycardia.

Identification of atrial activity. During sinus rhythm or an ectopic supraventricular rhythm, identification of distinct atrial activity initiating ventricular depolarization, regardless of how deformed the QRS complex may appear, establishes the diagnosis of supraventricular rhythm with QRS aberration. A causal relationship between the P and QRS complexes may be demonstrated in one or more of the following ways, depending on the nature of the supraventricular rhythms:

1. P waves with a normal contour precede and maintain a constant relationship to each QRS complex during sinus rhythms.
2. Interventions that alter the sinus rate, such as carotid sinus massage or exercise, secondarily alter the ventricular rate in exactly the same manner and maintain the same, or nearly the same, PR interval. This indicates that ventricular activation follows as a consequence of atrial discharge. Atrial pacing can be employed to alter the atrial rate during a tachycardia characterized by wide QRS complexes, and a diagnosis of ventricular tachycardia is considered likely when fusion and capture complexes result.
3. When atrial flutter, atrial fibrillation, or atrial tachycardia exists, carotid sinus massage, digitalis, verapamil, or edrophonium chloride (Tensilon) administration produces characteristic slowing of the ventricular response (at times also normalizing the QRS complex); during PSVT the rhythm may remain unchanged or terminate and allow sinus rhythm to resume.
4. Atrial and ventricular rhythms may be so related as to suggest dependency of the latter on the former, during typical AV Wenckebach cycles, for example.

5. When atria and ventricles are dissociated, finding ventricular captures that have the same contour as the QRS of the tachyarrhythmia in question indicates a supraventricular rhythm.

6. Bursts of an intermittent tachycardia that are always initiated by a premature atrial complex provide indirect evidence supporting a supraventricular diagnosis. However, it is important to remember that, under certain circumstances, a premature atrial complex can initiate a ventricular tachycardia.

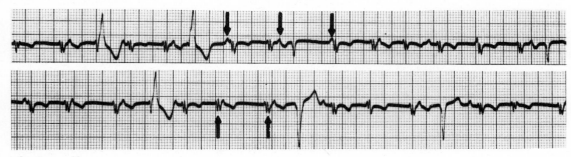

Continuous V₁

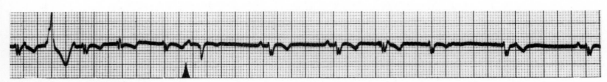

Carotid sinus massage V₁

Fig. 8-73. Nonparoxysmal AV junctional tachycardia with intermittent atrial captures producing functional right and functional left bundle branch block. The nonparoxysmal junctional tachycardia discharges at a slightly irregular rate and accounts for the W-shaped QRS complexes (*upright arrows*). Intermittent sinus captures (P waves indicated by inverted arrows) shorten the cardiac cycle and result in either a normal, W-shaped QRS complex, functional right bundle branch block, or functional left bundle branch block. Carotid sinus massage (in the bottom tracing at the arrowhead) slows both the sinus and junctional discharge rates. This tracing was recorded from a 13-year-old boy with no heart disease other than the cardiac arrhythmia. Therapy with digitalis slowed the junctional rate sufficiently so that the patient remained asymptomatic and had resting rates of 70 to 80 beats/minute with a normal response to exercise.

Rate: Atrial, approximately 88 beats/minute but varying; ventricular, approximately 88 beats/minute but varying.

Rhythm: Irregular; incomplete AV dissociation.

P waves: Normal.

PR interval: 0.14 second when premature capture does not occur.

QRS: Normal, functional right and functional left bundle branch block with a duration of 0.12 second.

7. During retrograde atrial capture the RP interval is of too short a duration to be explained by retrograde conduction from a ventricular focus (about 0.10 second or less).

8. If the rate and rhythm of abnormal QRS complexes are the same as the rate and rhythm of a known supraventricular tachycardia, this provides some support in favor of aberration.

9. The presence of AV dissociation during a wide QRS tachycardia is much more consistent with ventricular than supraventricular tachycardias.

Analysis of QRS contours and intervals. The following clues suggest aberrant ventricular conduction initiated by a supraventricular impulse:

1. The contour of the QRS is a triphasic rsR' in V_1. RBBB patterns occur more frequently than LBBB patterns because, at a slower heart rate, the right bundle branch appears to require more time to repolarize than the left. Therefore premature discharge is more likely to encounter a refractory right bundle branch and produce RBBB.

2. Monophasic or diphasic complexes in V_1 or an LBBB pattern favor the diagnosis of ventricular tachycardia, as does a frontal QRS axis that is directed superiorly and to the right.[30]

3. Faster rates speed repolarization, whereas slower rates retard it; the refractory period is proportional to the preceding cycle length. Therefore the heart takes longer to repolarize following a long cycle than it does after a short cycle. Because of this, when an early beat succeeds a long cycle, the early beat may encounter refractory tissue and conduct aberrantly. A comparison of such long-short cycle sequences aids in determining aberrant conduction.

4. During atrial flutter or fibrillation or a series of premature atrial complexes, aberrantly conducted beats persist in runs rather than maintain a bigeminal pattern and then lack a compensatory pause after their termination.

5. The initial vectors of aberrant and normal beats are similar during functional RBBB, since RBBB preserves the normal initial forces.

6. Aberrantly conducted supraventricular QRS complexes are not wildly bizarre or lengthened, most of the QRS prolongation occurring in the latter portion of the beat. QRS complexes with a duration exceeding 0.14 second are more likely to indicate ventricular tachycardia.

7. A fixed coupling interval between the normal and aberrant beats is absent during atrial flutter or atrial fibrillation. Conversely, fixed coupling during atrial flutter or fibrillation favors ventricular ectopy.

8. The aberrant beats are not excessively premature.

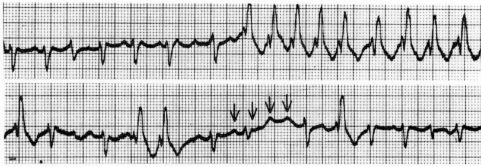

V₁—continuous

Fig. 8-74. Functional right bundle branch block. At first glance the tracing appears to be sinus rhythm interrupted by a burst of ventricular tachycardia and intermittent premature ventricular systoles. Closer inspection reveals flutter waves *(arrows)* when the ventricular rate slows slightly and suggests that the widened QRS complexes may be aberrantly conducted supraventricular beats. These beats conform in all respects to criteria established to differentiate supraventricular aberration from ventricular tachycardia. (See text.) The patient requires digitalis to slow the ventricular rate rather than lidocaine to suppress ectopic ventricular discharge.

Rate: Atrial, 280 beats/minute; ventricular, 90 to 200 beats/minute.
Rhythm: Atrial, regular; ventricular, irregularly irregular.
P waves: Flutter waves *(arrows)* can be seen when the ventricular rate slows and can be marched out with regularity.
PR interval: Flutter-R interval varies.
QRS: Varying contour between normal and functional right bundle branch block.

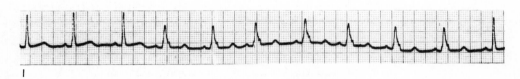

I

Fig. 8-75. Rate-dependent aberrancy of the left bundle branch block type. Gradual acceleration of the sinus rate results in a functional left bundle branch block that remains until the sinus rate slows sufficiently at the end of the tracing. This type of aberrancy is much more commonly of the left bundle rather than the right bundle branch block type and is more apt to be associated with cardiac disease than is functional right bundle branch block.

Rate: 60 to 78 beats/minute.
Rhythm: Slightly irregular.
P waves: Normal.
PR interval: Normal and constant, 0.14 second.
QRS: Varies between normal and functional left bundle branch block.

9. The QRS configuration appears the same as that resulting from known supraventricular conduction at similar rates. Conversely, if the QRS contour is the same as that resulting from known ventricular conduction, the tachycardia is probably ventricular in origin.

10. Vagal maneuvers remain a most important differentiating point, since vagal discharge does not usually affect ventricular tachycardia, whereas it slows the ventricular rate in most supraventricular mechanisms. However, ventricular tachycardia terminated by vagal discharge has been reported recently.

11. The presence of fusion and capture beats (see p. 229), as stated earlier, provides the most important evidence in favor of ventricular tachycardia.

None of the aforementioned features can be used to establish unequivocally the diagnosis of ventricular tachycardia, and in many instances invasive electrophysiologic studies must be performed.

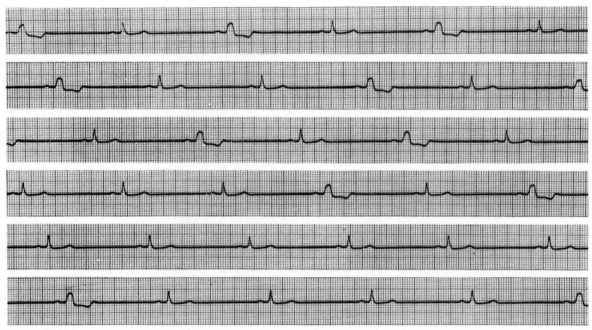

Continuous lead I

Fig. 8-76. Bradycardia-dependent left bundle branch block. In this unusual tracing the patient has a sinus bradycardia. When the sinus cycle *slows*, the P wave conducts with a left bundle branch block. Shorter sinus cycles are ended with a normally conducted QRS complex. Very small changes in the sinus rate account for these differences.

Rate: 34 to 38 beats/minute.
Rhythm: Fairly regular.
P waves: Normal and precede each QRS complex.
PR interval: 0.19 second.
QRS: Normal and left bundle branch block, 0.14 second.

ELECTROLYTE DISTURBANCES

Potassium (Figs. 8-77 and 8-78). During induced hyperkalemia in animals, the ECG correlates closely with the potassium blood level. The T wave peaks when potassium concentration reaches about 5.5 mEq/L; the corrected QT interval is normal or shortens initially but may prolong as the QRS complex widens. The QRS complex may widen when the external potassium concentration exceeds 6.5 mEq/L; about 7.0 mEq/L, P wave amplitude diminishes, and P wave and PR interval duration are prolonged. About 8.0 to 9.0 mEq/L, the P wave frequently disappears. Sometimes ST segment deviation, both elevated and depressed, occurs and stimulates an injury pattern. Clinically occurring potassium alterations do not correlate as well as during these experimental changes, probably because the patient has multiple abnormalities that may influence the ECG differently. For example, in some studies less than 25% of patients with hyperkalemia developed the characteristic tall, narrow, peaked T waves. It is believed that extracellular potassium concentration accounts for the ECG patterns rather than changes in total body potassium or intracellular potassium concentration.

During hypokalemic states the ST segment becomes depressed, the U wave is exaggerated, and the T wave amplitude is decreased without changing the actual duration of QT interval (as long as it can be measured accurately). Actually, it is the QU interval that becomes prolonged. The P and QRS amplitude and duration may increase, and the PR interval may be prolonged. Clinical hypokalemia does not normally slow AV conduction significantly; however, isolated cases have been reported demonstrating varying degrees of PR prolongation. Intraventricular conduction in adults seldom lengthens by more than 20 msec, but it may be more prolonged in children.

Spontaneous hyperkalemia rarely, if ever, produces more advanced AV block than simple PR prolongation; large doses of potassium administered rapidly may produce further advanced forms of AV block, however. Often the P wave disappears, which precludes the diagnosis of AV block. As the plasma potassium level continues to rise above 6.5 and 7.0 mEq/L, slowed intraventricular conduction results, manifested by uniform widening of the QRS complex. Areas of intraventricular block may occur and lead to ventricular fibrillation.

Potassium may potentiate the slowing effects of digitalis on AV conduction, particularly if plasma potassium level rises rapidly. However, if AV conduction is also hampered by a rapid atrial rate, slowing the atrial rate with potassium actually may improve AV conduction and offset any direct depressing effects of potassium. Fortunately, potassium administration to patients with digitalis-induced arrhythmias suppresses ectopic discharge at a much lower blood potassium level than that which further depresses AV conduction.

Low blood potassium levels encourage spontaneous ectopic pacemaker discharge, presumably by enhancing automaticity and also possibly by slowing dominant pacemakers or producing conduction defects. Low potassium levels may initiate ventricular fibrillation in humans. Reduced potassium concentration may precipitate arrhythmias in animals and humans receiving digitalis at plasma potassium levels that ordinarily do not produce ectopic beating in the absence of

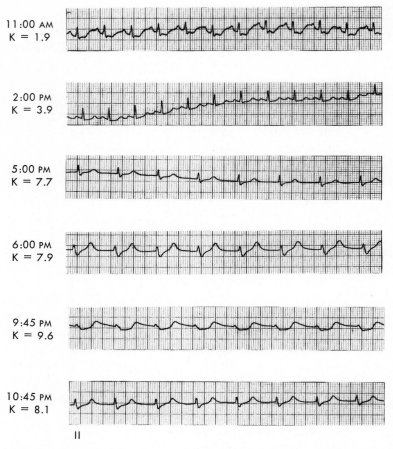

Fig. 8-77. Serial ECG tracings in a patient with marked changes in serum potassium level. In the 11:00 AM tracing the depressed ST segment and low amplitude T wave blending into a probable U wave (this cannot be seen with clarity because of the superimposed P waves) indicate the presence of hypokalemia. Following the administration of potassium the 2:00 PM tracing becomes relatively normal. Continued potassium administration results in hyperkalemia with the disappearance of atrial activity on the ECG and some prolongation of the QRS complex. By 7:00 PM the QRS complex is more prolonged, and by 9:45 PM the QRS complex is greatly prolonged. Secondary ST-T wave changes are present. Improvement follows the administration of bicarbonate, glucose, and insulin at 10:45 PM with reduction in serum potassium level; improvement in the ECG results.

digitalis. Possibly the synergistic effects of digitalis and reduced potassium on automaticity and conduction make animals and humans receiving digitalis particularly prone to arrhythmias precipitated by hypokalemia.

The antiarrhythmic effects of potassium administration may suppress varied rhythms, regardless of cause and whether or not hypokalemia exists. Digitalis-induced ectopic discharge generally responds to potassium therapy at sufficiently low doses to avoid further AV conduction delay. Many believe that potassium remains the drug of choice for ectopic rhythms produced by excessive digitalis.

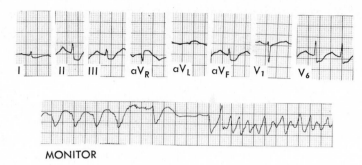

Fig. 8-78. Hypokalemia-induced ventricular tachycardia and fibrillation. The ECG demonstrates the characteristic changes of hypokalemia: depressed ST segment, low-amplitude T wave, and large U wave, blending into the following P wave. In the monitor lead a ventricular tachycardia briefly stops and then degenerates into ventricular fibrillation that was reversed with DC shock.

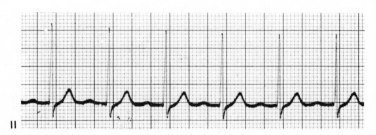

Fig. 8-79. The effects of hypercalcemia on the ECG. Serum calcium level, 14.0/100 ml. The ST segment and QT interval are shortened, and the PR interval is slightly prolonged (0.22 second).

Animals and humans with elevated potassium levels may tolerate large doses of digitalis without developing ectopic arrhythmias, whereas reduced potassium level predisposes to ectopic activity indigitalized animals or patients. Also, a low level of potassium may worsen the depression of AV conduction produced by digitalis.

Sodium. In general the magnitude of sodium change necessary to produce ECG alterations is not compatible with life, making clinical electrocardiographic manifestations of sodium derangements rarely seen, if ever.

Calcium (Fig. 8-79). In the ECG, low calcium level prolongs the duration of the ST segment and QT interval without prolonging the duration of the T wave, although the T wave may reverse polarity. Elevated calcium level shortens the ST segment and QT interval; the QRS duration may be prolonged during severe hypercalcemia, and AV block may develop. High calcium level opposes the effects of high potassium level, whereas low calcium level opposes the effects of low potassium. If the calcium level varies in a direction opposite that of potassium level, the effects of the latter are enhanced.

HIS BUNDLE ELECTROCARDIOGRAPHY (Figs. 8-80 to 8-83)

The technique of His bundle electrocardiography involves passing an electrode catheter that is introduced percutaneously into the femoral vein, in a cephalad direction up the inferior vena cava, and positioning the catheter tip near the septal leaflet of the tricuspid valve. The His potential (H) appears as a well-defined, most often bipolar spike between the low right atrial (A) and ventricular (V) electrograms. The interval between the earliest onset of the surface P wave or a high right atrial deflection (P) and the low right atrial deflection (PA interval) is a measure of intraatrial conduction. The AH interval is a measurement of the conduction across the AV node and varies in duration from 55 to 130 msec, depending on the cycle length and autonomic influences. The interval from H to V (HV interval) is determined by the interval between the His deflection and the earliest ventricular activity recorded in any lead. The HV interval is a measure of conduction through the His bundle distal to the recording electrode, the bundle branches, and the Purkinje system up to the point of ventricular activation. In contrast to a relatively wide range of values for the AH interval, the HV interval is fairly constant, measuring 30 to 55 msec, with an average value of 45 msec. In some patients, discharge of the right bundle branch may be recorded.

The ability to separate AV nodal and His-Purkinje conduction has enhanced our understanding of normal and abnormal AV conduction. Abnormal AV conduction may be caused by prolongation of P-A, A-H, or H-V intervals or all three. In addition, intra-His block has been demonstrated. During type I (Wenckebach) AV block in a patient with a normal QRS complex the conduction disturbance occurs at the AV node, proximal to the His bundle (Fig. 8-80). Type II AV block in a patient with a bundle branch block virtually always results distal to the His bundle (Fig. 8-81). Thus in type I AV block the blocked P wave is not followed by a His spike, whereas in type II AV block the blocked P wave is followed by a His spike.

His bundle electrocardiography has been useful in differentiating ventricular tachycardia and aberrant ventricular conduction, in understanding the nature of many supraventricular and ventricular tachycardias and other arrhythmias, in evaluating patients with the preexcitation syndrome or AV block, and in other areas as well, such as precipitating tachyarrhythmias in susceptible patients (Figs. 8-82 and 8-83). Further discussion is beyond the scope of this text, and the reader is referred to other sources.[10] The utility of His bundle electrocardiography as a routine clinical tool necessary to the care of patients with heart disease is not yet completely defined. In most instances, however, a carefully analyzed surface ECG clearly provides the necessary information required to make clinical therapeutic decisions.

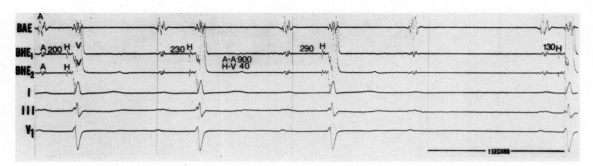

Fig. 8-80. Type I (Wenckebach) AV nodal block. Simultaneous recordings of electrograms from the high right atrium (*BAE*) and His bundle (*BHE₁, BHE₂*) and scalar leads I, III, and V₁ are displayed during normal sinus rhythm. The PR interval progressively lengthens until the fourth P wave fails to conduct. The conduction delay is due to AH prolongation that increases from 200 msec in the first beat shown (not the first beat in this Wenckebach series) to 290 msec just prior to the block. The AH interval then shortens to 130 msec in the first beat of the next Wenckebach series. The nonconducted P wave blocks proximal to the His bundle.

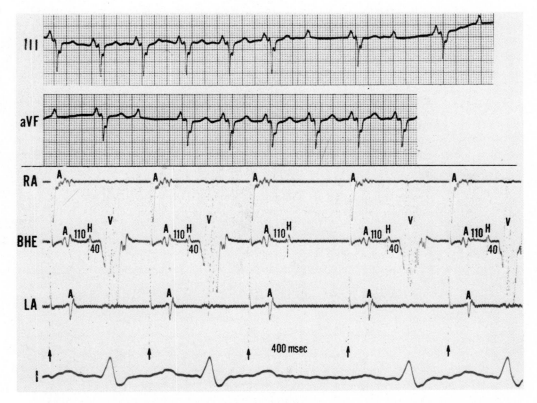

Fig. 8-81. Type II AV block. The scalar recordings in the top portion of the figure (leads III and AV_F) demonstrate type II AV block characterized by a fixed PR interval preceding the nonconducted P wave. During the electrophysiologic study (*bottom*), right atrial pacing at a cycle length of 400 msec resulted in a fixed AH interval of 110 msec and HV interval of 40 msec. The third P wave (*A*) blocked distal to the His bundle recording site, characteristic of type II AV block. *LA*, Left atrial electrogram. Arrows point to stimuli delivered to right atrium.

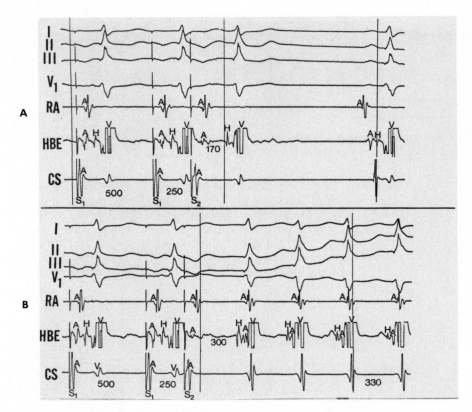

Fig. 8-82. Precipitation of AV nodal reentrant, supraventricular tachycardia. **A,** Recordings were obtained simultaneously from scalar leads I, II, III, and V_1 and intracavitary recordings from the right atrium *(RA)*, His bundle area *(HBE)*, and coronary sinus *(CS)*. The coronary sinus was stimulated at a fixed cycle length of 500 msec (S_1 to S_1) and then stimulated prematurely (S_2) at a cycle length of 250 msec. The AH interval lengthened slightly to 170 msec, but tachycardia did not result. **B,** Premature stimulation at the same coupling interval produced an AH interval of 300 msec and precipitation of a supraventricular tachycardia caused by AV nodal reentry at a cycle length of 330 msec (rate, 182 beats/minute). Findings are consistent with "dual AV nodal" pathways.

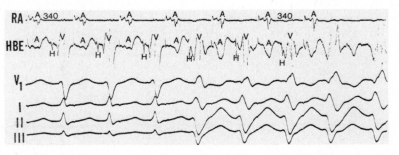

Fig. 8-83. Precipitation of ventricular tachycardia during right atrial pacing. In the left portion of the tracing the right atrium was paced at a cycle length of 340 msec. After the third normally conducted QRS complex, ventricular conduction becomes abnormally prolonged. The HV interval shortens, AV dissociation results, and the ventricular tachycardia continues, following cessation of atrial pacing *(top right)*. These findings are consistent with a ventricular tachycardia initiated during atrial stimulation. The tracing was recorded in an 18-year-old man who had exercise-induced ventricular tachycardia.

ARTIFACTS (Figs. 8-84 and 8-85)

Electronic instrumentation has provided vast dividends to the care of patients with heart disease. However, because we now rely so heavily on various types of monitoring devices, one must constantly be alert and recognize artifacts that mimic arrhythmias. A tracing that resembles ventricular fibrillation *must* be artifactual if the patient is found sitting up in bed in no distress, reading a newspaper!

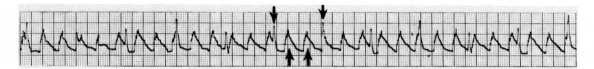

Fig. 8-84. Toothbrush tachycardia. This tracing was recorded from a patient brushing his teeth with an electric toothbrush at a rate of 188 brushes/minute. Note the regularly occurring artifacts *(upright arrows)* that do not influence the QRS complexes *(inverted arrows)*.

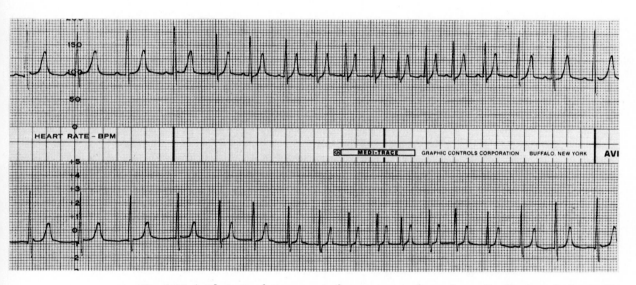

Fig. 8-85. Artifact simulating onset of supraventricular tachycardia. During playback of a tape-recorded ECG rhythm, the rate of revolutions per minute of the tape slowed and simulated the onset of a supraventricular tachycardia. The diagnosis of artifact is easily made, since, in addition to shortening of the RR interval, the PR, QRS, and QT intervals all decrease markedly. Both leads recorded simultaneously.

Arrhythmia test section

It is suggested that the reader use this section to test his knowledge of arrhythmias. Cover the interpretations in each legend, calculate intervals and irregularities as previously discussed, and determine the diagnosis. Consider also the significance of each arrhythmia and what form of treatment would most likely be employed. There may be disagreements in interpretation of rhythm strips, but the essential point is to make your diagnosis by using the analytic method described in this chapter. This approach offers a justification for your interpretation.

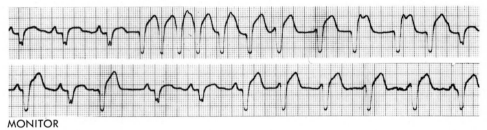

MONITOR

Fig. 8-86

Rate:	Atrial	78 beats/minute.
	Ventricular	Varies between 78 and 180 beats/minute.
Rhythm:	Atrial	Regular.
	Ventricular	Varying.
P waves:		Normal when visible.
PR interval:		0.16 second preceding the normally conducted QRS complexes. Not measurable in front of the ventricular ectopy.
QRS:		Normal for the sinus-conducted beats (0.09 second); prolonged for the ventricular ectopy (0.14 second).
Arrhythmia:		Paroxysmal ventricular tachycardia coexisting with an accelerated idioventricular rhythm.

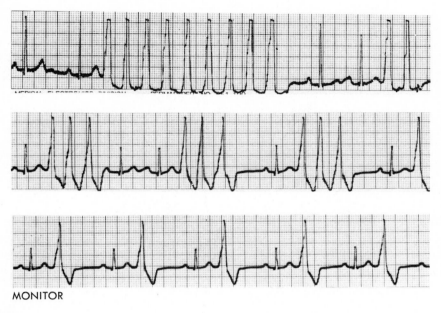

MONITOR

Fig. 8-87

Rate:	Atrial	60 to 75 beats/minute.
	Ventricular	170 to 210 beats/minute.
Rhythm:	Atrial	Slightly irregular.
	Ventricular	Irregular because of bursts of ventricular ectopy.
P waves:		Normal for the sinus-initiated QRS complexes.
PR interval:		Normal for the sinus-initiated QRS complexes, 0.16 second.
QRS:		Normal for the sinus-initiated complexes; wide, bizarre, prolonged (0.12 second) for the ventricular ectopy.
Arrhythmia:		Paroxysmal ventricular tachycardia gradually decreasing in frequency to bigeminy and then complete disappearance. This result followed administration of lidocaine, 50 mg IV in a patient with an acute myocardial infarction.

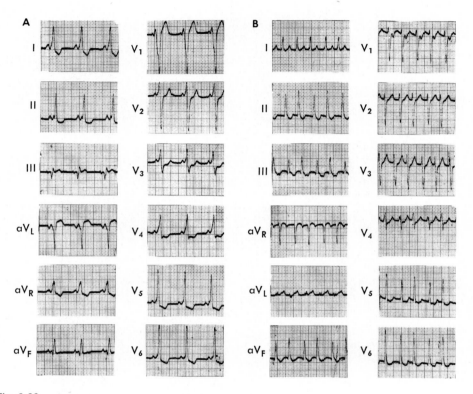

Fig. 8-88

Rate:	**A,** 82 beats/minute; **B,** varying between 150 and 180 beats/minute.
Rhythm:	**A,** regular; **B,** slight variation in RR intervals with long cycles alternating with short cycles.
P waves:	**A,** Normal; **B,** retrograde; see V₁.
PR interval:	**A,** 0.08 second; **B,** RP interval 0.12 second.
QRS:	**A,** Prolonged 0.12 second; **B,** normal 0.08 second.
Arrhythmia:	**A,** Normal sinus rhythm during preexcitation syndrome, type B; **B,** paroxysmal supraventricular tachycardia in the same patient.

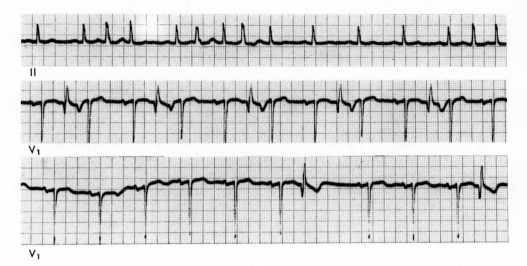

II

V₁

V₁

Fig. 8-89

Rate:	75 beats/minute, with premature systoles.
Rhythm:	Irregular because of premature systoles.
P waves:	Normal and precede each of the normal QRS complexes.
PR interval:	Prolonged following the premature systoles.
QRS:	Normal for the sinus-initiated systoles; prolonged to almost 0.12 second for the premature systoles.
Arrhythmia:	Interpolated premature ventricular systoles in the top and middle tracings. In the bottom tracing, premature ventricular systoles produce a compensatory pause and are therefore no longer interpolated.

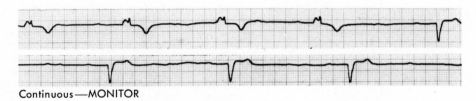

Continuous—MONITOR

Fig. 8-90

Rate:	Atrial	86 beats/minute.
	Ventricular	Upright complexes 38 beats/minute; negative complexes 28 beats/minute.
Rhythm:	Atrial	Regular.
	Ventricular	Fairly regular.
P waves:		Normal and have no relationship to the QRS complexes. Clear P waves cannot be seen throughout the entire tracing.
PR interval:		Not measurable.
QRS:		Abnormal; upright complexes 0.14 second, negative complexes 0.12 second.
Arrhythmia:		Complete AV block with a ventricular escape rhythm. The simultaneous change in ventricular contour and rate probably indicates a shift in the ventricular escape focus site.

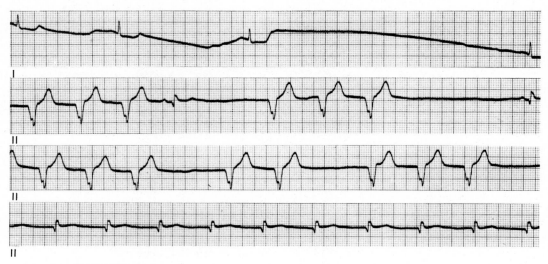

I

II

II

II

Atropine, 0.75 mg IV

Fig. 8-91

Rate:	Top tracing, slow with periods of asystole. Second and third strips 75 beats/minute with periods of asystole. Bottom tracing 65 beats/minute.
Rhythm:	Top three tracings, irregular; bottom tracing, regular.
P waves:	Normal contour, preceding the sinus-initiated QRS complexes in lead II but are hard to see in lead I.
PR interval:	Normal for the sinus-initiated P waves, not present for the other QRS complexes. In the bottom tracing no P wave or PR interval is apparent.
QRS:	Normal for the sinus-initiated QRS complexes, prolonged (0.13 second) for the ventricular ectopic beats.
Arrhythmia:	Various arrthymias recorded in a patient with an acute inferior myocardial infarction. Top tracing, marked sinus bradycardia and periods of sinus arrest. Middle two tracings, an accelerated idioventricular rhythm, slightly irregular. The duration of the pauses in the third strip appears to be a multiple of the basic idioventricular cycle length, thus suggesting the possible presence of an intermittent exit block. Bottom tracing, a junctional rhythm following atropine administration, suppresses the ventricular ectopy.

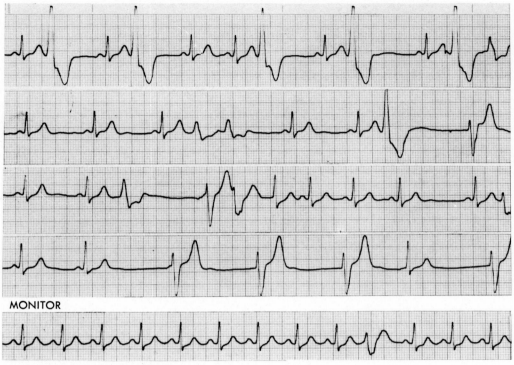

MONITOR

Atropine, 0.5 mg IV—MONITOR

Fig. 8-92

Rate:	45 to 125 beats/minute.
Rhythm:	Irregular.
P waves:	Normal and present before each of the sinus-initiated QRS complexes. Intermittent sinus slowing occurs.
PR interval:	Normal and constant before each of the sinus-initiated QRS complexes (0.14 second).
QRS:	Normal for the sinus-initiated QRS complexes, prolonged (0.14 second) for the ventricular systoles.
Arrhythmia:	Frequent multiformed ventricular systoles occurring singly and in pairs in a patient with an acute myocardial infarction. Sinus bradycardia results in the emergence of a slow idioventricular rhythm (fourth strip). Atropine (bottom tracing) produced a sinus rhythm and suppressed the ventricular ectopy.

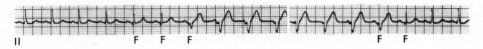

Fig. 8-93

Rate:	94 to 105 beats/minute.
Rhythm:	Fairly regular.
P waves:	Normal and precede each of the sinus-initiated QRS complexes. They do not precede the ventricular ectopic systoles.
PR interval:	Normal for the sinus-initiated P waves.
QRS:	Normal for the sinus-initiated P waves; prolonged (0.14 second) for the abnromal QRS complexes. Fusion beats labeled *F*.
Arrhythmia:	Accelerated idioventricular rhythm that becomes manifest because of gradual sinus slowing.

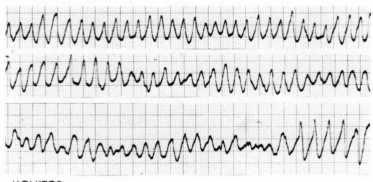

MONITOR

Fig. 8-94

Rate:	300 to 500 beats/minute.
Rhythm:	Grossly irregular.
P waves:	None seen.
PR interval:	Not measurable.
QRS:	Wide, bizarre, irregular.
Arrhythmia:	Ventricular flutter that becomes ventricular fibrillation in the bottom tracing. The ventricular fibrillation then seems to organize and merge into ventricular flutter or possibly ventricular tachycardia in the terminal portion of the tracing.

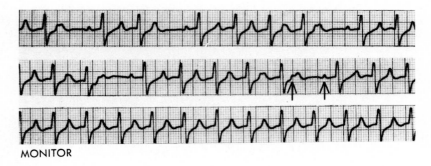

MONITOR

Fig. 8-95

Rate:	Atrial	115 beats/minute.
	Ventricular	Varying, depending on the degree of block.
Rhythm:	Atrial	Regular.
	Ventricular	Irregular.
P waves:		Precede each of the QRS complexes *(arrows)*.
PR interval:		Progressively lengthens until one P wave fails to conduct (Wenckebach AV block).
QRS:		Normal (0.08 second).
Arrhythmia:		Atrial tachycardia with varying block. Note the varying T wave contour as P waves fall during different portions of the antecedent T wave. In the bottom tracing 1:1 AV conduction occurs.

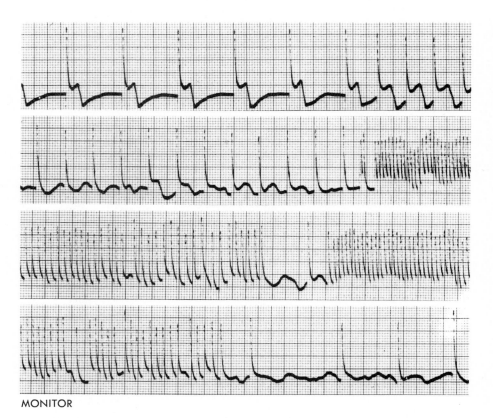

MONITOR

Fig. 8-96

Rate:	Ventricular	74 beats/minute to very rapid rates.
Rhythm:	Ventricular	Periods of regularity replaced by gross irregularity.
P waves:		None seen.
PR interval:		Not measurable.
QRS:		Wide, distorted, initiated by pacemaker spikes.
Arrhythmia:		Runaway pacemaker discharging at irregular and, at times, extremely rapid rates and finally initiating ventricular fibrillation. The pacemaker rate sped from 71 beats/minute to approximately 145 beats/minute and then greater than 1000 stimuli/minute.

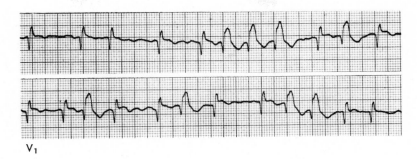

V₁

Fig. 8-97

Rate:	Ventricular	73 to 180 beats/minute.
Rhythm:	Ventricular	Grossly irregular.
P waves:		None seen.
PR interval:		Not measurable.
QRS:		Normal (0.08 second) and abnormal (0.12 second) with a right bundle branch block contour.
Arrhythmia:		Atrial fibrillation with a rapid ventricular response. QRS complexes, which demonstrate a right bundle branch block, terminate a short cycle (or a series of short cycles) that follows a long preceding cycle. The development of functional right bundle branch block caused by cycle length changes in this fashion is called the "Ashman phenomenon."

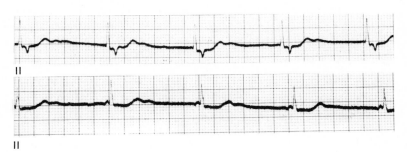

II

II

Fig. 8-98

Rate:	Top, 52 beats/minute; bottom, 48 beats/minute.
Rhythm:	Regular.
P waves:	Retrograde.
PR interval:	Bottom, 0.06 second.
RP interval:	Top, 0.08 second.
QRS:	Normal (0.06 second).
Arrhythmia:	AV junctional rhythm recorded on two occasions in the same patient. In the top tracing, retrograde P waves followed the QRS complex; in the bottom tracing, retrograde P waves preceded the QRS complex.

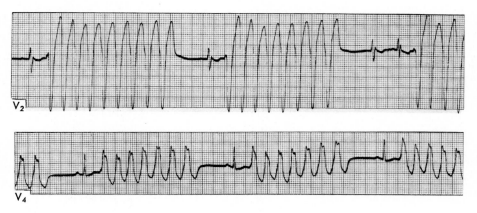

Fig. 8-99

Rate:	Ventricular	250 beats/minute.
Rhythm:	Ventricular	Regular in a recurrent paroxysmal fashion.
P waves:		Precede the normally conducted QRS complexes.
PR interval:		Normal for the normally conducted QRS complexes.
QRS:		Normal for the sinus-initiated QRS complexes. QRS prolonged for the ventricular ectopic systoles (0.14 seconds).
Arrhythmia:		Repetitive intermittent paroxysmal ventricular tachycardia. The lack of fusion or capture beats and precise determination of atrial activity during the tachycardia prevent an unequivocal diagnosis of ventricular tachycardia from this tracing, although the diagnosis is highly suggestive.

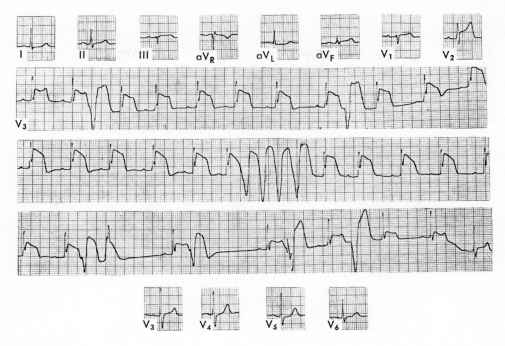

Fig. 8-100

Rate:	During V₃, approximately 75 beats/minute, interrupted by ventricular ectopy.
Rhythm:	Fairly regular except when interrupted by ventricular ectopy.
P waves:	Normal and precede each of the normally conducted QRS complexes.
PR interval:	Normal (0.16 second) and constant.
QRS:	Note abrupt ST segment elevation between V₁ and V₂ and during the V₃ rhythm strip. Then V₃ at the bottom shows a normal ST segment. Abnormal complexes have a QRS duration greater than 0.12 second.
Arrhythmia:	Atypical (Prinzmetal) angina pectoris characterized by ST segment *elevation*. Premature ventricular systoles trigger a short run of ventricular tachycardia in the midportion of the tracing. ST segments return to the base line as the chest pain abates and the ectopic ventricular activity ceases.

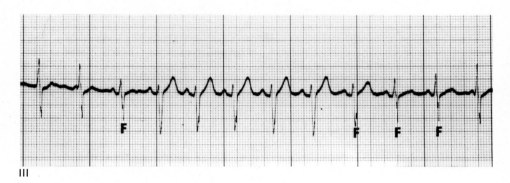

III

Fig. 8-101

Rate:	107 beats/minute.
Rhythm:	Regular.
P waves:	Normal and precede each of the QRS complexes in the midportion of the tracing.
PR interval:	Constant (0.16 second) for the QRS complexes in the midportion of the tracing.
QRS:	Normal duration (0.08 second) for both types of QRS complexes. Fusion QRS complexes indicated by *F*.
Arrhythmia:	Nonparoxysmal AV junctional tachycardia at beginning and end of tracing, which generates QRS complexes with a slightly different contour than during sinus tachycardia that occurs in the midportion of the tracing. The supraventricular origin of the tachycardia is suggested by the QRS duration (<0.12 second). However, recent data suggest that such a tachycardia actually may be ventricular, originating in the upper portions of the fascicular system and generating a QRS complex with a duration *less* than 0.12 second. The presence of fusion beats (*F*) supports this conclusion. In any event, during the tachycardia at the beginning and end of the ECG, QRS complexes are not related to atrial activity. Thus AV dissociation is present because of nonparoxysmal AV junctional (or ventricular) tachycardia. In the midportion of the tracing, slight acceleration of the sinus rate allows the sinus node to regain capture of the ventricles, suppress the nonparoxysmal AV junctional tachycardia, and eliminate the periods of AV dissociation.

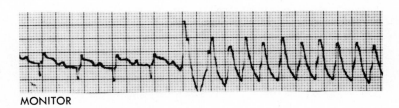

MONITOR

Fig. 8-102

Rate:	Atrial	110 beats/minute.
	Ventricular	230 beats/minute.
Rhythm:		Regular.
P waves:		Precede the normal QRS complexes but not seen during the tachycardia to the right.
PR interval:		0.24 second, preceding the normal QRS complexes; not measurable during the tachycardia.
QRS:		Normal (0.07 second) for the sinus-initiated QRS complexes; prolonged (0.14 second) during the tachycardia.
Arrhythmia:		Ventricular tachycardia that began, in this patient who experienced an acute myocardial infarction, *without* preexisting or precipitating ventricular extrasystoles. Although it is possible that the P wave preceding the widened QRS complex initiates a supraventricular tachycardia with aberration, it is unlikely.

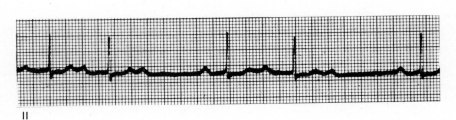

II

Fig. 8-103

Rate:	Atrial	75 beats/minute.
	Ventricular	3:2 conduction, average 50 beats/minute.
Rhythm:	Atrial	Regular.
	Ventricular	Irregular.
P waves:		Normal and precede each QRS complex.
PR interval:		Progressively lengthens prior to the nonconducted P wave.
QRS:		Normal (0.06 second).
Arrhythmia:		Second-degree AV block, type I (Wenckebach).

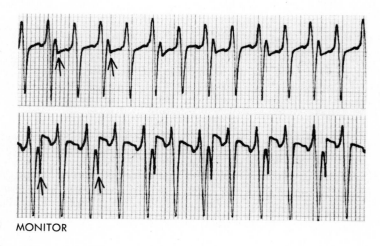

MONITOR

Fig. 8-104

Rate:	Atrial	120 beats/minute.
	Ventricular	240 beats/minute.
Rhythm:		Regular.
P waves:		Follow alternate QRS complexes.
PR interval:		0.08 second.
QRS:		Normal (0.10).
Arrhythmia:		Nonparoxysmal AV junctional tachycardia with 2:1 retrograde block to the atrium. Arrows indicate P waves. Top tracing, monitor lead; bottom tracing, intracavitary right atrial lead.

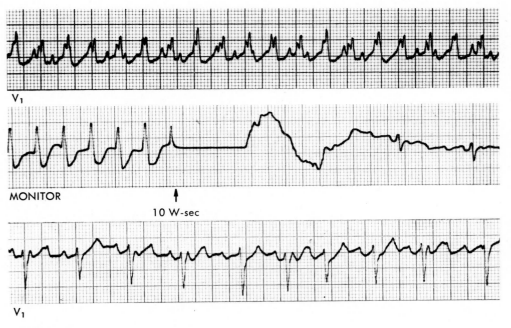

V₁

MONITOR

10 W-sec

V₁

Fig. 8-105

Rate:	Atrial	300 beats/minute (top panel).
	Ventricular	200 beats/minute (top panel).
Rhythm:	Atrial	Regular.
	Ventricular.	Regular.
P waves:		Atrial flutter.
PR interval:		Completely variable.
QRS:		Wide, prolonged (0.12 second).
Arrhythmia:		Atrial flutter and ventricular tachycardia in top tracing. Thus complete AV dissociation is present. In the monitor recording (middle tracing) the left portion reflects the same activity seen in V₁ above. However, the particular monitor lead fails to reveal the atrial flutter waves. Direct current cardioversion (*arrow*, 10 watt-seconds) terminates the ventricular tachycardia but allows the atrial flutter to persist, seen more clearly in V₁ below. The atrial flutter at this point is not as precisely regular at it was prior to the cardioversion.

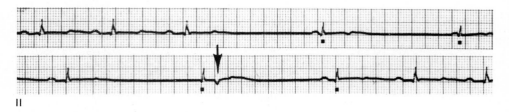

II

Fig. 8-106

Rate:	30 to 50 beats/minute.
Rhythm:	Fairly irregular.
P waves:	Precede and conduct to the QRS complexes that do not have dots beneath them. Those with dots beneath them are junctional escape beats.
PR interval:	Prolonged (0.26 second) and constant for the QRS complexes that do not have a dot beneath them.
QRS:	Normal duration and contour (0.08 second). Dots indicate AV junctional escape beats. The third AV junctional escape beat (lower tracing) retrogradely activates the atrium *(arrow)*.
Arrhythmia:	Sinus bradycardia with intermittent sinus arrest and AV junctional escape beats, the "sick sinus syndrome."

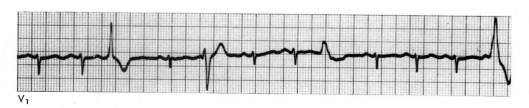

V₁

Fig. 8-107

Rate:	98 beats/minute.
Rhythm:	Irregular because of premature ventricular systoles.
P waves:	Normal and precede each sinus-initiated QRS complex.
PR interval:	Normal for the sinus-initiated QRS complexes (0.14 second).
QRS:	Normal for the sinus-initiated QRS complexes (0.08 second). Premature systoles are characterized by varied contour and a duration greater than 0.12 second.
Arrhythmia:	Multiformed premature ventricular systoles with four different contours.

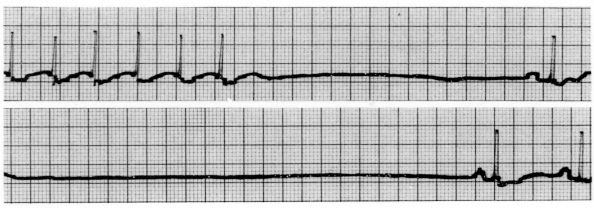

MONITOR

Fig. 8-108

Rate:	140 beats/minute, abruptly slowing following carotid sinus massage. Two periods of asystole are finally terminated by sinus rhythm.
Rhythm:	Regular, followed by asystole, an atrial escape beat, and then sinus rhythm.
P waves:	Can be seen when tachycardia terminates.
PR interval:	Normal (0.18 sec) in those beats preceded by P waves.
QRS:	Normal.
Arrhythmia:	Abrupt termination of paroxysmal supraventricular tachycardia by carotid sinus massage (at beginning of recording). A lengthy period of asystole results when the tachycardia stops, before sinus rhythm resumes.

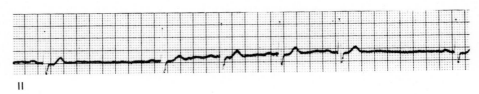

II

Fig. 8-109

Rate:	33 to 66 beats/minute.
Rhythm:	Irregular.
P waves:	Normal contour. Long PP cycles are exactly twice the short PP cycles.
PR interval:	Normal (0.20 second).
QRS:	Normal (0.08 second).
Arrhythmia:	2:1 sinus exit block.

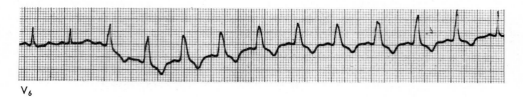

V₆

Fig. 8-110

Rate:	Gradually accelerates from 105 to 115 beats/minute.
Rhythm:	Fairly regular.
P waves:	Normal and precede each QRS complex.
PR interval:	Normal (0.14 second) and constant.
QRS:	Normal at the slower rates; left bundle branch block (0.12 second) at the faster rates.
Arrhythmia:	Rate-dependent aberration with functional left bundle branch block.

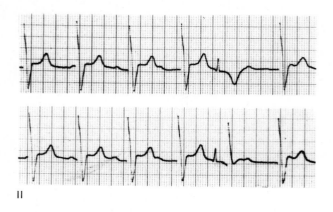

II

Fig. 8-111

Rate:	68 beats/minute.
Rhythm:	Fairly regular.
P waves:	Normal contour but have no consistent relationship to ventricular depolarization.
PR interval:	Completely variable.
QRS:	All but the fifth QRS complex in each panel are initiated by a pacemaker spike and have a duration of 0.16 second. The fifth QRS complexes represent supraventricular captures with a duration of 0.07 second.
Arrhythmia:	Left panel, ventricular inhibited pacemaker; right panel, conversion of ventricular inhibited pacemaker to a continuously discharging, asynchronous pacemaker by holding a magnet over the pacemaker. Note that the fifth QRS complex in right panel no longer suppresses pacemaker discharge. The ventricles are still refractory at the time of pacemaker discharge, and no QRS complex is generated.

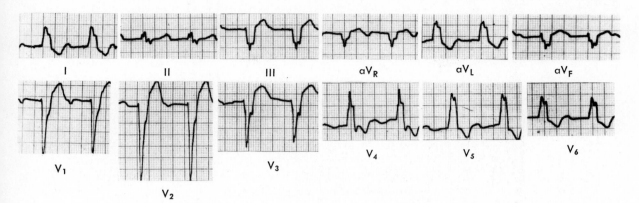

I II III aV_R aV_L aV_F

V_1 V_2 V_3 V_4 V_5 V_6

Fig. 8-112

Rate:	72 beats/minute.
Rhythm:	Regular.
P waves:	Hidden within the preceding T waves.
PR interval:	Prolonged (0.04 second).
QRS:	Wide (0.16 second).
Arrhythmia:	Normal sinus rhythm with left bundle branch block and first-degree AV block.

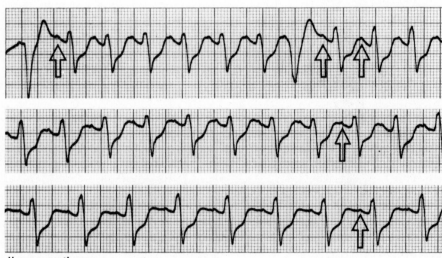

II—noncontinuous

Fig. 8-113

Rate:	125 beats/minute in top tracing; gradually slows to 100 beats/minute in bottom tracing.
Rhythm:	Regular.
P waves:	Normal, but hidden by preceding T waves (*arrows*).
PR interval:	0.16 second.
QRS:	Abnormal, prolonged (0.14 second) because of the presence of a preexisting left bundle branch block.
Arrhythmia:	Sinus tachycardia. Patient has a preexisting bundle branch block. Clear P waves (*arrows*) can be seen in the pause that follows the two ventricular extrasystoles (top tracing). The heart rate gradually slowed following edrophonium (Tensilon) administration (middle and bottom tracings).

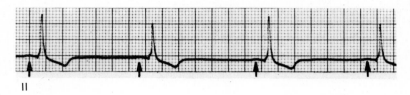

II

Fig. 8-114

Rate:	41 beats/minute.
Rhythm:	Fairly regular.
P waves:	Precede each QRS with a normal contour.
PR interval:	0.16 second.
QRS:	Borderline prolonged (0.11 second).
Arrhythmia:	Sinus bradycardia. Patient is receiving methyldopa for hypertension. Normal rate was restored following discontinuation of methyldopa therapy. Low-amplitude P waves indicated by arrows.

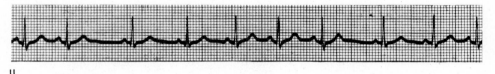

II

Fig. 8-115

Rate:	Sinus rate increases with inspiration and decreases with expiration (70 to 110 beats/minute).
Rhythm:	Irregular with a repetitive phasic variation in cycle length according to respiratory cycles. Cycle lengths vary by more than 0.16 second. Breath-holding eliminates the rate variations.
P waves:	Precede each QRS with a normal, fairly constant contour.
PR interval:	0.12 second.
QRS:	Normal (0.08 second).
Arrhythmia:	Respiratory sinus arrhythmia. The phasic variation corresponds to a respiratory rate of approximately 18 per minute.

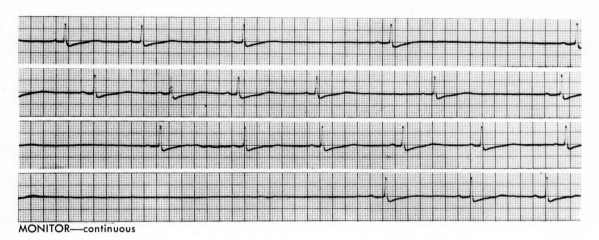

MONITOR—continuous

Fig. 8-116

Rate:	Varying, slow (maximum rate of 55 beats/minute).
Rhythm:	Irregular; periods of asystole not a multiple of basic sinus cycle length.
P waves:	Precede each QRS with a normal contour; may be altered by escape beats.
PR interval:	Slightly prolonged (0.21 second).
QRS:	Normal (0.09 second).
Arrhythmia:	Sinus arrest. Patient also has an acute inferior myocardial infarction. Asystolic intervals are not interrupted by escape beats.

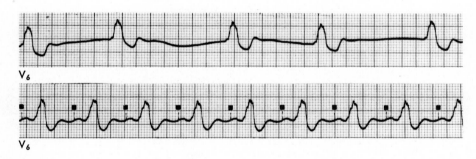

V_6

V_6

Fig. 8-117

Rate:	Varying, slow (36 to 50 beats/minute) (top); normal (81 beats/minute) (bottom).
Rhythm:	Irregular (top); regular (bottom).
P waves:	Not seen (top); follows pacemaker stimulus (bottom).
PR interval:	Not measurable (top); 0.16 second (bottom).
QRS:	Left bundle branch block (0.20 second).
Arrhythmia:	Sinus arrest (*top*) and right atrial pacing (*bottom*). Patient also has a left bundle branch block. A supraventricular escape focus controls the rhythm in the top panel, but atrial activity is not apparent. Atrial pacing (stimuli indicated by filled squares, bottom tracing) results in atrial capture, producing a P wave and an unchanged QRS contour.

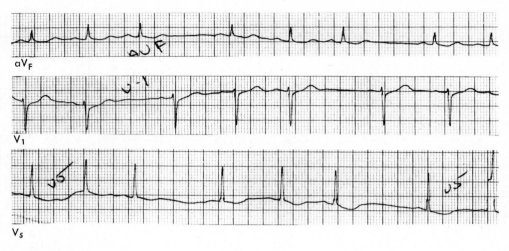

Fig. 8-118

Rate:	Varying, slow (50 to 88 beats/minute).
Rhythm:	(1) A pause in atrial activity occurs. (2) The PP interval progressively shortens up until the pause. (3) The duration of the pause is less than twice the shortest PP interval. (4) The PP interval following the pause exceeds the PP interval preceding the pause.
P waves:	Contour normal, precede each QRS complex; intermittent loss of P wave.
PR interval:	Normal, constant (0.20 second).
QRS:	Normal (0.08 second).
Arrhythmia:	Sinoatrial (SA) exit block (type I or Wenckebach). The four characteristic rhythm changes of this tracing allow the diagnosis of a Wenckebach exit block from the sinus node.

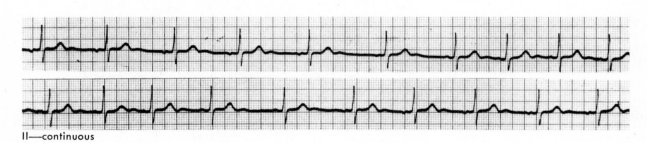

II—continuous

Fig. 8-119

Rate:	Varying, slow 47 to 75 beats/minute.
Rhythm:	Irregular with a repetitive phasic variation in cycle length as in sinus arrhythmia.
P waves:	Vary contour, indicating shift in pacemaker site. Become negative in lead II.
PR interval:	0.16 second.
QRS:	Normal, 0.08 second.
Arrhythmia:	Wandering atrial pacemaker. As the heart rate speeds, the P waves become upright and then gradually become inverted again as the heart rate slows.

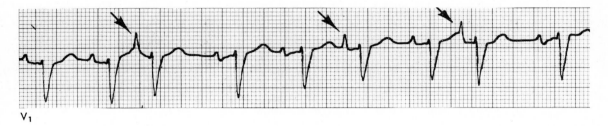

V₁

Fig. 8-120

Rate:	Varying.
Rhythm:	Irregular because of premature atrial systoles.
P waves:	Premature atrial systoles are sharply pointed *(arrows)*.
PR interval (of atrial systole):	0.16 second.
QRS:	Normal, 0.08 second.
Arrhythmia:	Premature atrial systoles depressing sinus node discharge. Sharply pointed P waves *(arrows)* represent premature atrial systoles that, when they occur early (first and third), delay return of sinus node. Contour of P waves following earlier premature atrial systoles differs from normal P wave, indicating a shift in pacemaker focus or a change in intraatrial conduction.

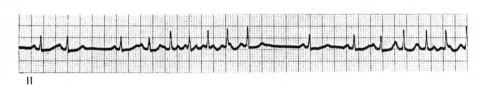

II

Fig. 8-121

Rate:	Varying.
Rhythm:	Irregular because of premature atrial systoles.
P waves:	Premature atrial systoles have different contour; some are buried in preceding T wave.
PR interval (of atrial systole):	0.14 second.
QRS:	Generally normal; may be aberrantly conducted (normal, 0.08 second).
Arrhythmia:	Single and multiple premature atrial systoles can be seen hidden within preceding T waves and appear to initiate short bursts of an atrial tachyarrhythmia, probably atrial flutter-fibrillation.

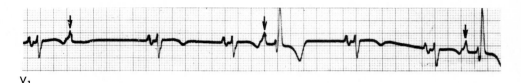

V₁

Fig. 8-122

Rate:	Slow, because of nonconducted premature atrial systoles.
Rhythm:	Irregular.
P waves:	Premature atrial systoles have different contour and are buried in preceding T wave *(arrows)*.
PR interval (of premature atrial systoles):	First two premature atrial systoles are completely blocked; third and fourth premature atrial systoles conduct with a prolonged PR interval 0.21 second.
QRS:	Third and fourth premature atrial systoles initiate aberrantly conducted QRS complex with a right bundle branch block pattern.
Arrhythmia:	Nonconducted premature atrial systoles and premature atrial systoles initiating functional right bundle branch block. Sinus-initiated P waves are abnormal and suggest left atrial enlargement. Premature atrial systoles *(arrows)* can be seen hidden in the preceding T waves. The first two premature atrial systoles are blocked and generate a pause in the ventricular rhythm. The second two premature atrial systoles conduct to the ventricle with a prolonged PR interval and initiate a functional right bundle branch block.

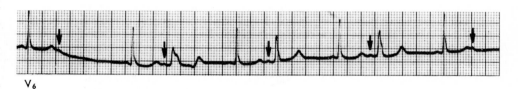

V₆

Fig. 8-123

Rate:	Varying.
Rhythm:	Irregular because of premature atrial systoles.
P waves:	Premature atrial systoles have different contour and look like U waves *(arrows)*.
PR interval (of premature atrial systole):	Later premature atrial systoles (second, third, and fourth) conduct whereas early premature atrial systoles (first, fifth, and sixth) fail to reach the ventricles.
QRS:	Second, third, and fourth premature atrial systoles produce varying degrees of left bundle branch block.
Arrhythmia:	Nonconducted premature atrial systoles and premature atrial systoles that produce a functional left bundle branch block. Premature atrial systoles can be seen in the terminal portion of the preceding T waves and look like a U wave *(arrows)*. Fairly early premature atrial systoles block whereas slightly later premature atrial systoles conduct to the ventricles with an increase in PR interval and varying degrees of left bundle branch block.

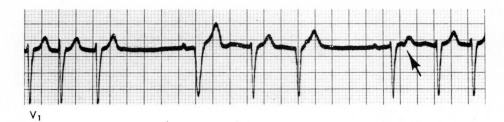

V₁

Fig. 8-124

Rate:	150 beats/minute.
Rhythm:	Varying.
P waves:	Not seen consistently.
PR interval:	Cannot determine.
QRS:	0.08 second.
Arrhythmia:	Paroxysmal supraventricular tachycardia. Paroxysmal supraventricular tachycardia suddenly terminates, begins briefly, stops, and then restarts again following a premature atrial systole *(arrow)* that conducts with a prolonged PR interval.

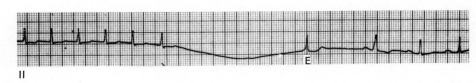

II

Fig. 8-125

Rate:	130 beats/minute.
Rhythm:	Regular, except at termination.
P waves:	Not seen during tachycardia.
PR interval:	0.20 second during sinus rhythm.
QRS:	0.06 second.
Arrhythmia:	Paroxysmal supraventricular tachycardia. PSVT suddenly terminates following carotid sinus massage and produces a short period of asystole that is ended by an AV junctional escape beat *(E)*. Sinus rhythm then returns.

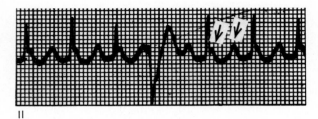

II

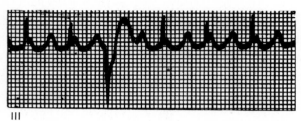

III

Fig. 8-126

Rate:	Atrial	280 beats/minute.
	Ventricular	140 beats/minute.
Rhythm:	Atrial	Regular.
	Ventricular	2:1.
P waves:		Flutter waves with regular oscillations resembling a sawtooth pattern.
PR interval:		Flutter-R interval is constant.
QRS:		Normal (0.08 second).
Arrhythmia:		Uncommon form of atrial flutter. Flutter waves indicated by arrows. A single premature ventricular systole occurs in each lead. The conduction ratio is 2:1; that is, flutter waves are conducted alternately to the ventricle.

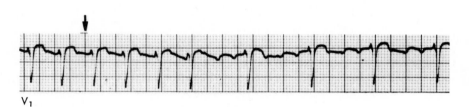

V₁

Fig. 8-127

Rate:	Atrial	300 beats/minute.
	Ventricular	150, decreasing to 75 beats/minute.
Rhythm:	Atrial	Regular.
	Ventricular	Regular.
P waves:		Flutter waves clearly seen after carotid sinus massage (arrow) decreases the ventricular response.
PR interval:		Flutter-R interval fairly constant.
QRS:		Normal (0.08 second).
Arrhythmia:		Atrial flutter. Atrial flutter with a 2:1 ventricular response is present in the left portion of the tracing but cannot be clearly diagnosed from this lead. At the arrow, carotid sinus massage increases the degree of AV block to 4:1 and clearly exposes the atrial flutter waves.

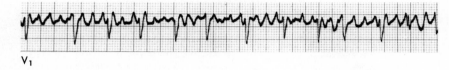

V₁

Fig. 8-128

Rate:	Atrial	300 to 500 beats/minute.
	Ventricular	72 to 150 beats/minute.
Rhythm:	Atrial	Irregular.
	Ventricular	Irregular.
P waves:		Variability in the contour and spacing of the flutter-fibrillation waves.
PR interval:		Nonmeasurable.
QRS:		Normal (0.09 second).
Arrhythmia:		Impure atrial flutter (coarse atrial flutter or flutter-fibrillation). Impure atrial flutter is characterized by a faster atrial rate than pure atrial flutter, and more variability shows in the contour and spacing of the flutter waves.

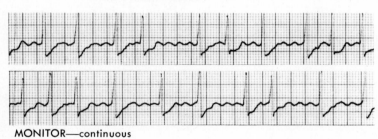

MONITOR—continuous

Fig. 8-129

Rate:	Atrial	350 to 600 beats/minute.
	Ventricular	75 to 160, average 130 beats/minute.
Rhythm:	Atrial	Irregularly irregular.
	Ventricular	Irregularly irregular.
P waves:		Irregular rapid base-line undulations called fibrillatory (F) waves.
PR interval:		Not measurable.
QRS:		Normal 0.09 second.
Arrhythmia:		Atrial fibrillation. Atrial activity is present as the undulating, wavy base line.

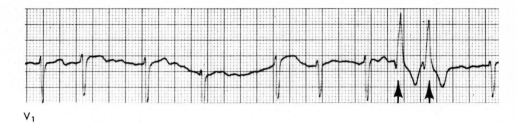

V₁

Fig. 8-130

Rate:	Atrial	350 to 600 beats/minute.
	Ventricular	65 to 160 beats/minute.
Rhythm:	Atrial	Irregularly irregular.
	Ventricular	Irregularly irregular.
P waves:		Irregular rapid baseline undulations indicate fibrillatory atrial activity.
PR interval:		Not measurable.
QRS:		0.08 second; two complexes indicated by arrows are functional right bundle branch block QRS complexes with a duration of 0.13 second.
Arrhythmia:		Atrial fibrillation. A long ventricular pause followed by a short ventricular pause precedes the QRS complex with a right bundle branch block contour *(arrow)*; this QRS complex is followed after a short interval by a second QRS complex, also with right bundle branch block *(arrow)*. The aberrant QRS pattern indicates functional right bundle branch block (Ashman phenomenon).

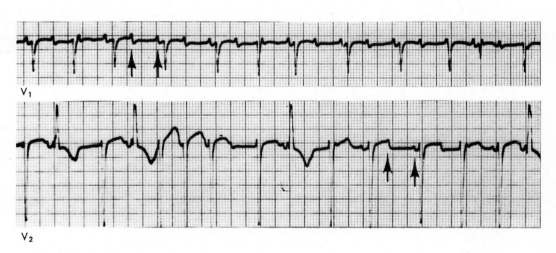

V₁

V₂

Fig. 8-131

Rate:	Atrial	167 beats/minute.
	Ventricular	Varies according to the degree of AV block (83 to 120 beats/minute).
Rhythm:	Atrial	Regular.
	Ventricular	Irregular (2:1, 3:2, and 4:3).
P waves:		Contour differs from sinus-initiated P waves.
PR interval:		Wenckebach cycles.
QRS:		0.08 second; functional right bundle branch block in lower tracing with a duration of 0.12 second.
Arrhythmia:		Atrial tachycardia with AV block. In the lower tracing, long-short QRS intervals, which follow longer intervals, set the stage for aberrant ventricular conduction that is manifest as a functional right bundle branch block. Arrows indicate P waves.

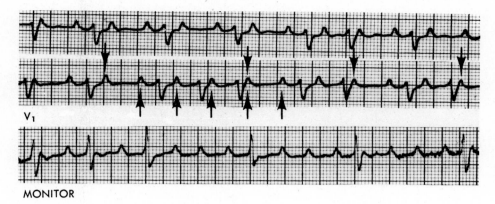

MONITOR

Fig. 8-132

Rate:	Atrial	150 beats/minute, top; 193 beats/minute, bottom.
	Ventricular	83 to 125 beats/minute, top; 50 to 94 beats/minute, bottom.
Rhythm:	Atrial	Regular.
	Ventricular	Irregular (2:1, 3:1, 4:1, 4:3, etc.)
P waves:		Contour differs from sinus-initiated P waves.
PR interval:		Wenckebach cycles.
QRS:		0.09 second.
Arrhythmia:		Atrial tachycardia with AV block caused by digitalis toxicity. Top two tracings recorded on admission. In the bottom tracing, continued digitalis administration increased the atrial rate to 193 beats/minute and increased the degree of AV block. Upright arrows indicate P waves; inverted arrows indicate nonconducted P waves.

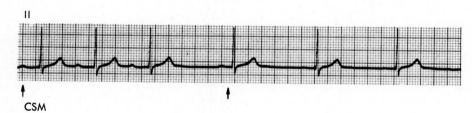

CSM

Fig. 8-133

Rate:	Atrial	75 beats/minute initially; atrial activity not apparent during the junctional rhythm.
	Ventricular	48 to 50 beats/minute during the junctional rhythm.
Rhythm:		Ventricular, generally regular.
P waves and PR interval:		Relationship between P and QRS as explained under premature AV junctional systoles. (P waves not apparent). PR interval not determinable during junctional rhythm.
QRS:		Normal (0.08 second); may be conducted with slight aberration.
Arrhythmia:		AV junctional rhythm. Carotid sinus massage (*CSM*, between arrows) produces significant sinus slowing to allow the escape of an AV junctional rhythm (fifth QRS). Note unchanged QRS complexes. Atrial activity to the right of the last arrow is not apparent and may be caused by the AV junctional rhythm with retrograde capture of the P wave, lost within the QRS complex.

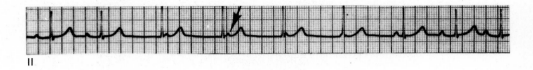

II

Fig. 8-134

Rate:	Atrial	45 to 70 beats/minute.
	Ventricular	58 to 70 beats/minute.
Rhythm:	Atrial	Slowing.
	Ventricular	Slowing but fairly regular.
P waves:		Normal.
PR interval:		See premature AV junctional systoles (AV dissociation in this tracing).
QRS:		Normal (0.08 second).
Arrhythmia:		AV junctional rhythm. Transient, spontaneous sinus slowing allows the escape of an AV junctional rhythm. P waves can be seen to occur just after the onset of the QRS complex *(arrow)* and represent normal sinus-initiated P waves. Gradual acceleration of the sinus rate reestablishes sinus control fo the ventricular activity at the end of the tracing and thus terminates the period of AV dissociation in the midportion of the tracing. The PR interval is prolonged.

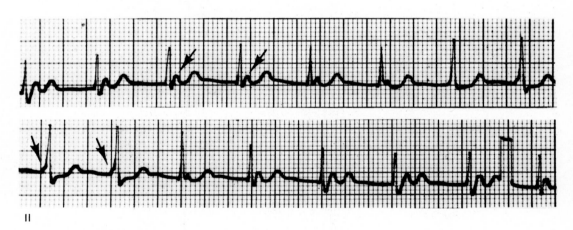

II

Fig. 8-135

Rate:	Atrial	100 beats/minute.
	Ventricular	100 beats/minute.
Rhythm:	Atrial	Regular
	Ventricular	Fairly regular.
P waves:		Normal.
PR interval:		Varying.
QRS:		0.08 second.
Arrhythmia:		Nonparoxysmal AV junctional tachycardia. Atrial activity *(arrows)* follows, then slightly precedes, and then once again follows the inscription of the QRS complex. Therefore AV dissociation is present because of the accelerated AV junctional discharge. This type of AV dissociation is called "isorhythmic."

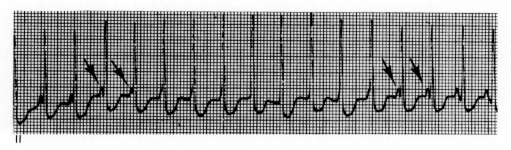

II

Fig. 8-136

Rate:	Atrial	166 beats/minute.
	Ventricular	166 beats/minute.
Rhythm:	Atrial	Regular.
	Ventricular	Regular.
P waves:		Normal.
PR interval:		Varying.
QRS:		0.06 second.
Arrhythmia:		Nonparoxysmal AV junctional tachycardia. Atrial activity *(arrows)* at a very similar rate and rhythm to the QRS can be seen to precede, then occur simultaneously with, and once again precede the onset of the QRS complex. This type of AV dissociation is called "isorhythmic."

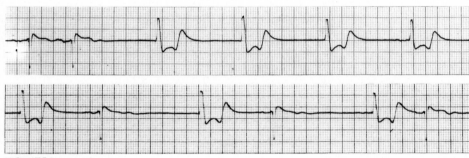

MONITOR—continuous

Fig. 8-137

Rate:	Atrial	Intermittent sinus arrest.
	Ventricular	43 beats/minute.
Rhythm:	Atrial	Irregular.
	Ventricular	Regular.
P waves:		Normal.
PR interval:		Varying.
QRS (of ventricular escape rhythm):		0.13 second.
Arrhythmia:		Ventricular escape beats. Intermittent sinus arrest produced periods of asystole terminated by ventricular escape beats that are characterized by a prolonged, abnormal QRS complex. Intermittent return of sinus node activity establishes periods of supraventricular capture. The reason why AV junctional escape beats did not terminate the asystolic periods is not known.

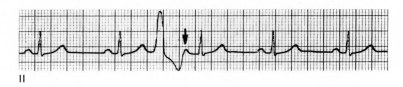

II

Fig. 8-138

Rate, rhythm, and P waves:	As in Fig. 8-42.
PR interval:	Prolonged following the interpolated premature ventricular extrasystole (0.20 second).
QRS:	0.14 second.
Arrhythmia:	Interpolated premature ventricular systole. A sinus-initiated P wave (↓) immediately following the premature ventricular systole conducts to the ventricles with a long PR interval. The PR interval following the premature ventricular systole is prolonged owing to incomplete recovery of the AV node because of partial retrograde penetration by the interpolated ventricular systole.

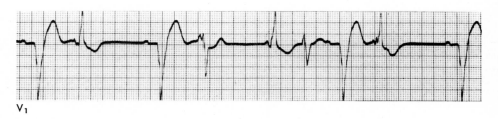

V₁

Fig. 8-139

Rate, rhythm, P waves, and PR interval:	As in Fig. 8-41.
QRS:	Wide, bizarre, greater than 0.12 second with varying contours and coupling intervals.
Arrhythmia:	Multiform premature ventricular systoles. The normally conducted QRS complexes have a left bundle branch block morphology. The PR interval is slightly prolonged (0.24 second). Premature QRS complexes with varying contours and coupling intervals are present and called *multiform* ventricular extrasystoles.

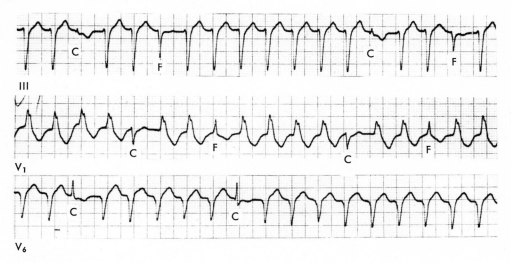

Fig. 8-140

Rate:	Atrial	Clear P waves not seen.
	Ventricular	150 beats/minute.
Rhythm:	Atrial	Regular.
	Ventricular.	Regular.
P waves:		Atrial activity is probably under independent control of sinus node.
PR interval:		Not measurable.
QRS:		0.14 second.
Arrhythmia:		Ventricular tachycardia. QRS complexes with a prolonged duration and a right bundle branch block morphology occur at a regular interval and are occasionally interrupted by QRS complexes with a normal contour (*C*, capture) or QRS complexes with an intermediate contour (*F*, fusion). Atrial activity cannot be seen; most likely, the atria are discharging independently to produce intermittent QRS captures and fusion beats. Therefore the most reasonable diagnosis is a ventricular tachycardia with AV dissociation.

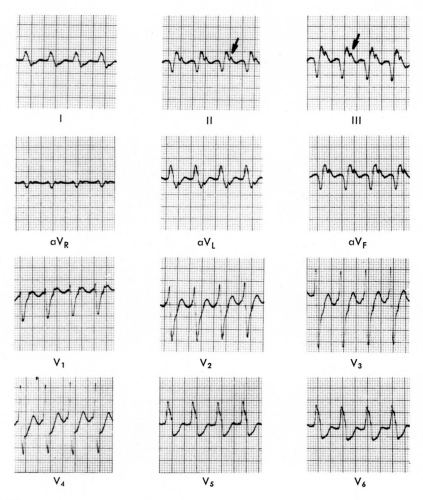

Fig. 8-141

Rate:	Atrial	150 beats/minute.
	Ventricular	150 beats/minute.
Rhythm:	Atrial	Regular.
	Ventricular	Regular.
P waves:		Retrograde P waves inverted in 2, 3 (*arrows*), and aV$_F$.
RP interval:		0.16 second.
QRS:		0.12 second.
Arrhythmia:		Ventricular tachycardia with retrograde atrial capture. Ventricular tachycardia cannot be diagnosed with certainty from this surface ECG because all the features of this arrhythmia can be mimicked by a supraventricular tachycardia with aberrant ventricular conduction of a left bundle branch block type. His bundle electrocardiography proved that this was a ventricular tachycardia, however. The importance of the illustration lies in demonstrating 1:1 retrograde conduction to the atrium. Retrograde atrial activity indicated by arrows. Thus AV dissociation is *not* present during this ventricular tachycardia.

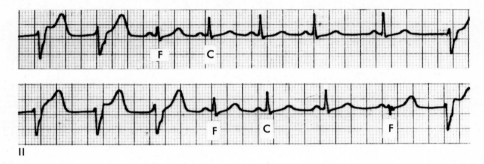

Fig. 8-142

Rate:	Atrial	70 to 90 beats/minute.
	Ventricular	72 beats/minute.
Rhythm:	Atrial	Regular.
	Ventricular	Regular.
P waves:		Independent.
PR interval:		Not measurable during accelerated idioventricular rhythm.
QRS:		0.14 second; fusion beats and capture beats often present (labeled *F* and *C*).
Arrhythmia:		Accelerated idioventricular rhythm. An accelerated idioventricular rhythm is present at the beginning and termination of the top and bottom strips. In the midportion of each tracing, slight sinus node acceleration reestablishes sinus node control by capturing the ventricles (*C*) and suppresses the accelerated idioventricular rhythm. When the sinus node slows, the accelerated idioventricular rhythm escapes. Fusion beats (*F*) may occur in the beginning and end of such arrhythmias because sinus and ventricular foci have similar rates.

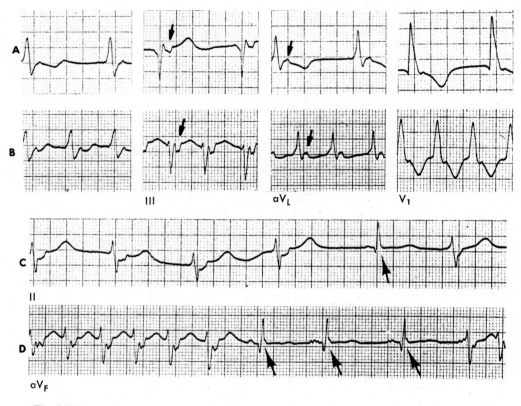

III   aVL   V₁

II

aVF

Fig. 8-143

Rate:	Accelerated idioventricular rhythm (60 beats/minute). Ventricular tachycardia (varying slight, 150 beats/minute).
Rhythm:	Accelerated idioventricular rhythm (regular). Ventricular tachycardia (regular).
P waves:	Retrogradely captured.
PR interval:	0.14 second.
QRS:	0.14 second.
Arrhythmia:	Accelerated idioventricular rhythm and ventricular tachycardia. An accelerated idioventricular rhythm and a ventricular tachycardia occurred at different times in this patient. **A** illustrates leads, I, III, aV$_L$, V$_1$, and V$_6$ during the accelerated ventricular rhythm, whereas **C** (lead II) illustrates the onset of the accelerated idioventricular rhythm. **B** illustrates the ventricular tachycardia in leads I, III, aV$_L$, V$_1$, and V$_6$, whereas **D** (aV$_F$) illustrates the onset and termination of the ventricular tachycardia. Retrograde atrial capture (↓) occurred during both tachycardias. Normally conducted QRS complexes present in **C** and **D** (↑). Note identical QRS contours for both tachycardias (aV$_L$, V$_1$, and V$_6$ in **A** were recorded at different standardization), indicating that they arose at same or similar areas of the ventricle.

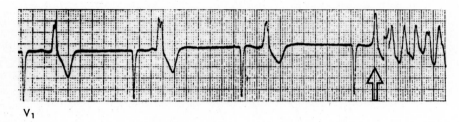

V₁

Fig. 8-144

Rate:	Atrial	60 to 100 beats/minute; any independent atrial arrhythmia may exist or the atria captured retrogradely.
	Ventricular	400 to 600 beats/minute.
Rhythm:	Atrial	Regular; may be irregular if the atria are retrogradely captured.
	Ventricular	Grossly irregular.
P waves:		Generally cannot be seen.
PR interval:		Generally not measurable.
QRS:		Base-line undulations without distinct QRS contours.
Arrhythmia:		Ventricular fibrillation. Premature ventricular systoles occurred in a bigeminal pattern with a decreasing coupling interval. The fourth premature ventricular systole discharged during the vulnerable period of the antecedent T wave and precipitated ventricular fibrillation (*arrow*).

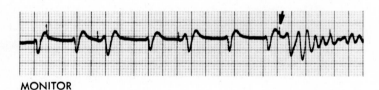

MONITOR

Fig. 8-145

Rate, rhythm, P waves, PR interval and QRS:	As in Fig. 8-144.
Arrhythmia:	Ventricular fibrillation. Pacemaker spikes (*arrow*) from a malfunctioning pacemaker fall randomly throughout the cardiac cycle at a slightly irregular interval. When the pacemaker spike discharged during the vulnerable period of the antecedent T wave (*arrow*), it precipitated ventricular fibrillation. Ventricular rhythm preceding onset of ventricular fibrillation is probably slightly irregular, accelerated idioventricular rhythm.

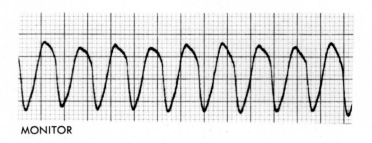

MONITOR

Fig. 8-146

Rate:	Atrial	P waves not seen.
	Ventricular	195 beats/minute.
Rhythm:	Ventricular	Regular.
P waves:		Cannot be seen.
PR interval:		Not measurable.
QRS:		0.16 second.
Arrhythmia:		Ventricular flutter. Sine wave with regular large oscillations. The QRS complex cannot be definitely distinguished from the ST segment or T wave.

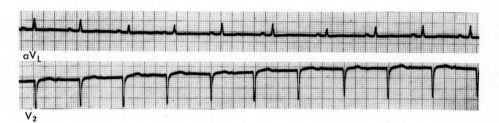

aV$_L$

V$_2$

Fig. 8-147

Rate:	62 to 71 beats/minute in aV$_L$; 78 beats/minute in V$_2$.
Rhythm:	Regular.
P waves:	Normal contour and precede each QRS complex.
PR interval:	0.22 in aV$_L$; 0.42 in V$_2$.
QRS:	Normal (0.08 second).
Arrhythmia:	First-degree AV heart block. Leads aV$_L$ and V$_2$ were recorded during the course of a 12-lead ECG in this patient. An increase in heart rate may have caused further abnormal lengthening of PR interval (V$_2$) in this patient with abnormal AV conduction.

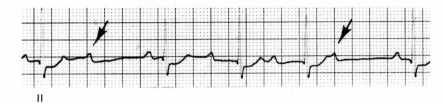

II

Fig. 8-148

Rate:	Atrial	Normal (83 beats/minute).
	Ventricular	Depends on degree of AV block, which may vary between 2:1, 3:2, 4:3, 5:3, etc.
Rhythm:	Atrial	Regular.
	Ventricular	Varying, depending on the degree of AV block.
P waves:		More numerous than QRS complexes but are related to ventricular beats in a consistent, repetitive fashion.
PR interval:		Progressive PR prolongation preceding the nonconducted P wave. Finally, one P wave is blocked, and the cycle then repeats.
QRS:		Normal; RR interval gradually shortens until the blocked P wave occurs; the cycle then repeats.
Arrhythmia:		Second-degree AV heart block (type I Wenckebach). AV Wenckebach is characterized by progressive PR prolongation preceding the nonconducted P wave. Wenckebach AV block, in the presence of a normal QRS complex, is virtually always at the level of the AV node. Conduction ratios (that is, the number of P waves to the number of QRS complexes) are 2:1, 4:3, and 3:2 in this tracing. Because the increment in conduction time is greatest in the second cycle of the Wenckebach group and then decreases progressively over succeeding cycles, the following characteristics are also present: (1) the interval between successive RR cycles prior to the nonconducted P wave progressively decreases; (2) the duration of the pause produced by the nonconducted P wave is less than twice the shortest cycle, which is generally the cycle immediately preceding the pause; (3) the duration of the RR cycle following the pause exceeds the duration of the RR cycle preceding the pause. These features can be seen in the middle 4:3 grouping. Blocked P waves indicated by arrows.

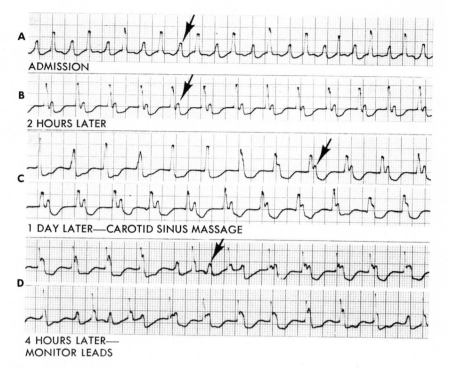

A
ADMISSION

B
2 HOURS LATER

C
1 DAY LATER—CAROTID SINUS MASSAGE

D
4 HOURS LATER—
MONITOR LEADS

Fig. 8-149

Rate:	**A,** 108 beats/minute; **B,** 115 beats/minute; **C,** 105 beats/minute; **D,** atrial rate, 115 to 120 beats/minute.
Rhythm:	Regular except for ventricular rhythm in **D.**
P waves:	Generally normal (slightly increased in amplitude); precede each QRS.
PR interval:	Prolonged to greater than 0.20 second (varying in the different tracings; **A,** 0.26 second; **B,** 0.42 second; **C,** 0.56 second; **D,** Wenckebach AV block).
QRS:	Normal (0.08 second).
Arrhythmia:	First-degree and second-degree (type I, Wenckebach) AV heart block in a patient with acute myocardial infarction. P waves indicated by arrows. On admission, **A,** first-degree heart block was present. Two hours later, **B,** the heart rate sped and lengthened the PR interval. In the tracing recorded the following day, **C,** atrial activity was not apparent. Two possibilities exist: first, an AV junctional rhythm could be present with normal sinus retrograde atrial activity hidden within the QRS complex; second, the patient may have developed a further lengthening of the PR interval so that the sinus-initiated P wave was hidden within the QRS complex and conducted with a very long PR interval to the following QRS complex. The PR interval then would be approximately 0.56 second in duration. Carotid sinus massage, by slowing the sinus rate and the RR interval as well, proves that the latter possibility is the correct diagnosis. Following release of carotid sinus massage (midportion of the second strip in panel C) the sinus rate speeds back to its previous rate. Four hours later, **D,** AV conduction has worsened slightly with the development of type I (Wenckebach) second-degree AV block. Some variations in the QRS complex occur.

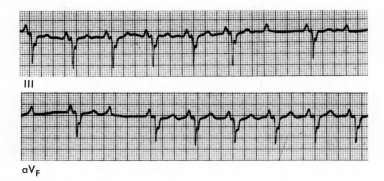

III

aV_F

Fig. 8-150

Rate:		86 beats/minute.
Rhythm:	Atrial	Regular
	Ventricular	Varying, depending upon the degree of AV block.
P waves:		Normal.
PR interval:		Normal, constant (0.12 second) with sudden failure of conduction.
QRS:		Prolonged; right bundle branch block and left anterior hemiblock (0.12 second).
Arrhythmia:		Second-degree AV heart block, type II. Right bundle branch block (not readily apparent in leads III and aV$_F$) along with left anterior fascicular block is present in this patient. Sudden failure of AV conduction results without antecedent PR prolongation. The PR interval for the conducted beats is normal, as it often is during type II second-degree AV heart block.

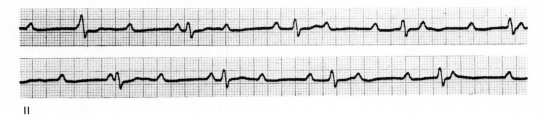

II

Fig. 8-151

Rate:	Atrial	85 beats/minute.
	Ventricular	38 beats/minute.
Rhythm:	Atrial	Regular
	Ventricular	Regular
P waves:		Normal
PR interval:		Completely variable.
QRS:		Prolonged (0.12 second).
Arrhythmia:		Third-degree (complete) AV heart block. Complete AV dissociation is present *resulting from* complete heart block. The abnormal QRS complexes (prolonged duration) indicate a ventricular origin for the escape rhythm.

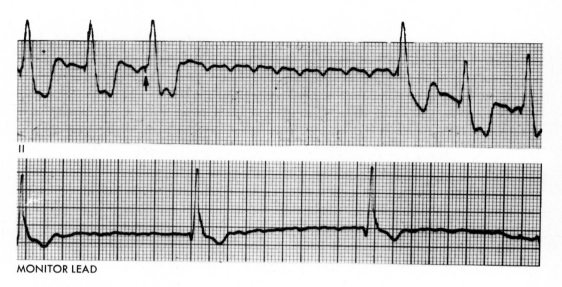

II

MONITOR LEAD

Fig. 8-152

Rate:	Atrial	Top tracing, 250 beats/minute; bottom tracing, 400 to 600 beats/minute.
	Ventricular	Top tracing, 100 beats/minute; bottom tracing, 32 beats/minute.
Rhythm:	Atrial	Top tracing, regular; bottom tracing, irregular.
	Ventricular	Top tracing, regular; bottom tracing, regular.
P waves:		Top tracing, atrial flutter; bottom tracing, atrial fibrillation.
PR interval:		Totally variable or nonmeasurable.
QRS:		Top tracing, ventricular paced beats (0.16 second); bottom tracing, 0.14 second.
Arrhythmia:		Complete (third-degree) AV heart block during atrial flutter and atrial fibrillation. In the top tracing a ventricular pacemaker controls ventricular activity (arrow indicates pacemaker artifact). In the midportion of the tracing the ventricular pacing was temporarily discontinued, and one can easily see the atrial flutter waves that fail to conduct to the ventricle. In the terminal portion of the tracing the ventricular pacemaker was turned on once again. In the bottom tracing the undulating baseline indicates the presence of atrial fibrillation. The regular ventricular rhythm establishes that none of the atrial fibrillatory impulses conduct to the ventricles; thus complete AV block is present during atrial fibrillation.

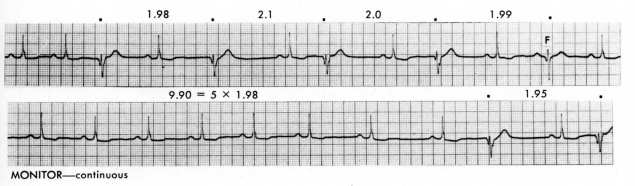

1.98   2.1   2.0   1.99   F

9.90 = 5 × 1.98   1.95

MONITOR—continuous

Fig. 8-153

Rate:	Atrial	Approximately 60 beats/minute.
	Ventricular parasystole	30 beats/minute.
Rhythm:	Atrial	Regular.
	Ventricular parasystole	Regular; interrupted by exit block or ventricular refractoriness.
P waves:		Normal.
PR interval:		During normally conducted beats, normal.
QRS (of ventricular parasystole):		Prolonged (0.13 second).
Arrhythmia:		Ventricular parasystole. The interval between ectopic ventricular systoles ranges between 1.98 and 2.1 seconds. The coupling interval varies between the sinus-initiated QRS complex and the parasystole complex. A ventricular fusion beat is labeled *F*. Ventricular refractoriness prevents the emergence of the ventricular parasystole during the long interval in which it is absent. This interectopic interval equals 9.90 seconds and is five times the normal interectopic interval. The dark marks above the tracing indicate the parasystolic ventricular systoles.

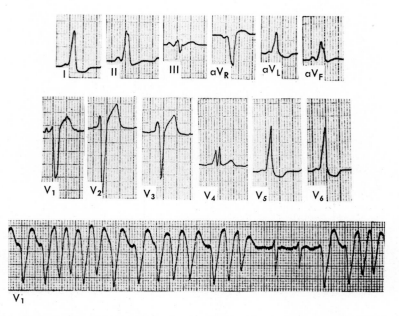

Fig. 8-154. Arrhythmia: twelve-lead ECG illustrating the preexcitation (Wolff-Parkinson-White) syndrome, type B. The lower recording (V₁ half standard) demonstrates an extremely rapid ventricular rate during atrial fibrillation in this same patient. The grossly irregular ventricular rhythm, extremely rapid rate, and gradations in QRS contour from normal to prolonged (as conduction changes from the normal AV nodal pathway to the anomalous route) help distinguish this arrhythmia from ventricular tachycardia. Bypass of the safety valve features provided by normal AV nodal delay accounts for the rapid ventricular rate that, less commonly, may actually cause the ventricles to fibrillate and result in sudden death.

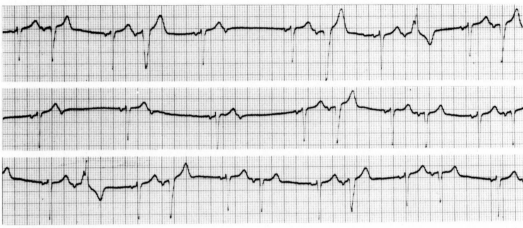

V_1—continuous

Fig. 8-155

Rate:	Determined by the number of premature atrial systoles.
Rhythm:	Irregular because of premature atrial systoles.
P waves:	Both sinus-initiated and premature atrial systolic P waves are abnormal.
PR interval:	Normal (0.12 second) for the sinus-initiated P waves; prolonged following the premature atrial systoles. Some premature atrial systoles failed to conduct to the ventricle.
QRS:	Normal, following the sinus-initiated P waves; functional left bundle and functional right bundle branch block following the premature atrial systoles.
Arrhythmia:	Functional right and left bundle branch block following atrial premature systoles. Premature atrial systoles occur at varying coupling intervals. When they occur with a very short RP interval, they fail to reach the ventricle and are therefore nonconducted atrial systoles. At slightly longer RP intervals, they conduct with both functional right and functional left bundle branch block. Differences in the duration of the preceding long cycle and in the duration of the short cycle account for whether functional right or left bundle branch block results.

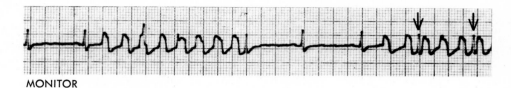

MONITOR

Fig. 8-156. Artifact. Regularly moving a loose electrode creates an artifact that mimics ventricular tachycardia. However, careful scrutiny uncovers the fairly regularly occurring normal QRS complexes *(arrows),* each preceded by a P wave. The question of ventricular tachycardia may be eliminated and the diagnosis of artifact established by observing that the QRS complexes continue uninterrupted and unaffected by the apparent ventricular tachycardia.

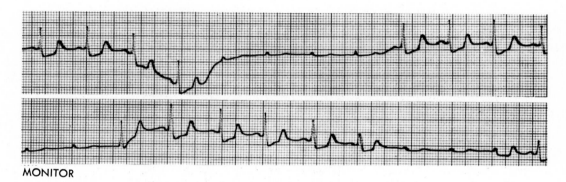

MONITOR

Fig. 8-157. Artifact simulating AV block. These tracings were recorded in a patient who presented with an acute anteroseptal myocardial infarction and 1 day later developed left anterior fascicular block. The monitored recording was interpreted as illustrating the development of advanced AV block with sequentially blocked P waves. Temporary transvenous pacemaker insertion was deemed immediately necessary. However, careful observation of the tracing reveals that the nonconducted P waves are artifactual in origin. In reality the "nonconducted P waves" are QRS complexes with a grossly diminished amplitude caused by intermittent poor ECG lead contact. The diagnosis is established by noting QRS complexes with intermediate amplitudes, by noting T waves that follow the diminutive QRS complexes and by "marching out" the QRS complexes and finding that they occur at the same time as the apparent P waves.

Electrocardiogram test section

This section provides a series of ECG tracings of various conditions that have been previously discussed. It is suggested that you cover the interpretations at the end of each legend and attempt to identify the abnormal patterns in each ECG.

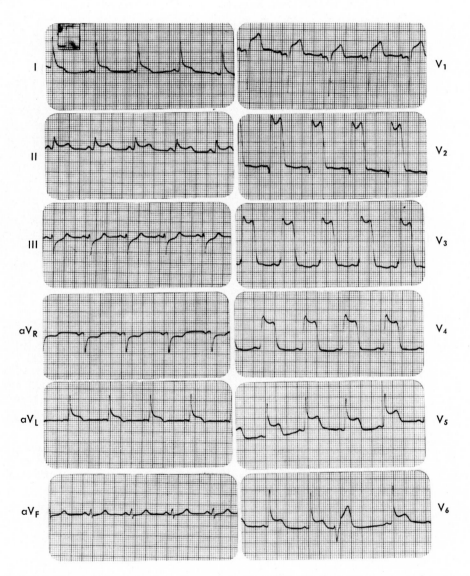

Fig. 8-158. Normal sinus rhythm. Q waves in V_1 and V_2. Marked ST segment elevation in leads I, II, aV_L, and V_1 through V_6. T waves have not yet inverted.

Electrocardiogram: *Hyperacute anterolateral, possibly apical, myocardial infarction.*

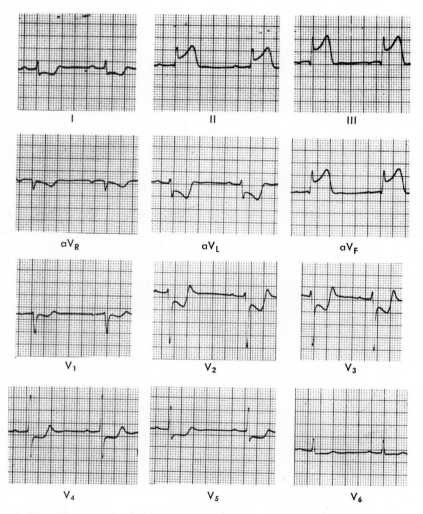

Fig. 8-159. Normal sinus rhythm. No pathologic Q waves have developed. Marked ST segment elevation in leads II, III, and aV_F, with reciprocal depression in leads I, aV_L and the anterior precordium. T waves are still upright.

Electrocardiogram: *Hyperacute inferior (diaphragmatic) myocardial infarction.*

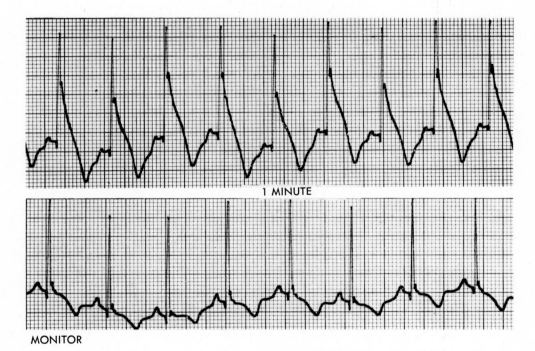

1 MINUTE

MONITOR

Fig. 8-160. Top tracing demonstrates marked ST segment elevation and T wave inversion. One minute later (bottom tracing) the ST segments have returned to base line. The T waves are still inverted.

Electrocardiogram: *The rapid ST changes from elevation to normal are characteristic of atypical (Prinzmetal) angina pectoris.*

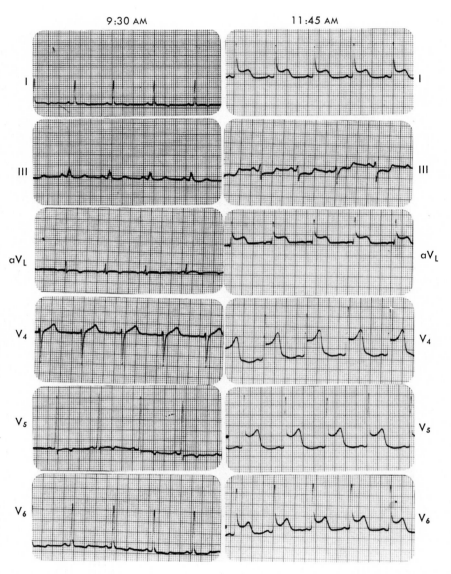

9:30 AM   11:45 AM

I

III

aV_L

V_4

V_5

V_6

Fig. 8-161. Normal sinus rhythm. Tracing at 9:30 AM, normal; tracing at 11:45 AM (after the patient developed more chest pain) demonstrates ST segment elevation in leads I, aV_L, and V_4 through V_6. The T waves are still upright, and no pathologic Q waves have developed.

Electrocardiogram: *Hyperacute lateral myocardial infarction.*

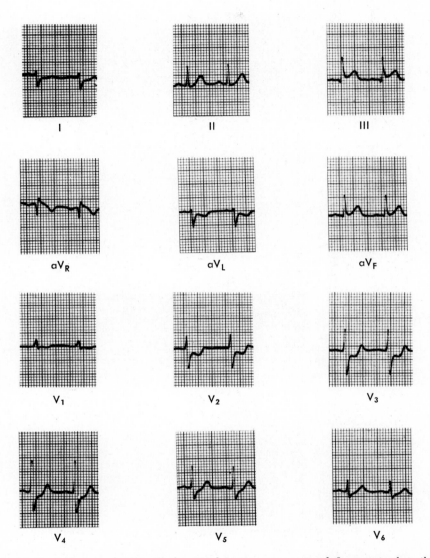

Fig. 8-162. Normal sinus rhythm. Right axis deviation suggesting left posterior hemiblock. ST segment elevation in lead III and slight ST segment elevation in lead aV$_F$. Large R wave in V$_1$, with slight ST segment depression in V$_1$, more marked in V$_2$ and V$_3$. T waves are still upright except for diphasic T waves in leads V$_1$ and V$_2$.

Electrocardiogram: *Acute posteroinferior myocardial infarction.*

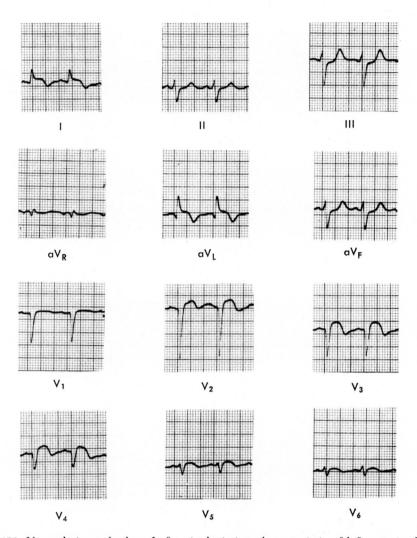

Fig. 8-163. Normal sinus rhythm. Left axis deviation characteristic of left anterior hemi-block. ST segment elevation in leads I, aV$_L$, and V$_2$ through V$_6$. Abnormal Q wave in V$_1$ through V$_4$, with small R waves in V$_5$ and V$_6$. T wave inversion in leads I and aV$_L$ and terminal T wave inversion in V$_2$ through V$_5$.

Impression: *Acute anterolateral myocardial infarction and left anterior hemiblock.*

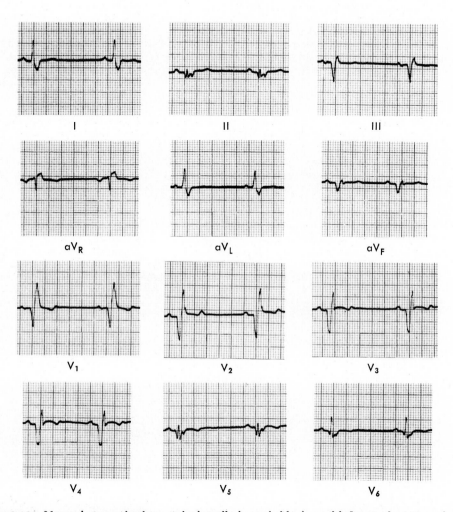

Fig. 8-164. Normal sinus rhythm, right bundle branch block, and left axis deviation characteristic of left anterior hemiblock. ST segments are normal. There are nonspecific T wave changes. A pathologic Q wave is present in leads II, III, aV$_F$, and V$_1$ through V$_4$ and makes the diagnosis of left anterior hemiblock difficult.

Electrocardiogram: *Right bundle branch block, possible left anterior hemiblock, and anteroinferior myocardial infarction, probably old.*

REFERENCES

1. Rosenbaum, M.B.: The hemiblocks: diagnostic criteria and clinical significance, Mod. Concepts Cardiovasc. Dis. **39**:141, 1970.
2. Jalife, J., and Moe, G.K.: A biologic model of parasystole, Am. J. Cardiol. **43**:761, 1979.
3. Anzelovitch, C., Jalife, J., and Moe, G.K.: Characteristics of reflection as a mechanism of reentrant arrhythmias and its relationship to parasystole, Circulation **61**:182, 1980.
4. Zipes, D.P.: New approaches to antiarrhythmic therapy (editorial), N. Engl. J. Med. **304**:475, 1981.
5. Zipes, D.P., Bailey, J.C., and Elharrar, V.: The slow inward current and cardiac arrhythmias, The Hague, 1980, Martinus Nijhoff.
6. Zipes, D.P.: Cardiac arrhythmias. In Conn, H.F., editor: Current diagnosis, Philadelphia, 1977, W.B. Saunders Co.
7. Zipes, D.P., Watanabe, A.M., and Besch, H.R.: Clinical electrophysiology and electrocardiography. In Wilkerson, J.T., and Sanders, C.A., editors: The science and practice of clinical medicine, New York, 1977, Grune & Stratton, Inc.
8. Zipes, D.P.: Tachycardia. In Conn, H.F., editor: Current therapy, Philadelphia, 1975, W.B. Saunders Co.
9. Pick, A., and Langendorf, R.: Interpretation of complex arrhythmias, Philadelphia, 1979, Lea & Febiger.
10. Josephson, M.E., and Seidco, S.F.: Clinical cardiac electrophysiology, Philadelphia, 1979, Lea & Febiger.
11. Nattel, S., and Zipes, D.P.: Clinical pharmacology of old and new antiarrhythmic drugs, Cardiovasc. Clin. **11**:221, 1980.
12. Rinkenberger, R.L., and others: Effects of intravenous and chronic oral verapamil administration in patients with supraventricular tachyarrhythmias, Circulation **62**:996, 1980.
13. Heger, J.J., Prystowsky, E.N., and Zipes, D.P.: New drugs for treatment of ventricular arrhythmias, Heart Lung **10**:475, 1981.
14. Fisher, J.D.: Role of electrophysiologic testing in the diagnosis and treatment of patients with known and suspected bradycardias and tachycardias, Prog. Cardiovasc. Dis. **24**:25, 1981.
15. Pick, A., and Dominguez, P.: Nonparoxysmal AV nodal tachycardia, Circulation **16**:1022, 1957.
16. Lie, K.I., Wellen, H.J.J., and Durrer, D.: Characteristics and predictability of primary ventricular fibrillation, Eur. J. Cardiol. **1**(4):379, 1974.
17. Bigger, J.T., Jr.: Management of arrhythmias. In Braunwald, E., editor: Heart disease: a textbook of cardiovascular medicine, Philadelphia, 1980, W.B. Saunders Co.
18. Josephson, M.E., and others: Recurrent ventricular tachycardia. I. Mechanisms, Circulation **57**: 431, 1978.
19. Zipes, D.P., and others: Clinical transvenous cardioversion of recurrent life-threatening ventricular tachyarrhythmias: low energy synchronized cardioversion of ventricular tachycardia and termination of ventricular fibrillation in patients using a catheter electrode (abstract), Am. J. Cardiol. **103**:789, 1982.
20. Horowitz, L.N., and others: Ventricular resection guided by epicardial and endocardial mapping for treatment of recurrent ventricular tachycardia, N. Engl. J. Med. **302**:589, 1980.
21. Zipes, D.P., Heger, J.J., and Prystowsky, E.N.: Sudden cardiac death (editorial), Am. J. Med. **70**:1151, 1981.
22. Ruskin, J.N., DiMarco, J.P., and Garan, H.: Out-of-hospital cardiac arrest: electrophysiologic observations and selection of long-term antiarrhythmic therapy, N. Engl. J. Med. **303**:607, 1980.
23. Coff, L.A., Werner, J.A., and Trobough, G.B.: Sudden cardiac death. I. A decade's experience with out-of-hospital resuscitation, Mod. Concepts Cardiovasc. Dis. **49**:31, 1980; II. Outcome of resuscitation management and further directions, Mod. Concepts Cardiovasc. Dis. **49**:37, 1980.
24. Zipes, D.P.: Second-degree atrioventricular block, Circulation **60**:465, 1979.
25. Hindman, M.C., and others: The clinical significance of bundle branch block complicating acute myocardial infarction, Circulation **58**:689, 1978.
26. Fisch, G.R., Zipes, D.P., and Fisch, C.: Bundle branch block and sudden death, Prog. Cardiovasc. Dis. **23**:187, 1980.
27. Prystowsky, E.N., Heger, J.J., and Zipes, D.P.: The Woff-Parkinson-White syndrome: diagnosis and treatment, Heart Lung **10**:465, 1981.
28. Gallagher, J.J., and others: The preexcitation syndromes, Prog. Cardiovasc. Dis. **20**:285, 1978.
29. Zipes, D.P., DeJoseph, R.L., and Rothbaum, D.A.: Unusual properties of accessory pathways, Circulation **49**:1200, 1974.
30. Wellens, H.J.J., Bärf, W.H.M., and Lie, K.I.: The value of the electrocardiogram in the differential diagnosis of a tachycardia with a widened QRS complex, Am. J. Med. **64**:27, 1978.

SUGGESTED READINGS

Bigger, J.T., Jr.: Mechanisms and diagnosis of arrhythmias: management of arrhythmias. In Braunwald, E., editor: Heart disease: a textbook of cardiovascular medicine, Philadelphia, 1980, W.B. Saunders Co.

Dubin, D.: Rapid interpretation of electrocardiograms, ed. 3, Tampa, Fla., 1974, Cover Publishing Co.

Goldman, M.J.: Principles of clinical electrocardiography, ed. 10, Los Altos, Calif., 1979, Lange Medical Publications.

Kennedy, H.L.: Ambulatory electrocardiography, Philadelphia, 1981, Lea & Febiger.

Lindsay, A.E., and Budkin, A.: The cardiac arrhythmias, ed. 2, Chicago, 1975, Year Book Medical Publishers.

Mandel, W.J.: Cardiac arrhythmias, Philadelphia, 1980, J.B. Lippincott Co.

Marriott, H.J.L.: Practical electrocardiography, ed. 6, Baltimore, 1977, The Williams & Wilkins Co.

McFarland, M.B.: Interpreting cardiac arrhythmias, New York, 1975, Springer Publishing Co. Inc.

McLachlan, E.M.: Fundamentals of electrocardiography, Oxford, England, 1981, Oxford University Press.

Nanda, O.S.: Cardiac arrhythmias, Baltimore, 1979, The Williams & Wilkins Co.

Phillips, R.E., and Feeney, M.K.: The cardiac rhythms: a systematic approach to interpretation, Philadelphia, 1980, W.B. Saunders Co.

Schamroth, L.: An introduction to electrocardiography, ed. 5, Philadelphia, 1976, J.B. Lippincott Co.

Schamroth, L.: Diagnostic pointers in clinical electrocardiology, Bowie, Md., 1979, Charles Press.

Schamroth, L.: The disorders of cardiac rhythm, ed. 2, Mead, Oxford, England, 1980, Blackwell Scientific Publications.

Watanabe, Y., and Dreifus, L.S.: Cardiac arrhythmias, New York, 1977, Grune & Stratton Inc.

Wenger, N.K., Mock, M.B., and Ringqvist, I.: Ambulatory electrocardiographic recording, Chicago, 1981, Year Book Medical Publishers.

9

SUDDEN CARDIAC DEATH

Eric N. Prystowsky
James J. Heger
Douglas P. Zipes

Sudden cardiac death is an enormous health care problem that accounts for approximately 1000 deaths in the United States every day.[1] Since most of the victims have significant coronary artery disease, as judged by postmortem evaluation[2-4] and catheterization data,[5] the ideal epidemiologic approach to prevent sudden death would be to decrease the incidence of atherosclerosis. In this regard, physicians and other health care personnel should instruct patients to stop smoking cigarettes and to maintain normal systemic arterial blood pressure, normal body weight, and normal plasma lipids. Moreover, prevention of atherosclerotic heart disease must start at a young age, and medical personnel as well as school systems must teach children and adolescents the value of an appropriate diet and life-style.

The wide-scale prevention of atherosclerotic heart disease will take years to accomplish, and until that time we must seek alternative methods to decrease the frequency of sudden cardiac death. One way is to teach cardiopulmonary resuscitation techniques to emergency personnel and to the general public. For example, in Seattle, Washington, Cobb, and co-workers[6] in association with the Seattle Fire Department, developed an emergency care system with various levels of medical expertise. Since patient survival depends on the rapidity with which cardiopulmonary resuscitation is initiated, it is notable that the average response time from dispatch until the first unit arrives is 2.9 minutes.[6] Many times, a bystander begins cardiopulmonary resuscitation before arrival of the emergency care team.

Early results from emergency care systems were not promising, and only approximately 15% of sudden death victims were resuscitated successfully *and* discharged from the hospital.[6,7] However, recent data from Seattle demonstrate improved survival statistics.[6] In 1978, 60% of 290 patients were successfully resuscitated from out-of-hospital ventricular fibrillation and about half of these patients (30% of total group) were discharged; still, the majority of patients did not survive. Furthermore, about 80% of patients who have out-of-hospital ventricular fibrillation do not have associated acute myocardial infarction; the 1-year risk of recurrent sudden death is 22% in these patients.[8] Therefore we need means to identify patients who are at risk for sudden death with the hope that appropriate therapy for these patients can prevent the occurrence of sudden death.

This chapter deals with the pathophysiology and risk factors of sudden death as well as the use of electrophysiologic testing to determine efficacy of antiarrhythmic drug therapy.

Pathophysiology of sudden cardiac death

Ventricular fibrillation is the most common arrhythmia recorded at the onset of cardiopulmonary resuscitation in patients who have out-of-hospital cardiac arrest.[6,7,9] In one study[9] bradyarrhythmias were present in nearly one third of the patients, a frequency much higher than that found in other studies.[6,7] Since bradyarrhythmias commonly occur when there has been delay in initiating emergency care,[6] it is unclear how often bradyarrhythmias actually cause sudden death. For example, combined data from eight monitored patients who did not have evidence of acute myocardial infarction showed that ventricular fibrillation caused sudden death in seven patients and severe bradyarrhythmias in only one patient.[10-12] An example from another patient of ours is shown in Fig. 9-1. More information is needed to define the role of bradyarrhythmias in sudden death.

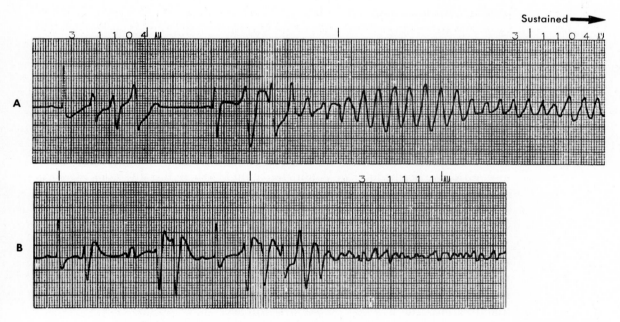

Fig. 9-1. Ventricular fibrillation recorded during ambulatory monitoring. These electrocardiographic tracings occurred during an in-hospital, 24-hour, ambulatory recording on a patient who had a previous out-of-hospital cardiac arrest. Tracing **A** shows the onset of rapid (approximately 300 beats/min) ventricular tachycardia that degenerated into ventricular fibrillation; the patient was successfully defibrillated to sinus rhythm. Seven minutes later (tracing **B**) a second episode of ventricular fibrillation occurred after a short run of ventricular tachycardia; defibrillation again restored sinus rhythm.

In contrast, ample data exist in support of ventricular tachyarrhythmias as the cause of sudden cardiac death.[10-14] Lie and co-workers[13] continuously monitored 262 patients who had an acute myocardial infarction (excluding patients with congestive heart failure or shock). All 20 patients requiring resuscitation had ventricular fibrillation, and in four patients ventricular tachycardia preceded ventricular fibrillation (Fig. 9-2). In another study Lie and co-workers[14] continuously monitored for 6 weeks 47 patients who had a recent myocardial infarction associated with bundle branch block. Out of 47 patients, 17 had cardiac arrest, and in all patients the arrhythmia was ventricular fibrillation. In this group, 14 out of 17 episodes of ventricular fibrillation were preceded by ventricular tachycardia. These two studies clearly show that ventricular tachyarrhythmias are the cause of sudden death in the vast majority of patients who have had a recent myocardial infarction and live long enough to be admitted to the hospital. Although it is not proven, ventricular arrhythmias are the most likely cause of sudden death in patients who have an acute myocardial infarction but die before being hospitalized.

Most patients who have coronary artery disease and develop sudden cardiac death demonstrate no recent thrombi in the coronary arteries at postmortem examination.[15,16] Moreover, the majority of patients successfully resuscitated from sudden death do not have an acute myocardial infarction.[17] In patients who are resuscitated from out-of-hospital sudden death, the presence of an acute myocardial infarction has important prognostic significance: of 424 survivors of ventricular fibrillation, the 1-year mortality in patients who had an acute myocardial infarction was 2%, and in patients who did not have an infarction the mortality was 22%.[8] These data confirm the observation that occurrence of ventricular fibrillation in the coronary care unit in patients who have an acute myocardial infarction does not increase the risk of sudden death in these patients after hospital discharge.[18]

The difference in long-term survival after resuscitation between patients who had and did not have an acute myocardial infarction may be explained in part as follows. Transient electrophysiologic and biochemical alterations occur in the ventricle during an acute myocardial infarction, and these alterations may result in ventricular fibrillation.[19,20] When the acute phase of the infarction resolves, the propensity for ventricular fibrillation becomes less because the patient's heart no longer has the electrophysiologic/anatomic capability to develop and/or sustain ventricular arrhythmias; these patients have a low recurrence rate of ventricular fibrillation. In contrast, patients who have ventricular fibrillation without infarction experience a relatively high risk of recurrent ventricular fibrillation. The high recurrence rate in those patients may be related to the fact that the "arrhythmogenic" area of the ventricle does not become infarcted and is still capable of initiating or sustaining ventricular arrhythmias.[21]

Although an acute myocardial infarction does not occur in most patients who have out-of-hospital ventricular fibrillation, acute myocardial ischemia may still be an important factor in the genesis of ventricular arrhythmias in these patients. Recently a patient who had a history of angina pectoris served to exemplify this point. During continuous electrocardiographic monitoring the patient had chest pain associated with ST segment elevation, and nonsustained ventric-

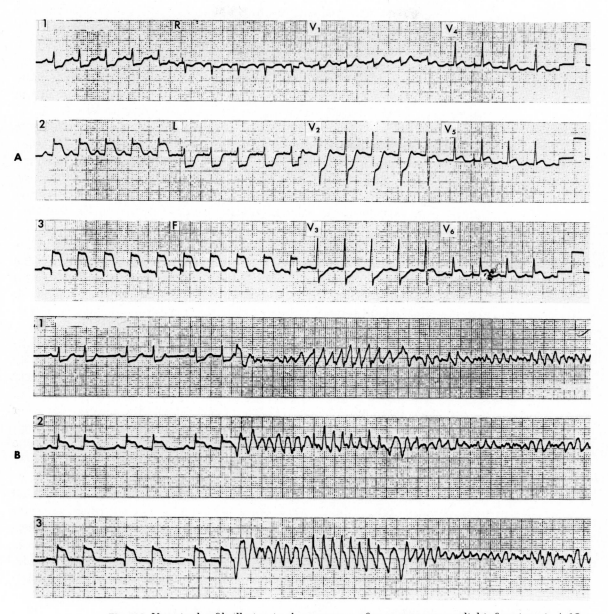

Fig. 9-2. Ventricular fibrillation in the presence of an acute myocardial infarction. **A,** A 12-lead ECG demonstrating a current of injury pattern (that is, ST elevations) in leads II, III, aV_F, and V_4 to V_6. This patient later developed Q waves in these leads. In both **A** and **B** the three leads arranged vertically were recorded simultaneously (for example, I, II, and III). **B** is a rhythm strip taken simultaneously for leads I, II, and III. Wenckebach AV block occurs on the left, and rapid ventricular tachycardia that degenerates into ventricular fibrillation is seen on the right.

ular tachycardia occurred with the episode of ischemia (Fig. 9-3). Subsequent coronary angiography demonstrated diffuse vasospasm as the cause for angina. Since few patients have had electrocardiographic recordings during out-of-hospital ventricular fibrillation, the frequency of ventricular arrhythmias induced by ischemia versus other causes remains to be defined.

Although sudden cardiac death occurs most often in patients who have coronary artery disease, it also occurs in patients with a variety of other cardiac conditions.[22-29] In a recent report about sudden death in 29 young athletes, 14 had hypertrophic cardiomyopathy, and five had concentric hypertrophy; only three had obstructive coronary artery disease, but three others had an anomalous origin of the left anterior descending coronary artery.[23] In our experience of 330 patients who had ventricular tachycardia/fibrillation, 161 (49%) did not have coronary artery disease (Table 9-1). Of note, 44 patients had primary electrical disease, that is, the presence of cardiac arrhythmias but no other cardiac abnormalities identified during physical examination, echocardiography, or cardiac catheterization.

An interesting group associated with an increased risk of sudden death is the prolonged QT entity.[24] The prolonged QT syndrome may occur in patients who are deaf[25] or who hear normally.[26,27] These patients are prone to develop ventricular tachycardia/fibrillation; the predisposition to ventricular arrhythmias may result from abnormalities in ventricular repolarization.[30] A recent study by Crampton[31] suggests that prolonged QT intervals in some of these patients result from either excessive activity of the left stellate ganglion, subnormal activity of the right stellate ganglion that creates "unopposed" left stellate ganglion activity, or both. Inflammation of epicardial ganglia has been reported in several patients who had QT prolongation syndrome and sudden death.[32]

An association of prolonged QT interval and sudden death has been demonstrated dramatically in patients receiving a liquid protein diet.[28,29] Singh and co-workers[28] described three young women who had lost 36 to 41 kg of body weight in 3 to 5 months. All had prolonged QT intervals and syncope caused by ventricular tachycardia/ventricular fibrillation; only one patient survived. Isner and co-workers[29] reported clinical and pathologic data in 17 patients who died suddenly while taking this diet. Twelve patients had ECGs recorded during dieting, and in nine patients the corrected QT interval was prolonged. Four of these nine patients had an ECG done before dieting, and the corrected QT interval was normal in three. Ventricular tachycardia was documented in all 11 patients who died in-hospital. Pathologic examination of 16 patients demonstrated no signifi-

Table 9-1. Ventricular tachycardia patient population

Coronary artery disease	169
Cardiomyopathy	52
Primary electrical disease	44
Mitral valve prolapse	40
Other	25
TOTAL	330

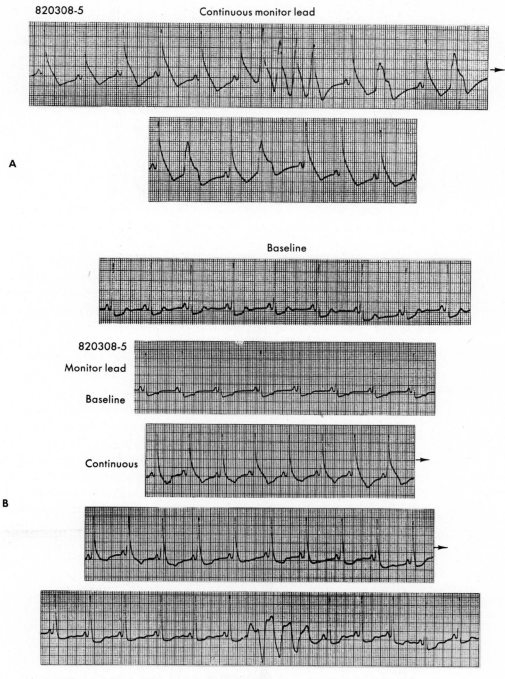

Fig. 9-3. Ventricular tachycardia during transient myocardial ischemia. Both are taken from the same patient. In the top of **A** the monitor lead recording shows ST elevations associated with a short run of nonsustained ventricular tachycardia. The lower tracing demonstrates the baseline QRST complex. In **B** the nonsustained run of ventricular tachycardia occurred *after* the elevated ST segment returned to baseline.

cant coronary artery disease, nor were myocardial abnormalities found by visual inspection. Some patients showed thinned left ventricular myocardial fibers consistent with starvation, but only one patient had histologic evidence of myocarditis. The cause for QT interval prolongation in these patients is unknown, but its frequent association with ventricular tachycardia suggests that ventricular tachycardia occurring in patients taking the liquid protein diet may be caused by abnormalities of ventricular repolarization. Whether the QT prolongation in this group of patients, in those receiving various drugs (*vide infra*), or in the congenital group relates to the same or similar electrophysiologic factors is not known.

Risk factors for sudden death
PREMATURE VENTRICULAR COMPLEXES

Premature ventricular complexes (PVCs) are ubiquitous. In patients who have no structural heart disease, PVCs occur commonly and do not seem to predict subsequent sudden death. In a group of apparently healthy medical students, 50% had isolated PVCs, 12% had multiform PVCs, 6% had R-on-T phenomenon, and one patient had nonsustained ventricular tachycardia.[33] In another study,[34] 25 patients who had no evidence of coronary artery disease demonstrated frequent PVCs during continuous electrocardiographic recording. The mean PVC frequency was 559/hour, and approximately 60% of the patients had couplets, although no ventricular tachycardia occurred. In fact, ventricular tachycardia occurred only after quinidine therapy in one patient who had no previous history of ventricular tachycardia. Hinckle, and co-workers[35] showed that PVCs were prevalent in patients whether or not they had heart disease, but PVCs were associated with an apparent increased risk of sudden death only in heart disease patients. Finally, Kostis and co-workers[36] studied 101 patients who had normal hearts determined by both noninvasive and invasive testing. During a 24-hour ambulatory electrocardiographic recording, 39 patients demonstrated at least one PVC. Thirty patients had their heart rhythms recorded for 72 hours, and only 5 of those thirty (17%) had no PVCs noted at the end of the recording period. Since these authors excluded patients who were referred to them for having PVCs or palpitations, it is likely that their study underestimated the incidence of PVCs in patients who have no structural heart disease.

Many investigators have studied the association between PVCs and the risk of subsequent sudden death in patients who have coronary artery disease.[37-48] Unfortunately, large differences in experimental design preclude accurate comparisons between studies. For example, although there appears to be a relatively high frequency of sudden death within the first 2 months after myocardial infarction,[43] in the study of Ruberman and co-workers[42] 50% of the patients were entered into the study at least 3 months after their myocardial infarction. Drug administration, which conceivably could alter the incidence of sudden death, was not controlled for in the majority of the studies.

Earlier studies[37-39] did not differentiate types of PVCs, but most of the later studies[40-48] used the Lown modified grading system[49] to classify PVCs as complex or simple. Minor differences in PVC classification occurred, but most often simple

PVCs were defined as uniform PVCs that occurred infrequently, and complex PVCs generally included those that occurred frequently and were multiform, bigeminal, paired, and early-cycle (that is, R-on-T phenomenon). Recent data have shown that the detection of high PVC rates or complex PVCs varies logarithmically with duration of electrocardiographic recording,[50] and that, although 95% of high PVC rates were detected during 12 hours of recording, recording for 18 hours was necessary to detect at least 95% of couplets or ventricular tachycardia. In another study, the maximal PVC grade (Lown classification) in patients who had coronary artery disease was recorded in 74% of patients during 24 hours of ECG recording but required 36 hours of recording to document maximal PVC grade in 95% of patients.[51]

Despite the necessity for prolonged electrocardiographic recording times to detect complex PVCs, most of the studies employed short recording periods. For example, duration of electrocardiographic recording used to detect arrhythmias included a single 12-lead ECG[37-39] and continuous electrocardiographic recording for 1 hour,[42,47,48] 6 hours,[43,44] and 8 to 12 hours.[45,46] Only two studies used recording times of 24 hours.[40,41] Thus, in some studies with short electrocardiographic recording times, the increased frequency of sudden death in patients who had complex versus simple PVCs may be more apparent than real, since the patients who had simple PVCs might have demonstrated complex PVCs if longer electrocardiographic recording times had been used.

Most of the studies state the highest Lown PVC grade detected in a patient and do not examine whether more than one type of PVC grade exists. Bigger and Weld[52] recently showed that this hierarchical type of PVC grading system has shortcomings regarding stratification of patients at risk for death after myocardial infarction. These authors prospectively studied 400 patients who were treated for acute myocardial infarction. All patients had a 24-hour electrocardiographic recording between 10 and 20 days after hospital admission, and the average follow-up was 30 months. Seventy-eight patients died during follow-up (the authors do not separate patients into sudden and nonsudden death). Of note, the authors found that the occurrence of paired PVCs and ventricular tachycardia led to a greater risk for subsequent cardiac death than R-on-T PVCs. Furthermore, the frequency of PVCs was a significant additional risk factor for cardiac death in patients who had repetitive PVCs or R-on-T PVCs. More studies are needed to corroborate these very interesting observations.

A more important issue is whether there is any value in subdividing PVCs into simple and complex forms. The premise for this subdivision appears to have originated during the early years of coronary care units when higher grades of PVCs were thought to represent "warning arrhythmias," that is, rhythms that presaged the occurrence of ventricular tachycardia and/or ventricular fibrillation.[49] However, in a recent study of 262 patients who had an acute myocardial infarction Lie and co-workers[13] showed that many patients have ventricular fibrillation without warning arrhythmias, and many patients who have warning arrhythmias do not have ventricular tachyarrhythmias. Thus there does not appear to be value in grading PVC severity in patients who have acute myocardial infarction.

In patients who have angina but no history of myocardial infarction, PVCs are associated with an increased risk of sudden death; but there is no difference in risk between simple and complex PVCs.[47] After myocardial infarction, patients who have complex PVCs appear to have a greater risk of subsequent sudden death than patients who have simple or no PVCs.[40-43,45,46] The presence of complex PVCs also is associated with an increased risk of nonsudden cardiac death,[42] and the prevalence of complex PVCs varies directly with the severity of coronary artery disease and left ventricular dysfunction.[41,53-55] In one study, patients who had an elevated left ventricular end-diastolic pressure and multiple zones of asynergy demonstrated by cardiac catheterization had the largest yield of high-grade complex PVCs.[53] Thus patients who have advanced atherosclerotic heart disease tend to have a higher frequency of complex PVCs; whether the PVCs are merely associated with or actually cause sudden death is unclear. If a causal relationship can be established, hope for decreasing sudden death by prophylactically treating patients who have PVCs becomes more realistic.

Lown assigned the highest PVC grade to those PVCs that interrupt the T wave of the previous QRS complex, that is, R-on-T phenomenon.[49] Repolarization of the ventricles accounts for the T wave on the surface ECG, and experimental work has shown that stimulation of the heart during early repolarization appears to be arrhythmogenic.[56,57] For example, in 1921 deBoer[56] demonstrated in the frog heart that a stimulus applied near the end of ventricular refractoriness could cause ventricular fibrillation. This observation was confirmed in dogs by Wiggers and Wegria[57] in 1940. These authors demonstrated that electrical stimuli of equal strength produced ventricular fibrillation when applied during the time of the T wave but induced only premature ventricular complexes when the stimuli occurred later in diastole. In 1960 Smirk and Palmer[58] reported a high occurrence of sudden death in patients who had R-on-T PVCs recorded on a 12-lead ECG. Notably however, approximately 90% of these patients had significant heart disease, and 25% had congestive heart failure.

Although there is no question that R-on-T PVCs can initiate ventricular fibrillation,[59] most recorded episodes of ventricular tachyarrhythmias result from midcycle rather than R-on-T PVCs.[13,60-64] In 52 patients who had acute myocardial infarction, 27 had a total of 131 episodes of paroxysmal ventricular tachycardia; early PVCs initiated only 12% of these episodes.[61] Furthermore, in 25 patients who did not have ventricular tachycardia, 13% of the PVCs were of the R-on-T variety. Winkle, and co-workers[62] recorded 94 episodes of ventricular tachycardia during ambulatory electrocardiographic recording in 23 patients, and only 14 episodes of ventricular tachycardia were induced by an early PVC. In another study 339 patients had 24-hour electrocardiographic recording, and only 5.6% of the PVCs recorded were early PVCs.[63] Forty-five episodes of ventricular tachycardia occurred, but only 16% of the patients who had early PVCs had ventricular tachycardia.[63] Finally, in a recent study by Follansbee, and co-workers[64] only 7 of 37 patients had ventricular tachycardia initiated by early PVCs. From all this data we conclude that R-on-T PVCs infrequently occur and in most patients do not induce ventricular tachycardia/fibrillation, and that most episodes of ventricular tachycardia/fibrillation are not initiated by early PVCs.

To summarize, in patients who have coronary artery disease, simple and complex PVCs commonly occur, the prevalence of complex PVCs increases directly with the number of diseased coronary arteries and with the severity of left ventricular dysfunction,[41,53,55] and complex PVCs increase the risk of subsequent sudden death, although most patients who have complex PVCs do not die suddenly.

VENTRICULAR TACHYCARDIA

Ventricular tachycardia probably should be placed in a class by itself, although Lown[49] has considered it part of a general classification of PVCs. A small subset of patients who have ventricular tachycardia and no apparent structural heart disease are not at increased risk for subsequent sudden death.[65] However, our experience with over 300 patients who were referred for control of ventricular tachycardia/fibrillation, as well as recent studies,[10,13,14] suggests that ventricular tachycardia often initiates or degenerates into ventricular fibrillation (Figs. 9-1 and 9-2). Follansbee and co-workers[64] reported that 10 of 37 patients who had self-terminating, asymptomatic, nonsustained ventricular tachycardia diagnosed from a 24-hour electrocardiographic recording died suddenly during follow-up, giving a yearly mortality of 17%. It is likely that, in these patients, sustained ventricular tachycardia or ventricular fibrillation caused sudden death (Fig. 9-4). Of note, 9 of the 19 patients (47%) who had congestive heart failure died suddenly, whereas only 1 of 18 patients (6%) who did not have congestive heart failure succumbed to sudden death, demonstrating the increased risk factor provided by myocardial dysfunction.

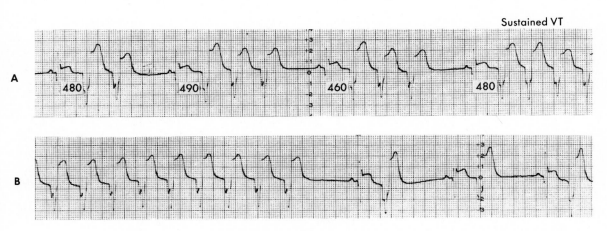

Fig. 9-4. Nonsustained ventricular tachycardia preceding the onset of sustained ventricular tachycardia. Tracings **A** and **B** were recorded during ambulatory monitoring and are not continuous. In **A** there are two episodes of nonsustained ventricular tachycardia followed by sustained tachycardia. The coupling interval between the sinus complex and the first complex of ventricular tachycardia is variable, and the shortest coupling interval, 460 msec, does not induce sustained tachycardia. **B** demonstrates the termination of the sustained ventricular tachycardia.

In a retrospective study Lie and co-workers[14] determined patients at high risk for the development of late in-hospital ventricular fibrillation after myocardial infarction. The authors demonstrated that the high-risk patients were those who had an anteroseptal myocardial infarction complicated by right or left bundle branch block. In a prospective study this same group[14] continuously monitored in the hospital for 6 weeks 47 high-risk post-myocardial infarction patients. Seventeen patients (36%) developed ventricular fibrillation, and in 14 of these 17 patients ventricular tachycardia preceded the ventricular fibrillation. In our experience ventricular tachycardia precedes by seconds to several minutes almost all episodes of ventricular fibrillation induced in the electrophysiology laboratory (Fig. 9-5). Thus patients who have ventricular tachycardia appear to have a significant risk of sudden death, although the prevalence and natural history of asymptomatic ventricular tachycardia in the general population remain unknown.

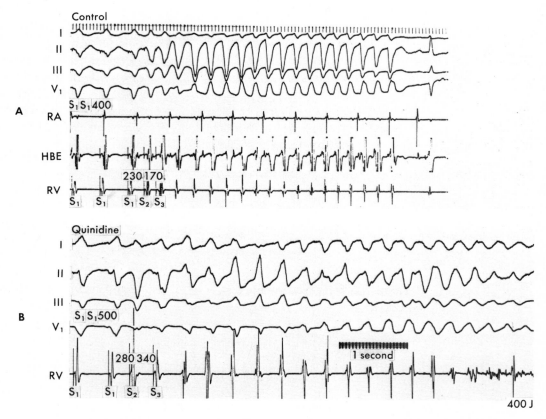

Fig. 9-5. Induction of nonsustained and sustained ventricular tachycardia during programmed ventricular stimulation. For both panels the top four tracings are ECG leads I, II, III, and V₁. Intracardiac electrograms were recorded from the right atrium (*RA*), right ventricle (*RV*), and His bundle area (*HBE*). During control study, nonsustained ventricular tachycardia (*VT*) was induced by two premature stimuli induced during ventricular pacing (panel **A**). A repeat electrophysiology study (panel **B**) was performed while the patient was receiving oral quinidine. Ventricular tachycardia was initiated, and within 5 seconds the VT degenerated into ventricular fibrillation.

LEFT VENTRICULAR DYSFUNCTION AND OTHER RISK FACTORS

Patients who have coronary artery disease and left ventricular dysfunction demonstrate an increased risk of sudden cardiac death.* In 425 survivors of out-of-hospital ventricular fibrillation, 340 patients had no acute transmural myocardial infarction, and 169 of these 340 had no evidence of remote myocardial infarction.[8] In these 169 patients the 1-year risk for subsequent sudden death was 30% (7 out of 23) for patients who had congestive heart failure and 11% (16 out of 46) for those who did not have heart failure.[8] Patients who have an acute myocardial infarction are at increased risk of developing subsequent sudden death if they have congestive heart failure while still in the coronary care unit[18,67] or have a low cardiac ejection fraction (determined by radionuclide angiography) prior to hospital discharge.[41] As noted in the previous section, complex PVCs commonly occur in patients who have myocardial dysfunction, and the two abnormalities appear additive as a risk for sudden death.[42] For example, the risk of sudden death is greatest in patients who have congestive heart failure and complex PVCs, but the risk is less for patients who have only congestive heart failure or complex PVCs.[42]

Many varied and seemingly unrelated factors appear to increase the risk of sudden death. Weinblatt and co-workers[68] reported that in men who had similar traditional risk factors and similar arrhythmias there was a relationship between a low educational level and subsequent sudden death in the posthospitalization period following myocardial infarction. The authors noted that patients with less than 8 years of schooling had a threefold increase in risk of sudden death compared with better educated men. It is unclear why patients who had a lower socioeconomic background are at increased risk for sudden death, but the availability of medical care does not appear to be a major factor.[68]

Bigger and co-workers[18] analyzed multiple variables in postmyocardial infarction patients. At 6 and 12 months there was a 15% and 19% mortality, respectively, and most of the deaths were sudden. Of note, serum BUN ($\geq$20 mg/dl), creatinine ($\geq$1.4mg/dl), and uric acid ($\geq$7.0 mg/dl) levels were higher risk factors for death than the occurrence of congestive heart failure in the coronary care unit, and more than one variable increased the risk for death.

There has been recent interest in the role of repolarization abnormalities recorded on the surface ECG and subsequent sudden death.[69-71] In 55 patients who had a myocardial infarction 2 months to 6 years in the past, the QT interval (corrected by Bazett's formula) was prolonged in 5 of 27 patients who survived and in 16 of 28 patients who died suddenly; this suggests that patients who survive myocardial infarction and have prolonged QT intervals may be at risk for subsequent development of sudden death.[69] Kentala and Repo[70] measured the corrected QT interval in patients 6 to 8 weeks after myocardial infarction and correlated these data with data about subsequent sudden death. The QT intervals were measured from ECGs recorded when the patient was resting in the supine position before and 5 minutes after exercise, and when the patient was in the upright position before starting exercise. Twenty-one patients died suddenly dur-

*References 5, 8, 18, 41, 42, 44, 54, 55, 66, 67

ing follow-up, and in this group the mean QT_c interval when the patients were upright before exercise was significantly longer than the resting supine QT_c value. There was no significant change in QT_c values in the upright versus supine position for the nonsudden death group and survivors. Furthermore, when the patients were upright before exercise, the mean QT_c interval was significantly longer in the sudden death group than in the nonsudden death group and survivors. Thus, although the supine resting QT interval did not differentiate patients at risk for subsequent sudden death, a prolonged ($\geq$440 msec), corrected QT interval recorded in the upright position occurred more frequently in patients who had subsequent sudden, as opposed to nonsudden, death. The abnormally prolonged QT intervals recorded from patients in an upright position may reflect the inability of the patients' autonomic nervous systems to respond normally to changes in cardiovascular tone. Since abnormalities of the autonomic nervous system may cause QT prolongation and may increase the risk for subsequent sudden death, future efforts to decrease the incidence of sudden death should include more detailed research on the autonomic nervous system and other factors that influence ventricular repolarization.[30] It is of particular interest that practolol,[72] alprenolol,[73] and timolol[74] appear to decrease the risk of sudden death; these results may be explained in part by the effects of the drugs on the autonomic nervous system. More recent studies with propranolol[75] and metoprolol[76] demonstrate a decrease in mortality of patients receiving these drugs, although a decrease in sudden death was not specified.

Treatment of ventricular arrhythmias

Ventricular tachyarrhythmias may be controlled by one or more of a variety of therapies that include drugs, pacemakers, and surgery. Probably the most difficult task in caring for patients who have ventricular arrhythmias is deciding *whether* to treat them, rather than which treatment modality to use. Since the risk of sudden death is not the same for all ventricular arrhythmias, treatment to suppress ventricular arrhythmias should be guided by the relative risks of sudden death in a particular arrhythmia (Fig. 9-6). The assumption, although often hard to prove, is that abolition of the arrhythmia will prevent death; obviously, the decision to treat a patient must be made from the data obtained on that patient and sound clinical judgment. Fig. 9-6 demonstrates that the lowest risk of sudden death occurs in patients who have PVCs but no structural heart disease, and the highest risk occurs in patients who have sustained ventricular tachycardia and severe congestive heart failure; as a rule, the former group should not receive antiarrhythmic therapy (assuming that the patient is asymptomatic), whereas the latter group requires therapy. In general, patients who have sustained ventricular tachycardia and patients who have heart disease and nonsustained ventricular tachycardia usually should be treated. If nonsustained ventricular tachycardia causes symptoms in patients who do not have structural heart disease, one should attempt to suppress the arrhythmia; if the arrhythmia occurs in otherwise healthy individuals, treatment may not be necessary, but careful follow-up of these patients is imperative. These broad guidelines must be interpreted according to specific clinical situations.

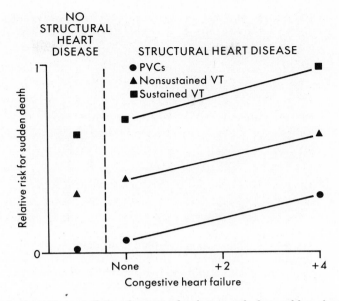

Fig. 9-6. Schematic concept of the theoretical relative risk for sudden death of various ventricular arrhythmias. See text for further detail.

One interesting group of patients who do not appear to require therapy if they are asymptomatic and have no structural heart disease are those who have repetitive monomorphic ventricular tachycardia (RMVT).[65] This form of tachycardia is identified electrocardiographically by frequent, recurrent bursts of ventricular tachycardia exhibiting uniform contour, and separated by sinus complexes that conduct with a normal QRS contour (Fig. 9-7). We evaluated 16 patients who had RMVT documented for 1 month to 16 years (mean 5.2 ± 4.8 years). Five patients who were asymptomatic were not treated and have remained asymptomatic during 8 years (mean) of follow-up. Of note, only one of seven patients had his arrhythmia induced during electrophysiologic study, suggesting but not proving that the mechanism responsible for the arrhythmia was automaticity rather than reentry.

The largest group of patients who have ventricular arrhythmias are those who have heart disease and PVCs. Furthermore, it is this group of patients for whom treatment is most controversial. For example, the risk of sudden death in these patients is greater than in patients who do not have heart disease but do have PVCs, and the risk of sudden death increases with decreasing myocardial function.[42] However, the overall risk of sudden death does not appear great, and there are no controlled studies to suggest that treating these patients with antiarrhythmic therapy decreases the incidence of sudden death. In fact, prospective studies of patients after myocardial infarction show that neither phenytoin,[77] procainamide,[78] nor aprindine[79] significantly decreases the incidence of sudden death as compared with control groups, although patients treated with aprindine and procainamide had fewer ventricular arrhythmias than the placebo-treated

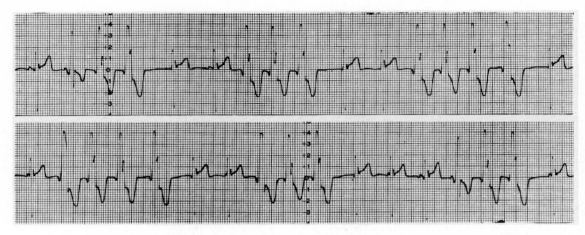

Fig. 9-7. Repetitive monomorphic ventricular tachycardia. The electrocardiographic tracings are not continuous. Note the recurrence of short episodes of nonsustained ventricular tachycardia with a uniform morphology and the normal intervening sinus complexes.

groups. The nonsignificant decrease in incidence of sudden death in patients treated with procainamide may be related to the low dosage of procainamide (500 mg every 6 to 8 hours) the authors prescribed.[78] In studies testing the effectiveness of therapy with beta-blocking drugs[72-74] a significant decrease in sudden death occurred in patients treated with alprenolol, practolol, and timolol compared with control patients. The apparent beneficial effect of beta blockers may be due to the drugs' antisympathetic properties, membrane-active properties, antiischemic effects, or a combination of multiple actions.

If antiarrhythmic drugs caused minimal side effects and had a high therapeutic-to-toxic ratio, their use to prevent sudden death, albeit of unproven value, would not be unreasonable. However, antiarrhythmic drugs commonly cause side effects[78] and in some patients can cause ventricular tachycardia and sudden death.[34,80,81] For example, in a recent study[81] 71 patients who had atrial fibrillation or flutter but no history of ventricular arrhythmias were given quinidine sulfate. Four patients developed ventricular fibrillation and two ventricular tachycardia, and there was no significant difference in the degree of QT prolongation or serum quinidine concentration between these patients and the patients who did not develop ventricular arrhythmias. In other patients, administration of type I antiarrhythmic drugs (for example, quinidine, procainamide, or disopyramide) may cause marked prolongation of the QT interval and result in a specific form of ventricular tachycardia, known as torsade de pointes.[82,83] (Fig. 9-8).

Because of the known adverse actions of conventional antiarrhythmic drugs, and because a decrease in the incidence of sudden death in treated patients has not been demonstrated, antiarrhythmic drug therapy for all patients who have coronary artery disease and complex or simple PVCs appears unwarranted at this time. A prospective controlled study is needed to determine if conventional antiarrhythmic drugs, for example, quinidine, disopyramide, or procainamide, administered at doses that result in "therapeutic" serum drug levels, can prevent

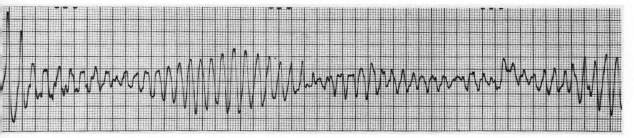

Fig. 9-8. Torsade de pointes. This specific type of ventricular tachycardia usually occurs in the presence of a prolonged QT interval and is characterized by a QRS morphology that appears repeatedly to change its axis by 180 degrees.

sudden death in patients who have coronary artery disease. According to Prineas,[84] as many as 2000 patients may be necessary for the study, making a multicenter cooperative study required. Such a trial, sponsored by the National Institutes of Health, tested the efficacy of propranolol to decrease the incidence of cardiac death and sudden death in patients after myocardial infarction. Preliminary results from this trial show a decrease in mortality in those patients who were treated with propranolol.[75]

Although some physicians may feel it unethical to initiate such a trial, since they believe that patients after myocardial infarction who have complex PVCs benefit from antiarrhythmic therapy, most believe that the efficacy of treating these patients has not been adequately tested. Knowledge of the total PVC count in such a trial would be of interest; however, one must remember that daily PVC counts vary considerably,[85] and, more important, the ability to suppress PVCs may not predict accurately the future occurrence of ventricular tachycardia/ventricular fibrillation.[79,86-88] Myerburg and co-workers studied survivors of out-of-hospital cardiac arrest.[86] Sixteen patients were treated with procainamide or quinidine and followed-up after hospital discharge. All eight patients who died within 1 year of follow-up had unstable drug plasma levels that were often subtherapeutic, and only two of the survivors had unstable subtherapeutic plasma drug levels. Of note, no significant difference in PVC counts occurred between patients who survived and those who had recurrent sudden death. Recently, Myerburg and co-workers[89] demonstrated in the same patients that suppression of spontaneous ventricular tachycardia requires significantly lower doses of procainamide than suppression of 85% of PVCs does. However, follow-up time was short, and these data should be considered preliminary at this time.

Other forms of therapy such as sulfinpyrazone[90] appear to be effective in specific circumstances but require more intensive investigation before widespread use can be recommended.

Electrophysiologic testing

The usual method employed to assess efficacy of drug therapy in the suppression of spontaneous ventricular tachycardia/fibrillation is to monitor for variable time periods the patient's heart rhythm during therapy under normal activity and often during stress testing. If no ventricular arrhythmias occur during the monitoring period, usually 2 to 4 days, the patient is discharged and further follow-up is done out-of-hospital. In many patients ventricular tachyarrhythmias are episodic, which precludes accurate assessment of drug efficacy by noninvasive monitoring techniques only; unfortunately, out-of-hospital sudden death is not an uncommon sequela in these patients.

Electrophysiologic testing using programmed electrical stimulation to induce ventricular tachycardia has been used to judge more accurately the ability of drugs to prevent ventricular arrhythmias.[91-97]

Thus patients who have ventricular tachycardia induced before but not after drug therapy usually have no recurrence of ventricular tachycardia if they continue to take the dosage of the antiarrhythmic drug that prevented induction of ventricular tachycardia at electophysiologic study. We routinely use electrophysiologic testing as part of our current treatment protocol (Fig. 9-9) and find that combined use of continuous electrocardiographic monitoring and electrophysiologic testing enables us to detect ventricular tachycardia in almost all patients referred for evaluation.[96] For example, of 46 patients who had a history of ventricular tachycardia, in the drug-free control period 32 had ventricular tachycardia induced during electrophysiologic study, and 33 had ventricular tachycardia detected during prolonged continuous electrocardiographic recording[96]; of note, only two patients did not demonstrate ventricular tachycardia during either electrocardiographic monitoring or electrophysiologic testing.

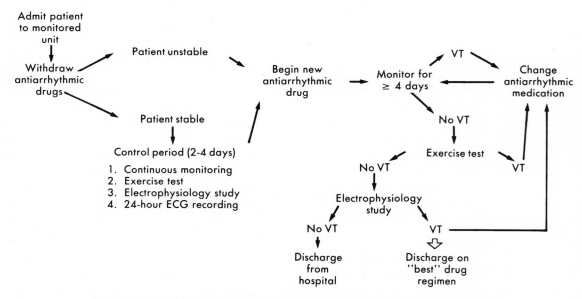

Fig. 9-9. Ventricular tachycardia treatment protocol. See text for details.

Our present protocol for treating ventricular tachycardia is outlined in Fig. 9-9. Patients are admitted to an intensive care unit, and all antiarrhythmic drugs are withheld. If stable, the patient is monitored continuously for 48 to 96 hours, and during this time a treadmill exercise test, a 24-hour electrocardiographic recording, and a base-line electrophysiologic study are performed. To induce ventricular tachycardia during electrophysiologic testing the following protocol is used:

1. Incremental (pacing at progressively faster rates) left and/or right atrial pacing starting at rates just faster than the spontaneous sinus rate and progressing until AV block occurs.
2. Premature left and/or right atrial stimulation during sinus rhythm and atrial pacing.
3. Incremental right ventricular pacing to rates $\geqslant$240 msec until ventriculoatrial block occurs or until limited by patient symptoms.
4. Premature right ventricular stimulation during sinus rhythm and during right ventricular pacing (S_1), with induction of one (S_2), two (S_2, S_3), and occasionally three (S_2, S_3, S_4) premature stimuli. Premature ventricular stimulation is performed at three pacing cycle lengths (usually 600, 500, and 400 msec, that is, 100, 120, and 150 per minute, respectively) and at two right ventricular sites (usually the apex and outflow tract) until ventricular tachycardia reproducibly is induced.
5. If no ventricular tachycardia occurs during premature ventricular stimulation, 3 to 10 ventricular paced complexes are induced at multiple rates $\leqslant$250/minute (RV burst pacing). In selected patients programmed electrical stimulation of the left ventricle is performed.

Using this pacing protocol in patients who have spontaneous ventricular tachycardia, we found that the frequency of ventricular tachycardia induction prior to drug therapy depends on the patient's type of heart disease and history of sustained versus nonsustained tachycardia[97] (Fig. 9-10). For example, in patients who have a history of sustained ventricular tachycardia we induced ventricular tachycardia in 56 of 59 (95%) who had coronary artery disease but induced ventricular tachycardia in only 27 of 39 (69%) patients who had no coronary artery disease (Fig. 9-10). These data are important, for they can help one decide which patients are best suited for serial electrophysiologic drug testing.

The majority of patients who have ventricular tachycardia and are referred to us suffer from ventricular arrhythmias that were not controlled by conventional antiarrhythmic drugs, or the patient was intolerant of the drugs. Thus most patients are treated with an investigational drug (Table 9-2). If the patient spontaneously develops ventricular tachycardia during drug therapy while being monitored continuously (Fig. 9-9), a new drug is tried. When a drug results in total suppression of ventricular tachycardia during continuous electrocardiographic monitoring, treadmill stress testing, and a 24-hour electrocardiographic recording, a repeat electrophysiologic study is performed. If programmed electrical stimulation does not induce ventricular tachycardia, the patient is discharged and followed-up closely in our outpatient arrhythmia clinic. In our experience many patients who have no ventricular tachycardia observed during noninvasive testing

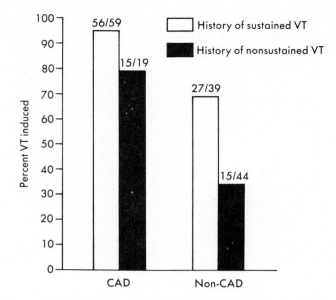

Fig. 9-10. Induction of ventricular tachycardia as a function of type of spontaneous tachycardia and type of heart disease in 161 patients. See text for further details. *CAD,* Coronary artery disease; *non-CAD,* patients who have no obvious structural heart disease or structural heart disease other than CAD; *VT,* ventricular tachycardia.

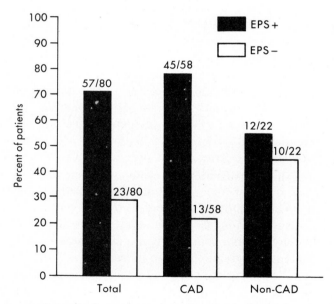

Fig. 9-11. Frequency of ventricular tachycardia induction at electrophysiologic study (EPS) in patients who received antiarrhythmic drugs and demonstrated no spontaneous tachycardia during prolonged (≥2 days) continuous electrocardiographic monitoring (CECG). Of 58 patients, 45 (78%) who had CAD had ventricular tachycardia induced (EPS +), even though drug therapy suppressed the occurrence of spontaneous tachycardia; 13 patients had no inducible tachycardia (EPS −). In the non-CAD group 12 of 22 patients (55%) had inducible ventricular tachycardia, and in 10 patients tachycardia was not induced.

Table 9-2. Experimental drug therapy for 219 patients with ventricular tachycardia

Drug	Number treated	Number taking drug
Amiodarone	93	65
Aprindine	159	47
Encainide	132	36
Mexiletine	42	11
Tocainide	12	2
TOTAL	438	161 (76%)

still have ventricular tachycardia induced during electrophysiologic testing[96] (Fig. 9-11). When tachycardia is induced, we change the antiarrhythmic drug and continue this process until either no ventricular tachycardia is induced during electrophysiologic testing or the best drug or drug combination is found, based on its ability to alter markedly the ventricular tachycardia (for example, no spontaneous ventricular tachycardia noted during noninvasive testing and induction of a ventricular tachycardia that is markedly slower than the tachycardia induced prior to drug therapy). The patient is discharged receiving the drug(s) that prevented or altered ventricular tachycardia and then is followed-up closely in our outpatient arrhythmia clinic.

Follow-up results of our initial 71 patients who had spontaneous sustained ventricular tachycardia and who underwent repeat electrophysiologic testing during one or more drug trials (that is, serial electrophysiologic testing) are noted in Fig. 9-12. We no longer could induce ventricular tachycardia in 15 patients during drug therapy, and 13 of 15 have had no recurrence of ventricular tachycardia for a mean of 16 months. One patient had recurrent ventricular tachycardia when his drug dosage was decreased, and another patient had tachycardia during an episode of congestive heart failure. In 56 patients no drug or drug combination prevented initiation of tachycardia during electrophysiologic study, although in almost all patients the rate of the induced ventricular tachycardia was markedly slower compared with control, and in many patients the ventricular tachycardia became nonsustained. Seventeen patients had recurrent ventricular tachycardia, but only 3 of 56 patients died suddenly. Of note, 36 of 56 patients (64%) have not had recurrent symptomatic ventricular tachyarrhythmias, and 29 are receiving amiodarone therapy, many in combination with other experimental drugs. Thus, in patients receiving amiodarone therapy, induction of ventricular tachycardia in the laboratory does not appear to predict recurrence of spontaneous ventricular tachycardia.[98] The full reason for this discordance is not clear, but it is possible that in certain patients amiodarone virtually eliminates PVCs and therefore prevents spontaneous initiation of ventricular tachycardia. It is unknown whether other investigational drugs can prevent the occurrence of spontaneous ventricular tachycardia in patients in whom ventricular tachycardia is induced during electrophysiologic testing.

The use of electrophysiologic testing to guide antiarrhythmic therapy in patients who have ventricular tachycardia or ventricular fibrillation is still experimental, and it should be performed only by physicians who have special training

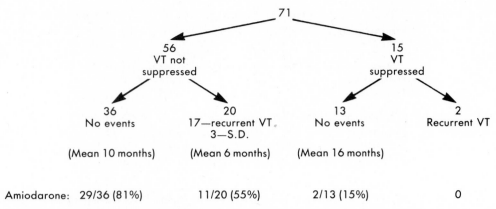

Fig. 9-12. Follow-up results in 71 patients who had sustained ventricular tachycardia and underwent serial electrophysiologic drug testing. See text for further detail.

in clinical electrophysiology. Many issues concerning electrophysiologic testing are not resolved. Previous reports[92-95] have suggested that patients who have ventricular tachycardia induced during control study but not during drug therapy have no recurrence of ventricular tachycardia. In general, our results support these data: 13 of 15 patients who had no ventricular tachycardia induced during drug therapy have had no recurrence of arrhythmias (Fig. 9-12). However, in certain patients changes in cardiac function over time (for example, the development of congestive heart failure) may preclude accurate predictions of drug efficacy as determined during electrophysiologic testing. Furthermore, some patients in whom ventricular tachycardia is induced during drug therapy may have no recurrence of spontaneous symptomatic ventricular tachycardia (Fig. 9-12). It is probable that, although these patients can sustain ventricular tachycardia, as demonstrated during electrophysiologic testing, they may still not have a symptomatic recurrence as long as the drug suppresses the event(s) that initiates the tachycardia.[22] Thus a good clinical result may occur in certain patients in whom ventricular tachycardia is still induced in the laboratory, and more data are needed to determine which patients can be discharged with minimal risk of recurrent arrhythmias.

Many questions remain unanswered. For example, in patients who have frequent episodes of ventricular tachycardia prior to drug therapy but who have no ventricular tachycardia during drug therapy, it is not known whether the drug should be discontinued because ventricular tachycardia is induced during electrophysiologic testing. Second, it is not clearly established which patients who have ventricular tachycardia should have electrophysiologic testing. Patients usually undergo electrophysiologic testing if (1) they have a history of syncope and/or out-of-hospital ventricular fibrillation, (2) ventricular tachycardia results in substantial hemodynamic compromise, (3) ventricular tachycardia has not been controlled by multiple antiarrhythmic drugs, and (4) the patient's arrhythmia does not occur often enough to evaluate drug efficacy. Many patients fulfill the last criterion, in our experience.

Electrophysiologic testing offers the additional advantage of enabling the physician to determine the patient's hemodynamic response to the ventricular arrhythmia that might recur, since the arrhythmia induced in the electrophysiology laboratory usually is the arrhythmia the patient develops during follow-up if that patient has recurrent tachyarrhythmias. For example, in 11 patients in whom drug therapy suppressed ventricular tachycardia as judged by noninvasive tests, sustained ventricular tachycardia often causing severe hypotension was induced during repeat electrophysiologic testing.[99] If the patients had been discharged receiving the drugs associated with induction of sustained ventricular tachycardia, it is possible that in some patients a recurrent episode of ventricular tachycardia might have resulted in sudden death.

In summary, electrophysiologic testing in selected patients who have ventricular tachycardia/fibrillation is an important adjunct to test drug efficacy. Ideally, the patient should be discharged, receiving the antiarrhythmic drug(s) that totally suppresses ventricular tachycardia/fibrillation during electrophysiologic testing. Practically, total suppression of ventricular tachycardia during electrophysiologic testing is not accomplished in many cases, and nonsustained or sustained ventricular tachycardia can still be induced. If patients continue to have hemodynamically unstable ventricular arrhythmias with all drug combinations, they should be considered for alternative therapy, for example, surgery, pacemaker implantation, or other electrical devices.[100-106]

We thank Nancy S. Lineback for her expert secretarial assistance and Jacqueline O'Donnell, M.D., Krannert Institute of Cardiology, for referring the patient demonstrated in Fig. 9-3.

REFERENCES

1. Lown, B.: Sudden cardiac death: the major challenge confronting contemporary cardiology, Am. J. Cardiol. **43**:313, 1979.
2. Kuller, L., Lilienfeld, A., and Fisher, R.: Epidemiological study of sudden and unexpected deaths due to arteriosclerotic heart disease, Circulation **34**:1056, 1966.
3. Liberthson, R.R., and others: Pathophysiologic observations in prehospital ventricular fibrillation and sudden cardiac death, Circulation **49**:790, 1974.
4. Reichenbach, D.D., Moss, N.S., and Meyer, E.: Pathology of the heart in sudden cardiac death, Am. J. Cardiol. **39**:865, 1977.
5. Weaver, W.D., and others: Angiographic findings and prognostic indicators in patients resuscitated from sudden cardiac death, Circulation **54**:895, 1976.
6. Cobb, L.A., Werner, J.A., and Trobaugh, G.B.: Sudden cardiac death. I. A decade's experience with out-of-hospital resuscitation, Mod. Concepts Cardiovasc. Dis. **49**:31, 1980.
7. Liberthson, R.R., and others: Prehospital ventricular defibrillation: prognosis and follow-up course, N. Engl. J. Med. **291**:317, 1974.
8. Cobb, L.A., Werner, J.A., and Trobaugh, G.B.: Sudden cardiac death. II. Outcome of resuscitation; management, and future directions, Mod. Concepts Cardiovasc. Dis. **49**:37, 1980.
9. Myerburg, R.J., and others: Clinical, electrophysiologic, and hemodynamic profile of patients resuscitated from prehospital cardiac arrest, Am. J. Med. **68**:568, 1980.
10. Lahiri, A., Balasubramanian, V., and Raftery, E.B.: Sudden death during ambulatory monitoring, Br. Med. J. **1**:1676, 1979.
11. Gradman, A.H., Bell, P.A., and DeBusk, R.F.: Sudden death during ambulatory monitoring: clinical and electrocardiographic correlations: report of a case, Circulation **55**:210, 1977.
12. Denes, P., and others: Sudden death in patients with chronic bifascicular block, Arch. Intern. Med. **137**:1005, 1977.
13. Lie, K.I., and others: Observations on patients with primary ventricular fibrillation complicating acute myocardial infarction, Circulation **52**:755, 1975.
14. Lie, K,.I., and others: Early identification of patients developing late in-hospital ventricular fibrillation after discharge from the coronary care unit: a 5½-year retrospective and prospective study of 1,897 patients, Am. J. Cardiol. **41**:674, 1978.

15. Spain, D.M., and Bradess, V.A.: The relationship of coronary thrombosis to coronary atherosclerosis and ischemic heart disease (a necropsy study covering a period of 25 years), Am. J. Med. Sci.**240**:701, 1960.

16. Myers, A., and Dewar, H.A.: Circumstances attending 100 sudden deaths from coronary artery disease with coroner's necropsies, Br. Heart J. **37**:1133, 1975.

17. Baum, R.S., Alvarez, H., III, and Cobb, L.A.: Survival after resuscitation from out-of-hospital ventricular fibrillation, Circulation **50**:1231, 1974.

18. Bigger, J.T., and others: Risk stratification after acute myocardial infarction, Am. J. Cardiol. **42**:202, 1978.

19. Elharrar, V., and Zipes, D.P.: Cardiac electrophysiologic alterations during myocardial ischemia, Am. J. Physiol. **233**:H329, 1977.

20. Opie, L.H., Nathan, D., and Lubbe, W.F.: Biochemical aspects of arrhythmogenesis and ventricular fibrillation, Am. J. Cardiol. **43**:131, 1979.

21. Warren, J.V.: Di si dolce morte: it may be safer to be dead than alive, Circulation **50**:415, 1974.

22. Pedersen, D.H., and others: Ventricular tachycardia and ventricular fibrillation in a young population, Circulation **60**:988, 1979.

23. Maron, B.J., and others: Sudden death in young athletes, Circulation **62**:218, 1980.

24. Moss, A.J., and Schwartz, P.J.: Sudden death and the idiopathic long QT syndrome, Am. J. Med. **66**:6, 1979.

25. Jervell, A., and Lange-Nielsen, F.: Congenital deaf-mutism, functional heart disease with prolongation of the QT interval, and sudden death, Am. Heart J. **54**:59, 1957.

26. Romano, C., Gemme, G., and Pongiglione, R.: Aritimie cardiache rare dell'eta pediatrica, Clin. Pediatr. (Bologna) **45**:656, 1963.

27. Ward, O.: A new familial cardiac syndrome in children, J. Irish Med. Assoc. **54**:103, 1964.

28. Sigh, B.N., and others: Liquid protein diets and torsade de pointes, J.A.M.A. **240**:115, 1978.

29. Isner, J.M., and others: Sudden, unexpected death in avid dieters using the liquid-protein modified-fast diet: observations in 17 patients and the role of the prolonged QT interval, Circulation **60**:1401, 1979.

30. Zipes, D.P., and others: Roles of autonomic innervation in the genesis of ventricular arrhythmias. In Abboud, F.M., and others, editors: Disturbances in neurogenic control of the circulation, Baltimore, 1981, Williams & Wilkins Co.

31. Crampton, R.: Preeminence of the left stellate ganglion in the long QT syndrome, Circulation **59**:769, 1979.

32. James, T.N., and others: Cardiac ganglionitis associated with sudden unexpected death, Ann. Intern. Med. **91**:727, 1979.

33. Brodsky, M., and others: Arrhythmias documented by 24-hour continuous electrocardiographic monitoring in 50 male medical students without apparent heart disease, Am. J. Cardiol. **39**:390, 1977.

34. Kennedy, H.L., and Underhill, S.J.: Frequent or complex ventricular ectopy in apparently healthy subjects: a clinical study of 25 cases, Am. J. Cardiol. **38**:141, 1976.

35. Hinkle, L.E., Jr., Carver, S.T., and Stevens, M.: The frequency of asymptomatic disturbances of cardiac rhythm and conduction in middle-aged men, Am. J. Cardiol. **24**:629, 1969.

36. Kostis, J.B., and others: Premature ventricular complexes in the absence of identifiable heart disease, Circulation **63**:1351, 1981.

37. Chiang, B.N., and others: Relationship of premature systoles to coronary heart disease and sudden death in the Tecumseh epidemiologic study, Ann. Intern. Med. **70**:1159, 1969.

38. The Coronary Drug Project Research Group: Prognostic importance of premature beats following myocardial infarction: experience in the Coronary Drug Project, J.A.M.A. **223**:116, 1973.

39. Fisher, F.D., and Tyroler, H.A.: Relationship between ventricular premature contractions on routine electrocardiography and subsequent sudden death from coronary heart disease, Circulation **47**:712, 1973.

40. Vismara, L.A., Amsterdam, E.A., and Mason, D.T.: Relation of ventricular arrhythmias in the late hospital phase of acute myocardial infarction to sudden death after hospital discharge, Am. J. Med. **59**:6, 1975.

41. Schulze, R.A., Strauss, H.W., and Pitt, B.: Sudden death in the year following myocardial infarction: relation to ventricular premature contractions in the late hospital phase and left ventricular ejection fraction, Am. J. Med.**62**:192, 1977.

42. Ruberman, W., and others: Ventricular premature beats and mortality after myocardial infarction, N. Engl. J. Med. **297**:750, 1977.

43. Moss, A.J., and others: Ventricular ectopic beats and their relation to sudden and nonsudden cardiac death after myocardial infarction, Circulation **60**:998, 1979.

44. Moss, A.J., and others: The early posthospital phase of myocardial infarction: prognostic stratification, Circulation **54**:58, 1976.

45. Kotler, M.N., and others: Prognostic significance of ventricular ectopic beats with respect to sudden death in the late postinfarction period, Circulation **47**:959, 1973.

46. Vismara, L.A., and others: Identification of sudden death risk factors in acute and chronic coronary artery disease, Am. J. Cardiol. **39**:821, 1977.

47. Ruberman, W., and others: Ventricular premature complexes in prognosis of angina, Circulation **61**:1172, 1980.

48. Ruberman, W., and others: Ventricular premature complexes and sudden death after myocardial infarction, Circulation **64**:297, 1981.

49. Lown, B., and Wolf, M.: Approaches to sudden death from coronary heart disease, Circulation **44**:130, 1971.

50. Thanavaro, S., and others: Effect of electrocardiographic recording duration on ventricular dysrhythmia detection after myocardial infarction, Circulation **62**:262, 1980.
51. Kennedy, H.L., and others: Effectiveness of increasing hours of continuous ambulatory electrocardiography in detecting maximal ventricular ectopy, Am. J. Cardiol. **42**:925, 1978.
52. Bigger, J.T., and Weld, F.M.: Analysis of prognostic significance of ventricular arrhythmias after myocardial infarction: shortcomings of Lown grading system, Br. Heart J. **45**:717, 1981.
53. Calvert, A., Lown, B., and Gorlin, R.: Ventricular premature beats and anatomically defined coronary heart disease, Am. J. Cardiol. **39**:627, 1977.
54. Schulze, R.A., Jr., and others: Ventricular arrhythmias in the late hospital phase of acute myocardial infarction: relation to left ventricular function detected by gated cardiac blood pool scanning, Circulation **52**:1006, 1975.
55. Schulze, R.A., Jr., and others: Left ventricular and coronary angiographic anatomy: relationship to ventricular irritability in the late hospital phase of acute myocardial infarction, Circulation **55**:839, 1977.
56. deBoer, S.: On the fibrillation of the heart, J. Physiol. (Lond.) **54**:400, 1921.
57. Wiggers, C.J., and Wegria, R.: Ventricular fibrillation due to single, localized induction and condenser shocks applied during the vulnerable phase of ventricular systole, Am. J. Physiol. **128**:500, 1940.
58. Smirk, F.H., and Palmer, D.G.: A myocardial syndrome—with particular reference to the occurrence of sudden death and of premature systoles interrupting antecedent T waves, Am. J. Cardiol. **6**:621, 1960.
59. Hinkle, L.E., Jr., and others: Pathogenesis of an unexpected sudden death: role of early cycle ventricular premature contractions, Am. J. Cardiol. **39**:873, 1977.
60. Engel, T.R., Meister, S.G., and Frankl, W.S.: The R-on-T phenomenon: an update and critical review, Ann. Intern. Med. **88**:221, 1978.
61. DeSoyza, N., and others: Ectopic ventricular prematurity and its relationship to ventricular tachycardia in acute myocardial infarction in man, Circulation **50**:529, 1974.
62. Winkle, R.A., Derrington, D.C., and Schroeda, J.S.: Characteristics of ventricular tachycardia in ambulatory patients, Am. J. Cardiol. **39**:487, 1977.
63. Boudoulas, H., and others: Malignant premature ventricular beats in ambulatory patients, Ann. Intern. Med. **91**:723, 1979.
64. Follansbee, W.P., Michelson, E.L., and Morganroth, J.: Nonsustained ventricular tachycardia in ambulatory patients: characteristics and association with sudden cardiac death, Ann. Intern. Med. **92**:741, 1980.
65. Heger, J.J., and others: Repetitive ventricular tachycardia: clinical and electrophysiologic characteristics, Circulation **62**:(III)321, 1980.
66. Oberman, A., and others: Sudden death in patients evaluated for ischemic heart disease, Circulation **51** and **52**:(III)170, 1975.
67. Christensen, D., and others: Sudden death in the late hospital phase of acute myocardial infarction, Arch. Intern. Med. **137**:1675, 1977.
68. Weinblatt, E., and others: Relation of education to sudden death after myocardial infarction, N. Engl. J. Med. **299**:60, 1978.
69. Schwartz, P.J., and Wolf, S.: QT interval prolongation as predictor of sudden death in patients with myocardial infarction, Circulation **57**:1074, 1978.
70. Kentala, E., and Repo, U.K.: QT interval prolongation during somatomotor activation as predictor of sudden death after myocardial infarction, Ann. Clin. Res. **11**:42, 1979.
71. Haynes, R.E., Hallstrom, A.P., and Cobb, L.A.: Repolarization abnormalities in survivors of out-of-hospital ventricular fibrillation, Circulation **57**:654, 1978.
72. Green, K.G., and others: Improvement in the prognosis of myocardial infarction by long-term beta-adrenoreceptor blockade using practolol, Br. Med. J. **3**:735, 1975.
73. Wilhelmsson, C., and others: Reduction of sudden deaths after myocardial infarction by treatment with alprenolol: preliminary results, Lancet **2**:1157, 1974.
74. The Norwegian Multicenter Study Group: Timolol-induced reduction in mortality and reinfarction in patients surviving acute myocardial infarction, N. Engl. J. Med. **304**(14):801, 1981.
75. National Heart, Lung, and Blood Institute of Bethesda, Maryland: The β-blocker heart attack trial, J.A.M.A. **246**:2073, 1981.
76. Hjalmarson, A., and others: Effect on mortality of metoprolol in acute myocardial infarction: a double-blind randomized trial, Lancet **2**:823, 1981.
77. Lovell, R.R.H.: Arrhythmia prophylaxis: long-term suppressive medication, Circulation **51** and **52**(III): 236, 1975.
78. Kosowsky, B.D., and others: Long-term use of procaine amide following acute myocardial infarction, Circulation **47**:1204, 1973.
79. Hugenholtz, P.G., and others: One year follow-up in patients with persistent ventricular dysrhythmias after myocardial infarction treated with aprindine or placebo. In Sando, E., Julian, D.G., and Bell, J.W., editors: Management of ventricular tachycardia—role of mexiletine, Amsterdam, 1978, Excerpta Medica.
80. Selzer, A., and Wray, H.W.: Quinidine syncope: paroxysmal ventricular fibrillation occurring during treatment of chronic atrial arrhythmias, Circulation **30**:17, 1964.
81. Ejvinsson, G., and Orinius, E.: Prodromal ventricular premature beats preceded by a diastolic wave, Acta Med. Scand. **208**:445, 1980.
82. Dessertenne, F.: La tachycardie ventriculaire à deux foyers opposés variable, Arch. Mal. Coeur **59**:263, 1966.

83. Smith, W.M., and Gallagher, J.J.: "Les Torsades de Pointes": an unusual ventricular arrhythmia, Ann. Intern. Med. **93**:578, 1980.

84. Prineas, R.J.: Problems in design and evaluation of antiarrhythmia trials, Circulation **51** and **52**(III):249, 1975.

85. Morganroth, J., and others: Limitations of routine long-term electrocardiographic monitoring to assess ventricular ectopic frequency, Circulation **58**:408, 1978.

86. Myerburg, R.J., and others: Antiarrhythmic drug therapy in survivors of prehospital cardiac arrest: comparison of effects on chronic ventricular arrhythmias and recurrent cardiac arrest, Circulation **59**:855, 1979.

87. Herling, I.M., Horowitz, L.N., and Josephson, M.E.: Ventricular ectopic activity after medical and surgical treatment for recurrent sustained ventricular tachycardia, Am. J. Cardiol. **45**:633, 1980.

88. Krone, R.J., and others: The effectiveness of antiarrhythmic agents on early-cycle premature ventricular complexes, Circulation **63**:664, 1981.

89. Myerburg, R.J., and others: Relationship between plasma levels of procainamide, suppression of premature ventricular complexes, and prevention of recurrent ventricular tachycardia, Circulation **64**:280, 1981.

90. The Anturane Reinfarction Trial Research Group: Sulfinpyrazone in the prevention of cardiac death after myocardial infarction: the Anturane Reinfarction Trial, N. Engl. J. Med. **298**:289, 1978.

91. Naccarelli, G.V., and others: The repetitive ventricular response: prevalence and prognostic significance, Br. Heart J. **46**:152, 1981.

92. Fisher, J.D., and others: Serial electrophysiologic-pharmacologic testing for control of recurrent tachyarrhythmias, Am. Heart J. **93**:658, 1977.

93. Mason, J.W., and Winkle, R.H.: Electrode-catheter arrhythmia induction in the selection and assessment of antiarrhythmic drug therapy in recurrent ventricular tachycardia, Circulation **58**:971, 1978.

94. Horowitz, L.N., and others: Recurrent sustained ventricular tachycardia. 3. Role of the electrophysiologic study in selection of antiarrhythmic regimens, Circulation **58**:986, 1978.

95. Ruskin, J.N., DiMarco, J.P., and Garan, H.: Out-of-hospital cardiac arrest: electrophysiologic observations and selection of long-term antiarrhythmic therapy, N. Engl. J. Med. **303**:607, 1980.

96. Heger, J.J., and others: Comparison between results obtained from electrophysiology testing, exercise testing, and ambulatory ECG recording. In Wenger, N.K., Mock, M.B., and Ringquist, I., editors: Ambulatory electrocardiographic recording, Chicago, 1981, Year Book Medical Publishers, Inc.

97. Naccarelli, G.V., and others: Role of electrophysiologic testing in patients with ventricular tachycardia but without coronary artery disease (abstract), Clin. Res. **28**(4):714A, 1980.

98. Heger, J.J., and others: Amiodarone: clinical efficacy and electrophysiology during long-term therapy for recurrent ventricular tachycardia, N. Engl. J. Med. **305**:539, 1981.

99. Rinkenberger, R.L., and others: Drug conversion of nonsustained ventricular tachycardia to sustained ventricular tachycardia during serial electrophysiological studies: identification of drugs that exacerbate tachycardia and potential mechanisms, Am. Heart J. **103**:117, 1982.

100. Gallagher, J.J.: Surgical treatment of arrhythmias: current status and future directions, Am. J. Cardiol. **41**:1035, 1979.

101. Guiraudon, G., and others: Encircling endocardial ventriculotomy: a new surgical treatment for life-threatening ventricular tachycardias resistant to medical treatment following myocardial infarction, Ann. Thorac. Surg. **26**:438, 1978.

102. Josephson, M.E., Harken, A.H., and Horowitz, L.N.: Endocardial excision: a new surgical technique for the treatment of recurrent ventricular tachycardia, Circulation **60**:1430, 1979.

103. Mirowski, M., and others: Clinical treatment of life-threatening ventricular tachyarrhythmias with the automatic implantable defibrillator, Am. Heart J. **102**:265, 1981.

104. Fisher, J.D., Mehra, R., and Furman, S.: Termination of ventricular tachycardia with bursts of rapid ventricular pacing, Am. J. Cardiol. **41**:94, 1978.

105. Jackman, W.M., and Zipes, D.P.: Low energy synchronous cardioversion of ventricular tachycardia using a catheter electrode in a canine model of subacute myocardial infarction, Circulation **66**:187, 1982.

106. Zipes, D.P., and others: Clinical transvenous cardioversion of recurrent life-threatening ventricular tachyarrhythmias: low energy synchronized cardioversion of ventricular tachycardia and termination of ventricular fibrillation in patients using a catheter electrode, Am. Heart J. **103**:789, 1982.

10

CARDIOVASCULAR DRUGS

James J. Heger
Eric N. Prystowsky
Douglas P. Zipes

In this section we review selected aspects of the pharmacology of drugs used to treat cardiovascular disorders, emphasizing clinically important factors. Included are standard approved drugs and several new investigational drugs that show unique or promising clinical effects.

Clinical pharmacokinetics

A drug will exert its pharmacologic effects only when it reaches a critical concentration at a specific site of action. Metabolic processes of absorption, distribution, biotransformation, and elimination determine drug concentration at active sites. *Pharmacokinetics* is the quantitative study of these factors, and by applying mathematical models, pharmacokinetics provides a rational basis to determine the method of administration, dose strength, and dose timing.

Pharmacokinetic models[1]

Several mathematical models may be employed to describe drug pharmacokinetics in humans, but the simplest and most applicable are the one-compartment and two-compartment models depicted in Fig. 10-1. The one-compartment model assumes that a drug has rapid and homogenous distribution throughout the body. Although this is not actually the case, this model is a useful method to describe pharmacokinetics of some orally administered drugs during chronic dosing. In the two-compartment model there is a smaller central compartment, representing blood volume in highly perfused tissues, and a larger peripheral compartment with a slower rate of perfusion. A drug is administered into and eliminated from the central compartment, which also reaches equilibrium with the peripheral compartment.

The rate at which drug movement occurs to and from the central and peripheral compartments and the rate at which a drug is eliminated from this central compartment are the kinetics of drug action. Most drugs exhibit "first-order kinetics" (Fig. 10-2), which means that the rate at which a drug leaves a compartment is proportional to the amount of drug present in that compartment. Therefore, over a given time period, a larger quantity of drug is eliminated if the initial amount of drug is large rather than small.

359

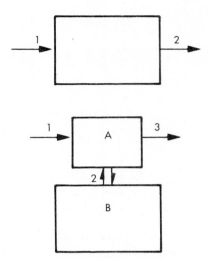

Fig. 10-1. *Top,* One-compartment model of drug pharmacokinetics. Drug is administered *(step 1)* and eliminated *(step 2)* from a large single compartment. Drug concentration in the single compartment is homogenous. *Bottom,* Two-compartment model of drug pharmacokinetics. Drug is administered *(step 1)* and eliminated *(step 3)* from a small central compartment *(A)*. The small central compartment reaches an equilibrium *(step 2)* with the larger peripheral compartment *(B)*.

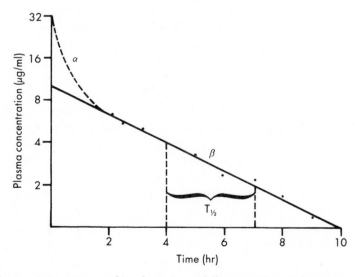

Fig. 10-2. Plasma concentration plotted over time following administration of a single dose of a drug exhibiting "first order" elimination kinetics. Distribution phase *(A)* is followed by elimination phase *(B)*. The time required to eliminate half of a given amount of drug is termed the *elimination half-life* ($T_{1/2}$).

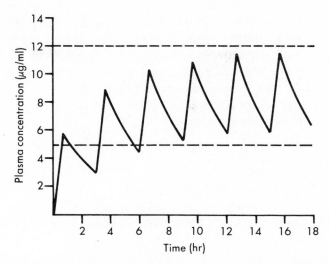

Fig. 10-3. Plasma concentration of a hypothetical drug administered at dosing intervals equal to an elimination half-life of 3 hours. Five half-lives are required to reach a steady-state level. A hypothetical range of effective plasma concentration is illustrated by hash lines.

Elimination half-life ($T_{1/2}$) is an important concept in pharmacokinetics; it refers to the amount of time required to eliminate half the drug load from a given compartment (Fig. 10-2). Because most cardiac drugs have a narrow toxic therapeutic ratio, it is desirable to maintain a narrow range of drug concentrations. In most cases this is best accomplished by timing each dose administration to approximate the half-life of the drug.

Loading dose refers to the amount of drug administered to initially achieve a given body load. As illustrated in Fig. 10-3, if a drug is begun by administering the usual maintenance dose, steady-state conditions will be reached after 4 or 5 elimination half-lives, which in the example would require 12 to 15 hours. Steady-state conditions are achieved more rapidly if an initial loading dose is given. Likewise, after an increase in a drug dose, the time required to reach a new steady-state level will be 4 or 5 elimination half-lives. The new steady state and the new concentration are achieved more rapidly if an additional loading dose is given. The *maintenance dosage* is the amount of drug administered to maintain the body load over a given time interval during steady-state conditions.

Each drug used in cardiac therapeutics has unique pharmacokinetics. However, a number of common variables modify therapy by affecting the relationship between drug dose and drug effects. These variables include age, weight, sex, nature of heart disease, route of administration of drug, patient tolerance, physiologic milieu (for example, acid-base balance, electrolytes, hypoxia), and concurrent medications.

The measured plasma concentration of a drug is often used to guide therapy, but this method must be interpreted and used according to the individual clinical situation. Plasma concentrations are especially useful to ascertain whether a toxic concentration is present and to determine whether an apparent drug failure is caused by unexpected low plasma levels. However, for a given patient, drug toxicity may occur at a drug concentration usually considered to be therapeutic, and a subtherapeutic effect of a drug may occur at a drug concentration considered to be toxic. Moreover, measurement of plasma drug concentration does not take into account the contribution of metabolites or changes in protein binding that may contribute to overall drug effect. Therefore plasma drug concentrations must be approached as any other laboratory test, that is, in light of the patient's entire clinical picture.

Digitalis

Digitalis preparations are the oldest and most widely used drugs in the treatment of heart disease. Many forms of digitalis are available, but at present digoxin and digitoxin are most often employed. The major use of digitalis is to treat congestive heart failure and supraventricular arrhythmias, especially atrial fibrillation.

Digitalis exerts positive inotropic effects that resemble those produced by catecholamines, but the effects are not affected by beta-adrenergic blocking drugs and occur in normal and failing hearts. The precise mechanism of positive inotropic actions of digitalis has not been clearly elucidated. However, it has been postulated that by inhibition of the Na^+-K^+ membrane pump, digitalis increases the intracellular pool of calcium ions available for excitation-contraction coupling.[2]

Although positive inotropic effects of digitalis are evident in normal and failing hearts, the net effect on myocardial oxygen consumption differs in these two conditions. Digitalis increases oxygen consumption in the normal, nonfailing ventricle. In the failing myocardium, however, the net effect of digitalis is to decrease ventricular size and reduce wall tension—changes that decrease myocardial oxygen consumption. Moreover, increased sympathetic tone often accompanies heart failure, so that withdrawal of sympathetic tone, coupled with the direct vagal effects of digitalis, may lower heart rate and further decrease myocardial oxygen consumption.

Digitalis produces electrophysiologic effects in myocardial tissues by direct actions on the heart and indirect actions that are mediated by the parasympathetic nervous system.[3] A major, clinically important antiarrhythmic action of digitalis is to prolong AV nodal refractoriness and conduction time. Digitalis also shortens atrial and ventricular refractoriness and generally depresses normal automaticity in Purkinje fibers but may produce abnormal forms of automaticity.

Digitalis has actions on the central nervous sytem and autonomic nervous system. Through direct vascular and sympathetic neural actions, digitalis produces vasoconstriction; but usually in patients treated with digitalis for heart failure, the increased cardiac output and reflex vasodilatation outweigh direct effects of vasoconstriction.

CLINICAL USES (Tables 10-1 and 10-2)

The positive inotropic effects of digitalis are utilized to increase contractility of the heart in congestive heart failure and states of low cardiac output. Clinical experience suggests that some forms of congestive heart failure respond differently to digitalis. For instance, when heart failure is caused by pressure overload, such as heart failure secondary to hypertension, or volume overload, such as heart

Table 10-1. Digitalis preparations for intravenous use

Agent	Initial dose	Subsequent dosage	Onset of action	Peak effect	Elimination half-life $T_{1/2}$
Ouabain (G-Strophanthin)	0.25-0.5 mg	0.1 mg every 30-60 min for total dose ≤ 1 mg/24 hr	5 min	30-60 min	21 hr
Lanatoside C (Cedilanid)	0.8-1.0 mg	0.4 mg every 2-4 hr for total dose ≤ 2 mg/24 hr	5-10 min	30-120 min	
Digoxin (Lanoxin)	0.5-1.0 mg	0.25 mg every 2-4 hr for total dose ≤ 1.5 mg/24 hr	10-15 min	30 min-4 hr	36 hr

Table 10-2. Digitalis preparations for oral use

Agent	Loading dose in 24 hr	Maintenance dose in 24 hr	Elimination half-life ($T_{1/2}$)	Principal route of elimination	Therapeutic serum levels
Digitoxin	0.7-1.2 mg	0.05-0.15 mg	4-5 days	Enterohepatic	14-24 ng/ml
Digoxin	1.0-1.5 mg	0.125-0.5 mg	36 hr	Renal	0.7-2.0 ng/ml

failure secondary to mitral regurgitation, inotropic effects appear to be more evident than those of heart failure caused by loss of myocardial tissue, as in chronic atherosclerotic heart disease. The positive inotropic effects of digitalis may aggravate hypertrophic cardiopmyopathy with obstruction by producing an increase in left ventricular outflow obstruction.

As an antiarrhythmic agent, digitalis is the drug of choice and is often the sole agent required to treat and prevent recurrences of PSVT and to control ventricular rate in atrial fibrillation or atrial flutter.

PRECAUTIONS

1. Each digitalis preparation has unique pharmacokinetics as outlined in Table 10-1. Therefore the route of administration, loading dose, and maintenance dosage must be determined for the individual patient and clinical situation.
2. Loading doses of digitalis are often not required for treatment of mild heart failure, since smaller amounts of the drug will produce a positive inotropic effect in an incremental manner.
3. Digoxin is excreted primarily by the kidneys, so the dosage must be adjusted during renal insufficiency.
4. Digitoxin is metabolized primarily by the liver, so the dosage must be adjusted in patients who have liver dysfunction.
5. Electrolyte disorders, especially hypokalemia, sensitize the myocardium to development of digitalis toxicity.
6. Thyroid status. Patients who have hyperthyroidism require large doses of digitalis to achieve clinical effects, such as a decrease in the ventricular rate during atrial fibrillation, and frequently require combined therapy with beta-adrenergic receptor blockers. Patients who have hypothyroid-

ism may require less than average doses of digitalis to achieve clinical response.

7. Concomitant medication. Quinidine, when added to digoxin and possibly digitoxin, causes a rise in serum digitalis levels.
8. Pulmonary disease. Arrhythmias in the setting of pulmonary disease are often difficult to control, and patients may exhibit increased sensitivity to development of digitalis toxicity.
9. Serum digitalis levels are often used to evaluate the presence of digitalis toxicity; however, efficacy of digitalis therapy is best guided by the clinical judgment that desired effects have been achieved without toxicity.
10. Electrocardiographic effects of digitalis on the ST segment and QT interval should not be confused with ECG manifestations of digitalis toxicity (Fig. 10-4).
11. The toxic manifestations of digitalis therapy, listed in Table 10-3, must be correctly identified.

Table 10-3. Digitalis intoxication

Cardiac	Neurologic	Gastrointestinal	Other
Changes in rhythm (effects on cardiac automaticity and conduction)	Mental depression and personality changes	Anorexia	Gynecomastia
Ventricular premature contractions, coupled rhythm (bigeminy)	Abnormal visual sensations	Nausea	Allergic manifestations such as skin rash
Ventricular tachycardia: precursor of ventricular fibrillation; may be mechanism of sudden death in digitalis intoxication	Color (especially brown, yellow, and green)	Vomiting	
Nonparoxysmal AV junctional tachycardia with or without AV block	Scotoma	Diarrhea	
Atrial tachycardia with or without block: most frequently seen in patients with associated potassium deficiency caused by concurrent use of thiazide diuretics	Blurred or dimmed vision		
Virtually *any* arrhythmia may be produced by digitalis excess	Photophobia		
Effect on conduction system	Cerebral excitation manifested as headache, vertigo, increased irritability, convulsions		
Prolonged PR interval	Peripheral neuritis		
Slow heart rates including sinus bradycardia and first-, second- (type I Wenckebach), and third-degree AV block	Generalized muscular weakness		
Cardiac failure			

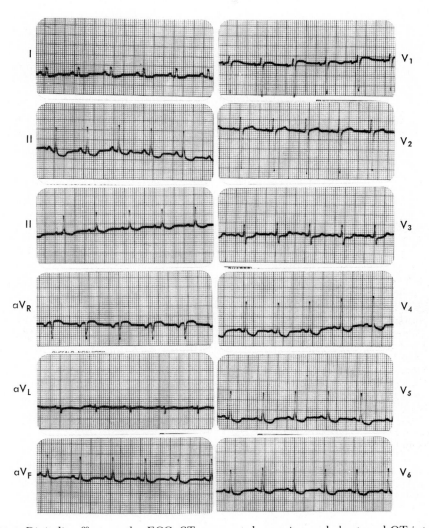

Fig. 10-4. Digitalis effect on the ECG. ST segment depression and shortened QT interval commonly occur with digitalization. This event should not be equated with digitalis intoxication. ST segment depression is present in leads I, II, III, aVF_F and V_3 to V_6. Note characteristic "sagging" of ST depression.

Dopamine (Intropin)

Dopamine, an endogenous catecholamine, is the immediate precursor in the synthesis of norepinephrine. The cardiovascular effects of dopamine result from actions mediated through dopamine-specific receptors and alpha-adrenergic and beta-adrenergic receptors.[4]

ACTIONS

1. The predominant cardiovascular effects of dopamine depend on the dosage administered.
2. At a dosage of less than 7 μg/kg/minute dopamine-specific and beta-adrenergic effects predominate. These effects include an increase in myocardial contractility, cardiac output, and renal blood flow but little or no peripheral vasoconstriction.
3. At a dosage greater than 7 μg/kg/minute alpha-adrenergic effects predominate, leading to peripheral vasoconstriction and an increase in mean arterial pressure.
4. Additional dopamine-specific effects include dilatation of mesenteric and renal vessels that results in an increased blood flow to these organs.

CLINICAL USES

1. The unique hemodynamic effects of dopamine make it an important agent to treat various forms of shock because it directly increases cardiac output and increases renal blood flow. Other catecholamines or inotropic agents do not exert this combination of effects.
2. Dopamine may be employed to treat cardiogenic, septic, or traumatic shock, and its use in these situations improves hemodynamics and short-term survival more than treatment with other catecholamines.
3. Low-dosage (0.5 to 2.0 μg/kg/minute) dopamine is used to treat chronic congestive heart failure that has been refractory to treatment with diuretics and digitalis. Such therapy, of course, is temporary and used only until more definitive long-term treatment can be formulated.

ADMINISTRATION

1. Dopamine is administered intravenously, preferably through a central venous line, since tissue necrosis may occur if there is local extravasation.
2. The dose is best administered by infusion pump to ensure precision.
3. Usual dosage is 0.5 to 20 μg/kg/minute although up to 50 μg/kg/minute is occasionally required.
4. The dose is titrated upward, beginning at 2 to 5 μg/kg/minute, until desired effects are achieved.

CONTRAINDICATIONS AND PRECAUTIONS

1. As with all inotropic agents, dopamine should be administered only after central blood volume and cardiac filling pressures are adequate.
2. Dopamine is contraindicated in the presence of uncontrolled arrhythmia.
3. Dopamine is contraindicated in the presence of pheochromocytoma.

4. Effects of dopamine may be increased in the presence of monoamine oxidase inhibitors, so dosage of dopamine must be reduced.

ADVERSE SIDE EFFECTS AND TOXICITY

1. Most serious adverse side effect of dopamine is the genesis or exacerbation of arrhythmia.
2. Dopamine, especially in a higher dosage may increase myocardial oxygen demands and cause further myocardial ischemia in the presence of coronary artery disease.
3. Occasionally, vasodilator effects of dopamine may produce hypotension.
4. Other side effects of dopamine include nausea, vomiting, and headache.

Dobutamine (Dobutrex)

Dobutamine is a synthetic sympathomimetic amine designed to achieve positive inotropic effects without the chronotropic and peripheral vascular effects of other sympathomimetic agents.[5]

ACTIONS

1. Dobutamine, by direct beta-adrenergic agonist effects, increases myocardial contractility and cardiac output.
2. At equivalent dosages dobutamine produces greater increase in cardiac output, less increase in heart rate, less increase in peripheral vascular resistance, and less cardiac arrhythmia than dopamine.[6]
3. These differences in actions are even more pronounced when dobutamine is compared with norepinephrine or isoproterenol.
4. Despite minimal vasodilator effects, dopamine increases peripheral and renal blood flow as a result of increased cardiac output.

CLINICAL USES

1. Dobutamine is the preferred agent for acute treatment of severe heart failure by various causes.
2. Dobutamine is useful in shock states due to direct myocardial decompensation.
3. When shock is due to vascular collapse and marked vasodilatation, as in anaphylactic shock, the absence of vasoconstrictor effects argues against the use of dobutamine.

ADMINISTRATION

1. Dobutamine is effective only as an intravenous preparation.
2. The usual dosage is 2.5 to 10.0 μg/kg/minute, but up to 40 μg/kg/minute may rarely be needed to achieve desired effects.

SIDE EFFECTS AND TOXICITY

1. Dobutamine may increase heart rate, blood pressure, and arrhythmia development, so constant monitoring of these parameters (and prompt dosage reductions if they occur) is mandatory.
2. Occasionally, nausea, headache, angina pectoris, and dyspnea may occur.

Potassium

Potassium is a major intracellular cation found principally in muscle, including cardiac tissue. The majority of total body potassium is located within the cells, and intracellular concentration is approximately 30 times the extracellular concentration. Despite this, extracellular or serum potassium concentration usually correlates well with total body potassium in stable, steady-state conditions. Renal function provides the major regulation of body potassium. Certain metabolic diseases, kidney diseases, diarrhea, vomiting, diuretic therapy, or infusions of potassium-free fluids that increase extracellular fluid volume all may reduce serum levels of potassium. Elevated serum levels of potassium are due to acidosis, renal failure, massive tissue necrosis, major catabolic states, and inadvertent administration of potassium.

ACTIONS

Potassium plays a major role in the maintenance of normal cellular excitability and conduction.[7] Hypokalemia prolongs recovery of excitability, manifested as a prolonged QU interval on the ECG, and slows AV and intraventricular conduction time. PVCs and disorders of AV conduction may occur. Hyperkalemia increases the rate of repolarization (shortened QT interval on the ECG) and at progressively higher levels initially increases and then decreases excitability and conduction velocity. Therefore potassium administration may initially facilitate conduction but later produce AV conduction delay and slow intraventricular conduction.

Factors other than potassium's serum concentration influence its cardiac effects. Slow increase of potassium depresses automaticity and leads to asystole, whereas rapid increases of potassium may transiently increase automaticity and lead to ventricular ectopy and fibrillation. Associated electrolyte and acid-base disturbances are important, since acidosis and hyponatremia augment the changes produced by hyperkalemia. Hypokalemia is synergistic with digitalis in producing arrhythmias. Elevated calcium concentration mitigates the effects of hyperkalemia, whereas reduced calcium concentration enhances them. Conversely, reduced calcium mitigates the effects of hypokalemia, and elevated calcium concentration enhances them.

CLINICAL USES AND ADMINISTRATION

Maintenance of potassium balance during diuretic and digitalis therapy involves the use of potassium salts and dietary adjustments. For treatment of severe potassium deficiency or arrhythmia secondary to digitalis toxicity, intravenous potassium may be required.

1. For patients receiving digitalis and diuretics, the routine prophylactic administration of 30 to 60 mEq of potassium chloride is recommended. (10 mEq KCl = 750 mg KCl).
2. Since potassium loss in the urine parallels to some degree sodium loss, the restriction of dietary sodium will help mitigate potassium loss.
3. Potassium chloride, which also replenishes chloride ions lost during diuresis and sodium chloride restriction, is the preferred salt for oral administration.

4. Potassium supplements are also available in some salt substitutes and foods such as bananas and citrus fruits.
5. Intravenous potassium is administered at a dosage of 30 to 60 mEq KCl in 500 to 1000 ml D5W and at a rate no more than 30 to 40 mEq/hour.

SIDE EFFECTS AND TOXICITY

1. Rapid potassium infusion produces sinus bradycardia, depression of intrinsic pacemakers, and slowing of AV conduction to the point of block.
2. Adverse symptoms reported with potassium therapy are nausea, vomiting, diarrhea, and abdominal discomfort.
3. Hyperkalemia may occur following administration of potassium, especially in the presence of impaired renal function. Hyperkalemia may manifest in weakness, paresthesias, decreased blood pressure, and electrocardiographic changes. Cardiac arrhythmias ranging from heart block to cardiac arrest caused by ventricular fibrillation or ventricular asystole may occur.
4. Electrocardiographic manifestations of hyperkalemia include a peaked, narrowed T wave and shortened QT interval. As toxicity increases, the QRS complex widens, the PR interval lengthens, and P wave may diminish in size or disappear.
5. ECG manifestations of hypokalemia are decreased T wave amplitude, depression of the ST segment, appearance of prominent U waves, and prolonged QU interval. Symptoms of hypokalemia include muscular weakness, lassitude, and emotional lability.

PRECAUTIONS

In the presence of potassium depletion the myocardium is sensitive to sudden increases in potassium concentration, so appropriate precautions should be taken.
1. Potassium administration to control arrhythmias in the presence of normal serum potassium concentrations may lead to potassium excess and intoxication.
2. Intravenous infusion of potassium chloride may cause burning or pain at the infusion site.
3. In the presence of known or expected cardiac toxicity of potassium, electrocardiographic monitoring is mandatory.

CONTRAINDICATIONS

1. The presence of second-degree AV block is generally a contraindication to the use of potassium. However, in digitalis-induced atrial tachycardia with AV block, potassium administration may slow the atrial rate and restore sinus rhythm without worsening the AV block.
2. Potassium is contraindicated in patients who have severe renal impairment, untreated Addison's disease, acute dehydration, heat cramps, acidosis, and preexisting hyperkalemia of any cause.

Calcium

Calcium is a major body cation of prime importance in bone metabolism, muscle contraction, and many cellular membrane actions. Over 90% of the body stores of calcium are in bone structures, so changes in serum calcium concentration often do not reflect changes in total body calcium. Nevertheless, changes in serum calcium concentration may have profound electrical and mechanical effects on the heart.

ACTIONS

1. Calcium flow into the myocardial cell during systole accounts for a portion of phase II, or plateau phase, of the cardiac action potential. This slow inward calcium current plays an important physiologic role in impulse formation and conduction in SA nodal and AV nodal cells and in other cells under pathologic conditions.[8]
2. Calcium directly increases myocardial contractility by interacting with the myofibrillar proteins in the coupling of excitation with muscle contraction.
3. Hypercalcemia shortens the plateau phase of the action potential, which is reflected as a shortened QT interval on the ECG, primarily by a shortening of the ST segment.
4. Hypocalcemia produces opposite effects and prolongs the interval from Q wave to onset of T wave with a flattening and prolongation of the ST segment.
5. Calcium excess may result in sinus bradycardia, AV conduction block, and ectopic arrhythmias. These are usually seen only when digitalis is also present.

CLINICAL USES

In cardiovascular therapy calcium administration is usually employed in the setting of cardiac arrest. If ventricular fibrillation has not responded to one or more electrical countershocks, initial CPR measures have restored circulation and ventilation, and epinephrine infusion has not been effective, intravenous calcium is indicated. A dose of 3 to 5 ml of 10% calcium chloride (3.4 to 6.8 mEq calcium) is employed. Stated but undocumented effects of calcium in this setting are to increase myocardial tone, convert fine fibrillation to coarse fibrillation, and enhance the success of electrical countershock.

PREPARATIONS AND PRECAUTIONS

1. Calcium chloride is usually given IV in a concentration of 5% to 10%. Injection rate should be slow (not to exceed 1 to 2 ml/minute). This drug is irritating to tissue and causes painful sloughing if extravasation occurs during intravenous therapy.
2. Calcium gluconate can be given intramuscularly or intravenously. Although lower in ionized calcium content than calcium chloride, calcium gluconate is less irritating to subcutaneous tissue. For parenteral use it is administered intravenously as a 10% solution (5 to 30 ml).
3. Calcium injection may produce a moderate fall in blood pressure caused by peripheral vasodilatation.

Sodium bicarbonate

Sodium bicarbonate is a major extracellular buffer that acts to provide physiologic control of acid-base balance. Bicarbonate metabolism is regulated primarily by the kidney; the bicarbonate system is one of many acid-base buffer systems.

CLINICAL USES

1. Sodium bicarbonate is employed to correct metabolic acidosis, especially lactic acidosis, and is specifically indicated to treat acidosis caused by cardiogenic shock or ventricular fibrillation.
2. Sodium bicarbonate is administered at a dosage of 1 mEq/kg every 10 minutes during cardiopulmonary resuscitation until circulation is restored. When possible, administration should be guided by repeated measurements of arterial blood pH.

PRECAUTIONS

1. Treatment of acidosis with sodium bicarbonate does not alter the underlying defect that caused the acidosis, such as cardiogenic shock.
2. Overdosage of sodium bicarbonate will produce a metabolic alkalosis.
3. The large sodium load administered with sodium bicarbonate may worsen preexisting congestive heart failure.

Atropine

Atropine blocks activity in portions of the parasympathetic nervous system by inhibiting the action of acetylcholine. In the heart, atropine principally increases the rate of automatic discharge of the SA node and shortens the refractory period and conduction time of the AV node. These effects lead to an increase in the ventricular rate during sinus mechanisms or many supraventricular tachycardias. A lesser effect, particularly in the atria, may be to increase contractility.

CLINICAL USES AND DOSAGE

1. Atropine is indicated to block unwanted effects of vagal tone such as symptomatic sinus bradycardia, sinus bradycardia associated with increased ventricular ectopy during acute myocardial infarction, or AV block caused by increased vagal tone.
2. Atropine is administered intravenously, usually in an initial dose of 0.5 to 0.8 mg by rapid injection. Additional increments of 0.3 to 0.5 mg are administered until desired effects are achieved, unwanted side effects occur, or a total dose of 2.0 to 2.5 mg is reached.
3. Smaller doses or slower administration of atropine may evoke a vagomimetic effect that produces SA node slowing and AV conduction delay.
4. Intramuscular atropine may be effective, but since absorption is slow compared to intravenous doses, drug concentrations in the serum and at the site of action may be low; thus a larger dosage, usually twice the intravenous dosage, is required.

5. Cardiac effects of intravenous atropine persist for about 2 hours, and systemic effects may last for up to 24 hours; so chronic therapy with intravenous atropine is usually not indicated because of its cumulative systemic effects.

SIDE EFFECTS AND TOXICITY

1. Adverse side effects of atropine are usually caused by effects of acetylcholine inhibition in extracardiac organs and are related to the total dosage of atropine.
2. Usual side effects are urinary retention, dryness of the skin, mucous membranes, and bronchial secretions, pupillary dilatation, acute glaucoma, mental confusion, and delirium.
3. Atropine-induced SA node acceleration during acute myocardial infarction may precipitate further ischemia, and atropine may have direct effects on ventricular myocardium. Either or both factors may lead to an emergence of ventricular arrhythmia and ventricular fibrillation following atropine administration during acute myocardial infarction.

Edrophonium (Tensilon)

Edrophonium is a cholinergic drug that acts by inhibiting the action of acetylcholinesterase, the enzyme that degrades acetylcholine. Cardiac effects of edrophonium are similar to those produced by enhanced vagal tone. Edrophonium decreases SA nodal discharge rate, increases refractoriness and conduction time of AV node, and decreases myocardial contractility.

CLINICAL USES AND DOSAGE

1. Edrophonium is primarily used to terminate episodes of PSVT when other vagal maneuvers, such as carotid sinus massage or Valsalva maneuver, are ineffective.
2. Edrophonium is administered as a 5- or 10-mg intravenous bolus. A test dose of 3 to 5 mg may be given initially.
3. Effects of edrophonium begin within 30 to 60 seconds after administration and may last as long as 10 minutes.
4. A continuous infusion of 0.25 to 2.0 mg/minute may be employed if longer lasting effects are desired.

SIDE EFFECTS AND TOXICITY

1. Enhanced vagal tone may aggravate preexisting conditions of intestinal obstruction, bronchial asthma, or urinary obstruction; edrophonium should be avoided in these circumstances.
2. Side effects relate mostly to results of vagal overactivity and may include nausea, perspiration, salivation, bronchial spasm, slow pulse, and hypotension.
3. To counteract any potential life-threatening complications, atropine should be immediately available when edrophonium is employed.

Adrenergic pharmacology

Adrenergic pharmacology includes the study of the sympathetic nervous system with its principal neurotransmitter, norepinephrine; the naturally occurring catecholamines, epinephrine and norepinephrine, secreted by the adrenal medulla; and the effects of drugs that stimulate (agonist) or block (antagonist) the sympathetic receptors.

The effects of neurotransmitters, hormones, or drugs on a specific end organ are mediated by the interaction of the agent with specific receptors on the end organ membrane. Adrenergic receptors have been classified into two major subgroups, alpha and beta, based on the observation by Ahlquist of differences in the physiologic actions and relative potency of effects of different catecholamines.[9]

For the cardiovascular system, alpha receptors are located in the smooth muscle of arterioles, where stimulation results in arteriolar constriction. Beta receptors are located in the heart, arterioles (primarily skeletal muscle arterioles), and lungs. Stimulation of beta receptors increases heart rate and contractility, decreases AV nodal conduction time and refractoriness, dilates arterioles of skeletal muscle beds, and dilates bronchioles.

SUBCLASSIFICATION OF BETA-ADRENERGIC RECEPTORS

The response of beta-adrenergic stimulation or inhibition may be further subclassified into $beta_1$ and $beta_2$ action.[10] This division is not complete, since there is overlap in activity of drugs on $beta_1$ and $beta_2$ receptors. However, differences in the relative potency of drugs to stimulate (agonist activity) or inhibit (antagonist activity) either beta receptor subtype allow more selective use of drugs.

$Beta_1$ receptors are located in the heart, where stimulation increases heart rate and contractility and shortens AV nodal conduction time and refractoriness. $Beta_2$ receptors are located in blood vessels and lung, where stimulation dilates arterioles and bronchioles.

SUBCLASSIFICATION OF ALPHA-ADRENERGIC RECEPTORS

The alpha-adrenergic receptors have also been subclassified into $alpha_1$ and $alpha_2$ receptors.[11] Although subpopulations of beta receptors appear to be tissue specific in that $beta_1$ receptors are present in the heart and $beta_2$ receptors in arterioles and lung, the situation is different for alpha receptors whose subclassification is not the same as that of beta receptors.

As depicted in Fig. 10-5, the adrenergic neural terminal is composed of the presynaptic sympathetic neuron, the synaptic cleft, and the postsynaptic effector cell. Alpha- and beta-adrenergic receptors are located on the membrane of the effector cell and the sympathetic neuron. Alpha receptors, located on the effector cell are termed *postsynaptic receptors*, or *$alpha_1$ receptors*. Receptors on the nerve terminal are *presynaptic*, or *$alpha_2$ receptors*.

Stimulation of the $alpha_1$ receptor mimics the effects of norepinephrine on the effector cell, whereas inhibition of the $alpha_1$ receptor antagonizes these

PRESYNAPTIC   POSTSYNAPTIC

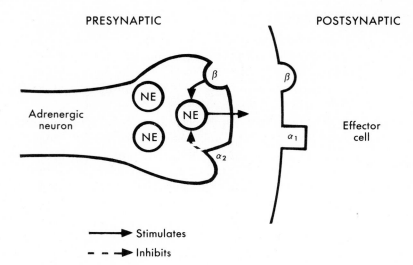

Fig. 10-5. Diagram of the adrenergic nerve terminal illustrating alpha₁-, alpha₂-, and beta-adrenergic receptors in presynaptic and postsynaptic positions. The effector cell contains alpha₁- and beta-adrenergic receptors, which interact with norepinephrine to produce end organ effects. The presynaptic alpha₂- and beta-adrenergic receptors interact with norepinephrine to stimulate (beta receptor) or inhibit (alpha₂ receptor) further norepinephrine release.

effects. On the other hand, the alpha₂ receptor serves an autoregulatory function. Stimulation of the alpha₂ receptor inhibits norepinephrine release from the nerve terminal, thus diminishing the effects of norepinephrine on the effector cell, and inhibition of the alpha₂ receptor stimulates release of norepinephrine.

Drugs that are alpha-adrenergic agonists or antagonists may affect alpha₁ or alpha₂ receptors. Furthermore, clinical effects may not be identical to the effects determined in isolated tissue preparations.

ALPHA- AND BETA-ADRENERGIC RECEPTOR-STIMULATING DRUGS
Epinephrine (Adrenalin)

Action. Epinephrine acts directly on beta₁ (cardiac) receptors to increase heart rate and contractility. In the peripheral circulation, epinephrine in lower doses produces beta₂ receptor stimulation that results in vasodilatation of skeletal muscle vessels, and larger doses activate both alpha₁ and alpha₂ adrenergic receptors to elevate peripheral resistance and blood pressure.

Cardiovascular uses

1. Epinephrine is most often employed clinically during cardiac arrest to stimulate cardiac pacemaker activity and increase contractility; it has been said to render the fibrillating heart more responsive to DC electrical shock.
2. Epinephrine is often the drug of choice in the immediate treatment of anaphylaxis.

Administration. The usual dose of epinephrine is 0.5 to 1.0 ml of 1:1000 solution or 5 to 10 ml of 1:10,000 solution administered by intravenous or intracardiac injection.

Side effects

1. Epinephrine may exacerbate ventricular arrhythmia.
2. Disturbing reactions of fear, anxiety, and tension may occur.
3. Epinephrine may precipitate myocardial ischemia because of the inability of coronary blood flow to meet increased myocardial oxygen requirements.
4. Epinephrine may produce headache, tremor, and weakness.
5. Renal blood flow, glomerular filtration rate, and sodium excretion are usually reduced after administration of epinephrine.

Norepinephrine (levarterenol [Levophed])

Actions. Norepinephrine exerts a greater alpha-adrenergic stimulating effect (alpha$_1$ and alpha$_2$) than does epinephrine, but its cardiac (beta$_1$) stimulating effect is approximately equivalent. Norepinephrine increases systolic and diastolic arterial pressure and total peripheral resistance. Cardiac output usually remains unchanged or decreased because of the increased peripheral resistance and slowed heart rate, which results from reflex vagal activation. Coronary blood flow increases whereas renal, cerebral, visceral, and skeletal muscle blood flow diminishes.

Clinical uses. Norepinephrine is used to treat hypotension and shock, but it has largely been replaced in clinical practice by the newer agents, dopamine and dobutamine. Norepinephrine may be especially useful when hypotensive states are accompanied by low peripheral vascular resistance and normal or slightly elevated cardiac output.

Administration. Dosage requirements vary widely and require careful titration. The usual dosage ranges from 2 to 20 μg/minute administered by intravenous infusion. A solution containing 4 to 8 mg of norepinephrine per 1000 ml of D5W is administered with an infusion pump.

Side effects

1. Anxiety, respiratory difficulty, and transient headache may result.
2. Overdosage may cause severe hypertension with headache, photophobia, angina, intensive sweating, and vomiting.
3. Cardiac arrhythmias may be produced or exacerbated.

Precautions

1. Blood pressure should be monitored frequently. The optimum method is by intraarterial pressure recording.
2. Norepinephrine is best administered by infusion into a large, central vein. If peripheral vein administration is employed, the site of administration should be observed frequently. Extravasation of drug at the infusion site may cause tissue sloughing as a result of local vasoconstriction. Local phentolamine (Regitine) infiltration (10 mg) may prevent tissue loss should extravasation occur.

BETA-ADRENERGIC RECEPTOR-STIMULATING DRUGS
Isoproterenol (Isuprel)

Actions. Isoproterenol has nearly exclusive beta-adrenergic receptor-stimulating activity and acts on beta$_2$ (smooth muscle, bronchioles) and beta$_1$ (heart) receptors. Isoproterenol relaxes smooth muscle of bronchi, skeletal muscle vasculature, and alimentary tract. In the heart, isoproterenol increases heart rate and contractility. Isoproterenol lowers peripheral vascular resistance and decreases diastolic arterial pressure. The net hemodynamic effect is to elevate cardiac output and systolic pressure and to decrease mean and diastolic arterial pressure. Furthermore, myocardial oxygen consumption rises with isoproterenol administration. In conditions of hypovolemia, isoproterenol may also decrease systolic pressure.

Cardiovascular uses

1. Isoproterenol is most often used to enhance pacemaker activity and improve AV conduction during episodes of sinus bradycardia or AV block.
2. In certain cardiogenic shock states, isoproterenol may be used to increase cardiac output and decrease peripheral vasoconstriction. Isoproterenol is not indicated to treat cardiogenic shock caused by acute myocardial infarction.
3. In bronchospastic lung disease isoproterenol may be used to produce bronchodilatation but is nearly always employed as a local inhalant for this purpose.

Administration. In emergency situations, isoproterenol is usually administered by intravenous injection of 0.02 to 0.06 mg. Intravenous infusions of 0.5 to 4.0 μg/minute are titrated to achieve the clinical response.

Side effects

1. Isoproterenol increases myocardial oxygen consumption and may precipitate myocardial ischemia.
2. Cardiac arrhythmias including sinus tachycardia, premature ventricular complexes, ventricular tachycardia, or ventricular fibrillation may result.
3. In the presence of hypovolemia, the vasodilating effects of isoproterenol may produce hypotension.
4. Headache, flushing of the skin, angina, nausea, tremor, dizziness, weakness, and sweating may result.

ALPHA-ADRENERGIC RECEPTOR-STIMULATING DRUGS
Phenylephrine (Neo-synephrine) and methoxamine (Vasoxyl)

Actions. Phenylephrine and methoxamine are noncatecholamine drugs that have alpha$_1$-adrenergic receptor-stimulating properties. They vasoconstrict renal, splanchnic, cutaneous, and muscular vascular beds but generally do not change or only slightly increase coronary blood flow. The increased mean arterial pressure reflexly increases vagal tone, which decreases the heart rate. Moreover, direct alpha-adrenergic receptor-stimulating effects on the heart may slow the SA node discharge rate to a slight degree.

Clinical uses

1. Phenylephrine and methoxamine are most commonly employed to treat PSVT. The hypertensive response increases vagal tone and may terminate the arrhythmia.
2. Hypotension caused by peripheral vasodilatation, such as occurs with ganglionic blocking agents or spinal anesthesia, may be reversed by phenylephrine or methoxamine.
3. These agents are not indicated in the treatment of cardiogenic shock.

Administration. The doses of phenylephrine and methoxamine should be titrated by clinical response. Intravenous dosing is usually recommended.

1. Phenylephrine is administered as 0.5 to 1.0 mg intravenous or 5 to 10 mg intramuscular following an initial test dose of 0.1 mg.
2. Methoxamine is administered as 5 to 10 mg intravenous or 10 to 20 mg intramuscular.

Side effects. Excessive dosage may produce headache, excessive hypertension, marked bradycardia, and vomiting.

Precautions

1. To reduce the risk of excessive hypertension, systolic blood pressure should be continuously monitored during drug administration.
2. These agents should not be administered to hypertensive patients for treatment of PSVT.
3. In most cases safer and more effective methods for termination of PSVT now exist.

ALPHA-ADRENERGIC BLOCKING AGENTS

The alpha-adrenergic blocking agents directly and selectively block the stimulation of alpha-adrenergic receptors. Effects are most prominent in peripheral vascular beds where vasoconstrictor responses are inhibited and vasodilatation results. Alpha-adrenergic blocking agents may accelerate heart rate either by reflex effects from peripheral vasodilatation or direct effects resulting from cardiac alpha$_2$ receptor inhibition, which increases norepinephrine release. The alpha-adrenergic blocking agents discussed here are phenoxybenzamine (Dibenzyline) and phentolamine (Regitine). Prazosin (Minipress), the most commonly used and perhaps the most potent oral alpha-adrenergic blocker, is discussed in the section on vasodilators. Phenoxybenzamine and prazosin inhibit alpha$_1$ receptors, and phentolamine inhibits both alpha$_1$ and alpha$_2$ receptors.

Clinical uses

1. Alpha-adrenergic blocking agents are indicated to inhibit excessive alpha-adrenergic stimulation that occurs either from an endogenous source, as during treatment of pheochromocytoma, or from an exogenous source, as during administration of catecholamines to treat shock.
2. Alpha-adrenergic blockers also have been employed as direct vasodilators to reverse the peripheral vasoconstriction that accompanies low cardiac output states, systemic hypertension, and peripheral vascular insufficiency.

Administration. Phenoxybenzamine, although poorly absorbed, is effective orally and is usually administered at a dosage of 20 to 200 mg/day. Phenoxybenzamine and phentolamine may be used intravenously: phenoxybenzamine in a dosage of 1.0 mg/, infused over 1 hour in a glucose or saline solution; phentolamine in titrated doses of 5 mg.

Side effects and toxicity

1. As with all vasodilators, blood pressure may fall precipitously. Maintenance of adequate volume status minimizes part of this problem.
2. Other side effects of alpha-adrenergic blockers include acceleration of

heart rate, miosis (constriction of pupil), nasal stuffiness, inhibition of ejaculation, sedation, nausea, and vomiting.

3. Phentolamine has direct gastrointestinal actions that may cause abdominal pain and exacerbate peptic ulcer disease.

BETA-ADRENERGIC BLOCKING AGENTS

Beta-adrenergic blocking agents selectively inhibit the inotropic and chronotropic actions produced by beta-adrenergic stimulation. A variety of compounds are available that differ in having cardioselective activity, intrinsic agonist activity, or membrane-stabilizing effects.[12] Beta-adrenergic blocking agents also affect cardiovascular function by inhibiting renin release by the renin-angiotensin system. This effect contributes to the antihypertensive effects of beta-adrenergic blocker therapy. Finally, the beta-adrenergic blocking agents may be lipid soluble (lipophilic) or water soluble (hydrophilic). The potential importance of this property derives from the suggestion that hydrophilic compounds are less able than lipophilic compounds to cross the blood-brain barrier and enter the brain. Therefore, hydrophilic agents may have fewer central nervous system side effects than lipophilic agents. Propranolol is the most widely studied beta-adrenergic blocking agent and serves as the prototype.

The cardioselective effects of beta-adrenergic blockade refer to the selective inhibition of beta$_1$ receptors, which produces a decrease of heart rate, contractility, myocardial oxygen demands, and cardiac output. The automatic discharge rate of the SA node is decreased and the refractory period and conduction time of the AV node is prolonged. The cardiac manifestations of beta-adrenergic blockade depend on the underlying level of beta-adrenergic tone, so in normal patients, resting heart rate and cardiac output change slightly, but the response to exercise is markedly blunted.

Other properties peculiar to certain beta-adrenergic blockers include intrinsic agonist activity and membrane-stabilizing effects or quinidine-like activity. Intrinsic agonist activity refers to a modest degree of beta-adrenergic *stimulation* produced by some agents such as oxprenolol. Quinidine-like activity, or membrane-stabilizing effects, refers to the local anesthetic effects seen, for example, with propranolol, but only at doses well above those usually employed in cardiovascular therapy.

Clinical uses (Table 10-4). Beta-adrenergic blocking agents are used most often in the treatment of angina pectoris, cardiac arrhythmias, and systemic hypertension. Additional uses include treatment of hypertrophic cardiomyopathy, cardiovascular manifestations of hyperthyroidism, and anxiety states.

1. *Angina pectoris.* The goal in treatment is to decrease myocardial oxygen demands. This is accomplished primarily by lowering heart rate, but a decrease in myocardial contractility also plays a role. Clinical effects appear additive to those of nitrates. The usual goal is to lower the resting heart rate to 50 to 60 beats/minute and blunt the heart rate response to exercise.

2. *Arrhythmias.* Usual indications are to control the ventricular response to atrial flutter or fibrillation and to terminate and prevent recurrences of PSVT. Beta blockers are useful in treating selected ventricular arrhythmias,

Table 10-4. Clinical features of beta-adrenergic blocking drugs

| Drug | Usual dosage | Properties* | | | |
		Cardio-selective	Intrinsic agonist activity	Membrane-stabilizing effects	Hydrophilic
Propranolol (Inderal)	Oral: 40-480 mg/day in 2-4 doses Intravenous: up to 0.10-0.15 mg/kg given as 1-mg increments at 3- to 5-minute intervals	−	−	+	−
Metoprolol (Lopressor)	Oral: 50-100 mg twice a day	+	−	−	+
Nadolol (Corgard)	Oral: 40-160 mg once a day	−	−	−	+
Atenolol (Tenormin)	Oral: 50-100 mg once a day	+	−	−	+
Timolol (Blocadren)	Oral: 10-20 mg twice a day	−	−	−	+

*+, Present; −, absent.

such as some arrhythmias induced by exercise, and in treating some of the arrhythmias caused by digitalis toxicity.
3. One potential use suggested for certain beta-adrenergic blockers is in prevention of sudden cardiac death following myocardial infarction. Such a response has been shown with practolol[13] (withdrawn from clinical use because of side effects), alprenolol[14] (investigational in the United States), timolol[15] (recently approved for this indication), metoprolol[16] (Lopressor), and propranolol[17] (Inderal).

Side effects

1. Most prominent adverse side effects of beta-adrenergic blocking therapy are decreased myocardial contractility, heart failure, sinus bradycardia, asystole, AV block, bronchospasm, fatigue, insomnia, nightmares, and hypoglycemia in diabetics.
2. Propranolol rebound refers to a syndrome of an apparent increased sensitivity to catecholamines that follows discontinuation of beta-adrenergic blocking drugs. In patients who have ischemic heart disease, angina pectoris, myocardial infarction, and arrhythmias, it may occur following abrupt cessation of beta-adrenergic blocker therapy. It is unclear whether slowly decreasing the dosage of beta blocker prior to discontinuation would completely obviate this rebound syndrome.

Anticoagulants

Anticoagulants inhibit the action or formation of one or more of the clotting factors and are used to prevent and treat a variety of thromboembolic disorders. Heparin and warfarin sodium (Coumadin) are the most widely used anticoagulants.

Precise indications for anticoagulation in many clinical situations are unclear. For example, uncontrolled studies have suggested that anticoagulant therapy is beneficial during acute myocardial infarction, but data from well controlled studies have failed to show an improvement in mortality with use of anticoagulants.

It is clear, however, that anticoagulation reduces the incidence of venous thromboembolism especially in the presence of heart failure. Low-dose, subcutaneous heparin (10,000 units/day), which does not prolong clotting times, appears to decrease the incidence of venous thromboembolism and is currently recommended for most patients during the initial days of infarction when bed rest is prescribed.

Anticoagulant therapy in doses sufficient to significantly affect clotting factors is generally recommended for (1) demonstrated thromboembolism, either venous or arterial, (2) prevention of thrombosis and thromboembolic events in some patients after prosthetic valve surgery or prior to electrical cardioversion of atrial fibrillation, and (3) when chronic atrial fibrillation is accompanied by mitral valve disease or congestive heart failure.

HEPARIN

Heparin is a naturally occurring substance, but its physiologic role has not been completely elucidated. In pharmacologic doses, heparin predominantly affects blood coagulation and blood lipids. Heparin inhibits thrombin and fibrin formation by complex mechanisms and produces prolongation of clotting time, prothrombin time, and thrombin time. Heparin also inhibits platelet aggregation induced by thrombin. Heparin clears plasma lipids by activating lipoprotein lipase, although the clinical significance of this action is not fully established.

Clinical uses
1. Heparin is administered intravenously or subcutaneously. Oral administration is ineffective, and intramuscular administration is usually not recommended because it may produce local hemorrhage.
2. Anticoagulant doses of heparin are determined by clotting time or activated partial thromboplastin time, either of which is maintained at 1½ to 2½ times the control values. Continuous infusion of heparin is associated with fewer hemorrhagic side effects than intermittent injection, since with the former a more stable anticoagulant effect is maintained.

Administration. The dosage of heparin varies with the method of administration.
1. Continuous infusion: 20,000 to 40,000 units/day; infusion is begun after a loading dose of 5000 units, and an increase in dosage should be initiated by a loading dose.
2. Intermittent dose: 5000 to 10,000 units every 4 to 6 hours.
3. Low-dose heparin: 5000 units subcutaneously every 12 hours.
4. Heparin disappearance rate is proportional to the dose administered, since larger doses have a longer half-life. Anticoagulant effects of a single intravenous dose of heparin last an average of 3 to 4 hours.
5. Heparin is the preferred anticoagulant in pregnant or lactating women because it does not cross the placenta or appear in maternal milk.

Side effects and toxicity
1. Hemorrhage is the predominant side effect, and heparin is contraindicated in the presence of active bleeding or hemorrhagic tendencies. The occurrence of hemorrhage during heparin therapy should initiate a search for a pathologic bleeding site.

2. Other side effects include thrombocytopenia and, rarely, hypersensitivity or anaphylactic reactions.

3. Long-term heparin therapy has been associated with alopecia, osteoporosis, neuropathy, and priapism.

4. Anticoagulant effects of heparin are reversible by administration of protamine sulfate. Doses of 1.0 to 1.5 mg protamine antagonize each 100 units of heparin, but the dose requirements fall quickly as the last heparin dose increases. In most cases discontinuation of heparin is sufficient therapy to correct anticoagulant effects.

WARFARIN SODIUM (COUMADIN)

Warfarin acts in the liver to inhibit the synthesis of vitamin K–dependent clotting factors, especially prothrombin. Effects take 24 hours or more to occur, and anticoagulant effects of a single dose usually are not complete until at least 48 to 72 hours have elapsed.

Clinical uses and administration

1. When anticoagulation beyond a few days is required, warfarin is the preferred treatment because it is effective orally. Warfarin and heparin are often begun simultaneously, and then heparin is stopped once warfarin is effective.

2. The dosage of warfarin is individually determined based on the results of prothrombin time, which should be stabilized at 1½ to 2½ times control value. Usual dosages range from 2 to 15 mg/day.

3. Currently it is recommended that warfarin be given in a daily dose of 10 to 15 mg until therapeutic prolongation of prothrombin time occurs rather than administering a large initial loading dose.

4. Peak effects on prothrombin time require 36 to 72 hours, and duration of effect is 4 to 5 days.

Precautions

1. Drug and disease interactions are important features of warfarin therapy.

2. Anticoagulant effects of warfarin are enhanced in the presence of hepatic disease, vitamin K deficiency, heart failure, broad-spectrum antibiotics, salicylates, quinidine, anabolic steroids, chloral hydrate, clofibrate, phenylbutazone, thyroxine, indomethacin, tolbutamide, methyldopa, diazoxide, alcohol, allopurinol, and amiodarone, to name a few.

3. Anticoagulant effects are decreased by glucocorticoids, vitamin K, barbiturates, oral contraceptives, antacids, antihistamines, and other agents.

4. Warfarin crosses the placenta and appears in maternal milk, so there is danger of hemorrhage in utero or in nursing infants.

Side effects and toxicity

1. Hemorrhage occurs in 2% to 4% of patients who receive warfarin anticoagulation and may be life threatening. Hemorrhage from nearly any source is possible; cutaneous, oral, gastrointestinal, genitourinary, and central nervous system hemorrhages are the most common. All patients receiving warfarin need frequent monitoring and close surveillance of prothrombin time to detect changes in hepatic function or drug therapy that may affect prothrombin time or influence the metabolism of warfarin.

2. Hemorrhage is treated by reduction or withdrawal of warfarin dose and, if necessary, reversal of anticoagulant effects by intravenous vitamin K or fresh frozen plasma.
3. The existence of a rebound hypercoagulable state after rapid reversal of warfarin is controversial but should argue against the routine use of vitamin K to dissipate anticoagulant effects.

Thrombolytic agents

Anticoagulants prevent formation of new clot but do not dissolve formed thrombi. Thrombolytic agents act directly to lyse formed thrombi and appear to offer therapeutic advantages in certain situations. Two drugs are available: streptokinase, which is derived from enzymes of the streptococcus, and urokinase, a substance found in human urine. Both activate the fibrinolytic system. Urokinase is very expensive, and for the most part its use is limited to patients who are hypersensitive to or show intolerance of streptokinase.

CLINICAL USES

1. Thrombolytic agents are generally employed to treat established pulmonary embolism for which they are superior to heparin by itself in achieving resolution of emboli.
2. An indication for treatment is the presence of a large thromboembolism producing cardiopulmonary compromise, usually when there is significant coexisting cardiopulmonary disease. Treatment must begin within 24 to 36 hours after occurrence.
3. Therapy may also be applied when there is extensive, acute, deep vein thrombosis and a high risk of subsequent embolus.
4. Recently, intracoronary infusion of thrombolytic agents has been used to lyse coronary thrombi within the first hours of myocardial infarction.
5. There is evidence suggesting that streptokinase decreases and limits the extent of myocardial infarction, but this application is still experimental.

ADMINISTRATION

Dosage of each agent is as follows:
1. Streptokinase: loading dose is 250,000 units over 30 minutes followed by 100,000 units/hour.
2. Urokinase: loading dose is 2000 units/pound over 10 minutes followed by 200 units/pound/hour.
3. Therapy with either agent is guided by prolongation of thrombin time.
4. Both agents are effective only if given within 24 to 36 hours of the thromboembolic event.

SIDE EFFECTS AND TOXICITY

Bleeding from thrombolytic therapy is more frequent than with other anticoagulants. Allergic reactions to streptokinase are common.

Drugs affecting platelet function

Both the demonstrated and the hypothesized effects of platelets suggest that these blood elements play an important role in several cardiovascular disorders, including genesis of atherosclerotic plaque, coronary artery thrombosis, coronary spasm, and arterial thromboembolism. Therefore drugs that interfere with platelet function are potentially valuable therapeutic agents. Antiplatelet drugs include aspirin, sulfinpyrazone (Anturane), and dipyridamole (Persantine).

These agents, in part, prolong platelet survival and interfere with metabolism of prostaglandins and thromboxane, agents which affect ability of platelets to clump and initiate thrombosis. Effects on the prostaglandins contained in vascular endothelium may also influence the net result of antiplatelet drugs.

CLINICAL USES

1. Clinical observations and therapeutic trials have suggested that aspirin, sulfinpyrazone, and dipyridamole may have beneficial effects in certain arterial thromboembolic disorders.
2. Sulfinpyrazone may play a role in reducing mortality by sudden death in the first 9 months after myocardial infarction.[18]
3. Aspirin has decreased the incidence of thrombotic stroke in men who have carotid artery disease and is indicated to treat cerebral transient ischemic attacks.[19]
4. At present, other specific indications for antiplatelet agents cannot be made, but the next 5 years promise great advances in understanding the role of platelets and prostaglandins in cardiovascular disorders and should see the emergence of more indications for use of antiplatelet therapy.

Vasodilators
NITRATES

This category includes nitroglycerin and isosorbide dinitrate. Their pharmacologic actions are based on the property of nitrite to relax smooth muscle, especially in vascular beds.

Nitroglycerin

Nitroglycerin produces venodilatation, which decreases venous return to the heart and reduces ventricular filling pressure.[20] Nitroglycerin also produces arteriolar dilatation, but its effects on systemic arterial resistance are less marked than those of other vasodilators. Coronary artery dilatation also is seen after nitroglycerin administration.

Clinical uses
1. Because of its rapid onset of action and its effects of decreasing cardiac oxygen demands and dilating coronary vessels, nitroglycerin is the preferred drug in the treatment of acute episodes of angina pectoris. Sublingual doses of 0.2 to 0.6 mg (usually 0.4 mg) terminate typical anginal episodes.

2. Topical nitroglycerin, usually 1 to 2 inches of 2% nitroglycerin ointment, may be used to prevent angina, and effects last from 4 to 6 hours. Recently, several controlled-release topical nitroglycerin compounds have been introduced (Transderm, Nitrodur). Nitroglycerin blood levels and systemic effects are evident for 24 hours.

3. Controlled-release capsules that contain 2.5, 6.5, or 9 mg of nitroglycerin may be effective in preventing angina; these are administered every 12 hours.

4. Intravenous nitroglycerin provides a method to continually administer a titratable dose of nitroglycerin. It is especially useful in treating unstable angina pectoris. Initial dosage is usually 10 μg/minute, with the dose titrated to achieve desired results.

5. The hemodynamic effects of nitroglycerin produce a decrease in left ventricular filling pressure and little change in systemic vascular resistance. Nitroglycerin preparations thus tend to reduce pulmonary congestion associated with heart failure without major effects on systemic blood pressure.

Isosorbide dinitrate (Sorbitrate, Isordil)

Antianginal and hemodynamic effects of isosorbide dinitrate are similar to those of nitroglycerin, but their duration of action is longer.[20] Controversy has long existed concerning efficacy of oral nitrates because first-pass hepatic metabolism deactivates a large amount of the orally administered dose. However, when given in a sufficient dosage to prevent complete degradation, oral doses have effects similar to those of sublingual doses.

Clinical uses

1. Sublingual isosorbide may be effective in terminating acute episodes of angina, but nitroglycerin is usually the preferred drug.

2. Onset of action of sublingual isosorbide is 2 to 5 minutes, and the duration of action ranges from 1 to 2 hours.

3. Oral isosorbide has a duration of action from 1 to 4 hours.

4. Sustained-release preparations, designed to last 6 to 12 hours, are available but not completely studied.

5. Sublingual or oral isosorbide is generally employed as a prophylactic agent for angina pectoris and maintenance of hemodynamic effects for a longer duration than obtainable with nitroglycerin.

6. Sublingual dosage is 2.5, 5, and 10 mg every 2 to 3 hours; oral dosage is 10 to 40 mg every 3 to 4 hours.

Side effects and toxicity of nitrates

1. Postural hypotension, syncope, dizziness, headaches, nausea, and, rarely, drug rash are seen with nitrate therapy.

2. Abrupt withdrawal of chronic nitrate therapy may precipitate myocardial ischemia.

SODIUM NITROPRUSSIDE (NIPRIDE)

Sodium nitroprusside is a vasodilating agent that acts directly on vascular smooth muscle independent of autonomic innervation. Nitroprusside has an immediate onset and termination of action. Nitroprusside is stated to have a balanced effect, dilating arterioles and venules equivalently, and thus, decreasing both preload and afterload of the heart.[20] In the failing heart afterload reduction increases the cardiac output with no or minimal decrease in mean arterial blood pressure. Heart rate tends to remain unchanged or to increase slightly. Decreased preload, resulting from venodilatation, decreases pulmonary capillary wedge pressure. Beneficial hemodynamic effects are observed when filling pressures and systemic resistance are elevated and cardiac output is depressed, as occurs in the failing myocardium. In normal hearts, however, or when left ventricular filling pressure is normal or low, nitroprusside produces hypotension and tachycardia with little change in cardiac output.

Clinical uses

1. Nitroprusside is employed in the acute treatment of low cardiac output states and congestive heart failure, especially during acute myocardial infarction.
2. Because of the potent and potentially harmful effects of nitroprusside, most patients should have close hemodynamic monitoring with pulmonary artery and intraarterial pressure recordings.
3. Nitroprusside is infused intravenously, beginning at 10 μg/minute and increased until desired effects are obtained.
4. Therapy is usually guided by the level of the pulmonary wedge pressure or pulmonary end-diastolic pressure and the systemic arterial pressure.

Toxicity and side effects

1. Hypotension caused by excessive vasodilatation is treated by lowering the dosage or stopping the infusion.
2. Nitroprusside is metabolized to thiocyanate, which may produce fatigue, nausea, muscle spasm, psychotic behavior, and hypothyroidism. Thiocyanate level should be measured if large amounts of nitroprusside (100 μg/minute) are infused for more than 48 hours.

HYDRALAZINE (APRESOLINE)

Hydralazine directly relaxes vascular smooth muscle, to a greater extent in arterioles than veins. Vasodilatation is independent of sympathetic vasomotor tone but is augmented when vasomotor tone is absent. As a result of vasodilatation, systemic vascular resistance decreases, and renal, splanchnic, and hepatic blood flow increases.[20] Peripheral vasodilatation recruits a reflex increase in heart rate, but hydralazine also may have a slight degree of direct cardiac stimulation. Reflex tachycardia may be prevented by beta-adrenergic blocking agents such as propranolol.

Clinical uses and administration

1. Originally introduced and widely used as an antihypertensive agent, hydralazine is also employed as an oral vasodilator agent to treat congestive heart failure and low cardiac output states.
2. Hydralazine is administered orally in a dosage of 40 to 400 mg/day in two to four divided doses.
3. For chronic treatment a dosage of less than 200 mg/day is recommended to minimize toxicity, particularly drug-induced lupus erythematosus.

Side effects and toxicity
1. Reflex tachycardia may precipitate myocardial ischemia and angina pectoris. In some instances of congestive heart failure in which the beta-adrenergic reflex responses are blunted, reflex tachycardia may not occur.
2. More important, chronic hydralazine therapy may induce a syndrome of systemic lupus erythematosus, possibly caused by an immunologic response to a metabolite of hydralazine.
3. Other side effects include headache, nausea, drug fever, urticaria, skin rash, neuritis, gastrointestinal hemorrhage, anemia, and pancytopenia.

PRAZOSIN (MINIPRESS)

Prazosin, an orally effective alpha-adrenergic blocking agent, is discussed here because its clinical applications are similar to those of the other vasodilators mentioned. Prazosin selectively blocks alpha$_1$-adrenergic receptors to reduce peripheral vascular resistance, and hemodynamic studies suggest that the net effect of prazosin is to dilate arterioles and venules equivalently, similar to the effects seen with nitroprusside.[11,20] The cardiac acceleration following vasodilatation with hydralazine or after nonselective alpha receptor blockade with phentolamine does not occur with prazosin. As a result of decreased systemic resistance, cardiac output increases and blood pressure falls, both in hypertensive patients and in patients with congestive heart failure. The improvement in cardiac output, however, may not be maintained during chronic therapy, since tolerance to the effects of prazosin seems to develop.

Clinical uses
1. Prazosin is employed as a vasodilator to treat congestive heart failure and low cardiac output states.
2. Prazosin is also an antihypertensive agent.
3. By plasma concentration measurements, prazosin has a half-life of 3 to 4 hours, although its vasodilating effects persist considerably longer.
4. Dosage of prazosin is 1 mg initially and up to 28 mg/day in two or three divided doses.

Side effects and toxicity
1. Excessive hypotension may occur, especially following the initial dose of prazosin.
2. Other side effects are uncommon or mild. Syncope caused by postural hypotension may occur, especially if nitrates are coadministered. Headache, drowsiness, nausea, lethargy, fluid retention, skin rash, urinary incontinence, and polyarthralgia may also occur.

Antiarrhythmic agents (Tables 10-5 and 10-6)

The following sections present selected features relating to the use of both conventional and investigational antiarrhythmic agents. Emphasis will be on the clinical and pharmacologic features of each agent as applied to treatment of cardiac tachyarrhythmias. These tables summarize clinical electrophysiologic and pharmacologic properties of these antiarrhythmic drugs.

Table 10-5. Clinical electrophysiologic effects of antiarrhythmic agents*

| | Sinus rate | Intervals | | | | | ERP AV node | ERP His-Purkinje | ERP Atrium | ERP Ventricle |
		PR	QRS	QT	AH	HV				
Lidocaine	0	0	0	0	0, ↓	0	0, ↓	0, ↑	0	0
Quinidine	0, ↑	0, ↑	↑	↑	↓ ↑	0, ↑	↓ ↑	0, ↑	↑	↑
Procainamide	0	0, ↑	↑	↑	0, ↑	0, ↑	0, ↑	0, ↑	↑	↑
Disopyramide	0, ↑	0, ↑	↑	↑	↓ ↑	0, ↑	↓ ↑	0, ↑	↑	↑
Phenytoin	0	0	0	0, ↓	0	0	0, ↓	↓	0	0
Propranolol	↓	0, ↑	0	0, ↓	0, ↑	0	↑	0	0	0
Bretylium	0, ↓	0, ↑	0	0, ↓						
Aprindine	0, ↓	↑	↑	0, ↑	↑	↑	↑	↑	↑	↑
Amiodarone	↓	↑	0, ↑	↑	↑	0, ↑	↑	↑	↑	↑
Encainide	0	↑	↑	↑	↑	↑	↑	↑	↑	↑
Mexiletine	0	0	0	0	0, ↑	0, ↑	0, ↑	0, ↑	0	0
Tocainide	0	0	0	0, ↓	0	0	0, ↓	0	↓	↓

*ERP, Effective refractory period; ↑, increase; ↓, decrease; 0, no change.

Table 10-6. Clinical pharmacology of antiarrhythmic agents

	Administration	Dosage	Elimination (T₁/₂)	Therapeutic plasma concentration
Lidocaine	IV	Load: 2 mg/kg Maintenance: 40 μg/kg/min	100 min	2-6 μg/ml
Quinidine	IV, oral	IV: Load 6-10 μg/kg Oral: 1200-2400 mg/day	6-11 hr	3-5 μg/ml
Procainamide	IV, oral	IV: Load 10-12 mg/kg at 20 mg/min Maintenance: 2-4 mg/min Oral: 2000-8000 mg/day	3-4 hr	4-8 μg/ml
Disopyramide	Oral	400-1200 mg/day	4-8 hr	3-8 μg/ml
Phenytoin	IV, oral	IV: Load 12 mg/kg at 20 mg/min Maintenance: 300-400 mg/day Oral: 300-400 mg/day	24 hr (dose dependent)	10-20 μg/ml
Propranolol	IV, oral	IV: 100-150 μg/kg/min over 10 min Oral: 40-1000 mg/day	4 hr	>40 μg/ml
Bretylium	IV, oral	IV: initial 5-10 mg/kg Maintenance: 1-2 mg/min Oral: ?	8-10 hr	?
Aprindine	Oral	50-200 mg/day	24 hr	1-2 μg/ml
Amiodarone	Oral	200-800 mg/day	?	?
Encainide	Oral	100-300 mg/day	3-4 hr	?
Mexiletine	Oral	600-1200 mg/day	12 hr	0.5-2 μg/ml
Tocainide	Oral	1200-1800 mg/day	12 hr	6-12 μg/ml

LIDOCAINE

Ease of administration, wide range of clinical efficacy, and infrequent development of major adverse side effects make lidocaine the preferred drug for emergency treatment of ventricular tachyarrhythmias and prevention of recurrent ventricular tachycardia and ventricular fibrillation, especially during acute myocardial infarction and digitalis toxicity.

Electrophysiology.[21,22] Lidocaine is a local anesthetic agent with electrophysiologic actions that appear to be different depending on whether tissue is nonischemic or ischemic. Lidocaine decreases conduction velocity in ischemic Purkinje or myocardial tissue. In nonischemic tissue, lidocaine has little or no effect on conduction velocity but decreases action potential duration. Moreover, lidocaine alters the time course of recovery by prolonging the time required for maximal rate of depolarization to recover to steady state following depolarization. In other words, after the administration of lidocaine, premature impulses are less likely to conduct or will conduct more slowly.

Clinical pharmacokinetics.[23] Lidocaine undergoes extensive first-pass hepatic metabolism so that oral administration produces unpredictable and low plasma levels, whereas metabolic products of lidocaine frequently produce toxicity. Therefore lidocaine is only used parenterally. Hemodynamic parameters substantially affect the rate of lidocaine elimination, since metabolism of lidocaine is dependent on hepatic blood flow. Therefore hypotension, low cardiac output, or congestive heart failure prolongs lidocaine half-life, necessitating adjustment in steady-state infusion rates. In normal subjects, elimination half-life of lidocaine averages 100 minutes but may extend to 4 to 10 hours or even longer in the presence of heart failure or cardiogenic shock. Therapeutic plasma concentrations of lidocaine range from 2 to 6 μg/ml, and toxic effects most often occur at levels over 10 μg/ml.

Administration. The intravenous loading dose is 2 mg/kg, given in two divided doses at 20-minute intervals. Maintenance dosage is 40 μg/kg/minute, usually 2 to 4 mg/minute. Dosage requirements are decreased in the presence of congestive heart failure (as just mentioned) and in elderly patients.

Adverse side effects and toxicity. Central nervous system toxicity is the major adverse effect of lidocaine, manifested as paresthesia, slurred speech, confusion, tremors, and convulsions. In the presence of other antiarrhythmic drugs that possess local anesthetic effects, such as procainamide or mexiletine, additive effects on central nervous system toxicity may be evident. Lidocaine may further aggravate preexisting AV conduction disorders and depress SA node function in predisposed patients perhaps by affecting depressed tissues, as mentioned earlier. Negative inotropic effects of lidocaine are reported but rarely achieve clinical significance.

QUINIDINE

Quinidine is an effective agent for a variety of ventricular and supraventricular arrhythmias. Quinidine may be used to suppress or prevent serious ventricular arrhythmias during acute myocardial infarction, recurrent ventricular tachycardia, symptomatic premature ventricular complexes associated with chronic heart disease, recurrent atrial fibrillation or flutter, and recurrent PSVT. Quinidine may be effective in WPW syndrome by directly affecting antegrade and retrograde conduction over accessory bypass tracts.

Electrophysiology.[21,22,24] Quinidine produces direct cardiac effects, similar in part to those of other agents classified as "local anesthetic" agents; it also has indirect effects mediated through the autonomic nervous system.

Direct effects of quinidine, measured in isolated atrial, ventricular, and Purkinje cells, are to decrease rate of rise and amplitude of action potential, increase action potential duration, increase effective refractory period, and decrease rate of spontaneous diastolic depolarization.[23,24] In a human, quinidine prolongs the HV interval and refractoriness of atrium and ventricle and results in mild prolongation of the QRS interval. By direct effects, quinidine may also depress sinus node automaticity and prolong AV nodal conduction.

Indirect effects of quinidine are anticholinergic and alpha-adrenergic blocking properties. These properties may result in atropine-like effects on SA and AV nodes and produce peripheral vasodilatation.

Clinical pharmacokinetics.[23] Quinidine, well absorbed after oral administration, is primarily eliminated by hepatic metabolism, although a portion of quinidine and its cardioactive metabolites are excreted by the kidney. Therefore, in renal failure or hepatic failure, quinidine therapy may be hazardous and must be guided by close attention to plasma concentrations and electrocardiographic signs of quinidine effect. Elimination half-life of quinidine averages about 6 hours, although there is considerable variability among individual patients. Quinidine half-life is reported to be prolonged in patients who have heart disease and hepatic disease, but studies of quinidine pharmacokinetics are difficult to compare, in part because of variations in methods of plasma quinidine measurement. Therapeutic plasma concentration of quinidine is stated to range from 3 to 5 μg/ml.

Administration. Quinidine is best administered by oral or intravenous routes and is available as quinidine sulfate and quinidine gluconate.

The usual oral dose is 1200 to 2400 mg/day, as 300 to 600 mg every 6 to 8 hours; the intravenous loading dose is 6 to 10 mg/kg; maintenance is 10 to 30 mg/kg/minute.

Adverse side effects and toxicity. Chronic quinidine treatment may often be limited by adverse side effects that include nausea, diarrhea, cinchonism (headache, dizziness, ringing in ears), and allergic reactions of fever, skin rash, thrombocytopenia, hemolytic anemia, and anaphylaxis. Quinidine may induce or exacerbate ventricular tachycardia in the presence of low, therapeutic, or toxic plasma levels. *Quinidine syncope* refers to syncope in patients receiving quinidine that is probably caused by the occurrence of a multiform ventricular tachycardia, *torsade de pointes,* usually occurring in the setting of a prolonged QT interval that may be produced by quinidine. At toxic dosages, adverse cardiovascular effects of quinidine include prolongation of QRS interval, AV block, and ventricular arrhythmias. Alpha-adrenergic blocking effects of quinidine may result in hypotension, particularly in patients receiving vasodilators or diuretics.

More recently described have been interactions between quinidine and digoxin and possibly digitoxin that may lead to an increase in plasma digitalis levels.

The mechanism of this interaction is not firmly established. Although central nervous system and gastrointestinal signs of digitalis toxicity may appear, it is unclear whether cardiac toxicity occurs in this setting.

PROCAINAMIDE

Procainamide is a versatile antiarrhythmic agent useful in parenteral form for immediate treatment and in oral form for chronic treatment of supraventricular and ventricular arrhythmias. Electrophysiologic actions of procainamide are similar to direct actions of quinidine, and indications for procainamide are the same as for quinidine.

Clinical pharmacokinetics.[23] Procainamide metabolism has important clinical implications. Approximately half of a dose is excreted unchanged in the urine, and the remainder is metabolized by the liver with formation of an active hepatic metabolite, N-acetyl procainamide (NAPA), which is primarily excreted by the kidneys. Therefore levels of procainamide and NAPA rise significantly during states of decreased renal perfusion or renal failure, so careful dose adjustments are necessary. The elimination half-life of procainamide is 3 to 4 hours, and therapeutic plasma concentrations range from 4 to 8 μg/ml. The short elimination half-life necessitates dosing intervals of 4 hours or less to maintain relatively stable plasma concentrations. A recently introduced slow-release preparation of procainamide appears to allow dosing intervals of 6 hours.

Administration. The oral dosage is 2 to 8 g/day in divided doses every 4 to 6 hours; the intravenous loading dose is 10 to 12 mg/kg at 20 mg/minute, and maintenance is 2 to 6 mg/minute.

Adverse side effects and toxicity. Adverse cardiovascular effects of procainamide most commonly include prolongation of AV and intraventricular conduction time, negative inotropic effects, and precipitation of ventricular arrhythmias. During chronic oral therapy, procainamide may be associated with development of gastrointestinal intolerance, skin rash, and, rarely, agranulocytosis. Conversion to a positive antinuclear antibody titer occurs in 70% to 80% of patients during long-term therapy, whereas drug-induced lupus syndrome occurs in 10% to 20% of patients. This syndrome includes fever, arthralgias, and pleuropericarditis, but as with other drug-induced lupus syndromes, the kidneys and central nervous system are not involved.

DISOPYRAMIDE (NORPACE)

Since introduction into clinical practice in 1978, disopyramide has become a popular agent for oral treatment of ventricular arrhythmias. Clinical reports indicate that disopyramide has antiarrhythmic efficacy equal to quinidine and effectively prevents recurrent ventricular tachycardia during chronic therapy. Although not currently approved for this purpose, disopyramide appears effective in the treatment of supraventricular arrhythmia.

Electrophysiology. Direct electrophysiologic effects of disopyramide, as examined in isolated tissue preparations, are similar to those seen with procainamide or quinidine. In the intact heart, however, disopyramide has direct membrane effects and significant anticholinergic or atropine-like effects. Although the anticholinergic effects of disopyramide may modify its actions, the extent of this modification may be unknown in a given patient.

Clinical pharmacokinetics. Disopyramide is currently available in the United States only as an oral agent. The intravenous preparation is still being investigated. About 40% to 70% of a dose of disopyramide is excreted unchanged in the urine, making careful dosage adjustments necessary in the presence of renal insufficiency. Therapeutic plasma levels of disopyramide are stated to range from 2 to 4 μg/ml, with an elimination half-life ranging from 6 to 9 hours.

Administration. The oral dosage is 400 to 1200 mg/day in divided doses every 6 to 8 hours. Use of loading dose is not recommended.

Adverse side effects and toxicity. During clinical use, disopyramide has frequent and often clinically significant adverse side effects. Most common are anticholinergic effects of dry mouth, urinary hesitancy, and constipation. Of greater concern are adverse cardiovascular side effects. Negative inotropic effects of disopyramide are substantial and include instances of heart failure, hypotension, and electrical-mechanical dissociation. Administration of disopyramide in the presence of borderline cardiac compensation may result in further hemodynamic impairment. Disopyramide may also induce ventricular tachycardia/fibrillation, probably in a manner similar to that seen with "quinidine syncope." The adverse cardiovascular effects of disopyramide should lead to caution in its use, especially in the presence of renal insufficiency or congestive heart failure.

PHENYTOIN (DILANTIN)

Primarily an anticonvulsive agent, phenytoin has antiarrhythmic effects, especially in arrhythmias due to digitalis toxicity and less commonly in arrhythmias associated with ischemic heart disease.

Electrophysiology. Phenytoin possesses direct cardiac electrophysiologic effects similar to those of lidocaine but may also possess important antiarrhythmic effects through its indirect actions in the central nervous system, which include a decrease in sympathetic nerve activity.

Pharmacokinetics.[23] Phenytoin's pharmacokinetics are complex. Plasma half-life of phenytoin increases as plasma concentration increases so that small changes in dosage may produce large changes in plasma concentration and lead to unexpected drug toxicity. During long-term therapy, however, it appears that single daily doses of phenytoin are adequate to maintain stable plasma levels. Phenytoin is extensively metabolized by the liver, a process that may be slowed in the presence of liver disease or by the administration of dicumarol, phenothiazines, phenylbutazone, or other drugs that compete with phenytoin for hepatic enzyme sites. On the other hand, agents such as barbiturates that induce hepatic microsomal enzymes may increase the rate of phenytoin metabolism. Therapeutic concentration of phenytoin is 10 to 20 μg/ml.

Administration. The oral dosage is 300 to 400 mg/day as a single dose; the intravenous loading dose is 12 mg/kg at 20 mg/minute; maintenance is 300 to 400 mg/day.

Adverse side effects and toxicity. Phenytoin toxicity is usually manifested by central nervous system effects, its severity usually correlating with plasma drug concentration. Manifestations of toxicity include nystagmus, ataxia, drowsiness, lethargy, and, finally, coma. Chronic phenytoin therapy has been associated with skin rash, megaloblastic anemia, lymphoid hyperplasia, gingival hyperplasia, and drug-induced systemic lupus erythematosus.

BRETYLIUM (BRETYLOL)

Bretylium was originally and unsuccessfully introduced as an antihypertensive agent but subsequently was found to have antiarrhythmic effects. Bretylium is currently approved for emergency parenteral administration to treat patients who have life-threatening ventricular tachycardia/fibrillation. Oral therapy with bretylium remains investigational at this time. Clinical reports attest to the efficacy of bretylium in selected clinical situations, which include drug-induced conversion of ventricular fibrillation and successful treatment of recurrent ventricular tachycardia/fibrillation resistant to other antiarrhythmic drugs.

Electrophysiology.[25] The mechanism by which bretylium exerts its antiarrhythmic action is unclear, since the drug possesses both direct cardiac effects and effects on the autonomic nervous system. Adrenergic effects of bretylium include an initial release of norepinephrine from adrenergic nerve endings followed by a blockade of the uptake of released norepinephrine. Bretylium also prevents release of norepinephrine during nerve depolarization; therefore bretylium initially acts as an adrenergic agonist and then produces adrenergic blockade. In experimental models bretylium increases the threshold for ventricular fibrillation independently of its adrenergic blocking effects. In isolated Purkinje fibers, bretylium prolongs duration of action potential and effective refractory period to equal degrees, again unrelated to its adrenergic blocking function. Following an acute myocardial infarction, in canine models, bretylium reduces the disparity in refractory periods between infarcted and normal regions. The relative importance of these observations to the antiarrhythmic action of bretylium is unknown.

Pharmacokinetics. Only limited information on the pharmacokinetics of bretylium is available. Bretylium is primarily unchanged by the kidney with elimination half-life averaging from 6 to 8 hours. Therefore the dosage needs to be reduced in the presence of renal insufficiency.

Administration. Bretylium is usually administered in emergency situations with an initial dosage of 5 to 10 mg/kg, repeated in 30-minute intervals to a total dosage of 30 mg/kg. If maintenance therapy is required, doses may be repeated every 6 to 8 hours, or constant infusion may be administered at a rate of 1 to 2 mg/minute.

Adverse side effects and toxicity. The most common side effects of bretylium relate to its effects on adrenergic blockade. Since its initial action is to release stored norepinephrine, bretylium may initially increase blood pressure, heart rate, and inotropic state. Postural hypotension, caused by peripheral vasodilatation, results from subsequent adrenergic blockade. Other side effects of bretylium include nausea, vomiting, and, during oral administration, severe parotid pain.

AMIODARONE (CORDARONE)

Amiodarone, used extensively in Europe and South America for several years, is not currently approved for general use in the United States. Amiodarone was initially introduced as a vasodilating agent to treat angina pectoris and then was found to have antiarrhythmic properties.

Amiodarone has been a highly effective antiarrhythmic agent in the treatment of supraventricular and ventricular arrhythmias, often in patients resistant to other antiarrhythmic drugs. Our reported experience includes 45 patients who demonstrated chronic, recurrent ventricular tachycardia/fibrillation resistant to therapy with all conventional antiarrhythmic drugs as well as to other investigational agents. During a follow-up period that ranges from 3 to 36 months, amiodarone alone (17 patients) or when combined with another previously unsuccessful antiarrhythmic agent (13 patients) successfully prevented recurrent ventricular tachycardia/fibrillation in 30 of 45 patients.[26]

Amiodarone has also been successful in the treatment of recurrent atrial fibrillation and arrhythmias associated with the WPW syndrome.

Electrophysiology. Amiodarone possesses direct electrophysiologic effects as well as antiadrenergic effects. In isolated tissue studies amiodarone prolonged action potential duration of sinus node, ventricular muscle, and Purkinje fibers with little or no change in maximal rate of depolarization.[27] We have studied clinical electrophysiologic effects of amiodarone after 2 weeks of chronic oral therapy. Amiodarone significantly increased the refractory period of atrium and ventricle, prolonged AV nodal conduction time, and slowed spontaneous SA node discharge rate. Amiodarone also increased the effective refractory period and slowed conduction in the accessory pathway in patients with WPW syndrome.

Pharmacokinetics. Amiodarone appears to have unique pharmacokinetic properties. The elimination half-life of amiodarone is at least 30 days, and antiarrhythmic effects may persist for up to several weeks after discontinuation of the drug. In our experience, full antiarrhythmic effects of amiodarone may not be attained for as long as 2 or 3 weeks to several months after initiation of therapy.

Adverse side effects and toxicity. Although generally well tolerated for chronic use, amiodarone appears to have significant adverse side effects. Most frequent is the occurrence of corneal microdeposits; these were found in nearly all adult patients who underwent regular ophthalmologic examination during chronic therapy. No changes in visual acuity or in the retina have been described. Elevation of serum transaminase levels without further clinical evidence of hepatic dysfunction has occurred in half of the patients. The most serious side effect, identified in five of our patients who received amiodarone, was pulmonary fibrosis. Amiodarone also has been associated with neuromuscular side effects of weakness and fatigue, which diminished or disappeared after the dose of amiodarone was reduced. Amiodarone appears to have minimal cardiovascular toxicity. There is a slight negative inotropic effect, and patients with preexisting SA or AV nodal disturbances may develop further AV conduction delay or further SA nodal dysfunction. Two patients in our series required pacemaker therapy to relieve the exacerbation of preexisting SA nodal dysfunction following amiodarone therapy.

ENCAINIDE

Encainide is a new antiarrhythmic agent developed in the United States and currently undergoing clinical investigation. In preliminary clinical trials, encainide appears to be a potent antiarrhythmic agent in reducing the frequency of PVCs as judged by 5-minute ECG recordings. We have found that approximately 30% of patients referred for treatment of drug-resistant ventricular tachycardia/fibrillation have been successfully treated with encainide. Encainide also appears to have promise in the treatment of PSVT, including that associated with WPW syndrome.

Electrophysiology. Pharmacologic and electrophysiologic effects of encainide appear to vary with the route and chronicity of administration. Following intravenous administration encainide prolonged HV and QRS intervals with variable effects on QT interval and did not significantly affect AH interval or refractoriness of atrium, AV node, or ventricle. Following 4 or more days of oral administration, encainide significantly prolonged the atrial and ventricular effective refractory period, AH interval, HV interval, and the shortest atrial-paced cycle that conducted 1:1 to the ventricle, as well as PR, QRS, and QT intervals on the ECG. The differences between electrophysiologic effects of encainide following acute intravenous administration and those following chronic oral administration suggest either a time-dependent action of encainide on cardiac electrophysiology or the presence of one or more active metabolites of encainide.[28]

In electrophysiologic studies on isolated canine Purkinje fibers, encainide decreased the slope of phase 4 diastolic depolarization, decreased the maximal rate of rise of the action potential, and decreased action potential duration and refractory period.

Pharmacokinetics. Elimination half-life of encainide is reported to be 3 to 4 hours. However, in clinical use antiarrhythmic effects of encainide appear to allow dosing intervals of every 6 to 8 hours. Encainide appears to undergo extensive metabolism with little of the drug excreted unchanged in the urine. As just mentioned, encainide may possess an active metabolite that permits longer dosing intervals than expected, which makes interpretation of pharmacokinetic data difficult.

Adverse side effects and toxicity. Encainide has been well tolerated during acute and long-term therapy in the majority of patients. Adverse side effects include dizziness, diplopia, vertigo, paresthesia, leg cramps, and metallic taste in the mouth. Encainide prolongs PR, QRS, and QT intervals and has been associated with type I second-degree AV block as well as with the worsening of ventricular arrhythmias. Although no clinically significant negative inotropic effects of encainide have been reported, it has been our experience that some patients have marked hemodynamic compromise when ventricular tachycardia occurs while receiving encainide.

We have encountered two patients who developed increased frequency of ventricular tachycardia while taking encainide. In both cases, prior to encainide therapy, recurrent ventricular tachycardia/fibrillation was resistant to conventional antiarrhythmic therapy but had always been successfully treated by electrical cardioversion. While the patients received encainide, ventricular tachycardia recurred, usually at a slower rate than noted previously, but remained resistant to electrical cardioversion until over 6 hours after discontinuation of encainide.

APRINDINE (FIBOCIL)

Aprindine, currently available for general clinical use in most of Europe, has been undergoing clinical investigation in the United States for several years. Aprindine has successfully treated chronic stable ventricular arrhythmias, ventricular arrhythmias complicating acute myocardial infarction, chronic, recurrent ventricular tachycardia/fibrillation, and certain supraventricular arrhythmias including those associated with WPW syndrome. In our initial experience with 120 patients treated with aprindine for suppression of recurrent ventricular tachycardia/fibrillation that was resistant to conventional drugs, aprindine has been continued in 53 patients with successful prevention of arrhythmias. Aprindine was discontinued in 67 patients because of poor control of the arrhythmia or presence of intolerable adverse side effects.[29]

Electrophysiology.[27,29] Aprindine is a local anesthetic agent possessing electrophysiologic properties simliar to those of quinidine and lidocaine. In isolated Purkinje fibers aprindine shortened action potential duration and effective refractory period, decreased the maximal rate of rise of phase zero, and decreased conduction velocity. In ventricular muscle aprindine slightly decreased action potential duration and lengthened effective refractory period.

In the intact heart aprindine prolongs AH and HV intervals and QRS duration and increases refractoriness of atrium, AV node, and ventricle. Aprindine also lengthens refractory periods and slows or blocks conduction in the accessory pathway of patients who have WPW syndrome.

Pharmacokinetics. Aprindine has a prolonged elimination half-life, ranging from 20 to 30 hours with a mean of 24 hours, that permits once or twice daily dosing. In our experience full antiarrhythmic effects of arpindine may not be evident for several days, even after initial administration of a loading dose. This suggests that aprindine may possess rather complex pharmacokinetics not fully explained by the usual models. Aprindine largely undergoes hepatic metabolism, but the effects of hepatic or renal disease on aprindine administration are unclear. Therapeutic serum levels of aprindine range from 0.7 to 2.0 μg/ml. The usual dose of aprindine ranges from 50 to 200 mg/day. Most patients cannot tolerate more than 200 mg/day because of side effects.

Adverse side effects. Adverse side effects of aprindine are common and may often limit therapy. Most frequent are neurologic side effects that include tremors, ataxia, dizziness, memory impairment, hallucinations, nervousness, and seizures. Gastrointestinal symptoms include nausea and diarrhea. The combination of aprindine with other agents possessing local anesthetic properties should be undertaken cautiously, since central nervous system toxicity may be additive. Most seriously, aprindine has been associated with agranulocytosis and cholestatic jaundice, both thought to be idiosyncratic reactions. The life-threatening potential of agranulocytosis mandates a weekly monitoring of white blood cell count during the first 4 months of treatment. Adverse cardiovascular effects of aprindine include a mild negative inotropic effect as well as a potential for worsening preexisting AV conduction disorders.

MEXILETINE (MEXITIL)

Mexiletine is a new antiarrhythmic agent with structural and pharmacologic properties that resemble those of lidocaine. Mexiletine is available for general clinical use in Europe and Great Britain, while its clinical investigation is currently in progress in the United States. Although initial reports indicated that mexiletine effectively suppresses ventricular arrhythmias associated with acute myocardial infarction, we have found less encouraging results for the treatment of chronic, recurrent ventricular tachycardia with mexiletine, since only approximately 20% of patients have had effective control of the arrhythmia.[30]

Electrophysiology.[27] Electrophysiologic properties of mexiletine resemble those of lidocaine, to which it is structurally related. In normal patients mexiletine produces no change in sinus rate or atrial refractory period, although mexiletine may further depress sinus node function in the presence of preexisting abnormalities. Mexiletine may depress HV conduction in some patients, but this appears to be a variable finding. In isolated cardiac Purkinje fibers mexiletine reduces conduction velocity and maximum rate of depolarization with little effect on resting membrane potential and action potential duration.

Pharmacokinetics. Elimination half-life of mexiletine is prolonged in patients who have cardiac disease. In our study elimination half-life averaged 12 hours during steady-state conditions. Therapeutic plasma concentrations range from 0.75 to 2.0 μg/ml and are maintained with oral doses of 200 to 400 mg every 8 hours. Mexiletine is primarily eliminated by hepatic metabolism with only 8% of an administered dose excreted unchanged in the urine. Because of the pharmcokinetics of mexiletine and its large total volume of distribution, the total body loading dose should not be given as one dose, since this may result in a high incidence of toxicity.

Adverse side effects and toxicity. Adverse side effects of mexiletine are frequent, and 30% to 40% of patients may require a change in dosage or discontinuation of therapy because of drug toxicity. The most common are neurologic side effects, which include tremor, dysarthria, dizziness, paresthesia, diplopia, nystagmus, mental confusion, anxiety, and such gastrointestinal effects as nausea, vomiting, and dyspepsia. Cardiovascular side effects are most often seen after intravenous dosing and include hypotension, bradycardia, and exacerbation of arrhythmia. Adverse side effects of mexiletine appear to be dose related, and toxic effects appear at plasma concentrations only slightly higher than those necessary to achieve therapeutic efficacy. Therefore effective use of this antiarrhythmic drug requires careful titration of dose and monitoring of plasma concentration.

TOCAINIDE

Tocainide, a primary amine analog of lidocaine that is effective orally, is currently undergoing extensive clinical trials in the United States as an antiarrhythmic agent for ventricular arrhythmias. In acute drug studies tocainide has produced significant reduction of PVC frequency in patients who have chronic, stable PVCs, but it has been less effective in preventing chronic, recurrent ventricular tachycardia/fibrillation. The majority of treated patients have required additional antiarrhythmic drug treatment or reduction or discontinuation of tocainide because of adverse side effects. In our experience only one of eight patients who received tocainide to prevent recurrent ventricular tachycardia/ fibrillation that was resistant to conventional drug therapy has had a successful response.

Electrophysiology.[27] Clinical and experimental electrophysiologic effects of tocainide are very similar to those of lidocaine. In humans tocainide shortens the mean effective refractory period of atrium, AV node, and right ventricle but produced minimal changes in AV conduction.

Clinical pharmacokinetics. Elimination half-life of tocainide is 10 to 17 hours, with a mean of 13.5 hours. Administration of tocainide every 8 to 12 hours is thereby feasible. Approximately 60% of the drug undergoes hepatic metabolism, whereas 40% is excreted unchanged in the urine. Therapeutic plasma concentrations are reported as exceeding 6 μg/ml, usually achieved by a daily dosage of 1200 to 1800 mg.

Adverse side effects and toxicity. Tocainide therapy has been associated with frequent adverse side effects that, although mild and reversible, may often limit therapy. Most common side effects are nausea, vomiting, anorexia, tremulousness, memory impairment, skin rash, sweating, paresthesias, diplopia, dizziness, anxiety, and tinnitus. Side effects of tocainide are similar to those seen with lidocaine and are also dose related, often resolving with a decrease in tocainide dose.

Slow-channel blockers (calcium channel blockers)[31]

Calcium antagonists or slow-channel blocking drugs represent an exciting new field of cardiovascular physiology and pharmacology. Slow-channel blocking drugs affect electrophysiologic and mechanical properties of the heart and have vasodilator effects through actions on vascular smooth muscle. Electrophysiologic effects include a decreased discharge rate of sinus node and prolonged conduction and refractoriness of AV node. These effects are manifested as increase in sinus node cycle length and prolongation of PR interval. Slow-channel blockers have the potential to produce negative inotropic effects by interference with calcium flow into the cell and inhibition of excitation-contraction coupling.

In cardiovascular therapy slow-channel blockers have been used for the following indications:
1. Antiarrhythmic agents to terminate and prevent recurrences of PSVT and to control ventricular rate during atrial fibrillation/flutter
2. Antianginal agents, particularly for treatment of coronary artery spasm
3. Treatment of systemic hypertension
4. Treatment of hypertrophic cardiomyopathy

VERAPAMIL (ISOPTIN, CALAN, IPOVERATRIL)

Verapamil possesses electrophysiologic, hemodynamic, and vasodilator effects at doses commonly employed in clinical practice.

Clinical use. Verapamil has become the preferred agent to terminate acute episode of PSVT. In PSVT caused by AV junctional reentry or by reciprocating tachycardia with an accessory pathway, verapamil (5 to 10 mg IV) has terminated the arrhythmia in nearly all cases. Oral verapamil has also been effective in the treatment of coronary artery spasm and hypertrophic cardiomyopathy.

Dosage. The intravenous dosage is 5 to 10 mg IV bolus to terminate PSVT; the oral dosage is 80 to 160 mg/6 to 8 hours.

Onset of action of intravenous verapamil is within 2 minutes. Verapamil undergoes extensive first-pass hepatic metabolism, so oral doses need to be higher than intravenous doses.

Side effects and toxicity. Following intravenous administration verapamil may produce excessive slowing of sinus node discharge rate, AV nodal conduction block, negative inotropic effects, hypotension, edema, headache, and flushing. Its effects on AV conduction are additive to those of digitalis or propranolol, so close monitoring is recommended if these drugs are also administered, and concurrent administration of propranolol and intravenous verapamil is contraindicated.

NIFEDIPINE (PROCARDIA, ADALAT)

Nifedipine acts by a different mechanism than verapamil to produce slow-channel blockade. At usual clinical doses vasodilatation is the major effect with little, if any, prolongation of AV nodal conduction time or negative inotropic effects.

Clinical use. Nifedipine is used as a vasodilator to treat coronary artery spasm, chronic stable angina pectoris, and systemic hypertension. Nifedipine lacks the antiarrhythmic properties of verapamil.

Dosage. The oral dosage is 10 to 30 mg every 8 hours; nifedipine may be given sublingually. Nifedipine appears to be safe when combined with propranolol or digitalis.

Adverse side effects and toxicity. Vasodilator effects may produce hypotension, headache, flushing, nausea, vomiting, and dizziness.

DILTIAZEM (HERBESSOR, ANGINYL, CARDIEM)

Actions and clinical use. Diltiazem is an investigational slow-channel blocking agent that has coronary vasodilating effects approximately equal to those of verapamil and that also slows AV node conduction time but to a slightly lesser extent than verapamil.

Diltiazem has been employed chiefly in the treatment of coronary artery spasm and chronic stable angina pectoris but also possesses antiarrhythmic properties.

Dosage. The usual doasge is 30 to 90 mg administered orally every 8 hours.

Adverse side effects and toxicity. Vasodilator effects appear to be less frequent with diltiazem than with nifedipine or verapamil, and AV block is less frequent than with verapamil. However, the exact nature and prevalence of diltiazem's side effects need to be established by further clinical trials.

REFERENCES

1. Greenblatt, D.J., and Koch-Weser, J.: Drug therapy: clinical pharmacokinetics, N. Engl. J. Med. **293**:702, 964, 1975.
2. Smith, T.W., and Braunwald, E.: The management of heart failure: digitalis glycerides. In Braunwald, E., editor: Heart disease: a textbook of cardiovascular medicine, Philadelphia, 1980, W.B. Saunders Co.
3. Rosen, M.R., Wit, A.L., and Hoffman, B.F.: Electrophysiology and pharmacology of cardiac arrhythmias. IV. Cardiac antiarrhythmic and toxic effects of digitalis, Am. Heart J. **89**:391, 1975.
4. Goldberg, L.I.: Dopamine: clinical uses of an endogenous catecholamine, N. Engl. J. Med. **291**:707, 1974.
5. Sonnenblick, E.H., Frishman, W.H., and LeJemtel, T.H.: Dobutamine: a new synthetic cardioactive sympathetic amine, N. Engl. J. Med. **300**:17, 1979.
6. Stoner, J.D., Bolen, J.L., and Harrison, D.C.: Comparison of dobutamine and dopamine in treatment of severe heart failure, Br. Heart J. **39**:536, 1977.
7. Hoffman, B.F., and Cranefield, P.E.: Electrophysiology of the heart, New York, 1960, McGraw-Hill Book Co.
8. Cranefield, P.E.: The conduction of the cardiac impulse—the slow response and cardiac arrhythmias, Mt. Kisco, N.Y., 1975, Futura Publishing Co.
9. Ahlquist, R.P.: A study of adrenotropic receptors, Am. J. Physiol. **53**:586, 1948.
10. Lands, A.M., and others: Differentiation of receptor systems activated by sympathomimetic amines, Nature **214**:597, 1967.
11. Hoffman, B.B., and Lefkowitz, R.J.: Alpha-adrenergic receptor subtypes, N. Engl. J. Med. **302**:1390, 1980.
12. Frishman, W.H.: β-Adrenoceptor antagonists: new drugs and new indications, N. Engl. J. Med. **305**:500, 1981.
13. Multicentre International Study: Improvement in the prognosis of myocardial infarction by long-term beta-adrenoreceptor blockade using practolol, Br. Med. J. **3**:735, 1975.
14. Wilhelmson, C., and others: Reduction of sudden deaths after myocardial infarction by treatment with alprenolol, Lancet **2**:1156, 1974.
15. Norwegian Multicenter Study Group: Timolol-induced reduction in mortality and reinfarction in patients surviving acute myocardial infarction, N. Engl. J. Med. **304**:801, 1981.
16. Hjalmarson, A., and others: Effect on mortality of metoprolol in acute myocardial infarction: a double-blind randomised trial, Lancet **2**:823, 1981.
17. The β-blocker Heart Attack Trial Research Group: A randomized trial of propranolol in patients with acute myocardial infarction, J.A.M.A. **247**:1707, 1982.
18. The Anturane Reinfarction Trial Research Group: Sulfinpyrazone in the prevention of cardiac death after myocardial infarction, N. Engl. J. Med. **298**:289, 1978.
19. The Canadian Cooperative Study Group: A randomized trial of aspirin and sulfinpyrazone in threatened stroke, N. Engl. J. Med. **299**:53, 1978.
20. Parmley, W.W., and Chatterjee, K.: Vasodilator therapy. In Harvey, W.P., editor: Current problems in cardiology, Chicago, 1978, Year Book Medical Publishers, Inc.
21. Gettes, L.S.: On the classification of antiarrhythmic drugs, Mod. Concepts Cardiovasc. Dis. **48**:13, 1979.
22. Rosen, M.R., Wit, A.L., and Hoffman, B.F.: Electrophysiology and pharmacology of cardiac arrhythmias, Am. Heart J. **89**:526, 665, 804, 1975.
23. Harrison, D.C., Meffin, P.J., and Winkle, R.A.: Clinical pharmacokinetics of antiarrhythmic drugs, Prog. Cardiovasc. Dis. **20**:217, 1977.
24. Mason, J.W., and others: The electrophysiologic effects of quinidine in the transplanted human heart, J. Clin. Invest. **59**:481, 1977.
25. Koch-Weser, J.: Drug therapy: bretylium, N. Engl. J. Med. **300**:473, 1979.
26. Heger, J.J., and others: Amiodarone: clinical and electrophysiologic effects during long-term therapy for ventricular tachycardia or ventricular fibrillation, N. Engl. J. Med. **305**:539, 1981.
27. Zipes, D.P., and Troup, P.J.: New antiarrhythmic agents, Am. J. Cardiol. **41**:1005, 1979.
28. Jackman, W.M., and others: Electrophysiology of oral encainide and efficacy in patients who have supraventricular and ventricular tachyarrhythmias, Am. J. Cardiol. **49**:1279, 1982.
29. Zipes, D.P., and others: Studies with aprindine, Am. Heart J. **100**:1005, 1980.
30. Heger, J.J., and others: Mexiletine therapy in fifteen patients with drug resistant ventricular tachycardia, Am. J. Cardiol. **45**:627, 1980.
31. Henry, P.D.: Comparative pharmacology of calcium antagonists: nifedipine, verapamil, and diltiazem, Am. J. Cardiol. **46**:1047, 1980.

11

ARTIFICIAL CARDIAC PACEMAKER

Edwin G. Duffin, Jr.
Douglas P. Zipes

The artificial cardiac pacemaker is an electronic stimulator used in place of the natural cardiac pacemaker, the SA node, and/or the specialized AV conducting system in the diseased, congenitally malformed, or iatrogenically damaged heart. The pacemaker system is comprised of a power source, usually a battery, electronic circuitry for generating appropriately timed stimuli, and an electrode/wire system ("lead") used to complete the electrical connection between the circuitry and the myocardium. Pacemakers may be packaged for implantation totally within the body (permanent pacemakers), or they may be configured so that the electronics and power source remain outside the body (temporary pacemakers). The first completely implantable devices were reported in the late 1950s.[1,2] Currently there are an estimated 900,000 patients worldwide who have implanted pacemakers. Advances in technology have been rapidly applied to pacemaker systems, providing noninvasively programmable single- and dual-chamber pacemakers typically weighing 40 to 50 g and lasting an estimated 6 to 10 years. These highly reliable devices are dramatically different form the 250 g, asynchronous, 18-month devices of the early 1960s.

Indications
PERMANENT

The most common indication for permanent pacing is fixed or intermittent third-degree AV block,[3] its primary cause being sclerotic degeneration of the AV conducting system. This indication accounts for 50% of all implants. An additional 26% of pacemaker implants are for treatment of sick sinus syndrome.[3] This may be manifested as sinus arrest or block, severe sinus bradycardia, or alternating periods of bradycardia and supraventricular tachycardia (bradycardia-tachycardia syndrome). Further indications for permanent pacing include the following:
1. Mobitz type II second-degree AV block distal to the His bundle[4]
2. Hypersensitive carotid sinus syndrome causing symptomatic severe slowing of sinus rate and/or AV block[5]
3. Chronic atrial fibrillation with a slow ventricular response that results in symptoms[4]
4. Bifascicular block with prolonged His-ventricular (H-V) interval in patients who have syncope or presyncope and no other demonstrated cause of

syncope (Bifascicular block with prolonged H-V interval in asymptomatic patients is generally accepted as not being an indication for permanent pacing, although the issue is not entirely resolved.)[4]

5. Termination or overdrive suppression of supraventricular[6-9] and, less frequently, ventricular tachycardia[6-10] resistant to drug therapy and not amenable to surgical correction
6. Periods of bradycardia or asystole following abrupt termination (overdrive suppression) of supraventricular or ventricular tachycardia resistant to drug therapy and not amenable to surgical correction
7. Prophylactic implantation in patients after myocardial infarction complicated by advanced AV block during the acute stages of infarction; this indication also causes some controversy, and the issue is not completely settled
8. Prevention of tachyarrhythmia by providing rate maintenance in combination with drugs or by control of AV conduction through use of dual-chamber pacemakers[6,11,12]

TEMPORARY

Indications for temporary pacing include the following:
1. Maintenance of adequate heart rate and rhythm in patients during a variety of circumstances, such as postoperatively, during cardiac catheterizations or surgery, during administration of some drugs that might inappropriately slow the rate, and prior to implantation of a permanent pacemaker
2. Prophylaxis following open heart surgery[4]
3. Acute (generally anterior) myocardial infarction with type II second-degree or third-degree AV block[4]
4. Acute (generally anterior) myocardial infarction with concurrent onset of right bundle branch block with left axis deviation[13] or concurrent onset of left bundle branch block
5. Acute inferior myocardial infarction with third-degree AV block refractory to pharmacologic intervention and producing ventricular dysrhythmias and/or hemodynamic compromise[13]
6. Termination of PSVT, atrial flutter, or ventricular tachycardia[9]
7. Suppression of ectopic activity, atrial or ventricular[9]
8. Evaluation of SA node function,[14] AV conduction, and anomalous conducting pathways in arrhythmia analysis[15]
9. Evaluation of efficacy of therapeutic control of tachyarrrhythmias[16]
10. Stress testing by rapid atrial pacing in patients who have coronary artery disease[17]

Pacemaker modalities[5,6,18,19]
ICHD CODE

In 1974 the Inter-Society Commission for Heart Disease (ICHD) promulgated a three-position code[20] designed as a shorhand notation to identify the many varieties of pacing modes. The original code has recently been revised[21] to extend its flexibility. The newly proposed five-position code is given in Table 11-1.

Table 11-1. Five-position pacemaker code (ICHD)

I. Chamber paced II. Chamber sensed	III. Mode of response	IV. Programmability	V. Tachyarrhthmia functions
V = Ventricle A = Atrium D = Atrium and ventricle O = None	I = Inhibited T = Triggered D = Atrial triggered and ventricular inhibited R = Reverse O = None	P = Programmable rate and/or output M = Multiprogrammability O = None	B = Burst N = Normal rate competition S = Scanning E = External

This table provides a shorthand description of pacemaker operation. Symbols placed in the first two positions indicate the chambers in which the pacemaker functions; in the third position, the mode of operation of the pacemaker; in the fourth position, its programmable characteristics; and in the fifth position, its antitachycardia features. For example, if the pacing lead is inserted into the ventricle and the pulse generator is a demand ventricular type, then the chamber paced is the ventricle, and the first letter in the five-position code is V. The chamber sensed is the ventricle and therefore the second letter in the five-position code also is V. The mode of response of the pacemaker is to inhibit a pacing spike when spontaneous electrical activity is sensed, and therefore I is in the third position. If only the rate and/or output of the pulse generator can be programmed externally, P is in the fourth position. If the pacemaker is used to treat tachycardias, then the tachyarrhythmia function is indicated in the fifth position.

Pulse generators that pace or sense in both the atrium and ventricle are indicated by the designation D, meaning dual. If the pacemaker does not have a function in one of the classifications, O is used. Finally, some pacemakers have a "reverse" function in that they discharge when the rate becomes too fast (and are thus used to terminate tachycardias). These pacemakers are indicated by the letter R in the third position. The different types of tachyarrhythmia functions are discussed in the chapter.

ATRIAL AND VENTRICULAR ASYNCHRONOUS PACEMAKERS (AOO, VOO)

The first pacemakers simply stimulated the myocardium at a constant rate independent of any underlying cardiac rhythm; these pacemakers only paced and did not sense any spontaneous activity. If connected to the atrium the pacemaker was referred to as an asynchronous atrial pacemaker (AOO), and if applied to the ventricles it was referred to as a ventricular asynchronous pacemaker (VOO). Block diagrams and representative ECGs for these devices are shown in Fig. 11-1. Asynchronous pacemakers are rarely used today, since it is relatively simple to provide noncompetitive pacemakers that avoid the potential risks of pacing during spontaneous rhythms.

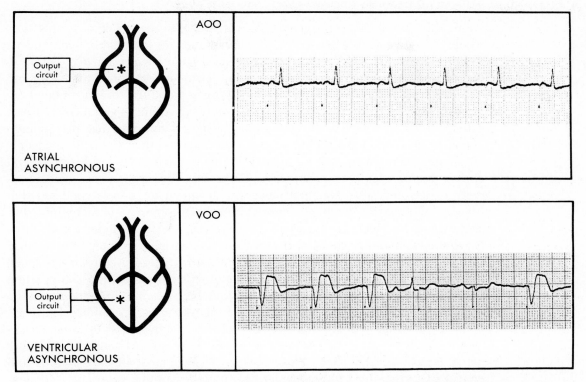

Fig. 11-1. Atrial and ventricular asynchronous pacemakers (AOO, VOO). On the left is a schematic diagram of the heart with the right and left atria on the top and the right and left ventricles on the bottom. The name of the type of pacemaker is given. The term *output circuit* connected to an asterisk indicates the chamber *stimulated* (see Fig. 11-2). A circle connected to an arrowhead labeled *amp* indicates the sensing portion of the pacemaker and identifies the chamber in which spontaneous acitivity is *sensed* (see Fig. 11-2). A circle surrounding an asterisk indicates that both pacing and sensing are performed in that chamber. The letters in the middle panel conform to the first three positions of the pacemaker code as indicated in Table 11-1. Panels on the right indicate an ECG example produced by that particular type of pacemaker.

In the top panel an example of an atrial asynchronous pacemaker (AOO) is displayed. In the left panel the asterisk indicates the atrium is paced. The ECG demonstrates pacemaker stimuli preceding each paced P wave. The asynchronous mode of operation cannot be seen in this ECG example, since spontaneous P waves do not occur.

The format in the bottom panel is the same. The asterisk indicates the ventricle is paced. On the right, ventricular asynchronous pacing is seen following the third paced QRS complex. A spontaneous QRS complex occurs, and yet a pacing stimulus falls in the ST segment of this complex. The next pacemaker stimulus occurs during the QRS complex of the following beat, producing a fusion complex. Finally, the last QRS complex is initiated by the pacemaker spike.

ATRIAL AND VENTRICULAR DEMAND PACEMAKERS (AAI, AAT, VVI, VVT)

In the early 1970s sensing circuits were added to pacemakers so that they would stimulate only when there was no appropriate underlying spontaneous rhythm. These pacemakers paced and sensed spontaneous activity. This prevented competitive pacing and the attendant risk of inducing fibrillation. Demand pacemakers are supplied in two versions, inhibited and triggered. Inhibited devices withhold the stimulus and reset their timing on sensing spontaneous cardiac activity. Triggered devices are activated to deliver a stimulus just after spontaneous depolarization into the refractory tissue and reset their timing immediately on sensing spontaneous cardiac activity. Both types deliver a stimulus at the end of their timing cycle (pacemaker escape interval) if no spontaneous cardiac activity is detected. The triggered mode was invented to address concerns that unipolar inhibited devices might allow a patient to become asystolic if extracardiac signals (for example, pectoral muscle potentials, electrical signals from radio transmitters, or power lines) were sensed, erroneously interpreted to be cardiac signals, and permitted to inhibit pacemaker output. Modern circuitry has reduced the likelihood of such occurrences, and the disadvantages of stimulating when not really necessary (ECG waveform distortion, high-power requirements for the pacemaker) have resulted in relatively little usage of the triggered mode. However, it can be of value to achieve termination of some tachycardias or to be certain diagnostically when or if the pacemaker sensed a spontaneous event; it is therefore generally available in modern pacemakers as an option. Block diagrams and typical ECGs for the ventricular demand inhibited (VVI), ventricular demand triggered (VVT), atrial demand inhibited (AAI), and atrial demand triggered (AAT) devices are shown in Fig. 11-2.

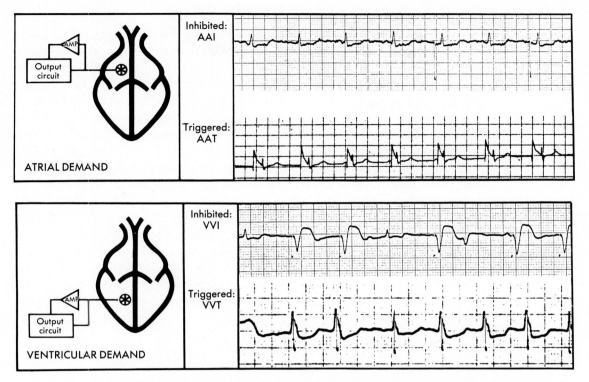

Fig. 11-2. Atrial and ventricular demand pacemakers (AAI, AAT, VVI, VVT). *Top left,* The asterisk and circle in the atrium indicate that the pacemaker stimulates the atrium and senses atrial activity. In the bottom panel the circle and asterisk in the ventricle indicate that the pacemaker stimulates the ventricle and senses spontaneous ventricular activity.

In the top ECG of the upper panel an example of an atrial inhibited (AAI) pacemaker is illustrated. Note that the pacing spike is inhibited from discharge until the fifth and seventh complexes, when the atrial rhythm slows slightly and allows escape of the atrial demand pacemaker. In the second ECG example each sensed P wave elicits a pacing spike delivered within the P wave (third, fourth, fifth P waves). A pacing spike initiates the P wave of the first, second, sixth, and seventh P waves. This is an example of AAT pacing.

In the bottom panel, upper ECG, an example of a ventricular demand pacemaker (VVI) is illustrated. Note that spontaneous ventricular activity inhibits pacemaker discharge, and pacing spikes are delivered only when the ventricular rate becomes slower than the escape interval of the pacemaker. In the lower ECG, pacing spikes are delivered into the QRS complex of each QRS complex (VVT).

ATRIAL SYNCHRONOUS VENTRICULAR PACEMAKERS (VAT, VDD)

To more closely approximate normal cardiac function, sophisticated dual-chamber (atrium and ventricle) "physiologic" pacemakers were developed. The atrial synchronous ventricular pacemaker (VAT) was designed for use in patients with normal sinus function and impaired AV conduction.[22] This device senses atrial activity by means of an electrode in the atrium and, after a suitable delay, paces the ventricles. It does not pace the atrium. This method of atrial sensing and ventricular pacing preserves the atrial contribution to ventricular filling and maintains sinus control of ventricular rate. Rate limits are designed into the pacemaker so that during atrial bradycardia the unit paces as an asynchronous ventricular pacemaker at a predetermined backup rate. During atrial tachycardia the pacemaker paces no faster than its upper rate limit, yielding an AV response to sensed atrial activity that is similar to type I or type II AV block. The VAT device has been refined by the addition of a ventricular sense amplifier, resulting in a new type of pacemaker called the atrial synchronous ventricular inhibited pacemaker (ASVIP), described in the ICHD code as VDD.[23] (The VDD pacemaker still does not pace the atrium but senses and paces the ventricle.) Block diagrams and ECGs for the VAT and VDD pacemakers are shown in Fig. 11-3.

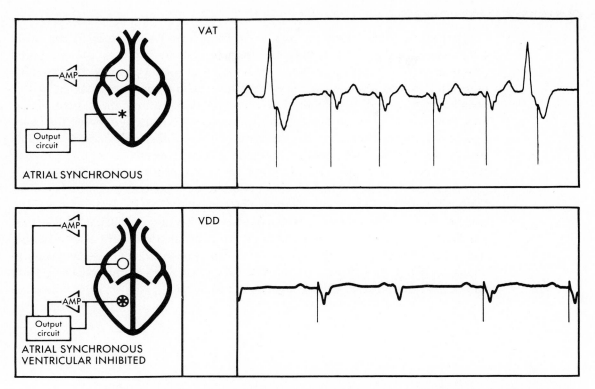

Fig. 11-3. Atrial synchronous pacemakers (VAT, VDD). For the VAT pacemaker (*top panel*) the circle in the atrium and the asterisk in the ventricle indicate that the pacemaker senses atrial activity and paces the ventricle. In the lower panel the circle in the atrium and the circle and asterisk in the ventricle indicate that the pacemaker senses both atrial and ventricular activity and paces the ventricle (VDD).

In the midportion of the top ECG the pacemaker delivers stimuli following each sensed P wave and produces a paced QRS complex. The first and last QRS complexes are spontaneous premature ventricular complexes (PVCs) that are *not* sensed by the pacemaker. The sinus P wave (hidden within the QRS complex) is sensed by the pacemaker and triggers it to deliver a pacing spike to the ventricle. Conceivably, such a response can deliver a stimulus into the T wave of the PVC. To avoid this problem, the VDD pacemaker has been equipped with a sensing circuit to sense spontaneous ventricular activity. Note in the lower ECG (VDD pacemaker) that the second P wave conducts to the ventricle with a PR interval shorter than the P-stimulus interval of the pacemaker. This conducted QRS complex is sensed by the pacemaker, and the pacing spike is inhibited, thus eliminating problems of pacemaker competition with spontaneous ventricular activity.

AV SEQUENTIAL PACEMAKERS (DVI)

In patients who have bradycardia and impaired AV conduction the atrial contribution to ventricular filling can be preserved by using an AV sequential pacemaker (DVI).[24] This pacemaker senses only ventricular activity but is capable of stimulating both the atrium and ventricle. Following ventricular sensed or paced events this device monitors the ventricular electrogram. If ventricular activity is not detected within a prescribed pacemaker escape interval, the pacemaker stimulates the atria. The pacemaker then waits long enough to allow passage of a normal AV interval and, if no ventricular activity occurs, paces in the ventricle. (Some AV sequential pacemakers are of the committed type; that is, they do not wait for normal AV conduction to occur but, instead, always deliver a stimulus to the ventricles following delivery of an atrial stimulus.)[25] Sensed ventricular activity inhibits the ventricular stimulus and resets all pacemaker timing. If the ventricular rate is sufficiently rapid, atrial stimuli are also inhibited. It is important to reemphasize that the DVI pacemaker does not sense spontaneous atrial activity. Fig. 11-4 contains the block diagram and representative ECG for the DVI pacemaker.

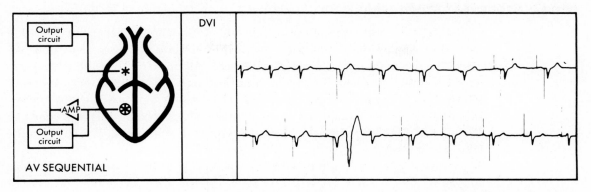

Fig. 11-4. AV sequential pacemaker (DVI). In the diagram the asterisk in the atrium and the asterisk and circle in the ventricle indicate that the pacemaker paces the atrium, paces the ventricle, and senses spontaneous activity in the ventricle. The ECG example demonstrates this operation. The first three sinus-initiated QRS complexes occur at a rate faster than the escape rate of the pacemaker, and the pacemaker is completely inhibited. At this point, SA node discharge rate slows and the pacemaker delivers a stimulus (*upper spike*) to the atrium. Because the paced P wave does not conduct to the ventricle within the escape interval of the pacemaker, the pacemaker then paces the ventricle (*downward directed spikes*). This occurs for three beats. Then the PR interval shortens slightly, inhibiting ventricular pacemaker discharge. The last two beats in the top strip and first three beats in the lower strip indicate pacing in the atrium and ventricle. Then a PVC occurs and is sensed, and pacemaker activity is inhibited. The pacemaker then resumes delivery of spikes to atrium and ventricle. In the terminal portion of this ECG the atrial rate speeds slightly. Since atrial activity is *not* sensed, pacemaker spikes "march" through the P wave but ventricular spikes are inhibited.

OPTIMAL SEQUENTIAL STIMULATION (DDD)

In 1977 came the first clinical implants of a dual-chamber pacemaker that functions in the atrial synchronous mode during normal sinus activity and provides AV sequential pacing during periods of bradycardia.[26] Thus the DDD pacemaker senses and paces the atrium and ventricle. This pacemaker, sometimes referred to as the Universal,* or Funke, pacemaker, operates in four modes, adapting to the underlying rhythm automatically according to the schema in Table 11-2. Fig. 11-5 shows a block diagram and representative ECGs for the DDD pacemaker.

A summary of each of the pacemaker modes described is presented in Table 11-3.

*The use of the term *Universal* is inappropriate, since DDD pacemakers are contraindicated in patients who have atrial tachycardias and in patients who conduct retrogradely to the atria with a long VA interval following ventricular stimulation.

Table 11-2. Operating modes of DDD pacemakers

Underlying rhythm	Pacemaker function
Normally conducted sinus rhythm	Totally inhibited
Normally conducted atrial bradycardia	Atrial pacing
Atrial bradycardia and prolonged or blocked AV conduction	AV sequential pacing
Normal sinus rhythm and prolonged or blocked AV conduction	Atrial synchronous ventricular pacing

Table 11-3. Summary of pacemaker modalities

Pacemaker type	ICHD Code	Senses		Paces	
		Atrium	Ventricle	Atrium	Ventricle
Atrial asynchronous	AOO			X*	
Ventricular asynchronous	VOO				X
Atrial demand	AAI, AAT	X		X	
Ventricular demand	VVI, VVT		X		X
Atrial synchronous	VAT	X			X
Atrial synchronous ventricular inhibited	VDD	X	X		X
AV sequential	DVI		X	X	X
Optimal sequential	DDD	X	X	X	X

*X, Pacemaker function.

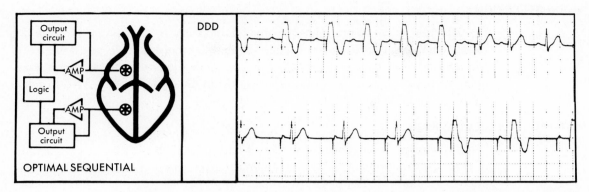

Fig. 11-5. Optimal sequential pacemaker (DDD). The diagram on the left indicates that the DDD pacemaker both senses and paces in the atrium and ventricle. The ECG on the right illustrates this feature. In the first five complete complexes, spontaneous atrial activity (P waves) is not followed by a spontaneous QRS complex within an appropriate PR interval. Therefore a pacemaker spike is delivered to the ventricle following each sensed P wave. The third QRS complex from the end occurs in time to be normally conducted from the P wave but not quite early enough to inhibit the pacemaker spike. The next QRS complexes follow a normal PR interval and thus inhibit pacemaker output. In the lower strip the development of sinus bradycardia triggers atrial pacemaker discharge, and pacemaker spikes precede the onset of P waves. Finally, in the bottom right portion, an atrial stimulus paces the atrium, and a ventricular stimulus paces the ventricle.

MODE SELECTION

Selection of an appropriate pacemaker modality in a given patient can be rather complex, requiring knowledge of the electrophysiologic performance of the SA node, AV conduction pathways, and hemodynamic status. When available, these data can be used with the algorithm illustrated in Fig. 11-6 to select the most suitable device type(s).

ANTITACHYCARDIA PACING[6,27-29]

Tachyarrhythmia control is achieved with pacemakers utilizing one or more of three broad approaches: rate maintenance, termination of tachyarrhythmias, and prevention of onset of tachycardia.

Some therapeutic approaches to control tachyarrhythmias result in symptom-producing bradyarrhythmias. Pacing can be combined with drug therapy in such situations to prevent the bradycardia. For example, digitalis or propranolol, given to treat the tachycardia component of the tachycardia-bradycardia syndrome, may aggravate the bradycardia, establishing the need for pacemaker implantation. Similarly, surgery to interrupt the AV conducting system in a patient who has drug-refractory supraventricular tachycardia with a rapid ventricular rate results in a bradycardia (caused by the AV block) that needs to be treated by pacing.[30]

Certain drug-refractory tachycardias, not amenable to surgical therapy, can sometimes be terminated by a pacemaker designed to produce an appropriate sequence of electrical stimuli. Some of the pacemakers are activated by the patient when perceiving the presence of a tachyarrhythmia,[7] whereas others automatically discharge when the pacemaker senses that a tachycardia is present.[31] Various cadences of stimuli can be delivered, including short bursts at high rates, stimuli that scan the cardiac cycle and automatically change rate[32] or shift the timing of one or more premature stimuli,[33] and coupled or paired stimuli. A *dual-demand* pacemaker is one that automatically delivers stimuli at a fixed, but relatively slow, rate (for example, 70 beats/minute) when it senses the presence of a bradycardia (for example, rates less than 70 beats/minute) or a tachycardia (for example, rates greater than 150 beats/minute).[34] The tachycardia is terminated when an appropriately timed stimulus occurs during a particular part of the tachycardia cycle; this is called *underdrive termination*.[34] Dual-chamber (DVI) pacemakers can be made to operate in the dual-demand mode and pace with short AV intervals for patients who have accessory bypass tracts.[35] Unique custom-built devices with characteristics tailored for specific patients can also be applied. Investigational trials have begun on a low-energy transvenous cardioverter[36] designed to increase the safety and efficacy of chronic electrical control of ventricular tachycardia, and an implantable defibrillator[37] for automatic termination of ventricular fibrillation also is undergoing clinical evaluation.

The preferred therapeutic approach to tachyarrhythmias is prevention. In some cases simply improving the patient's hemodynamic status[11] or restoring normal AV synchrony by means of an appropriate standard pacemaker[12] prevents the development of tachycardia. Some patients have bradycardia-dependent tachycardias (for example, ventricular tachycardia associated with complete AV block), and pacing at normal rates eliminates the ventricular tachycardia. In others

GIVEN: PATIENT NEEDS PACEMAKER
PROBLEM: DETERMINE MOST APPROPRIATE PACING MODALITY

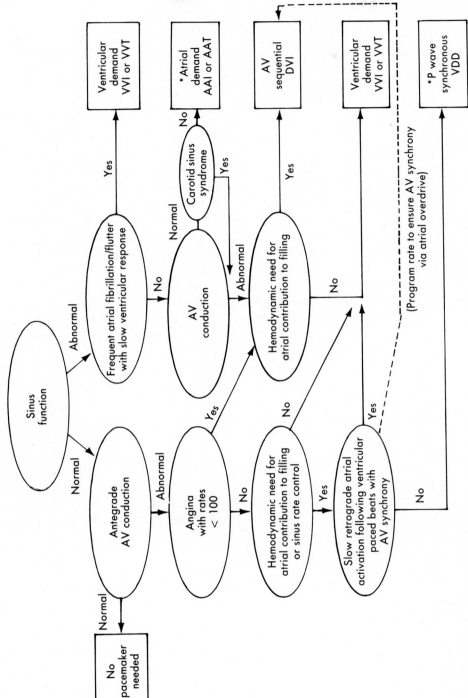

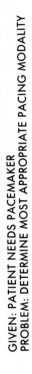

*DDD may be preferred if available.

Fig. 11-6. This "road map" indicates a method for selecting a particular type of pacemaker according to the individual patient's problem, to ensure that the most physiologic pacing modality is chosen. Beginning with the encircled term, *sinus function,* follow the arrows and establish the appropriate pacemaker modality. For example, if SA node function is abnormal (take the right fork) and if the patient has frequent episodes of atrial flutter or atrial fibrillation with a slow ventricular response (go to the right), then a demand ventricular (VVI) pacemaker is indicated. If, however, the patient has abnormal SA node function but does not have atrial flutter or atrial fibrillation and has abnormal AV nodal conduction (go straight down) with a hemodynamic need for atrial contribution to ventricular filling (go to the right), then an AV sequential (DVI) pacemaker is indicated.

pacing at moderately elevated rates suppresses ectopy that might otherwise precipitate tachycardias. In patients with accessory AV pathways use of an atrial synchronous or DDD pacemaker with a suitably short AV interval may preclude development of a reciprocating tachycardia while preserving normal sinus control of ventricular rate.[38]

Currently, pacing for tachyarrhythmia control accounts for less than 3% of all pacemaker implantations,[3] although it is anticipated that this indication will become increasingly frequent in the future.

Programmability[39-41]

The vast majority of permanent pacemaker implants today employ a programmable pacemaker. *Programmability* can be defined as noninvasive, reversible alteration of the electronically controlled performance of an implantable device such as a pacemaker. Use of a simple magnet to convert a demand pacemaker to its asynchronous mode generally is excluded from this definition, although it is in reality a simple form of programming. In the most advanced pacemakers many performance characteristics are programmable, including rate, stimulus output amplitude or duration, amplifier sensitivity, amplifier refractory period, hysteresis, pacing mode (for example, unipolar/bipolar, VVI/VVT/VOO), and operation of special information transfer channels (telemetry of intracardiac electrograms, programmed settings, and device operation indicators, such as "marker channel," battery status, and lead impedance). Furthermore, in dual-chamber pacemakers it is frequently possible to program AV intervals, atrial rate tracking limits, and the pacing mode (for example, DDD to DVI or VVI).

Programmability is of benefit to the clinician and patient in that it allows optimizing pacemaker function for specific patient needs, minimizes the need for invasive procedures to correct malfunctions or to revise the system to meet changing patient needs, and facilitates troubleshooting procedures. Table 11-4 indicates applications for many of the commonly available programmable parameters. It should be emphasized that programmability must be used with care, since it presents the risk of establishing inappropriate parameter settings (for example, insufficient output energy to maintain capture, dangerously high or low rates) and imposes a greater need for maintaining accurate records to prevent erroneous decisions based on lack of knowledge about the rationale for the current status of the programmed settings in a given patient.

Power sources

Nearly all pacemakers, with the exception of some research units, are battery powered. External pacemakers typically use standard alkaline or mercury batteries of the type used in common household appliances (such as transistor radios, flashlights), although an occasional external device uses a rechargeable or lithium battery.

Implantable pacemakers are powered by one of five broad energy sources: mercury zinc batteries, rechargeable batteries, nuclear batteries, lithium batteries, or radio frequency energy broadcast to the pacemaker from an external device called a transmitter.

Mercury zinc batteries were the standard power source for nearly all pacemakers manufactured during the 1960s and early 1970s. These batteries made the implantable pacemaker a practical reality, but they are heavy, they lose a significant amount of their capacity to internal intrinsic losses ("self-discharge"), so that pacer longevity is reduced (typically 24 to 42 months), and they produce hydrogen gas, making it impractical to hermetically seal the pacemaker from damaging body fluids. Virtually none of today's pacemakers use mercury zinc cells.

Rechargeable batteries have been used successfully in pacemakers, but they have never achieved wide acceptance because they require frequent attention from the patient or his family to maintain the battery in a charged state, and, more important, because the lithium battery (described later) has proven to be so effective and trouble free that it has become the present power source of choice.

In the early 1970s nuclear batteries were developed for use in implantable pacemakers. The most commonly employed nuclear battery converted the heat generated by the decay of radioisotopic plutonium into electrical energy. Pacemakers using these batteries have demonstrated the greatest actual longevity of any pacemaker to date, surpassing in performance even the lithium battery as a pacemaker power source. Unfortunately, governmental regulations imposed on the implanting physicians and on the manufacturers have made nuclear power sources unacceptable from an economic standpoint.

Virtually all current pacemakers are powered by one of the many varieties of the lithium battery. These batteries share certain characteristics that make them especially suitable for implantable use, yet they exhibit significant differences. Each of the lithium systems offers high-energy density and low internal losses caused by self-discharge. Most of the systems can be hermetically sealed to prevent ingress of body fluids and egress of damaging battery materials. Each system offers unique electrical characteristics and varying degrees of reliability.[44,45] The most commonly used lithium batteries are the lithium iodide, lithium cupric sulfide, and lithium silver chromate.

Reported performance characteristics of the major power sources show clearly the substantial progress made toward creating a pacemaker that will have sufficient longevity to prevent the need for replacement in the majority of patients. In 1981, survival probabilities were reported for large groups of pacemakers using

Table 11-4. Applications of programmable pacemaker parameters

Parameter	Patient/pacemaker optimization	Diagnostic applications	Correction of malfunctions
Rate	Improve cardiac output by allowing greater range of conducted sinus activity. Minimize angina by keeping the rate below that which produces pain. Suppress arrhythmias. Adapt pulse generator to pediatric needs (faster rates). Terminate tachycardias with short rapid bursts. Minimize "pacemaker syndrome" (caused by AV dissociation) by selecting low rate.	Suppress pacing to access underlying rhythm by ECG. Test AV conduction with an atrial pacemaker by determining rates at which AV nodal Wenckebach behavior occurs. Test sinus function with an atrial pacemaker by using bursts of rapid pacing to determine SA node recovery times. Confirm atrial capture by altering pacemaker rate and observing concomitant ventricular rate change.	
Output, amplitude, or duration	Maximize pulse generator longevity by selecting output energy that provides the minimal level of stimulation consistent with reliable maintenance of pacing. Provide increased energy for high threshold patients. Avoid extracardiac stimulation (pectoral muscle, phrenic nerve).	Evaluate pacing threshold.	Regain capture following threshold increases caused by infarcts, electrolyte disturbances, drugs. Eliminate diaphragmatic or pectoral muscle stimulation.
Amplifier sensitivity	Establish appropriate sensitivity to detect intracardiac electrogram while avoiding sensing of extraneous signals (pectoral muscle potentials, electromagnetic interference). Increase sensitivity for atrial sensing applications.	Alter sensitivity to evaluate possible sources of oversensing or undersensing.	Compensate for changes in intracardiac electrogram amplitude. Resolve oversensing of T waves, muscle potentials, electromagnetic interference.
Refractory period	Extend duration for atrial applications to avoid sensing conducted R waves. Shorten duration in ventricular applications to detect closely coupled ectopic events.	Alter duration to evaluate possible causes of over- or undersensing.	Lengthen duration to avoid T wave sensing. Shorten duration to eliminate failure to sense closely coupled ectopic events.
Hysteresis	Minimize pacemaker syndrome by allowing sinus rhythm over widest possible rate range while establishing adequately high pacing rate when needed.		
Unipolar/bipolar		Evaluate lead fracture (bipolar → unipolar). Enhance stimulus artifact visibility on ECG (bipolar → unipolar).	Convert to unipolar operation to regain capture in case of lead fracture. Change mode to adapt to altered electrogram causing sensing failure.

Table 11-4. Applications of programmable pacemaker parameters—cont'd

Parameter	Patient/pacemaker optimization	Diagnostic applications	Correction of malfunctions
Unipolar/bipolar—cont'd		Evaluate oversensing (unipolar → bipolar).	Convert to bipolar to eliminate sensing of myopotentials. Convert to bipolar to avoid extracardiac stimulation.
Mode	Select optimum mode (e.g., VDD for patients who have normal sinus function and impaired AV conduction). Alter mode if patient's needs change (e.g., VDD → DVI if patient develops sinus bradycardia).	Establish triggered mode to enable external control of pacemaker from chest electrodes and external stimulator to perform noninvasive electrophysiologic studies of sinus function, AV conduction, efficacy of antiarrhythmic agents. Confirm oversensing signal source by selecting triggered mode.	Change to backup mode (e.g., VVI) if atrial portion of dual-chamber system is nonfunctional (e.g., lead displacement). Prevent oversensing by selecting asynchronous mode.
AV delay	Maximize hemodynamic efficacy. Control or prevent tachyarrhythmias.		
Atrial-rate–tracking limit	Maintain widest range of sinus rate control without incurring angina. Control ventricular response to atrial arrhythmias. Prevent rapid synchronization to dissociated atrial activity during ventricular escape pacing in VDD mode. Prevent occurrence of retrograde atrial activity that would result from a long delay between the triggering event in the atrium and the resultant stimulus in the ventricle. This retrograde activity can continuously trigger the pacemaker causing "pacemaker tachycardia."	Select high rate limit for stress testing.	Reduce tracking rate limit if pectoral muscle activity triggers rapid pacing.
Telemetry		Compare programmed settings to actual device operation. Use marker channel indicators to determine which events pacemaker is causing and which events are being sensed. Use electrogram to evaluate causes of under- or over-sensing. Use electrogram to evaluate drug effects on myocardium.	

the power sources described.[45] A series of approximately 2000 mercury zinc pacemakers showed a cumulative survival probability of 40% at a longevity of 4 years. Six thousand lithium pacemakers showed a cumulative survival probability of 86% at a 6.8-year longevity, and a small series of 143 nuclear pacemakers exhibited a survival probability of 94% at a longevity of 6.8 years. These data reflect actual clinical results and clearly demonstrate the longevity advantages of nuclear and lithium power sources.

A very small group of special-purpose antitachycardia pacemakers is powered by radio frequency energy transmitted through the body to the implantable device. This is practical because these pacemakers are not required to pace constantly but are used to generate short bursts of rapid asynchronous stimuli to terminate episodes of tachycardia. These devices (Fig. 11-7) are manually activated by the patient who, when experiencing the symptoms induced by tachycardia, places a small, battery-powered transmitter over the implant site and presses a button, causing the transmitter to energize the implantable stimulator. This technique eliminates the need, caused by power source depletion, for pacemaker replacement and makes it possible to reduce the size and weight of the implantable generator.

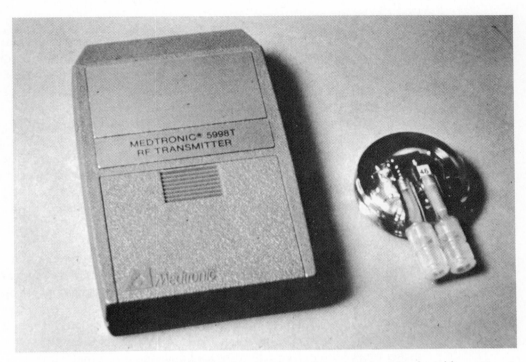

Fig. 11-7. Radio-frequency–powered antitachycardia pacemaker. Implantable portion is shown on the right and the external portion (RF transmitter), operated by the patient, is shown on the left.

Pacemaker electrode systems ("leads")[46,47]

The pulse generator is electrically connected to the heart by means of a wire and electrode system referred to as a *lead*. The electrodes may be unipolar or bipolar. In bipolar systems the positive and negative electrodes both are located within the cardiac chamber and are in contact with the endocardium or are on the heart. Unipolar systems place only the negative electrode at the heart and use a large area anode electrode, usually the metallic housing of the pulse generator, at a remote location. Either approach is clinically acceptable. Bipolar systems are less susceptible to extraneous electromagnetic interference (such as electrical signals generated by nearby power lines, automobile spark plugs, and radio transmitters), extracardiac myopotential interference, unwanted extracardiac stimulation, or threshold changes caused by defibrillatory currents.

TRANSVENOUS

Permanent pacing leads are designed for either transvenous or epicardial placement. Transvenous leads are usually implanted within the right ventricular apex for ventricular pacing and in the right atrial appendage or coronary sinus for atrial applications. The leads are typically inserted via the cephalic, subclavian, or external jugular veins, using fluoroscopy for visualization and stiff wires (stylets) inserted within the lumen of the lead for control during positioning. (The stylets must be removed following lead placement to avoid damaging the lead.) A rapid technique for lead placement in the subclavian vein with minimal trauma employs a simple venipuncture using a special percutaneous lead introducer.[48] This approach is gaining favor and involves minimal risk, although there is the possibility of inadvertently entering the pleural cavity or the arterial system. The newly introduced urethane-insulated leads have reduced diameters and a decreased coefficient of friction, making it possible to pass an atrial and a ventricular lead through a single vein, facilitating use of dual-chamber pacemakers.[49,50]

Transvenous leads come in a variety of designs, each purporting to ensure stable permanent positioning of the electrodes.[51-57] Fig. 11-8 includes examples of ventricular and atrial leads with flanges, tines, barbs, and screws for fixation. Many atrial leads also incorporate a J shape to aid in proper positioning within the atrial appendage. The transvenous approach is associated with very low morbidity and, with current lead designs, a very low rate of displacement.[51-52]

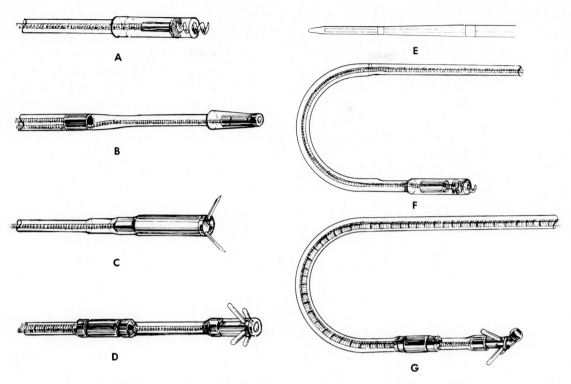

Fig. 11-8. Example of atrial and ventricular transvenous pacemaker electrodes. **A,** Unipolar endocardial urethane lead with a screw-in tip electrode for active fixation to the atrial or ventricular endocardial surface (Medtronic model 6957). **B,** Bipolar ventricular electrode utilizing flanged Silastic tip for positioning stability (Medtronic model 6901R). **C,** Unipolar ventricular electrode with extensible metallic barb that provides active fixation to the ventricular myocardium (Biotronic IE 65-I). **D,** Bipolar urethane ventricular electrode with flexible tines adjacent to the ring-tip electrode. The tines provide passive lead fixation by lodging within the trabecular structure of the ventricle (Medtronic model 6972). **E,** Bipolar Silastic lead designed for stable placement in the coronary sinus; the electrodes are shaped for atrial pacing applications (Medtronic 6992). **F,** Unipolar urethane lead with J shape and screw-in tip electrode for active fixation to the atrial endocardial surface (Medtronic 6957J). **G,** Bipolar urethane atrial lead with J shape and flexible tines adjacent to the tip electrode. The J shape and tines provide passive fixation of the electrode within the atrium (Medtronic model 6990U).

EPICARDIAL

Epicardial leads are used less frequently than transvenous systems, but they are of particular benefit in problem patients who have smooth, dilated right ventricles and in patients who have truncated right atrial appendages. The placement approach depends on the type of epicardial electrode used. A transthoracic approach (thoracotomy) is used to apply electrodes that are sutured to the myocardium. More commonly, for ventricular applications a sutureless corkscrew electrode is used, since this device can be applied with a transmediastinal approach avoiding entrance into the pleural cavity and reducing morbidity and discomfort.[58] Fig. 11-9 shows examples of myocardial electrodes.

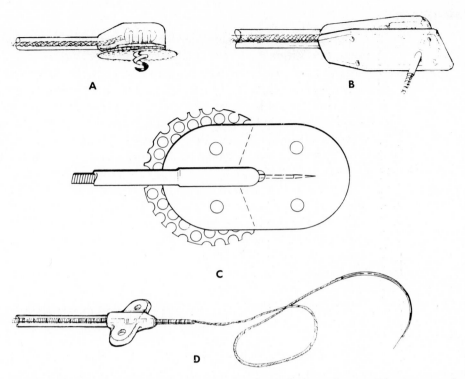

Fig. 11-9. Examples of atrial and ventricular epicardial electrodes. **A,** Silastic sutureless unipolar ventricular electrode with corkscrew tip. Positive fixation is achieved by screwing the electrode into the myocardium (Medtronic model 6917A). **B,** Silastic unipolar epicardial electrode designed to be sutured to either the atrial or ventricular myocardium (Medtronic model 5815A). **C,** Urethane unipolar epicardial barbed-hook electrode providing positive fixation (without sutures) to either the atrial or ventricular myocardium (Medtronic model 4951). **D,** Silastic unipolar electrode for atrial or ventricular use. The needle and suture material extending from the exposed stainless steel electrode are used to fasten the electrode directly to the myocardium (Teletronix 030-170).

TEMPORARY

Temporary pacing leads include transvenous catheter electrodes, wire electrodes, and, in extreme circumstance, precordial surface electrodes. Temporary transvenous catheter electrodes can be placed in a fashion similar to that used for permanent leads. Placement is facilitated by designing the catheters to be stiffer than would be acceptable for permanent use, and by sometimes incorporating additional aids such as inflatable balloons or cuffs that "float" the catheter in the bloodstream to the right ventricle. In the absence of fluoroscopy, ECG recordings from the catheter enable the user to determine the location of the electrodes (Fig. 11-10).

Heart wires are frequently placed in the atria and ventricles of patients at the time of open heart surgery. These stainless steel wires are used during the surgical procedure and during the postoperative recovery phase. In emergency situations wire electrodes can be inserted percutaneously into the heart by a pericardiocentesis (or similar) needle.

Similarly, during emergencies surface skin electrodes placed on the chest wall can be stimulated with very high (and quite painful) voltages to achieve cardiac pacing transthoracically. Such an approach should be used only until a transvenous catheter electrode can be positioned. Recently an improved technique for noninvasive pacing has been reported to be of minimal discomfort and suitable for prolonged use. Special, large surface area electrodes and external pulse generators with very wide (about 40 msec) stimulus pulse widths are required.[59] This may offer a viable approach if such equipment can be obtained readily.

For temporary and permanent pacing it is important to place the electrodes in a position that provides acceptably low stimulation thresholds and sufficiently large intracardiac signals to be sensed by the pulse generator. Generally this implies acute thresholds of less than 2 mA and 1.25 V, with ventricular electrograms greater than 4mV or atrial electrograms in excess of 2mV. Thresholds generally rise following acute positioning, reaching a peak two to four times the acute values within the first 2 to 6 weeks and then falling to intermediate values.[60] The electrogram typically decreases in amplitude by 15%; its rate of rise with respect to time (slew rate) decreases as much as 50% with maturation of the implant.[61] These factors must be considered when evaluating the appropriateness of a given lead position.

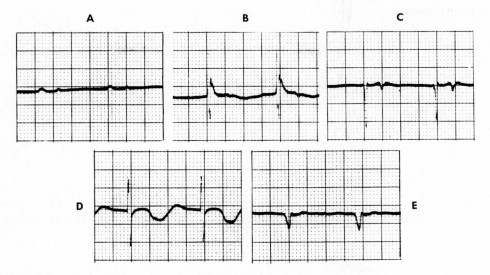

Fig. 11-10. Electrograms obtained when bipolar electrode is located in high superior vena cava **(A)**, superior vena cava/right atrium **(B)**, right atrium **(C)**, right ventricle **(D)**, and pulmonary artery **(E)**. All tracings calibrated at 1 mV/cm except **D**, which is recorded at half standard.

Postimplantation follow-up[62]

Despite the reliability demonstrated by current pacemakers, it is important to monitor the patient and the pacemaker system regularly after implantation. Such monitoring has four major goals: evaluate electrical function of the pacing system to detect malfunctions or imminent power-source depletion; evaluate the implant site for possible mechanical difficulties such as erosion or infection; detect progression of the patient's cardiac problems, which may necessitate reprogramming or revising the pacing system or accompanying drug regimen; and both provide patient reassurance that due concern and attention is being given his or her progress and offer an opportunity to discuss concerns that may arise.

The follow-up schedule should be arranged to provide close monitoring during the immediate postimplantation period, moderately frequent observation during the routine service life of the system, and increased surveillance as the system nears completion of its service life. A suggested schedule is 6 weeks after implantation, twice annually beginning 6 months after implantation, and monthly once initial signs of power-source depletion are observed (in almost all pacemakers this appears as a rate decrease when monitored with a magnet over the pulse generator). Given the longevity of modern systems, it may be counter-productive to attempt to stretch out the last few months of service by frequent monitoring since this will probably add but 5% to 10% to the total service life while increasing monitoring costs by 30% to 40%.

Follow-up visits should be scheduled in the physician's office or in a special pacemaker clinic where the patient can be seen in person. (Telephone monitoring of the patient's ECG, pacing rate, and pulse generator stimulus duration can be of value as a supplement between personal evaluations but should not replace office visits.) Each visit should include a recording of a 12-lead ECG with a rhythm strip showing that the pacemaker appropriately captures and senses, a measurement of pacemaker parameters with appropriate rate and pulse width measurement equipment, and a general physical examination including careful scrutiny of the pacemaker pocket. If a problem is evident or if the patient reports symptoms, an x-ray film may be obtained to evaluate the lead and its position, blood tests may help uncover threshold problems related to electrolyte imbalances, and long-term ambulatory monitoring may be indicated if intermittent failures are suspected. The results of the follow-up procedure should be carefully recorded,[63] since much of the required analysis depends on changes in operation rather than on absolute values of measured parameters. This record is especially important when following patients who have programmable pacemakers[64] and for whom changes may be totally innocuous if intentional (such as a rate change programmed to improve cardiac output) or may signify device-performance problems (such as a rate decrease caused by battery depletion).

Care should be exercised in selecting follow-up equipment, and data must be analyzed with full understanding and knowledge of the idiosyncrasies of the equipment used. For example, digital monitoring and recording systems frequently do not register the pacemaker stimulus artifact reliably and reproducibly because of its extremely short duration. As a result, the artifact may not always be recorded even if present, or its polarity and amplitude may vary markedly throughout the recording. On the other hand, such systems may substitute a standardized artifact for the real signal, eliminating diagnostic information in the process. As another example, some follow-up clinics perform waveform analysis using an oscilloscope or special ECG machine to display the waveshape of the pacemaker stimulus. One must be fully aware of the correct waveshape for each pacemaker to be evaluated. Modern pacemakers frequently produce much more complex stimulus pulse shapes than the traditional "square wave," and it is not unusual for such waveforms to be misread as signs of malfunction.

An often underestimated benefit of follow-up is a reduction in patient anxiety. A clear answer to a simple question can be extremely important to a patient's well-being. In recognition of this, some clinics have formed pacemaker clubs, which allow patients to meet periodically to compare notes and provide mutual support.

Troubleshooting[65-67]

Complex systems involving electrical, mechanical, and physiologic interactions will inevitably develop malfunctions, and pacemakers are no exception. Fortunately, the detection and correction of such problems are relatively straightforward for the knowledgeable user if appropriate equipment is available.

EQUIPMENT

The most useful troubleshooting tool is a *12-lead ECG machine*. This permits evaluation of pacemaker sensing, capture, and approximate rate, evaluation of electrode positioning (by vector analysis of ventricular activity), and confirmation of appropriate function for the mode of pacing employed. Multiple ECG leads are necessary for vector analysis of lead positioning and are frequently helpful in increasing visibility of small artifacts produced by bipolar systems or in evaluating atrial activity when dealing with dual-chamber or atrial demand pacemakers.

A *digital counter* is useful in obtaining accurate rate and pulse width information. These counters may be supplied as specialized patient monitors, built into pacemaker programmers, or purchased alone. Such devices are necessary when evaluating pacing rate and pulse width changes caused by battery depletion, component failure, or reprogramming.

A *magnet* should always be available for troubleshooting sessions. Nearly all pacemakers can be converted to asynchronous operation by the placement of a magnet over the generator site. This enables evaluation of capture when the patient's intrinsic rhythm inhibits the pacemaker and can be useful in diagnosing oversensing by disabling all sensing function. Magnet application should be used with care, since some pacemakers can be programmed by application of a suitable magnet, and there is always a definite but slight risk of inducing tachyarrhythmias when pacing asynchronously.

Carotid sinus massage or Valsalva maneuver may slow a patient's intrinsic rhythm and induce pacing. Such a procedure may be used to evaluate capture if a pacemaker fails to respond to magnet application because of either a component failure or a unique design having no asynchronous magnet mode.

Exercise may be used to speed the patient's spontaneous rate in the evaluation of sensing capability.

Chest wall stimulation with an external stimulator connected to precordial surface electrodes can be utilized to test sensing function and to determine rate tracking limits for atrial tracing pacemakers (VAT, VDD, DDD).

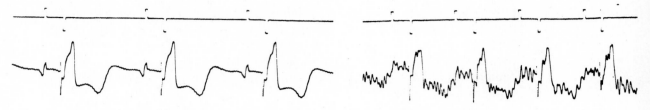

Fig. 11-11. Lower tracing is lead III surface ECG from patient with normally functioning Medtronic "Enertrax" atrial synchronous ventricular inhibited pacemaker. Upper tracing is marker channel transmitted by implanted pacemaker, indicating detection of atrial activity (small positive deflection) and pacing in ventricles (larger negative deflection). Right half of panel was recorded during exercise to show utility of marker channel in identifying atrial activity in presence of interference.

Manipulation of the pulse generator in its pocket can sometimes elicit electrocardiographic signs of a loose connection or damaged lead close to the generator site.

X-ray examination or fluoroscopy of the chest and pacemaker system in multiple views helps determine lead position, gross lead fractures, and disconnections at the generator. A base-line x-ray film should be obtained before the patient is discharged, following implantation of the system.

An *oscilloscope* or special ECG recorder designed to display the waveshape of the pacemaker stimulus is used by some centers to evaluate lead problems or unusual component failures.

A pacemaker *programmer* is an extremely useful troubleshooting tool in dealing with a programmable pacemaker, allowing the user to vary stimulus strength, amplifier sensitivity, rates, refractory periods, and pacing modes. This permits noninvasive threshold evaluation and, in some of the newer systems, permits the user to obtain noninvasive intracardiac electrograms to evaluate sensing operation. Many systems include digital telemetry of the programmed settings of the pacemaker allowing actual performance to be compared to expected performance. The most sophisticated systems provide a *marker channel,* a noninvasively telemetered ECG-like tracing, which in conjunction with a surface ECG clearly identifies pacemaker sensing and pacing operations (Fig. 11-11).

Invasive procedures are necessary if noninvasive approaches fail. A *pacing system analyzer* is the primary tool for invasive troubleshooting. This instrument typically can analyze the implantable pulse generator function (sensitivities, refractory periods, rates, pulse widths, and amplitudes), evaluate lead integrity and positioning, and provide electrophysiologic patient data (stimulation thresholds, electrogram amplitudes, AV conduction, sinus function).

In addition to the troubleshooting hardware, it is equally important to have detailed patient records, including prior ECGs and x-ray films, and full information on the characteristics of the implanted system. It is unfortunately common for a normally functioning pacemaker to be diagnosed as malfunctioning simply because of inadequate understanding of proper device operation. Systems with

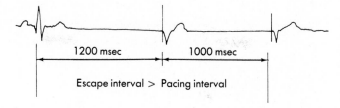

Fig. 11-12. Diagrammatic representation of operation of a VVI pacemaker incorporating hysteresis. The last beat of the patient's sinus rhythm is shown as the first complex on the left. Spontaneous sinus bradycardia results, and the pacemaker "escapes" at an interval of 1200 msec. The subsequent pacing interval is 1000 msec, however; thus the escape interval of the pacemaker exceeds the pacing interval (in other words, the initial escape rate of pacemaker discharge is *slower* than the subsequent rate of pacing) to allow the patient to remain in a normally conducted rhythm for as much of the time as possible.

hysteresis,* special antitachycardia pacemakers, and synchronous pacemakers are especially vulnerable to misdiagnosis.

Pacemaker-related problems fall into five broad cateogries: failure to pace, loss of sensing, oversensing, pacing at an altered rate, and undesirable patient/pacemaker interactions.

FAILURE TO PACE

Failure to pace implies nondelivery of a stimulus or delivery of an ineffective stimulus that fails to depolarize or "capture" the myocardium. Failure to deliver a stimulus can result from various factors: improper connection of the lead to the generator (as when set screws are not tightened); broken lead wires with no insulation defect; "crosstalk" between atrial and ventricular portions of dual-chamber pacemakers so that the atrial stimulus is sensed by the ventricular amplifier, inhibiting the ventricular stimulus (caused by improper electrode placement or incorrect electrode types); pulse generator component failure; or power source depletion. Occasionally, a misdiagnosis of failure to pace is made when a normally functioning pacemaker is merely inhibited by the patient's intrinsic rhythm. This is especially common with programmable pacemakers set at relatively low rates. (Inappropriate nondelivery of a stimulus also may be caused by oversensing, discussed later.)

Loss of capture may be caused by lead dislodgement (the most common cause), myocardial perforation with lead migration to an extracardiac position, failure of lead insulation and/or wire fracture; increased stimulation threshold caused by infarction, drug effects, electrolyte imbalances, or fibrosis at the electrode site, or inappropriate programming of pacemaker stimulus strength. Lack of capture when a stimulus is delivered during the myocardial refractory period is a frequent source of misdiagnosis.

*Pacemakers with hysteresis are designed to work as follows: the escape interval (before pacing) following the last sensed spontaneous activity exceeds the interval between subsequent consecutive pacing artifacts. This allows maintenance of normal sinus rhythm over a wide range of rates (pacemaker-inhibited) while ensuring an adequate pacing rate when needed. This type of operation is diagrammed in Fig. 11-12.

LOSS OF SENSING

A pacemaker may fail to sense intracardiac signals, resulting in competitive pacing or, in the case of atrial synchronous units, loss of AV synchrony. This may be caused by the following: lead dislodgement (the most common cause); inadequate amplitude or waveshape of the intracardiac electrogram caused by inappropriate lead placement, fibrosis, infarct, drugs, or electrolyte disturbances; inappropriate programming of amplifier sensitivity, refractory periods, or mode (for example, AOO, VOO); lead fracture or insulation defect; connector defect; or component failure (such as a stuck magnetic reedswitch).

Occasionally, a misdiagnosis of sensing failure is made when spontaneous activity occurs simultaneously with delivery of the pacemaker stimulus and results in fusion beats. The reason for this is as follows. Electrical activity may occur within the myocardium and be visible on the surface ECG record before it reaches the pacemaker electrode site. Concurrently, the pacemaker escape interval may elapse with resultant stimulation just before arrival of the spontaneous depolarization. This apparent failure to sense is, in fact, perfectly normal operation. Another cause of apparent sensing failure is reversion to asynchronous operation in the presence of electromagnetic interference—also a normal mode of operation for many pacemakers. Finally, closely coupled intracardiac signals may occur within the pacemaker refractory period and not be sensed. This is frequently seen with certain AV sequential (DVI) pacemakers, which initiate the ventricular sensing amplifier refractory period upon stimulating in the atrium. If the atrial response propagates to the ventricles, the pacemaker will not sense this conducted ventricular activity but will stimulate into the refractory tissue. This is normal operation for such "committed" DVI devices (Fig. 11-13).

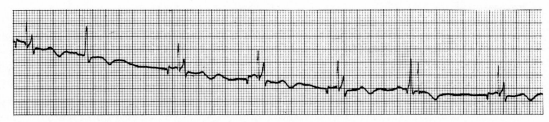

Fig. 11-13. Surface ECG (monitor lead) demonstrating an example of a "committed" mode DVI pacemaker. Note that the first, third, fourth, fifth, and seventh complexes are initiated by an atrial spike (small negative deflection) that paces the atrium and then a ventricular spike (large upright deflection) that paces the ventricle. The second QRS complex occurs sufficiently early to inhibit pacemaker discharge. However, the sixth QRS complex occurs early, but not early enough to inhibit the atrial discharge. Following the atrial spike (seen as the initial negative deflection preceding the onset of the QRS complex, after the P wave) a conducted QRS occurs. However, this QRS complex is not sensed by the pacemaker, which is committed into delivering a pacemaker spike (large upright spike following the QRS complex in the ST segment) regardless of spontaneous ventricular activity.

OVERSENSING

Occasionally a pacemaker will sense signals other than those cardiac signals that it is designed to detect, a phenomenon referred to as *oversensing*. Ventricular sensing pacemakers (DVI, VVI, VVT, VDD, DDD) may sense T waves if the amplifier is too sensitive or has too short a refractory period, or if the patient has unusually large or delayed T waves, as in hyperkalemia or hypocalcemia. A dislodged ventricular lead resting near the right ventricular outflow tract may cause inappropriate sensing of atrial activity. Conversely, atrial sensing pacemakers (AAI, AAT, VAT, VDD, DDD) may inappropriately sense ventricular activity if the atrial amplifier refractory period is too short, or if the atrial signals are too small to be sensed with consequent failure to initiate appropriate atrial refractory periods. Some AV sequential pacemakers (DVI) may sense delivery of an atrial stimulus and inhibit the ventricular stimulus ("crosstalk") if they are used with incorrectly spaced bipolar electrodes, or if the atrial and ventricular electrodes are not separated by a suitable distance (typically 4 cm, minimum).

Unipolar pacemakers may sense skeletal muscle potentials generated by contraction of the major pectoralis muscles, resulting in inappropriate inhibition (AAI, VVI, DVI, VDD, DDD) or triggering (AAT, VVT, VAT, VDD, DDD) of stimuli.

All pacemakers except asynchronous devices sense the voltage changes produced when a lead with a hairline fracture or loose connection makes intermittent contact or when two endocardial leads come into contact. Electromagnetic interference from power lines, radio or television transmitters, and other electrical noise sources may occasionally be sensed, especially by unipolar pacemakers. Sometimes this may result in inhibition or triggering, but it more commonly produces reversion to the asynchronous mode that provides the patient with continued pacing support. Very rarely, a pacemaker may sense the afterpotentials remaining on a lead following delivery of a stimulus. This is most commonly the result of using very wide pulse widths or excessively short refractory periods.

In all cases of suspected oversensing, placing the pacemaker in an asynchronous mode (with application of a magnet if it is a permanent pacemaker, or turning off the sensitivity if it is an external pacemaker) will abolish the symptoms caused by the pacemaker malfunction and confirm the diagnosis.

PACING AT AN ALTERED RATE

A fairly common cause for concern is apparent operation of a pacemaker at an unexpected rate. This can be an indication of a real problem with the pacemaker system but more frequently reflects a diagnostic error.

The possible true causes of unexpected pacing at an altered rate include the following: oversensing that induces rate slowing caused by inhibition or rate acceleration caused by triggering; rate drift, a gradual benign shift of the pacing rate caused by component aging or temperature effects (most commonly found in older pacemakers that do not use digital timing circuits); rate slowdown built into most pacemakers to indicate approaching power source depletion; and component failure (usually causing either no stimulus output or a rapid stimulation rate typically limited to less than 150 beats/minute by "runaway" protection circuits).

Frequent causes of pacing at an altered rate when there is no system failure include the following: presence of a rate hysteresis that produces a long escape interval following sensed activity; reprogramming of a programmable pacemaker without proper recording of the change in the patient records; tracking of spontaneous intrinsic cardiac rate accelerations with VVT, AAT, VAT, VDD, or DDD pacemakers; failure of the reader to note a nearly isoelectric atrial or ventricular complex in a single-lead ECG tracing so that the pacemaker appears to have a prolonged stimulus-to-stimulus interval; misinterpretation of nonpacemaker artifacts such as rapid spike potentials generated by muscle fasciculation or electrical noise in the ECG recording system; lack of familiarity with device operation (such as a DVI pacemaker perceived to be pacing the ventricles at a rate equivalent to its VA interval when it is, in fact, pacing atrially and appropriately inhibiting the ventricular stimulus in response to conducted ventricular activity).

UNDESIRABLE PATIENT/PACEMAKER INTERACTIONS

Occasionally, there can develop undesirable patient/pacemaker system interactions. The pacemaker pocket may become infected or develop hematomas, or the generator may erode through the pocket site. These problems occur less frequently with the current small, lightweight generators. Some patients exhibit "twiddler's syndrome," playing with their pulse generators and rotating them in their pockets, retracting the lead and producing total system failure.

Extracardiac stimulation of the pectoralis muscles or diaphragm may be observed. These problems are generally restricted to unipolar pacemakers, although they have been reported, in rare instances, with bipolar systems. Decreasing the pulse width, voltage, or current of the stimulus can be useful in eliminating or reducing such extracardiac stimulation.

Incorrect pacing mode selection for a given patient or changes in a patient's postimplantation status can have serious consequences. For example, atrial tracking pacemakers (VAT, VDD, DDD) may detect slowly conducted retrograde atrial activity (long RP interval) following ventricular stimulation, inducing "pacemaker tachycardia" with a rate equal to the pacemaker's upper rate limit. Patients may respond poorly to other specific pacing modes depending on their underlying hemodynamic and electrophysiologic substrates. In many such cases, the use of multiprogrammable pacemakers allows the clinician to alter the pacing system characteristics without resorting to invasive procedures.

AN ILLUSTRATIVE APPROACH

The following hypothetical example demonstrates how one troubleshoots a pacemaker malfunction, in this case intermittent loss of capture and failure to sense spontaneous ventricular activity (Fig. 11-14). The patient has a ventricular demand (VVI) pacemaker implanted 1 year ago.

The first step in troubleshooting is to list the likely causes of the symptoms. Since there are two malfunctions in this example, it is highly probable, although not absolutely certain, that there is a common cause. The most likely etiologies are these:

Lack of capture	Lack of sensing
Lead dislodgement, perforation	Lead dislodgement, perforation
Lead wire fracture	Lead wire fracture
Lead insulation failure	Lead insulation failure
Pulse generator failure	Pulse generator failure
Inappropriate programming of output energy	Inappropriate programming of amplifier sensitivity or refractory period
High threshold	Inadequate electrogram amplitude (caused by infarct, electrolyte disturbance, myocardial disease)
Misread ECG ("loss of capture" seen only when stimulus occurs during cardiac refractory period)	Electromagnetic interference–induced (EMI) reversion to asynchronous mode
	Stuck reed switch
	Misread ECG (fusion beats)

Analysis should begin by comparing a current 12-lead ECG to a base-line tracing predating occurrence of the problem. The current tracing should be carefully reviewed to prevent misinterpretation of fusion beats as sensing failure or pacing artifacts during the cardiac refractory period as lack of capture. EMI-induced reversion to the asynchronous mode can usually be eliminated as a cause if the problem of nonsensing persists in a 12-lead ECG that shows no signs of electrical interference. Comparison of the current and base-line ECGs establishes the presence or absence of lead position changes, including perforation, as evidenced by shifts in the paced QRS vector and pacing artifact vector.* An x-ray examination provides confirmation of significant dislodgements. Insulation defects in the lead will result in vector changes in the pacing artifact but usually not in the paced QRS complex.

Application of a magnet should result in pacing without sensing. In most pacemakers magnet application alters the pacing rate (sometimes by only a few milliseconds), confirming that the reed switch is functioning and allowing one to eliminate the possibility of nonsensing caused by a stuck reed switch.

If inappropriate programming is thought to be the problem, it is a simple matter to reprogram the amplifier sensitivity and refractory period to restore sensing and to increase the stimulus intensity to restore capture. If such reprogramming fails to resolve the problem or if the parameter settings required are not within normally accepted bounds, then inappropriate programming can be excluded.

*Digital ECG systems with low sampling rates cannot be used to determine pacemaker artifact vector's reliability.

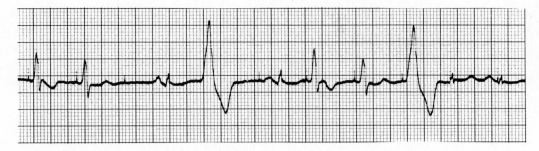

Fig. 11-14. Failure of a VVI pacemaker. Note that pacing stimuli occasionally fail to elicit a paced QRS complex and also occasionally fail to sense spontaneous electrical activity. Lead II.

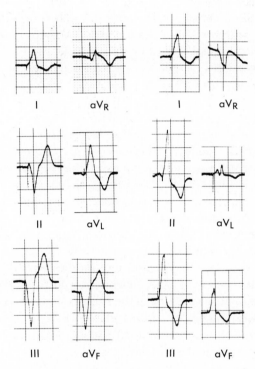

Fig. 11-15. ECG leads I, II, III, aV$_R$, aV$_L$, and aV$_F$ were recorded before *(left panel)* and after *(right panel)* pacemaker malfunction. VVI pacemaker developed sensing and capture problems. Note that the vector and amplitude of the spikes are different in the two 12-lead ECGs and that the generated QRS complexes also are different. This ECG example is most consistent with migration of the pacing electrode from its initial appropriate location in the right ventricular apex to a different position in the ventricle. This was the case, and the lead was repositioned.

Wire fracture can produce nonsensing and lack of capture, but it is generally accompanied by random resetting of the escape interval as the broken wire ends touch intermittently. An x-ray examination can sometimes be helpful in confirming wire fracture, but not all fractures are visible on the x-ray film. In this example the regularity of the escape intervals probably eliminates wire fracture as the cause of the problem.

At this point noninvasive procedures have been explored to evaluate the majority of potential causes for the reported malfunctions. Threshold elevation, inadequate electrogram characteristics, and pulse generator failure all require invasive evaluation, although some noninvasive determinations can be obtained if the patient has a sophisticated multiprogrammable pulse generator. Some of these devices can telemeter the intracardiac electrogram, facilitating evaluation of sensing problems. They also allow the user to obtain noninvasive threshold measurements. Nevertheless, correction of sensing and pacing failure due to any of these causes will require invasive procedures.

In the example cited, ECG evidence, shown in Fig. 11-15, indicates a lead dislodgement. Note the axis shift in the pacemaker stimulus artifact and in the paced QRS complexes. Lead displacement is the most common cause of sensing and capture failures.

Patient concerns

Although a pacemaker cannot cure the underlying disease, it can extend the patient's longevity and may greatly improve the quality of his or her life. Yet the patient has psychologic needs that must be considered if the therapy is to be of maximum benefit. The patient should understand why he has a pacemaker, how it works (in simple terms), and what it can and cannot do for him (many patients think that a pacemaker cures or makes the heart stronger). The patient should be told what, if any, life-style restrictions must be observed. If this is not explained, patients may become excessively apprehensive to the point even of avoiding bathing lest they "short-circuit" their pacemakers. The patient will be greatly concerned about his dependency on the pacemaker, the risks of its failing, the anticipated longevity of the system, and the severity of the replacement procedure. If these issues are addressed in lay terms with straight, clear, and concise answers, the pacemaker patient can fully enjoy the extra years and greater quality of life that a pacemaker makes possible.

REFERENCES

1. Elmquist, R., and Senning, A.: An implantable pacemaker for the heart, Proceedings of the second international conference of medical-electrical engineers, London, 1959, Iliffe and Sons Ltd.
2. Zoll, P., and Linenthal, A.: Long-term electrical pacemakers for Stokes-Adams disease, Circulation **22:**341, 1960.
3. Goldman, B.S., and Parsonnet, V.: World survey on cardiac pacing, PACE **2**(5):W1, 1979.
4. Furman, S.: Cardiac pacing and pacemakers. I. Indications for pacing bradyarrhythmias, Am. Heart J. **93**(4):523, 1977.
5. Sutton, R., Perrins, J., and Citron, P.: Physiological cardiac pacing, PACE **3**(2):207, 1980.
6. Citron, P., and Duffin, E.: Implantable pacemakers for management of tachyarrhythmias, Herz **4**(3):269, 1979.
7. Kahn, A., Morris, J., and Citron, P.: Patient-initiated rapid atrial pacing to manage supraventricular tachycardia, Am. J. Cardiol. **38:**200, 1976.
8. Cooper, T., MacLean, W., and Waldo, A.: Overdrive pacing for supraventricular tachycardia: a review of theoretical implications and therapeutic techniques, PACE **1**(2):196, 1978.
9. Waldo, A., and others: Temporary cardiac pacing: applications and techniques in the treatment of cardiac arrhythmias, Prog. Cardiovasc. Dis. **23**(6):451, 1981.
10. Hartzler, G.: Treatment of recurrent ventricular tachycardia by patient-activated radiofrequency ventricular stimulation, Mayo Clin. Proc. **54:**75, 1979.
11. Hyman, A.: Permanent programmable pacemakers in the management of recurrent tachycardias, PACE **2**(1):28, 1979.
12. Khan, M., and others: Management of recurrent ventricular tachyarrhythmias associated with QT prolongation, Am. J. Cardiol. **47**(6):1301, 1981.
13. Hindman, M.C., and others: The clinical significance of bundle branch block complicating acute myocardial infarction. II. Indications for temporary and permanent pacemaker therapy, Circulation **58:**689, 1978.
14. Scheinman, M., Strauss, H., and Abbott, J.: Electrophysiologic testing for patients with sinus node dysfunction, J. Electrocardiol. **12**(2):211, 1979.
15. Aranda, J., and others: His bundle recordings: their contribution to the understanding of human electrophysiology, Heart Lung **5**(6):907, 1976.
16. Fisher, J., and others: Cardiac pacing and pacemakers. II. Serial electrophysiologic-pharmacologic testing for control of recurrent tachyarrhythmias, Am. Heart J. **93**(5):658, 1977.
17. Robson, R.H., Pridie, R., and Fluck, D.C.: Evaluation of rapid atrial pacing in diagnosis of coronary artery disease, Br. Heart J. **38:**986, 1976.
18. Sutton, R., and Citron, P.: Electrophysiological and haemodynamic basis for application of new pacemaker technology in sick sinus syndrome and atrioventricular block, Br. Heart J. **41:**600, 1979.
19. Harthorne, J.: Indications for pacemaker insertion: types and modes of pacing, Prog. Cardiovasc. Dis. **23**(6):393, 1981.
20. Parsonnet, V., Furman, S., and Smyth, N.P.D.: Implantable cardiac pacemakers: status report and resource guideline, Circulation **50:**A21, 1974.
21. Parsonnet, V., Furman, S., and Smyth, N.P.D.: A revised code for pacemaker identification, PACE **4**(4):400, 1981.
22. Nathan, D., Center, S., and Wu, C.: An implantable synchronous pacemaker for the long-term correction of complete heart block, Am. J. Cardiol. **11:**362, 1963.
23. Kruse, I., Ryden, L., and Duffin, E.: Clinical evaluation of atrial synchronous ventricular inhibited pacemakers, PACE **3:**641, 1980.
24. Berkovits, B., Castellanos, A., and Lemberg, L.: Bifocal demand pacing, Circulation **39:**44, 1969.
25. Barold, S., and others: Characterization of pacemaker arrhythmias due to normally functioning AV demand (DVI) pulse generators, PACE **3**(6):712, 1980.
26. Funke, H.D.: Three years experience in optimized sequential cardiac pacing, Stimucoeur **9**(1):26,1981.
27. Wellens, H., and others: Electrical management of arrhythmias with emphasis on the tachycardias, Am. J. Cardiol. **41:**1025, 1978.
28. Haft, J.: Treatment of arrhythmias by intracardiac electrical stimulation, Prog. Cardiovasc. Dis. **16**(6): 539, 1974.
29. Batcheleder, J., and Zipes, D.P.: Treatment of tachyarrhythmnias by pacing, Arch. Intern. Med. **135:** 1115, 1975.
30. Giannelli, S., and others: Therapeutic surgical division of the human conduction system, J.A.M.A. **199:**123, 1967.
31. Neumann, G., and others: A new atrial demand pacemaker for the management of supraventricular tachycardias. In Meere, C., editor: Proceedings of the sixth world symposium on cardiac pacing, Montreal, 1979, Pacesymp.
32. Mandel, W.J., and others: Recurrent reciprocating tachycardias in the Wolff-Parkinson-White syndrome, Chest **69:**769, 1976.
33. Camm, A., and others: The clinical evaluation of tachycardia termination by utilizing autodecremental atrial pacing, PACE **4**(3):A84, 1981.
34. Curry, P., Rowland, E, and Krikler, D.: Dual-demand pacing for refractory atrioventricular re-entry tachycardia, PACE **2**(2):137, 1979.
35. Maloney, J., and others: Follow-up assessment of dual-demand, dual-chamber DVI-DVO pacing for automatic conversion, control, and prevention of refractory paroxysmal supraventricular tachycardia, PACE **4**(3):A57, 1981.
36. Jackman, W.M., and Zipes, D.P.: Transvenous low-energy cardioversion of ventricular tachycardia in a canine model of subacute myocardial infarction, Circulation **64**(suppl. IV):171, 1981.
37. Mirowski, M., and others: Termination of malignant ventricular arrhythmias with an implanted automatic

defibrillator in human beings, N. Engl. J. Med. **303**(6):322, 1980.

38. Leclercq, J.F., Attuel, P., and Coumel, P.: Les stimulateurs cardiaques destines a traiter les tachycardies paroxystiques, Stimucoeur **7**(1):8, 1979.

39. Parsonnet, V., and Rodgers, T.: The present status of programmable pacemakers, Prog. Cardiovasc. Dis. **23**(6):401, 1981.

40. Furman, S., and Pannizzo, F.: Output programmability and reduction of secondary intervention after pacemaker implantation, J. Thorac. Cardiovasc. Surg. **81**(5):713, 1981.

41. Hayes, D.L., and others: Initial and early follow-up assessment of the clinical efficacy of a multiparameter—programmable pulse generator, PACE **4**(4):417, 1981.

42. Parsonnet, V.: Cardiac pacing and pacemakers. VII. Power sources for implantable pacemakers, part 1, Am. Heart J. **94**(4):517, 1977.

43. Brennen, K.R., and others: A capacity rating system for cardiac pacemaker batteries, J. Power Sources **5**:25, 1980.

44. Hurzeler, P., and others: Longevity comparisons among lithium anode power cells for cardiac pacemakers, PACE **3**:555, 1980.

45. Bilitch, M., and others: Performance of cardiac pacemaker pulse generators, PACE **4**(4):479, 1981.

46. Greatbatch, W.: Metal electrodes in bioengineering, CRC Crit. Rev. Bioeng. **5**(1):1, 1981.

47. Smyth, N.P.D.: Techniques of implantation: atrial and ventricular, thoracotomy and transvenous, Prog. Cardiovasc. Dis. **23**(6), 435, 1981.

48. Littleford, P., Parsonnet, V., and Spector, S.: Method for the rapid and atraumatic insertion of permanent endocardial pacemaker electrodes through the subclavian vein, Am. J. Cardiol. **43**:980, 1979.

49. Parsonnet, V., and others: Transvenous insertion of double sets of permanent electrodes, J.A.M.A. 62, 1980.

50. Parsonnet, V.: Routine implantation of permanent transvenous pacemaker electrodes in both chambers: a technique whose time has come, PACE **4**(1):109, 1981.

51. Furman, S., Pannizzo, F., and Campo, I.: Comparison of active and passive adhering leads for endocardial pacing, PACE **2**(4):417, 1979.

52. Furman, S., Pannizzo, F., and Campo, I.: Comparison of active and passive adhering leads for endocardial pacing, part 2, PACE **4**(1):78, 1981.

53. El Gamal, M., and vanGelder, B.: Preliminary experience with the helifix electrode for transvenous atrial implantation, PACE **2**(4):444, 1979.

54. Bisping, H., Kreuzer, J., and Birkenheier, H.: Three-year clinical experience with a new endocardial screw-in lead with introduction protection for use in the atrium and ventricle, PACE **3**(4):424, 1980.

55. Mond, H., and Sloman, G.: Small tined ventricular pacemaker leads—reduction of lead complications, PACE **4**(3):A60, 1981.

56. Smyth, N.P.D., and others: Permanent pervenous atrial sensing and pacing with a new J-shaped lead, J. Thorac. Cardiovasc. Surg. **72**:565, 1976.

57. Messenger, J., and others: New permanent endocardial atrial J lead: implantation techniques and clinical performance, PACE **4**(3):A59, 1981.

58. deFeyter, P., and others: Permanent cardiac pacing with sutureless myocardial electrodes: experience in first one hundred patients, PACE **3**(2):144, 1980.

59. Zoll, P., Zoll, R., and Belgard, A.: External noninvasive electric stimulation of the heart, Crit. Care Med. **9**(5):393, 1981.

60. Furman, S., Hurzeler, P., and Mehra, R.: Cardiac pacing and pacemakers. IV. Threshold of cardiac stimulation, Am. Heart J. **94**(1):115, 1977.

61. Furman, S., Hurzeler, P., and DeCaprio, V.: Cardiac pacing and pacemakers. III. Sensing the cardiac electrogram, Am. Heart J. **93**(6):794, 1977.

62. Furman, S.: Cardiac pacing and pacemakers. VIII. The pacemaker follow-up clinic, Am. Heart J. **94**(6):795, 1977.

63. MacGregor, D., and others: Computer assisted reporting system for the follow-up of patients with cardiac pacemakers, PACE **3**(5):568, 1980.

64. Zipes, D.P.: Pacing 1980, PACE **4**(2):182, 1981.

65. Winner, J.: Pacemaker troubleshooting guide, Minneapolis, 1980, Medtronic, Inc.

66. Furman, S.: Cardiac pacing and pacemakers. VI. Analysis of pacemaker malfunction, Am. Heart J. **94**(3):378, 1977.

67. Cook, A.M., and Webster, J.G.: Therapeutic medical devices, Englewood Cliffs, N.J., 1981, Prentice-Hall Inc.

12

CARE OF THE CARDIAC PATIENT

Marguerite R. K   ey
Donna Rogers Packa
Martha E. Branyon
Linda J. Miers

Care of the cardiac patient is a multifaceted undertaking. Many aspects of the knowledge and expertise of health professionals are utilized in surveillance of the patient who has sustained a myocardial infarction. Health professionals have an opportunity to collect a variety of data concerning the patient while assessing, planning, implementing, and evaluating care. Subjective data are collected from the patient and the family in the form of the chief complaint, past health history, and family and social history (Chapter 4). Objective data are acquired from the physical examination, laboratory studies, observations of the patient, and information gathered from invasive and noninvasive techniques (Chapters 4 and 5).

At a time when modern technology and scientific research are expanding the ability of health professionals to diagnose and treat patients who have acute myocardial infarction, some investigators are questioning the necessity of admitting all patients to the coronary care unit (CCU). Before analyzing the actual care of the coronary patient, a brief discussion regarding the loca on for that care is appropriate.

Hospital versus home care

As health care costs rise and as private and governmental agencies investigate the validity of these rising costs, it is sm ll wonder that research teams have questioned the value of managing all patients with suspected acute myocardial infarction in hospital CCUs. The basic premise for CCUs seems sound. Early death related to myocardial infarction is usually caused by ventricular fibrillation. Advanced life-support techniques that are available in CCUs can be used to prevent or correct ventricular fibrillation. Mortality caused by myocardial infarction can be reduced if patients are entered into an emergency medical system and CCU as soon as possible after the onset of the illness. However, there are those who believe there is a lack of adequate randomized trials that support the long-term value of intensive coronary care.

Throughout the last few years several British researchers have conducted controlled randomized studies to determine whether the care provided in the CCU is any more beneficial than care provided by general practitioners and nurses

439

in the home.[1-4] The methods for patient selection and randomization for hospital or home care varied among the studies, but the mortality rates of all the groups were compared. In general the investigators found no significant statistical differences in the mortality rates of the two groups. The results led them to recommend reconsideration of the practice of admitting all patients with suspected acute myocardial infarction to a CCU.

The results of these studies have not been widely accepted in England or elsewhere. All of them are subject to criticism, since in each case the randomized sample was so small that the ability to generalize to a larger population is limited. In one study[3] the patients were accepted into the study up to 48 hours after the onset of their illness. Hypothetically, a substantial part of the mortality could have occurred before admission into the study was achieved.

In another study,[2] the researcher organized the most ideal situation for initial assessment and care in the home. A senior house officer and a CCU nurse equipped with an electrocardiograph, a defibrillator, resuscitation equipment, and appropriate drugs were sent to the patient's home. They provided necessary emergency treatment, recorded a history, and obtained an initial ECG. If the patient was considered to be suitable for the study, he was observed for 2 hours and then randomized to either home or hospital care. Patients were managed at home by their general practitioners, who visited them often enough to ensure adequate pain relief and who could send them to the hospital at any time if complications occurred. There is concern that the results that this methodology produced cannot be replicated in a more realistic and feasible home situation. As with the other study,[3] the time delay before randomization creates questions concerning the accuracy of the mortality rates.

The concept of caring for the patient with acute myocardial infarction in the home is one that merits consideration and a great deal more investigation. British studies related to this question may or may not be relevant in the United States or other countries, particularly in light of the differences in the health care system of various countries. Until more information is available from studies conducted in this country, we recommend that all patients with suspected acute myocardial infarction be admitted to a CCU as soon as possible after the onset of their illness.

Role of the health team

Scientific and technologic advances have created an increasingly complex environment for the care of the cardiac patient. In an effort to improve patient care services, newer or more specialized health practitioners have been introduced into the milieu of coronary care. Many units now employ monitor and/or cardiovascular technicians whose primary responsibility is for equipment used in patient care. A variety of therapists, such as respiratory, physical, and occupational, are available. Dietitians and pharmacists are often employed solely for the cardiac patient population. Cardiovascular nurse clinicians and cardiovascular clinical nurse specialists are commonplace in many CCUs and have varying responsibilities related to patient care and staff development. Physicians seek consultation from specialists who have advanced knowledge and skill in cardiovascular nuclear radiology, electrocardiography, echocardiography, and arteriography. Associated with these specialists are a variety of additional technicians who interact with the patient.

With the proliferation of health practitioners in coronary care comes the potential for fragmentation of patient care and loss of focus on the patient as a whole being. If this is to be prevented and if effective, efficient, holistic care is to be provided for the cardiac patient, collaboration and cooperation among all of these individuals are essential. The primary physician and nurse have the responsibility of seeking advice and assistance from the other health practitioners, the patient, and the family, as appropriate, and for utilizing their contributions as they make decisions concerning patient care. Together the physician and nurse need to develop a comprehensive plan that encompasses the goals and activities of all who interact with the patient.

The environment in which the cardiac patient is managed has made the process of treating and caring for the patient a complex one. However, by forming co-worker relationships, reaching decisions about the patient's needs and priorities can be made easier and more rewarding for all involved.

Care of the patient with a myocardial infarction

Goals for acute care of the patient who has a myocardial infarction include rapid management of existing problems, prevention and/or early detection of arrhythmias, and beginning rehabilitation.

ACUTE PHASE

The initial approach to the patient begins at the time of admission to the CCU. At this very critical time, health team members are collecting data about the patient and considering priorities in data collection and subsequent actions based on these data (see p. 442). The data collection process is discussed in Chapters 4 and 5. At this point the patient may or may not be physically able to describe any events except the presence of pain and/or shortness of breath.

PRIORITIES IN ADMISSION TO THE CCU

Immediate monitoring of cardiac rate and rhythm. *Rate meter alarms should always be set.* As electrodes are applied to the chest, a very brief explanation of the purpose of the electrodes should be given to the patient. Later, as he recovers, more information regarding the monitoring equipment may be discussed.

Establishment of a patent intravenous (IV) line. This is done with an indwelling catheter, preferably not a long catheter. This important line administering fluid and pain medication prevents the necessity of establishing an IV line in an emergency, when the task is much more difficult because of circulatory insufficiency or collapse. This line also allows for an immediate route to treat arrhythmias with IV medications. A butterfly-type needle should never be utilized in a patient who has had a myocardial infarction, since it is easily dislodged from the vein.

Relief of pain and anxiety. The patient should be given analgesic medication immediately if he continues to complain of pain on arrival to the unit. With pain there may be an elevation in pulmonary venous pressure. Although morphine is the drug of choice under these circumstances, it may be contraindicated or its

Example form for an admission note to the CCU

ADMISSION NOTE

Admission status: Clinic _____ ER _____ Date _____ Time _____

Married _____ Single _____ Widowed _____ Divorced _____

Race and nationality _____ Religion _____ Age _____

Patient history

Chest pain _____ Onset _____ Duration _____ Location _____

    Radiation _____ Subjective description _____

Associated acute events:

    Loss of consciousness _____ Duration _____ Cardiac arrest _____

    Palpitations _____ GI _____ Perspiration _____ Anxiety _____

    Dyspnea _____

Medications taken or administered and time _____

Medical history and risk factors (check those appropriate):

    Myocardial infarction _____ Angina _____ Obesity _____

    Weight loss _____ Cerebrovascular accident _____ Alcohol _____

    Respiratory _____ Hypertension _____ Glaucoma _____ Diabetes _____

    Smoking _____ Prostatic hypertrophy _____ Blood transfusion _____

    Gout _____ Surgery _____ Reaction to anesthesia _____ Other _____

Personal information

    Height _____ Weight _____ Dentures _____ Glasses _____ Contacts _____

    Sleeping habits _____ Usual diet _____

    Food, medication, environmental allergies _____

    Prosthesis _____ Family history _____

Physical examination

    General appearance _____ Mental status _____

    Vital signs: Temperature _____ Pulse _____ Respirations _____

    Blood pressure: Right _____ Left _____

    Lungs: Aeration _____ Wheezes _____ Rales _____

    Cardiovascular: Heart sounds _____ Quality _____ Rhythm _____

        Lifts _____ Heaves _____ Thrills _____ Murmur _____ Rub _____

        Gallop _____

    Pulses (all extremities) _____ Neck veins _____ Abdomen _____

    Skin: Color _____ Temperature _____ Cyanosis _____ Edema _____

    Clubbing _____ Other _____

        Signature _____

Insert ECG strip here.

dosage reduced if the patient has second-degree AV block or sinus bradycardia because of its vagotonic effects. If it is used and worsens the degree of AV block or sinus bradycardia, atropine may be administered to reverse its effects. Morphine also may decrease respiratory drive. Blood pressure, heart rate, and respiratory rate should be monitored for any untoward effects after morphine is given. The physician will usually write orders for analgesics and nitrates as needed for relief of pain. Pain and anxiety may potentiate the effects of each other and increase myocardial oxygen demands in an already compromised heart. Thus they should be alleviated as rapidly as possible. Explanations to the patient of all activities and equipment assist in relieving anxiety. Often families, although well intentioned, provoke anxiety. Visiting time should be terminated if such anxiety is noted. In other instances, however, the absence of families may produce excessive anxiety. Unit policies should be flexible enough to allow for individualization of care in each situation, as judged appropriate. Other policies and procedures should be explained to the patient as necessary measures in assisting the injured heart to heal. Such an explanation assists the patient in accepting that what is done is usual and necessary. Often a fact sheet with similar information for the family is helpful (see p. 444). Some physicians prescribe a mild sedative such as diazepam (Valium), which may help reduce stress and anxiety. However, opiates and sedatives should be given cautiously or not at all to confused and restless patients suffering from cerebral dysfunction caused by shock or heart failure.[5]

Supplemented oxygen. Oxygen is used to relieve dyspnea and thereby relieve anxiety. Even in patients with uncomplicated infarcts, hypoxemia caused by ventilation/perfusion abnormalities may exist. After an explanation of its use and the patient's need for it, humidified oxygen should be started at 1 to 2 L/minute with a binasal cannula. Frequent application of a lubricant or emollient to the nares will help to maintain skin integrity. Measurement of arterial blood gas levels 30 minutes after initiating oxygen therapy gives a base line of arterial oxygenation. Such measurements may be repeated as necessary to guide oxygen administration and maintain acid-base balance.

Decrease in myocardial work load. The myocardium requires time, oxygen, and nutrients to recover from the injury of infarction. Decreasing the amount of work, and therefore the oxygen demand of the heart, will assist the recovery of the myocardium. The methods used to decrease demand should be adequately explained to the patient and his family. Generally accepted methods of decreasing work load of the heart include the following:

1. Bed rest is recommended initially. After the early phase of the illness, progressive mobilization is considered advantageous in preventing complications. Many health care providers are now beginning rehabilitation while the patient is in the CCU and continuing until discharge. Whatever the activity level, it should be discussed and reinforced with the patient, since his cooperation is important.

2. In connection with bed rest, questions of self-feeding and methods of bladder and bowel elimination arise. Many physicians allow the patient to feed himself and to use the bedside commode with staff assistance. The physiologic stress that may result from these activities is thought to be

Example of fact sheet given to families of patients in CCU

CORONARY CARE UNIT INFORMATION

While you, a family member or friend, are in the CCU you may hear terms such as "coronary," "electrocardiogram" (ECG), or "congestive heart failure" and be uncertain as to what they mean about the patient's condition. This may be a time whenyou have a lot of questions and anxieties.

The CCU staff understands this and has prepared this information sheet to help you understand what goes on in a CCU. If you want to know more about heart disease, there is literature available in our unit on request. Also, we will be glad to try to answer any questions you may have.

The CCU Staff

Patient care

A CCU is for the "intensive" care of cardiac patients. This CCU has 11 beds and is attended 24 hours a day by registered nurses who are specially trained to read ECGs and recognize any early signs of complications. From the time a patient arrives in the unit until he is transferred to a room, there is a nurse near his bedside to render the care needed.

Because of the serious nature of heart disease, a patient is placed in the CCU during the critical phase of the heart's condition and remains there until this critical phase is over, usually 3 to 5 days. His progress is followed continuously with special monitoring equipment at each bedside and at the nurses' station to record the patient's ECGs. These indicate a person's heart rhythms.

While in the CCU patients need only their necessary personal belongings. Shaving equipment (razor with nurse's approval), cosmetics, toilet articles, eyeglasses, and small change may be kept in the bedside drawer. Male patients may wear pajama bottoms. Female patients do not need their gowns, since it is preferred that a hospital gown be worn. Patients may have a small radio and reading materials if approved by the doctor. Television, flowers, and suitcases are not allowed.

When the physician approves transfer out of the CCU, the patient is usually taken to a room on another floor. Transferring patients is usually done during the day, but if an emergency situation arises and a bed is needed in the unit during the night, a patient may have to be moved then.

Visiting is permitted from 10 AM to 8 PM by members of the patient's immediate family or significant others. Because of the nature of the patient's illness, no more than two visitors should be in the patient's room at one time.

If emergency situations exist, visitation may be refused.

Phone

There is a pay phone available. Direct calls to the unit are not permitted. Families may leave their phone numbers at the desk in the CCU.

Chaplain

This service is available on request at any time by contacting a CCU nurse or the chaplain's office.

Waiting rooms

The waiting room is open only until 8:30 PM. Those who wish to stay during the night must use the emergency room's waiting room.

less than the stress that results from almost total dependence on another person. The stress secondary to dependence is evident most frequently in male patients who find themselves dependent on females in a drastic reversal of roles. Maintaining some degree of independence can contribute significantly to the patient's psychologic state of self-worth and recovery. This, in turn, facilitates physical recovery.

Initially, a brief explanation by the nurse about the need for assistance in performing activities is sufficient. As the patient improves, additional information regarding the reasons for assistance in activity may be explained in greater depth to the patient and family.

OTHER INFORMATION

Other information necessary to complete the data base may be obtained after admission to the unit and includes the following subjective and objective data:

A. Patient history (see Chapter 4)

B. Physical examination (see Chapter 4)
  1. Inspection of skin for color, diaphoresis, and other abnormalities.
  2. Palpation of chest area for unusual movements, excursion, cardiac enlargement, apical impulse, and other signs.
  3. Percussion of chest for areas of dullness and of the liver for edge and size; cardiac borders are seldom defined by percussion.
  4. Auscultation of blood pressure, apical heart rate, normal heart sounds, gallops, and murmurs, especially the murmur of papillary muscle dysfunction, which may occur in the acute phase as a result of ischemia and/or infarction of the papillary muscle. The sound is the murmur of mitral regurgitation resulting when the injured papillary muscle fails to contract properly, allowing blood to regurgitate into the left atrium during systole. The murmur is often transient, but it may be permanent if the papillary muscle does not heal completely. A ventricular septal defect murmur may also be present, resulting from perforation of the septum. This murmur usually occurs during the first 10 days after infarct and is a very loud grade 4 or 5 systolic murmur. There is usually an accompanying systolic thrill, and the murmur is best heard along the lower left sternal border. The appearance of this murmur is an ominous event prognostically. It is also important to auscultate the lungs for the presence of rales, rhonchi, wheezes, and increased or decreased breath sounds. Also note the rate, character, and depth of respirations. These data are necessary to evaluate the presence or absence of congestive heart failure and are useful for comparison should this be a consideration at a later date.

C. Supportive data
  1. A 12-lead ECG (Chapter 6) should be performed initially in the emergency room or in the CCU. A copy should be maintained on the patient's chart for comparison with later tracings, which are performed daily for 3 days and with every exacerbation of chest pain and/or developing arrhythmia. Personnel in the CCU should be adept at obtaining and

interpreting the 12-lead ECG in a patient with myocardial infarction. (See ECG procedure.)

2. Serum cardiac isoenzyme levels (Chapter 5) should be measured initially and then daily for 3 days to document any abnormal increase in serum levels. Should the patient have a sudden exacerbation of pain with associated ECG changes, cardiac enzyme level measurements may be indicated to assist in determining whether the previous infarction has extended.

3. Arterial blood gas levels may be measured initially, then as needed (depending on the patient's condition) to determine the adequacy of oxygenation and acid-base balance.

4. Fluid and electrolyte balance should be monitored. It is imperative that fluid intake and output be accurately measured. Equally important is accurate daily weight of the patient taken at the same time each day on the same scale. This can help to determine the minimal weight gain in the early stages of heart failure or when other indicators, such as the chest x-ray film, are still normal. Personnel must be reminded to actually measure rather than estimate intake, just as all output is measured. It should also be remembered that fluids, such as tube feedings, those used to flush Swan-Ganz and arterial lines, and those from any other sources, must be included in the patient's total fluid-intake measurement. Output should include bleeding and drainage from any site, as well as urine and stool. The patient's state of hydration may also be evaluated by the skin tone.

5. Peripheral edema is a late sign of congestive failure and should be added to the data base already gathered regarding the fluid balance of the patient. The extent of peripheral edema should be measured by palpation once it appears, and comparative evaluations should be performed frequently to determine changes in edema noted in the periphery.

6. Dietary regimen, if altered from the patient's usual diet, should be explained to him and his family. Cardiac patients are usually placed on a low-sodium diet for several days. In some patients, sodium restriction may be unnecessary or impractical; these patients are given food with the usual sodium content. A soft diet is usually prescribed with frequent small feedings, although some physicians order clear liquids on the first day followed by full liquids on the second day. Since metabolic demands increase following ingestion of food, the quantity of food at each serving should be kept small. A recent study shows that hot and cold liquids are not detrimental, so their exclusion from diets, although routine in many CCUs, is questionable.[5] Coffee and tea are usually permitted.

All the data must be evaluated and intervention planned according to the goals that have been defined by the patient and the staff. If the goal has not been attained, revision of one or more components of the plan may be necessary to assist the patient in meeting the goals.

12-LEAD ECG PROCEDURE FOR CCU

A. Purpose: to record an ECG for diagnostic purposes (A graphic record of the electrical impulses causing heart action recorded by electrodes placed on the body surface.)

B. Equipment
1. ECG machine with five-lead cable (see Fig. 12-1, p. 451)
2. Four-limb electrode plates with rubber straps
3. One Welsh cup electrode
4. ECG electrode paste
5. Cotton or gauze
6. Alcohol sponges

C. Procedure
1. Instruct patient regarding procedure, and assure him that there is no discomfort associated with procedure.
2. Place patient in a comfortable position on back with legs and arms adequately supported. Feet should not touch the footboard of the bed, nor arms touch the sides of the bed.
3. Plug in ECG machine. Turn power switch to *on* position.
4. Plug in five-lead patient cable to top of recorder.
5. Select site for limb electrode placement on each extremity. Electrodes may be placed anywhere on the extremities from shoulder to hand or hip to foot. The electrode should be placed securely so that it does not rock back and forth or move as patient breathes.
6. Cleanse the skin area with alcohol; attempt to achieve a slight erythema by rubbing skin.
7. Apply electrode paste and rub with electrode. Fasten electrode to place with rubber strap. Apply just the amount of tension on the strap necessary to adequately hold electrode in place. A tight electrode strap might produce muscle tremors and create an artifact on the tracing. Electrodes should be placed in such a way that patient cable can be attached without overbending lead wire; that is, connectors on electrodes should be pointing down on arms and up on legs.
8. Attach each of the five-lead wires to the appropriate limb electrode. The cables are color coded and letter labeled for easy identification.
9. Before proceeding with recording, check the instrument controls.
   a. Check the grounding of the instrument by placing the lead selector on STD position. Using one finger, touch the top of the switch marked *test*. If the writing stylus vibrates, press the test button down. The test button is left in the position by which there is no vibration of the writing arm when the button is touched.
   b. Adjust the *position* control so that the writing is centered on the ECG paper.
   c. Adjust the *intensity* control to produce the necessary heat in the writing arm to give a firm, clear black line.
   d. Turn the power switch to *run* and check the standardization of the machine. When the button marked *STD (I MV)* is pushed, the

writing arm should be deflected exactly two large squares (10 mm) when the *sensitivity* indicator is on *I* (Chapter 6). Accurate standardization is important, since some diagnostic and measurement criteria are meaningless without a point of reference.

NOTE: ECGs are standardized with each lead change. ECGs are routinely run at standard *I*.

10. All ECGs must be identified by labeling beginning of tracing with patient's name, medical record number, date, and time.

11. A standard ECG consists of 12 separate leads. Each of these leads must be marked for the purposes of identification. This can be done by using the button labeled *marker* to create a mark in the upper margin of the paper. The following lead code is used for this purpose.

I _	V_1 __ _
II _ _	V_2 __ _ _
III _ _ _	V_3 __ _ _ _
aV_R __	V_4 __ _ _ _ _
aV_L __ __	V_5 __ _ _ _ _ _
aV_F __ __ __	V_6 __ _ _ _ _ _ _

12. To record the first six leads:
    a. Place the lead selector switch at *I*. Observe the writing arm; it should oscillate in the center of the strip.
    b. Turn the power switch to *run*.
    c. Push the *STD (I MV)* button once while the paper is running, and identify the lead by pushing the *lead marker* button. (Some machines mark automatically.)
    d. After recording 8 to 10 beats with a stable base line, turn power button to *on* position.
    e. Move the lead selector to lead II and proceed as above. Continue through and, including lead aV_F, move the lead selector to the next *dot* position on the lead selector dial.

    Some machines record 3 to 6 channels simultaneously.

13. To record the *V* leads of the ECG:
    a. Place the Welsh cup electrode on the lead marked *C* (for "chest").
    b. Expose the patient's chest.
    c. Locate the electrode positions of leads V_1 through V_6. Cleanse the areas with alcohol sponge, rubbing to produce a slight erythema. Place a small amount of ECG paste to mark position.
    d. The electrode positions are as follows:
       V_1—fourth intercostal space at right of sternal border
       V_2—same interspace at left of sternal border
       V_3—midway between position V_2 and V_4
       V_4—fifth interspace at midclavicular line
       V_5—same level as V_4 at anterior axillary line
       V_6—same level as V_4 at midaxillary line
    e. Rub the electrode paste on first chest lead (V_1) site, and secure Welsh electrode cup. Turn lead selector to *V* position and power

switch to *run*. Position stylus as necessary. Press *lead marker* to identify lead.

    f. Repeat the preceding step for each of the chest lead positions on chest.

14. Disconnect the electrodes from the patient, and reposition the patient for comfort. Wipe electrode paste off chest and extremities.

15. Be sure ECG is correctly labeled. See that ECG is mounted in the patient's chart.

DAILY APPROACH TO THE PATIENT

Data collection is again the first phase in the daily approach to the cardiac patient. Data are collected utilizing the same procedures discussed in the section concerning initial contact with the patient.

    A. Subjective data must consist of information obtained from the patient and his family. These data should supplement the subjective data obtained during the initial interview. The information may be gathered at any time and be added to the initial data base. It is appropriate for all health team members to contribute to the data base.

    B. These objective data are obtained by the parameters discussed under initial care:

        1. Physical examination—comparison of findings with previous findings.

        2. Supportive data—cardiac enzyme levels daily for 3 days and with chest pain; other laboratory work may be indicated, such as electrolyte-level measurements and arterial blood gas levels as needed to evaluate the status of acid-base balance.

In caring for the patient on a daily basis it is imperative that health care personnel, especially the primary nurse, be aware of and accurately document the function of all equipment in use. This includes the monitor, IV drip regulators, ventilators, crash cart, defibrillator, and any other equipment. In the event that legal questions arise at a later time, this documentation of appropriate functioning is extremely important.

POTENTIAL PROBLEMS

Following collection of data pertinent to the patient's current status, assessment is made regarding potential problems for which personnel should be alert. These problems include development of arrhythmias, myocardial dysfunction, and psychologic disturbances.

Arrhythmias. Staff in the CCU should be skilled in arrhythmia interpretation and treatment. Most CCUs have personnel trained to give lidocaine, atropine, and other medications useful in arrhythmia management by a preestablished protocol to patients who have ventricular arrhythmias. Currently there is a lack of agreement regarding the prophylactic use of lidocaine and other antiarrhythmic agents in patients admitted with sinus rhythm. However, it has been suggested that prophylactic use of antiarrhythmic agents *may* protect the myocardial infarction patient from developing ventricular arrhythmias.[5] See Chapter 10 for further discussion of drugs useful in arrhythmia management.

Staff should also be certified in skills of basic cardiac life support as defined by the American Heart Association or the American Red Cross. After certification in basic cardiac life support, staff must be trained to perform other procedures, including preparation of medication, recording times of events and medication given, and assisting as necessary with activities during the resuscitation effort. Commonly, nurses who are well prepared in resuscitation techniques successfully treat a patient who has had a cardiac arrest prior to the arrival of a physician.

Some community hospitals without full-time physician coverage now encourage other health care personnel to become certified in the skills of advanced cardiac life support, which includes all the skills of basic cardiac life support in addition to the techniques of endotracheal intubation, venipuncture, arrhythmia interpretation, and drug administration.

Cardioversion. Transthoracic cardioversion involves the delivery of electrical energy to the heart by means of metal paddles placed on the intact chest or placed directly on the heart when the chest is opened, as during cardiac surgery. This procedure depolarizes the excitable myocardium, thereby interrupting reentrant circuits and discharging automatic pacemaker foci to establish electrical homogeneity. Cardioversion successfully restores sinus rhythm if the sinus node becomes the automatic focus that fires first and fastest after the electrical shock and controls the cardiac mechanism. An exciting new development, transvenous cardioversion, involves delivery of electrical energy by a catheter electrode placed in the right ventricle and, using very low energies, permits cardioversion in an awake, unsedated patient.[6]

When a patient develops a tachyarrhythmia, slowing the ventricular rate represents the initial and frequently the most important therapeutic maneuver. The patient's clinical status and the nature of the arrhythmia determine the speed with which this must be accomplished. Pharmacologic therapy for tachyarrhythmias involves a time-consuming and potentially dangerous biologic titration of drugs such as digitalis or quinidine; exact therapeutic or toxic levels of these drugs cannot be predicted with absolute certainty, and side effects may occur. Electrical cardioversion eliminates many of these problems. Under conditions optimal for close supervision and monitoring, a precisely regulated "dose" of electricity can restore sinus rhythm immediately.

By synchronizing the capacitor to discharge during the downslope of the R wave or with the S wave, the ventricular vulnerable period (an interval of 20 to 40 msecs near the apex of the T wave) may be avoided. This minimizes, but does not completely eliminate, the danger of precipitating ventricular fibrillation with the DC shock. However, if synchronization cannot be established rapidly and immediate cardioversion is indicated, the shock is delivered asynchronously. Immediate cardioversion using maximum voltage without synchronization (defibrillation) is the mandatory treatment for ventricular fibrillation or ventricular flutter and for ventricular tachycardia if it produces cardiovascular collapse. If it is unsuccessful, drug therapy should begin with lidocaine, followed by procainamide IV.[5] However, if the tachyarrhythmia does not terminate properly, cardioversion or defibrillation should be performed. Short, self-limited bursts of ventricular tachycardia are treated medically. As a general rule, any supraventricular tachyarrhythmia that produces signs or symptoms such as hypotension, angina,

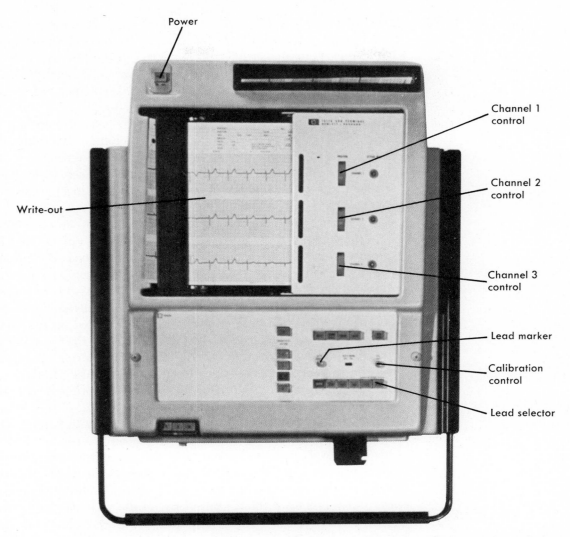

Fig. 12-1. Electrocardiograph machine showing components, including three channels that provide for display of three leads simultaneously. Lead selector allows choice of leads. Lead marker automatically marks which leads are being written. Calibration control allows choice of size of ECG complexes. (Reprinted with permission of Hewlett-Packard Co., Palo Alto, Calif.)

or congestive heart failure and does not respond promptly to medical therapy should be terminated electrically.

   A. *Elective cardioversion procedure.* An elective cardioversion may be carried out wherever resuscitative aids, such as suction and intubation equipment and medications, and experienced personnel trained in airway management are available. The steps followed are listed here.

      1. Explain the procedure to the patient and obtain written *informed* consent.

2. Withhold diuretics and short-acting digitalis preparations for 24 to 36 hours. However, some recent data suggest that discontinuing digitalis in nontoxic, normokalemic patients may not be necessary. If it is indicated, obtain a serum potassium or a serum digitalis level. Hypokalemia enhances electrical instability and may increase arrhythmias after cardioversion.[7]

3. Keep the patient fasting for 6 to 8 hours prior to cardioversion.

4. Perform a thorough physical examination, including vital signs, mentation, and palpation of pulse (see Chapter 4).

5. Obtain a 12-lead ECG before and after cardioversion, as well as a rhythm strip or oscilloscopic monitoring (or both) during procedure.

6. Maintain a reliable IV site.

7. Allow the patient to breathe 100% oxygen for 5 to 15 minutes before, and then immediately after, DC shock, if not contraindicated. This promotes myocardial oxygenation. During cardioversion the presence of oxygen with electrical arching may encourage combustion.

8. Remove patient's dentures if present.

9. Employ synchronous discharge mode on the defibrillator/cardioverter for elective procedures. The QRS complex recorded on the oscilloscope must be tall to ensure that it alone triggers the capacitor discharge. Determine the accuracy of synchronization by discharging several test shocks before applying the paddles to the patient.

10. Administer diazepam (Valium) or other medication ordered to produce transient amnesia or light sleep.

11. Apply electrode paste liberally but not excessively to the polished surface of the paddles, which are then placed in firm contact with the chest wall at points distant from the monitoring electrodes; or apply pads to chest. The paddles may be positioned (1) anteroposteriorly, in the left infrascapular region and over the upper sternum at the third interspace, or (2) anteriorly, to the right of the sternum second intercostal space and in the left midclavicular line at the fifth intercostal space.

12. Employing the minimally effective electrical energy level reduces complications; therefore the starting level for most arrhythmias is around 50 watt-seconds or less (Fig. 12-2). The energy necessary to terminate some arrhythmias, such as atrial flutter or ventricular tachycardia, may be considerably less. If unsuccessful, this initial level may be increased to 100 watt-seconds, and then by 100–watt-second increments until a level of 400 watt-seconds is reached. Make sure that all personnel have moved away from the patient and the bed before discharging the defibrillator.

13. Record the postshock rhythm to determine whether the procedure was successful. V_1 lead recording is preferable. An oscilloscopic interpretation is frequently unreliable.

14. Continue rhythm monitoring and close observation of cardiovascular and pulmonary status for 2 to 3 hours until stable after cardioversion.

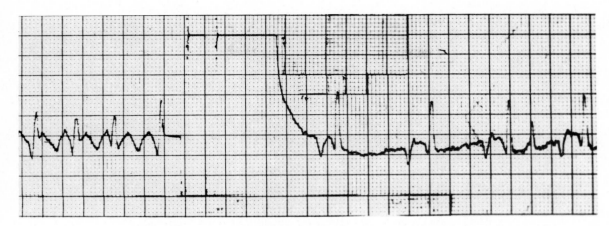

Fig. 12-2. Termination of atrial flutter. Direct current countershock was administered at 50 watt-seconds. The synchronized discharge occurred on R wave and terminated the flutter rhythm.

B. *Emergency cardioversion procedure.* The nature of an emergency clinical situation determines which of the steps listed must be omitted. Selected procedures range from immediate cardioversion using maximum voltage without any preamble for treating ventricular fibrillation to omitting the delay of 6 to 8 hours after the patient's last meal to cardiovert a less threatening arrhythmia.

C. Precautions
1. When digitalis excess is suspected, electrical cardioversion should be deferred and the arrhythmia treated with medication initially to prevent production of serious ventricular tachyarrhythmias and failure to terminate the digitalis-related arrhythmia.
2. Emergency drugs such as atropine, isoproterenol, and lidocaine and the emergency equipment needed for pacing, intubation, or suction must be available.
3. If using electrode paste, avoid coating the paddles excessively or placing them too near monitoring electrodes. This may allow a spark to jump and burn the skin. Local skin inflammation caused by the paddles is best treated with a topical steroid preparation.
4. Disconnect the patient from any other electrical apparatus.
5. Certain arrhythmias may occur after cardioversion; therefore monitoring the rhythm must continue for 2 to 3 hours. Other complications may include embolic episodes, which occur in 1% to 3% of patients cardioverted to sinus rhythm.

Resuscitation. Circulatory arrest is reversible if resuscitation begins during the first 3 to 4 minutes, before irreversible cerebral damage occurs. Ventricular fibrillation, rather than ventricular asystole, commonly precipitates the arrest; ventricular fibrillation occurs 25 times more commonly during the first 4 hours than it does the day after a myocardial infarction (see Chapter 9). A well-trained

CCU team initiates defibrillation procedures within 30 seconds of onset of the arrest. Prompt reversion to sinus rhythm often prevents the biochemical derangements that accompany ventricular fibrillation, eliminates the need for endotracheal intubation, and significantly increases the success rate of resuscitation attempts. After a successful resuscitation, measures must be taken to prevent recurrence of the cardiac arrest. Simple arrhythmias, such as premature ventricular systoles, may presage the occurrence of ventricular tachycardia/fibrillation. Early treatment of the former may prevent initiation of the latter.

The monitor alarm usually gives the first indication that a cardiac emergency has occurred. Occasionally personnel may observe the arrhythmia on the oscilloscope before the alarm sounds. At that time they must correlate the observed rhythm with the patient's clinical status by rapidly evaluating the patient's orientation, respirations, pupils, and carotid or femoral pulses. Loose leads can produce a rhythmic pattern simulating ventricular fibrillation. Moreover, a lidocaine reaction can mimic the disoriented state seen in tachyarrhythmias associated with inadequate cardiac output. The importance of careful diagnosis cannot be overemphasized.

A. Resuscitation procedure
   1. Establish unresponsiveness by shaking the patient and calling his name. If there is no response, call for help.
   2. Place the patient in a supine position with a board or firm mattress under the chest.*
   3. Open the patient's airway using the head-tilt and neck-lift method or head-tilt and chin-lift method. The chin-lift method is preferred.
   4. Look, listen, and feel for breathing. If the patient is breathing, keep the airway open, but do not begin other CPR techniques.
   5. Administer four rapid mouth-to-mouth ventilations, if the patient is not breathing. Pinch the nostrils and seal the mouth.
   6. Check the patient's carotid pulse. If it is present, do only breathing, one breath every 5 seconds.
   7. If the patient has no palpable pulse, begin cycles of five external cardiac compressions (at a rate of 60/minute) and one ventilation if two people are resuscitating, or cycles of 15 compressions (at a rate of 80/minute) and two ventilations if only one person is resuscitating the patient. Check for correct hand positioning.
   8. After four cycles of ventilation and compression check for return of the patient's pulse and spontaneous breathing. If there is no pulse or spontaneous breathing, repeat the process.
   9. Do not stop CPR for more than 5 seconds once it has begun. Pause every 4 or 5 minutes (after the initial pause noted in no. 8) to check for carotid pulse, spontaneous breathing, and pupillary reaction to light.

*For further information refer to the American Heart Association or the American Red Cross guidelines for cardiopulmonary resuscitation.

10. While one or more people provide cardiorespiratory support, someone else sets up the defibrillator, if the patient's rhythm is unknown or is known to be ventricular tachycardia or fibrillation. If only one person is present, he or she must decide between instituting cardiopulmonary resuscitation and attempting to defibrillate the patient. If the defibrillator is close at hand and the patient can be treated with it in 15 to 30 seconds, it is probably best for the single resuscitator to choose defibrillation rather than beginning cardiopulmonary resuscitation alone. (It is extremely critical that DC shock not be delayed when cardiopulmonary resuscitation has begun, an intubation attempted, an ECG recorded, or a physical examination [other than a brief palpation of pulses and so forth] performed. Rapid application of DC shock is usually the most important therapeutic maneuver in this situation.)

11. IV fluid is started if it is not already running.

12. It is helpful to have a drug list such as the one shown in Table 12-1 taped to the emergency cart. Those medications most likely to be needed are prepared at the first opportunity.

13. If there is time and a sufficient number of people and if the mechanism of the arrhythmia producing the cardiac arrest is unknown, an ECG may be done from resuscitative measures. If necessary, an ECG is done after DC shock. Certain defibrillators have monitoring capability; their paddles act as electrodes that record the rhythm disturbance immediately prior to defibrillation.

14. As soon as the defibrillator is made ready (this should take no more than 30 seconds), the patient is shocked with the paddles in the same location as for cardioversion, at a peak energy level: 400 watt-seconds (Fig. 12-3). If this is not successful, defibrillation is repeated; the shock may be repeated again after lidocaine or procainamide administration.

    NOTE: The energy level required for defibrillation is controversial. Some studies have suggested that lower levels of energy are successful in terminating potentially fatal arrhythmias. This decision should be made and a policy written so that all members know the procedure in an emergency situation.

15. Ventricular fibrillation and ventricular tachycardia producing cardiovascular collapse are defibrillated immediately. Failure to restore an effective rhythm after delivery of a properly administered shock at high intensity suggests that complicating problems such as hypoxia, acidosis, or drug toxicity may be present. If possible, these conditions should be corrected before the next shock is delivered. If the cardiac arrest continues after several shocks, sodium bicarbonate should be administered. Serial pH determinations should be performed to prevent overcorrection of acidosis (to alkalosis) and to determine whether enough sodium bicarbonate has been given.

Table 12-1. Essential emergency cardiac drugs*

Drug	How supplied	Dosage
Sodium bicarbonate	44.6 mEq/50 ml in prefilled syringe 50 mEq/50 ml in prefilled syringe	1 mEg/kg initially; thereafter based on arterial blood gas levels
Epinephrine	1 mg/10 ml (1:10,000 dilution) in prefilled syringe or 1 mg/1 ml (1:1,000 dilution in ampule)	0.5-1.0 mg (5-10 ml of 1:10,000 solution) may be given IV every 5 minutes during resuscitation
Atropine	1 mg/10 ml (0.1 mg/ml) in prefilled syringe 0.5 mg/5 ml (0.1 mg/ml) in prefilled syringe	0.5 mg IV as a bolus; repeated at 5-min intervals until pulse rate is greater than 60; total dose should not exceed 2 mg
Lidocaine	100 mg/5 ml (2%) in prefilled syringe 2 g/10 ml for dilution 100 mg/10 ml (1%) in prefilled syringe	50 to 100 mg (1 mg/kg) IV bolus with infusions of (2 g/500 ml dextrose in water) 1 to 4 mg/min (20-50 μg/kg/min)
Calcium chloride	1 g/10 ml (10%)	2.5 to 5.0 ml of 10% solution (200 to 500 mg), estimated from patient's weight, may be repeated every 10 min; repeated large doses may elevate blood levels of calcium with detrimental effect
Procainamide (Pronestyl)	1000 mg:100 mg/ml in 10-ml vials; 1000 mg:500 mg/ml in 2-ml vials	100 mg IV every 5 min at 20 mg/min until (1) dysrhythmia is suppressed, or (2) hypotension ensues, or (3) QRS complex is widened by 50% of original width, or (4) total of 1 g of drug is injected; maintenance rate is 1-4 mg/min
Bretylium tosylate	500 mg in 10-ml ampule	In ventricular fibrillation (VF): 5 mg/kg rapidly IV; if VF persists after defibrillation, 10 mg/kg repeated as necessary; in ventricular tachycardia (VT) 500 mg (10 ml) diluted to 50 ml and 5-10 mg/kg given IV over 8-10 min; if VT persists, 5-10 mg/kg given in 1-2 hr and repeated every 6-8 hr
Verapamil (Isoptin)	2.5 mg/ml in 2-ml ampule	*Adult:* single dose: 0.075-0.15 mg/kg body weight (max: 10 mg) given as IV bolus over 1 min; repeat dose: 0.15 mg/kg body weight (max: 10 mg) 30 min after first dose if initial response inadequate (total cumulative dose in 30 min should not exceed 15 mg) *Older patients:* IV dose given over 3 min
Morphine	2 mg/ml in 10-ml prefilled syringe; 8 mg/ml, 10 mg/ml, 15 mg/ml in 1-ml Tubex syringe	Titrate small IV dose at frequent intervals to achieve desired response starting with 2-5 mg IV every 5-30 minutes; 15 mg/ml diluted to 5 ml yields 3 mg/ml or dilute to 1 mg/ml for safe small IV increment dosage

*See Chapter 10 for in-depth discussion of drugs and *American Heart Association Textbook of Advanced Cardiac Life Support* for more detailed discussion of essential emergency cardiac drugs.

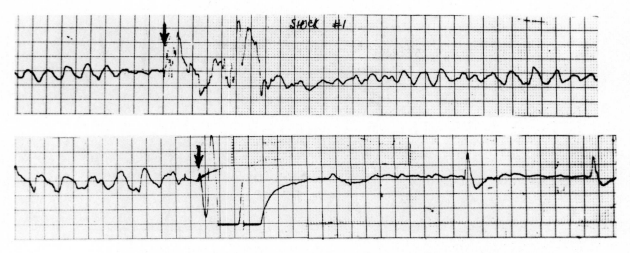

Fig. 12-3. Ventricular fibrillation was treated with application of countershock at 400 watt-seconds in top strip, noted by arrow. Since countershock was unsuccessful, as noted in continuous strip, countershock was again applied at 400 watt-seconds (arrow in second strip). Rhythm then converted to idioventricular mechanism.

NOTE: Sodium bicarbonate should not be given without adequate ventilations.[5] Cardiopulmonary resuscitation must be continued between defibrillations or other procedures, since even a short interruption results in inadequate perfusion and increased anoxia. These complications in themselves may prevent successful resuscitation.

16. Repetitive shocks may not be effective in the presence of fine fibrillatory waves on the ECG. Giving 5 ml of epinephrine 1:10,000 IV may convert these waves to large waves. In some cases lidocaine alone or in combination with epinephrine may assist in defibrillation. Propranolol (Inderal) IV and bretylium tosylate (Bretylol) may also be tried.[5]

17. After successful conversion to sinus rhythm, continuous infusion with lidocaine for maintenance arrhythmic therapy should be instituted.

18. If the rhythm is known to be ventricular asystole or slow idioventricular rhythm, atropine, 0.1 to 0.3 mg/kg, may be given IV. If the heart beat is not restored, cardiopulmonary resuscitation should be instituted (nos. 1 to 9).

19. Epinephrine, 5 ml of a 1:10,000 solution, is administered IV. If this is unsuccessful, isoproterenol (Isuprel) and calcium chloride may be administered.

20. Sodium bicarbonate should be given during the arrest, as described in no. 16.

21. Transvenous pacing equipment should be made ready for use. A direct percutaneous puncture of the heart may also be tried.

22. At the first opportunity an episode sheet (Fig. 12-4) is completed, and clinical events and a drug tally are recorded.

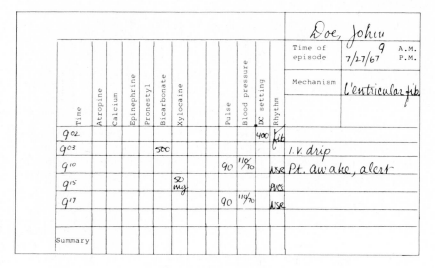

Fig. 12-4. CCU episode sheet.

B. Environment
1. Regulation of the environment facilitates the rapidity and efficiency of the resuscitation procedure. The corridor to the patient's room must be free from obstacles. The patient's room should have adequate lighting with electrical outlets visible from the door. Furniture should not block traffic from the room door to the patient's bed. Flowers, if allowed in the unit, should be set on a shelf away from the bed, so that they will not be knocked off the table during an emergency.

NOTE: A fully stocked, adequately maintained emergency cart is imperative in every unit. It should include all drugs and equipment needed in an arrest and should not be cluttered with unnecessary items.

C. Postresuscitative care
1. In the aftermath of a successful resuscitation it seems natural for unit personnel to relax. Yet, meticulous attention to the patient's hemodynamic status, blood gas levels, and electrolyte balance continues to be important in maintaining a clinical stability and in preventing recurrence. This is a time, too, during which the patient's family should be encouraged to visit when appropriate. The family should also be prepared for changes in the patient or new equipment in use, such as a ventilator.

MYOCARDIAL DYSFUNCTION

Myocardial dysfunction may be evaluated using several methods (Chapters 4 and 5). Measurements can be made through noninvasive techniques such as blood pressure, heart rate, ECG, echocardiogram, and myocardial scans. Invasive measurements include pulmonary artery pressure, pulmonary capillary wedge pressure, and cardiac output measurements and cardiac catheterization (Chapters 5 and 7).

PSYCHOLOGIC ALTERATIONS

Psychologic alterations may be noted at any point during the illness of the patient and should be evaluated on a continuing basis. The alterations and mechanisms of dealing with them are discussed in Chapter 13.

Components of daily care

Once potential problems have been assessed, daily care of the patient can be based on the data obtained. Important components in daily care of the patient include relief of anxiety and pain, monitoring of blood gas levels and fluids, decreasing of the myocardial work load, and continuation of dietary recommendations.

RELIEF OF ANXIETY AND PAIN

This aspect of care has been previously discussed and is applicable in daily care. If the patient experiences pain, it is important to note the frequency, duration, quality, quantity, location, associated factors such as diaphoresis and dyspnea, and alleviating factors. This information should be recorded on the patient's chart, accompanied by an ECG rhythm strip. Furthermore, a 12-lead ECG should be obtained and evaluated for changes from the initial ECG, and the patient's physician should be notified. If the physician has left orders for nitrates and analgesics, they should be given as ordered, making sure that the patient's vital signs and respiratory characteristics are being monitored. If the pain is not relieved, the physician should be notified so that the duration of pain and, thus, increased oxygen demand load of the heart can be decreased as soon as possible.

Methods of reducing anxiety are continuously applicable throughout hospitalization. See Chapter 13 for further discussion.

EVALUATION OF BLOOD GAS LEVELS

The need for supplemental oxygen, once established, should be evaluated often during the acute phase of the illness. Arterial blood gas samples should be drawn often to evaluate acid-base balance.

Flow sheets that record many values are useful in maintaining a graphic representation of the patient's progress (Fig. 12-5). Some units prefer a separate flow sheet for arterial blood gas levels, especially for people who require frequent arterial blood gas analysis.

REDUCTION OF MYOCARDIAL WORK LOAD

Decreasing myocardial work continues to be an important component of daily patient care. Activities should be gradually increased according to the plan of rehabilitation and the patient's stage of recovery. Patients are now being mobilized earlier than they used to be, since prolonged bed rest may not prevent but actually increase development of complications following myocardial infarction. The patient must, however, be assisted in all activities, especially during the acute phase of the illness.

CONTINUATION OF DIETARY RECOMMENDATIONS

Initial dietary recommendations are usually maintained throughout the acute phase of illness and often throughout hospitalization and convalescence.

		Date:						
		Time	7-3	3-11	11-7	7-3	3-11	11-7
Chest	Chest pain R$_x$ and response Gallops/murmurs Edema Jugular venous distention Breath sounds Rales Cough Dyspnea Cyanosis Other							
Abdomen	Nausea/vomiting Appetite/diet Bowels/guaiac Abdominal distention Hepatomegaly Other							
Rhythm	Basic rhythm Arrhythmias Conduction defect							
	Emotional status							
	Other							
Vital signs	Bath/activity level Temperature/weight Apical/radial pulse Respirations Blood pressure							
	Time							
Laboratory data	Enzymes Blood gases Other							

I and O	Intake Oral
	          IV
	          Total
	          Total 24 hours
	Output Urine
	            Emesis/Gomco
	            Total
	            Total 24 hours							

	Signature							

Stamp here with patient's Addressograph plate

Fig. 12-5. CCU summary flow sheet.

EVALUATION OF FLUID AND ELECTROLYTE BALANCE

Fluid and electrolyte balance is very important during the acute phase of the myocardial infarction, as previously discussed. Accurate measurement of intake and output levels, daily weight readings, evaluation of hydration, presence of pulmonary findings such as rales, and any edema are all very important components in the evaluation of fluid and electrolyte balance.

Each of these components should be evaluated and care planned accordingly. Goals should be set with the patient for his care. Reevaluation and further planning are performed in relation to changes in the patient's status.

COMPLICATIONS

The complications most frequently encountered in patients who had a myocardial infarction are congestive heart failure and arrhythmias. The following sections outline methods of preventing these complications. For further discussion, see Chapter 7.

Thromboembolic events
ANTICOAGULANTS

The need for anticoagulation therapy in patients who have a myocardial infarction continues to be controversial. Many physicians are not administering anticoagulants to patients in the acute phase following an infarction. However, if the patient has been given anticoagulants, partial thromboplastin times should be monitored while the patient receives anticoagulant therapy. Any tendencies toward bleeding should be noted and treated immediately. Once the patient is out of the intensive care unit, oral anticoagulants may be prescribed to replace heparin if anticoagulation therapy is to be continued.

EXERCISE PROGRAM

The exercise program is a very important part of the total rehabilitation effort. An exercise program can help prevent the complications engendered by inactivity and aid the patient psychologically. Exercise therapy helps prevent respiratory complications, venous stasis, joint stiffness from immobility, and the weakness resulting from loss of muscle tone. Furthermore, it promotes relaxation by decreasing tension.

An exercise program should be planned jointly with the patient for use throughout hospitalization and after discharge (see Chapter 4). Appropriate program goals and priorities for implementation should be planned with the patient. The exercise program should be structured in progressive stages and individualized according to the patient's tolerance. Initially the patient may be assisted in performing passive exercises. A footboard is useful for the patient to exercise his leg muscles. Tolerance to exercise at each stage should be observed, evaluated, and recorded. The first time the patient is out of bed, supine and standing blood pressures should be noted.

ELASTIC BANDAGES OR ELASTIC STOCKINGS

Elastic supports also may be used to prevent venous stasis. They must be applied with equal pressure from the foot to above the knee, checked frequently, and removed two or three times a day. Lotion or powder may be applied to the skin. The patient should be instructed not to cross his legs or ankles. Sometimes the elastic stockings roll down over the knee and create a tourniquet effect on the leg; if this occurs, it should be corrected promptly. The legs should be observed for redness, swelling, heat, red streaks and a positive Homans sign. This sign occurs as a slight pain at the back of the knee or calf when the ankle is forcibly dorsiflexed and is indicative of incipient or established thrombosis in the veins of the leg. Should any evidence of embolization be observed, the patient's physician should be notified.

Congestive heart failure

Techniques such as recording accurate intake and output measurements and daily weight are aimed to prevent and detect congestive heart failure early. Intake of routine I fluids should be kept to a minimum of 20 ml/hour in the patient who has had a myocardial infarction, unless dehydration is present. All fluids, except in an emergency, should be administered via microdrip, and drugs such as lidocaine should be placed in a reliable automatic drip-control device and checked frequently to ascertain whether the proper amount of fluid is being delivered. A heparin lock may be substituted when it is necessary to continue IV medications.

The patient should be assessed frequently to check for signs of possible congestive heart failure. The examination should include the following points:

1. Examine the heart, listening closely for the presence of a ventricular gallop (S_3) indicative of heart failure, and proceed with the other usual components of the cardiac examination. Special notice should also be given to the development of any tachyarrhythmias. These should be treated immediately after the physician has been notified.
2. Examine the lungs, listening for rales and, if present previously, comparing of their location, type, and amount. The presence of rhonchi that do not clear with coughing is important to note. Also, observe whether the patient is coughing (especially when lying flat), has Cheyne-Stokes respirations, or wheezes.
3. Search for peripheral edema or ascites. Although both of these are late signs, they can be correlated with other, earlier evidence of congestive failure.
4. Evaluate dyspnea. Congestive failure should be suspected in the patient who has had a myocardial infarction and then develops dyspnea without other known cause.
5. Evaluation of jugular veins may reveal signs of elevated jugular venous pressure. The neck veins also may become distended when sustained pressure is applied on the liver (hepatojugular reflux). Systemic venous pressure is often abnormally elevated and may be recognized most easily by observing t extent of distension of the jugular veins.

Arrhythmias

The improved management of arrhythmias constitutes a significant advance in the treatment of myocardial infarction. The prevention of serious and life-threatening arrhythmias depends on early recognition and aggressive management of their precursors. The most frequent arrhythmias noted in the acute phase of myocardial infarction are premature ventricular systoles, ventricular tachycardia, ventricular fibrillation, idioventricular rhythms, and AV blocks (see Chapter 8).

Psychosocial responses

Another aspect of preventive care and rehabilitation is the recognition and treatment of the patient's emotional responses to the myocardial infarction. After such an experience psychologic stress is normal and to be expected. Refer to Chapters 13 and 15 for discussion of these responses.

Equipment
MONITORING SYSTEM

The first equipment in the CCU with which the patient is likely to come in contact is the monitoring system. For a patient who has suffered a myocardial infarction or who has had a pacemaker implanted, careful monitoring of cardiac performance is the objective of preventive care. The cardiac monitor simplifies such care by continuously displaying the cardiac rhythm, blood pressure, and other parameters not readily followed by other means. Since most arrhythmias occur during the first 48 to 72 hours after infarction and 80% to 90% of patients who have myocardial infarctions experience arrhythmias, the need for constant surveillance is obvious.

Recurring arrhythmias compromise cardiac function by reducing cardiac output and coronary blood flow, increasing the myocardial need for oxygen, predisposing the patient to the development of more serious arrhythmias, and complicating therapy. Therefore prompt prevention and control of arrhythmias and the states predisposing to them (acidosis, electrolyte imbalance, early cardiac failure, pain, and anxiety) decrease the incidence of more serious arrhythmias and should improve the chances for survival after myocardial infarction. Awareness of these facts underscores the importance of detecting arrhythmias through the cardiac monitor.

Components. The cardiac monitor is an instrument that displays electrical activity during the cardiac cycle as a wave pattern across a screen. Since the components of particular monitoring systems vary widely, the basic components of most cardiac monitors are described in Fig. 12-6.

Oscilloscope. The screen on which the patient's electrocardiographic pattern appears is an oscilloscope.

Digital display. An electronic mechanism averages the number of ventricular complexes per minute, and this rate is shown on the rate scale indicator. Also, each QRS complex is indicated by an audible beep and flashing light. If the pulse rate can be relayed to a console at the nursing station, the bedside monitor beep should be silenced so that the patient does not hear it.

Rate meter. Integrated with the alarm system is the rate meter, which signals if the rate goes above or below predetermined limits. The limits vary according to the routine of a particular unit as based on the sensitivity of the electrodes and monitoring system. For example, the alarm may be triggered to sound at

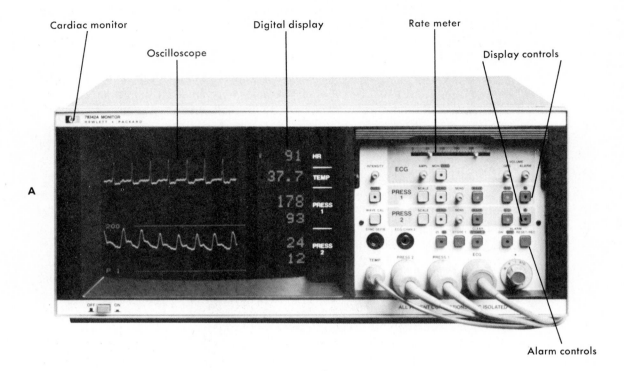

A

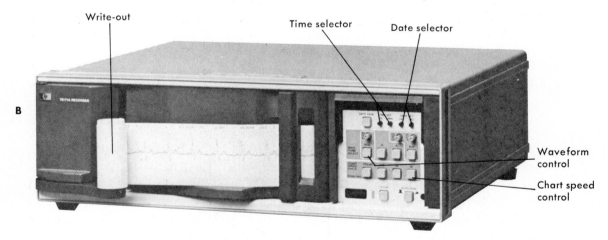

B

Fig. 12-6. Two sections of a cardiac monitor. **A** shows components: oscilloscope, digital display, rate meter, display control, and alarm control. **B** shows write-out, time selector, data selector, waveform control, and chart speed control. (Reprinted with permission from Hewlett-Packard Company, Palo Alto, California.)

either 25 beats above or below an individual patient's average heart rate, or it may be set automatically to sound at the high-low values of 150 and 50 beats/minute.

Alarm control system. When the heart rate falls below or rises above the preset levels, audio and visual alarms alert the staff. Each time an alarm is triggered, the staff must observe the patient and make a prompt decision regarding the cardiac rhythm.

When the CCU personnel depend on an alarm system for warning, the rate limit indicators and alarm system must be checked regularly—not only for accuracy but also to be sure that the system is operative. There are times when the limit settings are temporarily turned off in the patient's room. At these times personnel must depend on visual observation of the oscilloscope and the related clinical picture. For instance, the limit settings are turned off to prevent false alarms from electrical interference resulting from the use of a high-power machine (direct write-out ECG machine, portable x-ray machine, and so forth). False alarms may also be triggered by manipulation of the chest electrodes when repositioning the electrodes to other sites on the chest or when bathing the patient (see Chapter 8). The patient's welfare is endangered if the alarm limit settings remain off. It is essential to check these settings periodically.

When such an alarm system is not available, personnel must develop some other means of being alerted to changes in rhythm on the monitor oscilloscope. Only through an adequate method of observation can significant changes be identified and further rhythm disturbances prevented.

Sweep speed. The rate at which the electron beam sweeps across the screen can be controlled, and the sweep can be set at trace speeds of 25 mm/second (beam sweeps across standard screen in 6 seconds) or 50 mm/second (the 3-second sweep position). The 6-second position is generally used for routine monitoring. The 3-second position often provides for better interpretation of the rhythm or the pressure waveform by spreading the complexes.

Filter. The filter reduces extraneous muscular artifacts. However, when a 12-lead ECG is recorded from the monitor, the filter must be switched off, since it may distort the ST segment.

Central console. The individual bedside monitors in a CCU are connected to a central console at the nursing station. This permits continuous observation of the ECG patterns from all the monitors.

Additional components. Complementary parts can be added to the basic monitoring system as necessary. For example, a direct write-out ECG machine can be located in the central station; this is triggered to record the cardiac rhythm automatically during alarm situations or on demand. Such recordings may be used to demonstrate the patient's response to antiarrhythmic therapy.

Some monitor systems have memory tapes that store a predetermined duration of the patient's ECG, which can then be recalled at will. This allows a printing out of the cardiac rhythm recorded over the previous 60 seconds, for example. At the time of alarm some monitors write out memory storage and then the current rhythm from the time of trigger. Memory mechanisms, however, erase after a period of time; therefore, at the moment of an alarm personnel must decide whether to record the stored memory information or the current rhythm. Use of 24-hour tape monitoring simplifies this problem.

The monitoring system may also include multichannel recorders to monitor central venous, pulmonary artery, pulmonary capillary wedge, and arterial pressures and other physiologic parameters. In some research centers this information is coded for a computer where it can be stored and retrieved when needed. A pacemaking unit can be made an integral part of some monitors and can be set to trigger when the heart rate slows below a preset limit.

ELECTRODES

Topical electrode patches are commonly used for patient monitoring. The following steps are involved in preparing the skin and in applying the electrodes:
1. At the sites chosen for electrode placement, clean the skin thoroughly with alcohol to remove all residues. If necessary, shave the hair at these sites.
2. The skin of some patients may require abrasion at the electrode sites to obtain an adequate ECG signal. If this is the situation, abrade each site by rubbing the area with a gauze pad and abrasive electrode paste.
3. Apply adhesive electrode pads to the electrode, and press them against the skin at the prepared sites.
4. Electrodes may be secured in place with a strip of nonallergenic tape.

Placement of electrodes. The lead that best displays the QRS complexes and P waves (and pacing stimuli if pacing is used) is ideal for monitoring.

A positive, a negative, and a ground electrode are required to record one bipolar lead. The location for these electrodes determines the lead recorded by the monitor. For example, a modification of lead V_1 ($MC1_1$) is recorded by placing the negative electrode just under the outer quarter of the left shoulder and the ground electrode beneath the right clavicle, with the positive electrode being placed at the fourth right intercostal space at the right sternal border (the usual V_1 position).

To prevent their interfering with the physical examination, the chest electrodes should be placed away from the area near the apex of the heart. For long-term monitoring, chest leads are preferable to limb leads. Placement of the electrodes on the chest reduces motion and muscle artifact and allows the patient more freedom of movement than does limb-lead monitoring.

The modified V_1 chest lead has the added advantage over the other chest leads (often haphazardly positioned on the chest) of giving a maximum amount of information about rhythm disturbances and conduction. The $MC1_1$ provides an easily recognized recording of the sequence of ventricular activation and therefore furnishes maximum information to discriminate between right and left bundle branch block and between PVCs and aberrant supraventricular complexes.

Topical electrodes should be repositioned daily to prevent occurrence of local skin sores caused by prolonged contact of the hypertonic electrode paste with one point on the skin surface. When topical electrodes are changed, the used electrodes should be replaced with clean ones. (Many institutions use disposable electrodes.) The electrodes can be washed with soap and water. A pencil eraser may help remove dried paste from the electrode. Steel wool should not be used to clean electrodes, since it will leave grooves in the electrode surface that may generate recording artifacts.

The electrode wires from the patient are attached to a connecter unit pinned to the patient's gown. From this unit a cable leads to the monitor, where the electrode wires are connected to their respective terminals: positive wire to positive terminal, negative wire to negative terminal, and ground to ground. In certain machines the electrode terminals are specifically labeled. In other machines it is necessary to be familiar with the terminal connections. Incorrect matching of electrodes and terminals will change the lead that is to be monitored.

Interference with monitoring. Faulty techniques probably cause over 90% of the problems encountered in the course of cardiac monitoring. The common artifacts produced by electrical interferences can be prevented.

External voltage and/or patient movements generally are responsible for interference that occurs in a properly operating monitoring system. External voltage interference (alternating 60-cycle current) appears on the screen as a smooth thickening of the base line resulting from the 60 tiny peaks/second (Fig. 12-7, *A*). Inadequate grounding of the monitor and other equipment or improper electrode placement and connection may produce this type of interference.

Since the cardiac monitor registers muscle potential, any sudden voluntary or involuntary movement by the patient can cause interference. For example, coughing or turning over in bed may precipitate a wandering base line and erratic or irregular fluctuations on the oscilloscope (Fig. 12-7, *B*). Placing the electrodes in areas of limited muscular activity will reduce this problem.

In the tense, nervous, or cold patient the monitor may display a harsh, jagged, uneven oscillation about the base line. One must be careful not to interpret these base-line undulations as signifying fibrillatory waves.

Patient's feelings about the monitor. During the stay in CCU the patient is bound to experience significant psychologic stress. The intricate electronic equipment may contribute to these feelings. Patients should be encouraged to discuss their feelings about the monitor. Continued simple explanations and reassurance

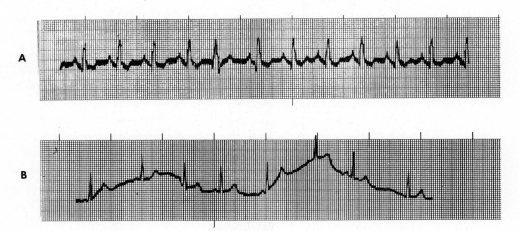

Fig. 12-7. A, ECG tracing that shows external voltage interference (alternating 60-cycle current) appearing as a smooth thickening of the base line as a result of the 60 tiny peaks per second. **B,** ECG tracing in which patient interference (coughing, turning, etc.) is shown by a wandering base line.

should help relieve anxiety. Families should be included, too, because they often share the patients' fears and increase their apprehension. The presence of the cardiac monitor is reassuring to most patients because it ensures constant surveillance. (See Chapter 13 for further discussion.)

ARTERIAL CATHETERS

The uses and purposes of the arterial catheter are discussed in Chapter 7. When monitoring arterial pressure directly, one must carefully observe the following precautions to obtain meaningful values:

1. Standardize, balance, and calibrate the monitoring equipment at least once every 8 hours and after position changes or movements that might alter the calibration. Instructions for this procedure accompany the individual manufacturer's equipment.
2. Alarms must be left on when an arterial line is in place.
3. Flush the arterial line every hour. If Intraflo catheters are used, flushing every 5 to 15 minutes is not necessary. A solution of D5W with heparin added is used for flushing. The catheter should be flushed manually every 1 to 2 hours to clear the line after blood is drawn, if blood is in the line for any reason. The pulse waveform will become dampened or flattened somewhat when impairment of flow occurs.
4. Prevent catheter displacement by fastening the arterial catheter securely to the skin. The catheter may be sutured to the skin after insertion.
5. Prevent blood from entering the transducer. Blood in the transducer will dampen the pressure reading and may damage the transducer.
6. Observe the extremity every 1 to 2 hours for bleeding and circulatory insufficiency. The arterial catheter should be observed frequently for leakage and proper stopcock position.
7. Apply a sterile dressing to the site, and change it at least once every 24 hours. When the dressing is changed, note the condition of the site and the surrounding area.
8. Observe the site for infection when dressings are changed. Should the catheter remain in the artery longer than 48 to 72 hours, observation of the site at least every 8 hours is imperative.
9. Immobilize the extremity to prevent accidental dislodgment of the catheter. If an armboard or wooden device is used, proper padding will prevent stasis changes of skin and increase comfort.
10. Exercise care when drawing blood from the catheter. The stopcock must be returned to the original position to ensure proper operation and prevent leakage.
11. After removing the catheter, apply direct pressure to the artery for 10 to 15 minutes or longer, until bleeding ceases. The site should be covered with a sterile dressing for 24 hours.
12. After the catheter is removed, observe the site for signs of bleeding, infection, and circulatory insufficiency until healing is complete. If any of these are noted, immediate attention should be given to correction of the condition.

SWAN-GANZ CATHETERS

The use of Swan-Ganz catheters to measure pulmonary arterial and pulmonary capillary wedge pressures is discussed in Chapter 7.

The use of the central venous pressure (CVP) to determine right atrial pressure (RAP) is no longer considered sufficiently accurate because the relationship between RAP and left ventricular end-diastolic pressure (LVEDP) is inconsistent. Therefore pulmonary artery end-diastolic pressure (PAEDP) and pulmonary capillary wedge pressure (PCWP), rather than CVP, should be accepted as major guides in the treatment of heart failure and shock.

PRESSURE MEASUREMENT

Pulmonary artery pressure. The pulmonary artery (PA) waveform evidences a sharp rise during ejection of blood from the right ventricle after the pulmonary valve opens. This pressure rise is followed by a slow decrease in pressure during the ejection of blood from the right ventricle until the pulmonic valve closes, indicated by the dicrotic notch. The pressure continues to decrease until systole occurs again.

Normal PA systolic pressure is 20 to 30 mm Hg, and normal PA diastolic pressure ranges from 5 to 16 mm Hg. The normal mean PA pressure ranges from 10 to 20 mm Hg. The PA systolic pressure normally equals the right ventricular pressure (Fig. 12-8). The PAEDP should be almost equal to the mean PCWP in the absence of pulmonary vascular disease.

Elevation of PA pressure may occur during (1) increased pulmonary blood flow, as in a left-to-right shunt resulting from atrial or ventricular septal defect, (2) increased pulmonary arteriolar resistance resulting from primary pulmonary hypertension or mitral stenosis, and (3) left ventricular failure resulting from any cause.

Pulmonary capillary wedge pressure. Since there is normally a direct relationship between PAEDP, PCWP, and LVEDP, an elevated PAEDP or PCWP reflects the elevated LVEDP that occurs when the left ventricle can no longer adequately pump the blood presented to it.

The PCWP is normally 4 to 12 mm Hg. PCWP exceeding 12 mm Hg may occur as a result of left ventricular failure, mitral stenosis, or mitral insufficiency, in addition to other possible causes.

Pulmonary artery end-diastolic pressure. Since the PAEDP is approximately equal to the PCWP, and since the PAEDP is an accurate reflection of LVEDP (Fig. 12-9), the PAEDP can be used as an alternative measurement of LVEDP in most patients, even in the presence of pulmonary venous hypertension. At the time of catheter insertion, the PAEDP can be compared with the PCWP. If the difference is less than 5 mm Hg, the PAEDP can be used as an accurate estimation of the LVEDP.[8]

Potential problems in use of Swan-Ganz catheters. There are several disadvantages to monitoring with a Swan-Ganz catheter. The major disadvantage is the need to reinflate the balloon each time a measurement is made. Pulmonary hemorrhage may result if the balloon is inflated when the catheter tip is in a small arterial branch; however, careful adherence to proper procedures for balloon

A

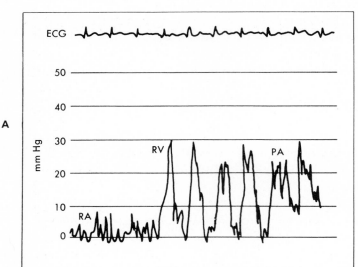

B

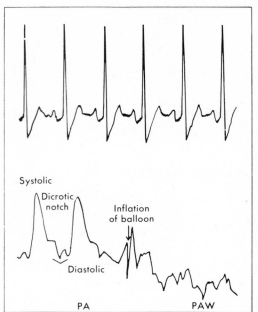

Fig. 12-8. A, After inflation of balloon at tip of Swan-Ganz catheter, intracardiac pressure identifies right atrium (*RA*), right ventricle (*RV*), and pulmonary artery (*PA*) as catheter is advanced. Right ventricle is characterized by higher systolic but similar diastolic pressure when compared to right atrial pressure. Pulmonary artery pressure shows same systolic value as that in right ventricle, but diastolic pressure is higher than that in either right ventricle or atrium. Catheter whip or artifact is produced by exaggerated motion of catheter with inflated balloon and usually disappears with deflation of balloon. **B,** PA pressure waveform via balloon-tip catheter. Note balloon inflation and subsequent change to PAW waveform. (**A** modified from Rackley, C.E., and Russell, R.O.: *Invasive techniques for hemodynamic monitoring,* Dallas, 1973, by permission of the American Heart Association. **B** modified from Daily, E.K., and Schroeder, J.S.: Techniques in bedside hemodynamic monitoring, St. Louis, 1976, The C.V. Mosby Co.)

inflation is likely to minimize this risk. The catheter tip may become wedged in a distal branch after repeated inflations, which may lead to a pulmonary infarction. When the catheter tip is withdrawn from the wedged position, it often recoils into the right ventricle or right atrium and must be repositioned.[8]

Measurement of PA pressure and PCWP. The method used to record PA pressure and PCWP from the standard strain-gauge pressure transducer differs among institutions. Special points to consider in maintaining the catheter and measuring pressures include the following:

A. Record readings.
   1. Record pressures at regular intervals as ordered and as necessary. Evaluate changes and report to the physician if not present when the reading is performed.
   2. Calibrate equipment before each reading.
   3. Irrigate line before each reading by pulling red rubber Intraflo plunger for 5 seconds (or manually if Intraflo is not used).

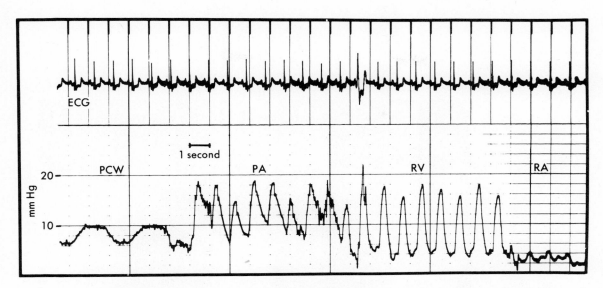

Fig. 12-9. Simultaneous recording of ECG and pulmonary capillary wedge (*PCW*), pulmonary arterial (*PA*), right ventricular (*RV*), and right atrial (*RA*) pressures. The pulmonary arterial catheter was initially in a wedged position, with the balloon inflated. The balloon was then deflated, and the catheter was slowly withdrawn through the right heart chambers. Note the cyclic respiratory effects in the pressure signals. The PCW and PA end-diastolic pressures are equal. (From Mantle, J.A., and others: Advances in the treatment of heart failure. In Rackley, C.E., editor: Critical care cardiology: Cardiovascular Clinics, 11/3, Philadelphia, 1981, F.A. Davis Co.)

       4. Patient should be in same position for each reading, and position should be recorded.

  B. Maintain catheter.

    1. Maintain patency of the catheter.

      a. Pressure bag at 300 mm Hg irrigates automatically with 3 ml of saline and heparin solution per hour, using an Intraflo catheter.

      b. Irrigate manually every hour by pulling the red rubber Intraflo stopper for 5 seconds.

      c. Count irrigating solution used at the end of each shift as part of IV intake.

      d. Change the dressing every 24 hours, clean the site with povidone-iodine (Betadine), and apply antibacterial ointment.

      e. Observe for signs of infection and/or phlebitis at the insertion site.

    2. Observe the complexes for changes in fluctuation.

      a. Flattened complexes: a possible wedging of catheter in a pulmonary arteriole, which could result in pulmonary infarction. Turn the patient and ask him to cough and take some deep breaths; this may dislodge a catheter stuck in wedge. The physician should be alerted.

      b. Irregular complex: an irregular fluctuation with no clear complex, denoting the need for irrigation with a 10-ml syringe. If this complex continues, the catheter is probably of no value and should be removed.

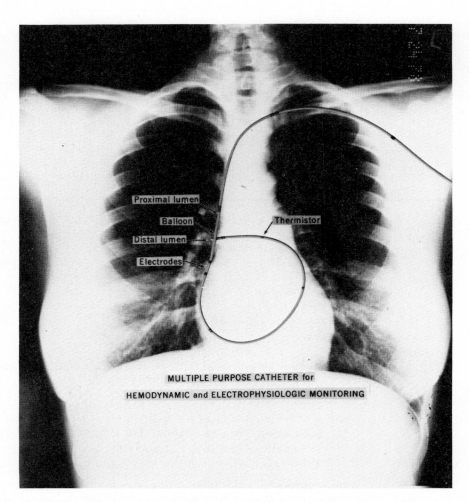

Fig. 12-10. The multiple-purpose pulmonary triple-lumen catheter with atrial electrodes is shown superimposed on a chest x-ray film. The distal lumen records the pulmonary arterial or wedge pressure and is a useful site for withdrawing blood samples. The balloon can be inflated to facilitate passage through the right side of the heart. The thermistor permits measurements of the cardiac output by the thermal dilution technique. The electrodes record the atrial electrogram and can be used for atrial pacing. The proximal lumen records the CVP and is a useful site for infusing fluids and medications. The catheter tip should be kept in the proximal pulmonary artery except when a wedge pressure is being recorded. (From Mantle, J.A., and others: Chest **72**:285, 1977.)

c. No complex: recalibration of the transducer needed.

Cardiac output. Most Swan-Ganz catheters are equipped with a thermistor in the distal portion, which permits measurement of the cardiac output by the thermodilution technique (Fig. 12-10). This technique is very reliable in producing cardiac outputs that closely approximate those of the other methods, such as the Fick method, used in cardiac catheterization. Data regarding the cardiac output, when combined with the LVEDP, are useful in determining the adequacy of left ventricular function.[8]

Measurement of cardiac output. Procedures for measuring cardiac output vary with the type of equipment used. Since the measurements are made with the Swan-Ganz catheter, care of the patient and equipment is unchanged.

Care of the patient and Swan-Ganz equipment

1. Following insertion of the Swan-Ganz catheter, a sterile dressing should be applied to the site and changed at least every 24 hours. The condition of the site, including presence of active bleeding and signs of infection, should be noted.
2. The extremity should be immobilized to prevent accidental dislodgment of the catheter. Taping the catheter to the extremity stabilizes the catheter. Padding of an armboard or wooden device promotes comfort and immobilizes the extremity.
3. The extremity should be checked for circulatory insufficiency and bleeding at least every hour.
4. The catheter should be observed frequently for leakage and proper stopcock position. Care should be taken to return the stopcock to the *off* position when drawing blood from the catheter.
5. The balloon should always remain deflated with a syringe attached, except when the PCWP is being read.
6. After the catheter is removed, the site should be observed closely for bleeding and infection until healing is complete. A sterile dressing should be applied to the site.

Electrophysiologic monitoring

A multipurpose flow-directed pulmonary arterial catheter permits monitoring of the bipolar atrial ECG, pulmonary arterial wedge pressure, CVP, and cardiac output, and also allows atrial pacing. The standard Swan-Ganz thermistor catheter is modified to include two ring electrodes on the shaft at the marks for 25 and 26 mm from the tip. This is the only visible difference between this catheter and the standard Swan-Ganz catheter. With the catheter in the right atrium at the junction of the superior vena cava, stable ECGs of high quality can be obtained. These high-fidelity ECGs allow rapid and accurate diagnosis of various complex arrhythmias. Because of the limited noise in the ECG signal, continuous quantitative interval measurements by a computerized system are possible. Moreover, the stable intracavitary electrode position provides a reliable atrial pacing site for converting supraventricular tachycardias, for maintaining an adequate rate during sinus bradycardia, and for suppressing ventricular premature beats by rapid atrial pacing rates.[8] This multipurpose catheter permits both hemodynamic and electrophysiologic monitoring, plus atrial pacing that is convenient and safe for long periods in patients with unstable cardiopulmonary problems.

Care of the patient and equipment is the same as in patients with Swan-Ganz catheters in place.

Intraaortic counterpulsation

The intraaortic balloon technique may be employed in patients with low output failure and is discussed in Chapter 7. Special points to be considered include the following:

1. Arrangement and preparation of equipment prior to insertion must be meticulous.
2. Pulses must be assessed prior to insertion to evaluate postinsertion complications.
3. The ECG is the triggering stimulus for balloon activation.
4. Antibiotic therapy must be adequate.
5. Anticoagulation therapy may be desirable.
6. Angina and/or acute back pain may herald complications of balloon insertion.
7. Timing of the balloon must be carefully monitored and adjusted as necessary.
8. A chest x-ray film may be used to verify the position of the balloon.
9. Strict aseptic technique must be maintained for dressing changes.

Computer systems

During the past 15 years computers have been developed that have been used primarily for acquiring, reporting, and storing electrocardiographic and hemodynamic data.

Computer-based arrhythmia systems have generally been limited to analysis of the shape and timing of the QRS complex. Detection of premature ventricular beats has become reasonably reliable, and variable levels of alarms allow for alerting the staff according to the degree of the arrhythmias' severity. The swallowable capsule electrode for esophageal monitoring of atrial activity makes possible the recognition of supraventricular arrhythmias as well.

Closed-loop computerized hemodynamic monitoring systems automatically regulate selected parameters based on sampled data and thereby contribute to early stabilization of the patient's condition. For example, nitroprusside may be infused by the computer based on a prescribed mean arterial pressure and is more effective than manual control.

The use of newer microprocessors should augment the applications of computer technology to patient care and may reduce the costs of these systems.

Electrical safety for patient and equipment operator

The varied electronic equipment in a CCU increases the potential of electrical shock hazard for both the patient and the equipment operator. Consequently, CCU personnel should have a basic understanding of the principles of current flow, current source, and grounding.

If all ground connections of equipment are not at the same potential (zero volts or a few millivolts above zero), leakage current may flow between the source and its ground. Current will flow through the patient if he serves as a link in this circuit. Skin offers resistance to current flow and therefore protects the heart from electrical shock. If the voltage is high enough or skin resistance has been lowered or eliminated, ventricular fibrillation may result. On some equipment, built-in isolation circuits isolate the patient from the ground and the power line, thus preventing any conductive pathways. However, an intracardiac catheter or fluid column bypasses the skin and the protection from current flow that it affords, making the patient highly vulnerable to electrical shock. Alternating current (AC) power-line current levels of only millionths of amperes, undetectable when applied to the skin, can induce ventricular fibrillation if contact with the myocardium is made.

Any AC power-line–operated device from which some of the current flows through the metal frame, case, or other exposed parts may serve as a current source. It may be an electric bed with a broken or missing ground connection or any device with two-wire power cords (two-pronged plugs) such as TV sets, bed lamps, or electric fans. The patient may lie in the path between the current source and ground directly, by touching the electrical device, or ground indirectly, by making physical contact with another person who touches the defectively grounded instrument. Either situation causes the patient to become a conductive pathway and allows current to flow through him to ground.

Equipment operators should be cautious when using electronic equipment near water, steam pipes, radiators, or plumbing fixtures. Such pipes and fittings are excellent electrical grounds. Consequently, any electrical device near them, including the power cords, plugs, and wall receptacles, that exposes the user to live current can be extremely hazardous if the operator simultaneously contacts both the device and a grounded pipe, faucet, and so forth. The operator then becomes the link between the current source and the ground that the current seeks. The resultant shock may not be fatal, but serious injury can result from violent muscular reaction in "letting go" (Table 12-2).

Ward personnel may detect tingling sensations when touching or brushing against a piece of electronic equipment. The voltage necessary to produce this sensation is only one thousandth of an ampere. Under ordinary circumstances this is harmless; however, this voltage is nearly 50 times the amount necessary to produce ventricular fibrillation if current flows directly to the patient's heart.

Table 12-2. Effects of electric current

60-cycle current (1-second duration) delivered through skin		60-cycle current (1-second duration) leading to heart	
Milliamperes	Effects	Microamperes	Effects
1	Threshold of perception; tingling	20 to 50	Ventricular fibrillation
16	"Let go" current; muscle contraction		
50	Pain; possible fainting; mechanical injury		
100-3000	Ventricular fibrillation		
6000 or greater	Sustained myocardial depolarization followed by normal rhythm; temporary respiratory paralysis; burns		

Clearly, many considerations are necessary to ensure electrical safety. Awareness of potential hazards, prompt correction of faulty equipment, and regular safety inspection checks are all needed. Personnel should be thoroughly briefed in the following rules for electrical safety in the CCU:

A. All equipment should be grounded. This means that a pathway of least resistance is available for the currents within the machine to flow to ground.

   1. All equipment must have three-pronged plugs (which connect the hospital ground to the equipment chassis).

   2. Adaptors fitting a three-pronged plug into a two-slot electrical outlet should not be used.

   3. Extension cords should not be used to connect electronic equipment. If extensions are necessary, use only three-pronged grounding-type cords.

B. Wet surfaces conduct current. Therefore such hazards as wet sheets and wet floors should be eliminated.

C. Safety inspection checks should be routine. A qualified electrical technician should check all equipment for faulty or missing ground connections and hazardous voltages. (Remember that equipment can still operate with defective ground connections.)

D. When two instruments are in use near a patient, connect them to the same power receptacle.

E. Never plug or unplug equipment, turn on a light, and so forth while any part of your body is in contact with water, steam pipes, radiators, or plumbing fixtures.

F. Prevent equipment cords from kinking, draping on pipes and plumbing, or lying on wet surfaces.

G. Report tingling sensations emitted from a bed frame, instrument case, and so forth. Unplug the equipment that is not necessary to life support of the patient; correct this condition immediately in equipment necessary for life support.

H. When using an intracavitary lead, connect the electrode catheter to the V lead of the ECG machine, since this circuit has a high electrical resistance in relation to ground. Anyone or anything electrically grounded must not touch the V-lead electrode terminals.

I. Additional precautions should be taken for patients with temporary cardiac pacemakers.

   1. The electrodes at the end of the pacemaker should be well insulated. On older models a rubber glove is used to cover the exposed terminals at the junction with the external power source. Most newer models are adequately insulated, however.

   2. When possible, use external battery pacemakers that are isolated from the power-line sources.

   3. Personnel should wear rubber gloves when connecting or disconnecting the battery pacemaker and when adjusting electrodes at the end of the catheter.

      4. Personnel should not wear leather-bottomed shoes on conductive or
         carpeted floors.
  J. Patients should wear bedroom shoes at all times on conductive floors.
  K. Patients should use battery-operated electric razors.

Transfer from CCU

Patients tend to become dependent on the CCU atmosphere during the acute phase of their illness. Comfort is derived from sophisticated equipment and the individualized care provided by personnel in constant attendance. The concern expressed by physicians, nurses, and other health personnel adds to the developing patient dependence on the CCU. Not unexpectedly then, the patient may have both emotional and physiologic reactions to transfer if adequate preparation and follow-up arrangements are not included in his care.

Schwartz and Brenner[9] reported a study in which two experimental groups and two control groups were used. The experimental groups contained subjects who were exposed to a family-centered nursing approach or to development of a staff nurse-patient relationship prior to transfer from the critical care unit. Patients in each experimental group scored lower than the control patients in patient stress as reported by the patient, family, and nurse, cardiovascular complications within 24 hours of transfer, and cardiovascular complications 24 to 72 hours after transfer. These data support the need for health care team involvement with the patient and family in preparation for and implementation of the patient's transfer from the unit.

Health personnel, especially the primary nurse, have a responsibility to ease the reaction of the patient in the transition from CCU to the intermediate care unit. Personnel should not force or attempt to impose desired behaviors on the patient, but should strive for a working relationship that allows the patient to rely on the nurse and other health personnel for assistance and information as progress in the adaptation process is made. Acting on behalf of the patients, guiding and teaching them in a supportive manner, and helping them to adjust to the physical changes in their new environment are all ways by which health personnel can ease patient transitions.

Acting on behalf of the patient. Health personnel should actively assist the patient once the transfer is anticipated. Calling the patient's family to notify them of the move is helpful to both, since the patient will know that he will not be "lost" to his family, and the family will not be unduly alarmed at finding an empty bed at the next visiting time.

During daily care in the CCU the nurse has an opportunity to discuss areas of concern with the patient. Financial concerns are often the first worries mentioned by the patient. Discussing these concerns and securing assistance for the patient, such as a visit from the social worker or other rehabilitation team member, can be helpful in alleviating emotional upset. The social worker and other appropriate personnel can assist in the transition phase by rechanneling the patient's energies toward adaptation and planning for recovery.

Guiding, supporting, and teaching the patient. Beginning in the early phase of CCU care, the nurse should prepare the patient for transfer by explaining that the CCU is an area in which he is to receive temporary care and that once he has improved sufficiently, care can be maintained in a unit that provides intermediate care. This explanation prepares the patient for the move well in advance and helps in the realization that improvement in condition is the primary determinant for the move.

Since the actual transfer may be planned or sudden, the patient should be informed about the elements of transfer prior to the anticipated time of transfer. The patient should be aware that staff in the intermediate care unit will be given a verbal report concerning his illness, progress, and potential problems for which they should be alert, in addition to charted information gathered throughout the CCU phase. The CCU nurse should accompany the patient to the intermediate care unit and introduce him to the primary nurse responsible for his care, so that he is familiar enough with the person to call should he need assistance. Any information that the patient requests regarding the new unit can then be answered by the intermediate care unit nurse.

Positive and realistic reinforcement of the patient's progress is a necessaary component in his adaptation. Information regarding his status and improvement should be discussed as his condition evolves. Reassurance by health personnel, along with factual information about his progress, assists the patient in looking forward to the transfer and his return to a normal life.

Assisting in the patient's adaptation to environmental changes. The possible dependence of the patient on the monitor has been mentioned previously. The use of the monitor and its limitations should be described to the patient initially and periodically thereafter. Patients have been known to think that their heart beat depended on the monitor. If such inaccuracies in the patient's perceptions can be dispelled early, potential anxieties related to discontinuation of the monitor may be prevented. If possible, the patient should be "weaned" from all equipment, including the monitor, before transfer.

Continuity in the plan of care for the patient should be discussed with the intermediate care unit staff. The patient should be made aware that such communication has taken place and that such continuity is planned. The clinical nursing specialist can be an asset in the coordination of planning and implementation to provide maximum continuity for the patient.

INTERMEDIATE PHASE

Studies have shown that some patients who suffer acute myocardial infarction continue to be at risk even after surviving the first few hazardous days after onset. In fact, mortality during the later in-hospital phase of the illness, when the patient is usually no longer being cared for in the CCU, may be as high as that in the CCU for some groups of patients. This fact is the basis for the concept of intermediate coronary care, whereby patients can be located in an area that is usually close to the CCU. This unit has monitoring and resuscitative equipment and is staffed with personnel sufficiently prepared to provide routine as well as cardiopulmonary emergency care.

Several terms have evolved to describe an area designed to allow closely supervised convalescence for patients who have transferred from the CCU. This area provides more intense observation and care than a routine medical ward but less than that provided in a CCU. Synonyms for this area include *step-down unit, liberalized cardiac unit,* and *intermediate care unit.* Regardless of the name selected, this unit has these multiple purposes:

1. Continued patient monitoring to allow for immediate recognition of cardiac arrhythmias and conduction disturbances
2. Immediate cardiopulmonary resuscitation
3. Safe, supervised, early mobilization
4. Reduction in costs of acute care practices in hospitalization
5. Environment conducive to psychologic and physical recovery
6. Education and reeducation concerning abilities and disabilities related to heart disease
7. Continuation of the planned rehabilitation program

The following groups of patients have been shown to be at increased risk of catastrophic cardiac events during hospitalization and after discharge from the CCU[10-12]:

1. Patients with anterior infarctions involving large portions of the left ventricle and interventricular septum
2. Patients who, while in the CCU, exhibit circulatory failure in the form of cardiogenic shock, pulmonary edema, and congestive heart failure
3. Patients with preexisting cardiovascular disease, prior infarction, and fascicular block
4. Patients who exhibit arrhythmias that are primarily ventricular in origin or are indicative of heart failure; for example, atrial fibrillation or flutter and/or persistent sinus tachycardia

Although current data support the fact that people who fall within the categories listed above have a two to six times greater chance of late in-hospital sudden death, this cannot be predicted with complete accuracy. However, these patients have had a slightly longer stay in the CCU (1 to 2 days longer) and tend to be 3 to 4 years older than their counterparts who survive hospitalization. These facts alone support the need for accurate assessment and interpretation of data to prevent and/or treat the complications that contribute to this high late in-hospital mortality.

RECEIVING THE PATIENT FROM THE CCU

The following suggestions will ease the patient's transition from the CCU to the intermediate care area:

1. Having the intermediate care area prepared with all the equipment needed by the patient and located close to bathroom facilities, nurses' station, and emergency equipment
2. Monitoring cardiac activity by telemetry to provide continuity and rapid detection of potential arrhythmic problems
3. Providing a proposed guideline for educational activities in which the patient participates during the remainder of hospitalization
4. Providing patient and family with information on routines appropriate to efficient operation of the unit, such as visiting policies, educational opportunities, activity routines, and purpose of specialized equipment

ASSESSMENT OF THE PATIENT

The evaluation process initiated on admission to the CCU should be continued in the intermediate care unit. This evaluation can be easily divided into three phases: initial or admission assessment, assessment of health needs, and preparation for discharge.

Initial assessment. Initially the person with primary responsibility for providing care to the patient should complete a health assessment. This entails collecting data, making a plan of care based on the assessment of the data, carrying out the plan, and, finally, evaluating the effectiveness of the care.

First, when the patient arrives at the intermediate care area, a brief history can be obtained by direct questioning. This limited interview provides a basis for a therapeutic relationship and yields information needed for making judgments about appropriate care. Additional information can be obtained from the clinical record and from CCU personnel.

Second, a brief physical examination concentrating on the cardiopulmonary system provides base-line information by which progress is evaluated.

Assessment of health needs. The second phase of evaluation involves assessment of the individual's health needs. Attention should be given to activity tolerance, educational strengths and deficits, and the physical and psychologic status of the individual.

One goal of intermediate care is supervised early mobilization. Consistent with this expectation is a gradual increase in physical activity during the remainder of hospitalization, enabling the patient to reach the activity levels required for self-care when he returns home. The activities allowed include progressively increased self-care, increasing time spent sitting up in a chair, and body motion and strength-building exercises. The patient should increase his ambulation daily until he can walk about the hospital unit without tiring.

These physical activities are alternated with rest periods. Exercise should always be avoided after meals, when a large percentage of cardiac output is diverted to digest food. Criteria for decreasing the level of activity include the following:

1. Chest pain or dyspnea
2. Heart rate exceeding 120 beats/minute
3. Occurrence of a significant arrhythmia
4. Decrease in systolic blood pressure of 20 mm Hg
5. Increased ST segment displacement on the ECG or monitor

Assessment of the patient's educational strengths and deficits should be determined soon after admission to the intermediate care unit so that planned teaching can be completed before discharge. In many instances personnel with special knowledge and skill in psychologic evaluation can be of tremendous assistance in determining how to best motivate patients and facilitate their learning. For some patients denial, depression, and despair are patterns of behavior that prevent optimal benefit from educational efforts. People who have psychologic expertise can be of particular assistance in dealing with these exceptional patients and their families. This period immediately following the CCU experience has been recognized as the time when patients are most receptive to changes in lifestyle. Lifelong habits can be changed at this point more easily than later, when the emotional impact of the acute event has subsided. The personnel must take full advantage of this receptive period.

Preparation for discharge. Preparing the patients and their families for the time when they leave the hospital should be a primary focus of care during the intermediate phase. All of the following items should be considered in a discharge planning program:

Intervention. Intervention should be aimed at the prevention and treatment of health problems, and personnel should be especially aware of the following potential complications.

ARRHYTHMIAS. Most patients often have some type of occasional premature systole. However, rhythms such as supraventricular and ventricular tachycardias warrant immediate and accurate diagnosis and instigation of appropriate therapy (see discussion of arrhythmias, Chapter 8).

HEART FAILURE. Heart failure is a frequent complication of myocardial infarction (see Chapter 7).

PULMONARY DYSFUNCTION. Pulmonary dysfunction is noted frequently as pulmonary embolism, chronic obstructive pulmonary disease (COPD), and/or pneumonia requiring early detection and intervention.

POSTMYOCARDIAL INFARCTION SYNDROME. As emphasized by Dressler, postmyocardial infarction syndrome occurs in a small percentage of patients. The cause is unknown, but it has been attributed to a hypersensitivity reaction in which the antigen is necrotic cardiac muscle. The disorder usually occurs a few weeks or months after myocardial infarction, but it has been observed within 1 week after infarction. The syndrome is characterized by pericardial-type pain, pericardial friction rub, and fever. It may last days to weeks and must be distinguished from a recurrent myocardial infarction, a pulmonary infarction, or congestive heart failure. The condition is treated with corticosteroids, aspirin, or indomethacin.

MYOCARDIAL ISCHEMIA AND/OR MYOCARDIAL INFARCTION. Some patients sustain further myocardial damage as a result of extension of a previous infarction or development of a new area of infarction. Personnel must be alert to this possibility and arrange for immediate transfer to the CCU for treatment of the acute episode. Although data reported in the literature provide some conflicting statistics, it is generally accepted that the following factors provide evidence for predicting the increased possibility of reinfarction[12-14]:

1. *Age*. The risk of reinfarction is generally greater for people over the age of 65 years.
2. *ECG readings*. Assessment of site and extent of infarction can help in anticipating further problems. Anterior infarctions carry a greater risk, especially when associated with bundle branch block. The larger the area of infarction, the greater the chance of reinfarction.
3. *Systolic blood pressure on admission*. People who have systolic blood pressures of 85 mm Hg or below and with clinical signs of shock and heart rates above 100 beats/minute are at increased risk of reinfarction.
4. *Heart size determined by x-ray film*. Cardiomegaly recognized as an increased cardiothoracic ratio usually reflects chronic heart disease.
5. *Degree of pulmonary congestion determined by x-ray film*. Acute left-sided heart failure noted as confluent lung densities in the central lung fields

and increased pulmonary vascularity denotes an increased risk of rein-farction.

6. *Previous history of cardiac ischemia.* The risk of reinfarction increases when a person has a history of angina pectoris and/or one or more myo-cardial infarctions.

Evaluation. Evaluation must be a part of care to ensure intervention that fa-cilitates reaching the goals established by the patient, his family, and health care personnel. Accurate assessment, planning, intervention, and evaluation during hospitalization will allow the discharge process to proceed with minimal problems.

Patient preparation for cardiac rehabilitation. Intervention is based on individual-ized prescriptions for care and includes activity, diet, and educational pursuits. It is important that the family be included in all planning. An in-depth discussion of cardiac rehabilitation is in Chapter 14.

ILLNESS. Help the patient gain insight into his illness of condition. Provide information about the disease process, risk factors, and symptoms.

MEDICATIONS. Explain prescriptions and details of the drug program to both the patient and the responsible family member; knowledge of the drugs' actions and side effects is helpful to patients. Prescriptions should be labeled. Help the patient adjust the medication schedule to the usual life-styles at home to ensure maxi-mum adherence to the regimen.

NUTRITION. Explain dietary modifications of calories, fats, and/or sodium. Dem-onstration of food preparation consistent with the dietary regimen and the pa-tient's eating preferences and habits is desirable.

PHYSICAL ACTIVITY. Prescribe recommendations related to the type and magnitude of exercise, based on the patient's prior level of activity and job requirements. It is the responsibility of the health team to prescribe and initially supervise the type of exercise, to determine its duration and schedule, and to warn against overexercising and describe its signs.

SMOKING. Health care personnel should set an example by not smoking. Clinics are offered by many communities to help people stop smoking.

SEXUAL ACTIVITY. This topic is frequently overlooked or glossed over when plan-ning for the cardiac patient's discharge; indeed, it is an area which is often not considered at any time during the patient's hospitalization.

The health team must remember that sexual desire and activity are not re-stricted to healthy individuals. The topic must be confronted and discussed openly and honestly with the patient. Begin at the time of admission to the CCU by explaining to the patient that normal sexual desires may be experienced but that expression of this desire should be postponed until transfer from the CCU because of the temporary effect of masturbation on the heart rate and blood pressure. Be alert to the fact that suppressed sexual desire may cause emotional stress for some patients, and that this factor may be responsible for temporary alterations in vital signs.

As part of the discharge planning process, obtain an in-depth precoronary sexual history. Renshaw[15] suggests that the history include questions about fre-quency, preferred position, intercoital masturbation, morning erections, alter-native sexual expressions, and the spouse's health, interest in sex, and cooper-ation. The influence of medications and alcohol is also important to note. The patient should be questioned about sexual self-expectations. Previous sexual problems, marital problems, anger, anxiety, or fear may inhibit postcoronary rehabilitation. After the history is obtained, work with the other health team members, the patient, and the sexual partner to develop a plan for the return to precoronary sexual activity.

COMMUNITY RESOURCES. The local heart association, vocational rehabilitation center, Veterans Administration, and other organizations may be of help to the patient. Other people, such as the social worker, public health nurses, dietitian, physical therapist, chaplain, occupational therapist, and psychologist may be asked to help in the planning. Many communities have developed "coronary clubs," in which interested postmyocardial infarction patients, their families, and health care workers meet at regular times for guidance in care and education. This offers an opportunity to teach basic cardiac life support to the former patient and his family. Guest speakers may discuss topics such as nutrition, exercise, sexuality, basic cardiac life support, and antismoking techniques.

Finally, assure the patient that help is readily available if it is needed again. Inform the patient about when to seek help and where to obtain it. This can be done by "reliving" with the patient the symptoms and the action taken prior to the last heart attack. Warning symptoms other than those previously experienced can be discussed. Explore alternative ways of reaching help. Direct family members in obtaining skills in basic life support.

DISCHARGE

The actual discharge process will require little time if the goals established for the patient during hospitalization have been met. To ensure that all points have been covered, a checklist that includes the following considerations should be initiated several days before actual discharge:

1. *Activity.* The prescription depends on the patient's psychologic and emotional limitations.
2. *Diet.* Dietary modifications, particularly of calories, fats, and sodium intake, should be recommended and recorded.
3. *Medications.* Information about the actual medication prescribed, including drug name, dosage, desired effects, and possible adverse effects, should be thoroughly explained to the patient.
4. *New or recurrent symptoms.* Chest pain is particularly important. Palpitation, shortness of breath, dyspnea, syncope, or presyncope should be looked for by the patient and reported to the health team. Intensive education instructing the patient to seek immediate medical care is mandatory to decrease deaths from recurrent myocardial infarction. Personnel should provide the family with a telephone number for assistance at any hour. Many communities have available the universal emergency number 911.
5. *Follow-up care.* An appointment should be given to the patient for a visit to his physician. A second appointment should be made to get the patient and family active in a "coronary club."
6. *Return to employment.* Studies show that a majority of people under the age of 65 years return to their former work after recovering from a myocardial infarction. For those unable to achieve their former level of physical

activity, special centers to evaluate the work capacity of the individuals are available in most medical complexes. In either event the goal of health personnel should be to restore the person to as full and useful a life as possible. A positive attitude on the part of the personnel and patient does much toward improving the patient's quality of life.

Summary

Increasing concern about the quality of life following myocardial infarction has resulted in increased scrutiny by health professionals of the cardiac environment, with assessment and intervention beginning in the CCU and continuing until the patient returns to his maximal functioning. Although many questions concerning the effects of secondary prevention programs on morbidity and mortality remain, reducing the level of invalidism following myocardial infarction seems a goal worthy of attention from health professionals.

REFERENCES

1. Colling, A., and others: Teeside coronary survey: an epidemiological study of acute attacks of myocardial infarction, Br. Med. J. **2**:1169, 1976.
2. Hill, J.D., Hampton, J.R., and Mitchell, J.R.A.: A randomized trial of home versus hospital management for patients with suspected myocardial infarction, Lancet **1**:837, 1978.
3. Mather, H.G., and others: Myocardial infarction: a comparison between home and hospital care for patients, Br. Med. J. **1**:925, 1976.
4. Mather, H.G., and others: Acute myocardial infarction: home and hospital treatment, Br. Med. J. **3**:334, 1971.
5. Gazes, P., and Gaddy, P.: Bedside management of acute myocardial infarction, Am. Heart J. **97**(6):782, 1979.
6. Zipes, D.P., and others: Transvenous cardioversion of ventricular tachycardia and termination of ventricular fibrillation in man (abstract), Am. J. Cardiol. (In press.)
7. Spence, M.: Cardioversion. In Millar, S., and others, editors: Methods in critical care, Philadelphia, 1980, W.B. Saunders Co.
8. Mantle, J.: Cardiovascular evaluation and therapy in unstable patients. In Kinney, M., and others, editors: AACN's clinical reference for critical care nursing, New York, 1981, McGraw-Hill Book Co.
9. Schwartz, L., and Brenner, Z.: Critical care unit transfer: reducing patient stress through nursing intervention, Heart Lung **8**(3):540, 1979.
10. Cosby, R.S., and others: Late complications of myocardial infarction, J.A.M.A. **236**:1717, 1976.
11. Thompson, P., and Sloman, F.: Sudden death in hospital after discharge from coronary care unit, Br. Med. J. **4**:136, 1971.
12. Vedin, A., and others: Prediction of cardiovascular deaths and nonfatal reinfarctions after myocardial infarction, Scand. J. Rehabil. Med. **201**:309, 1977.
13. Kjolley, E.: Long-term prognosis after acute myocardial infarction with special reference to long-term survival, the risks of reinfarction, and cardiac arrest, Dan. Med. Bull. **23**:238, 1976.
14. Hurst, J.W., and others: The heart, ed. 4, New York, 1978, McGraw-Hill Book Co.
15. Renshaw, D.C.: Sex and the cardiac patient, Compr. Ther. **4**(11):13, 1978.

SUGGESTED READINGS

American Heart Association: Textbook of advanced cardiac life support, Dallas, 1981, American Heart Association.

Kinney, M.R., and others, editors: AACN's clinical reference for critical care nursing, New York, 1981, McGraw-Hill Book Co.

Millar, S.G., and others, editors: Methods in critical care: the AACN manual, Philadelphia, 1980, W.B. Saunders Co.

13

PSYCHOLOGIC CONSIDERATIONS IN CORONARY ARTERY DISEASE

James A. Blumenthal
Helene Mau

There has been a radical change in the epidemiology of disease in the United States in the twentieth century. Morbidity and mortality are no longer related to the infectious diseases that were so prevalent 100 years ago. Chronic diseases are now the most prevalent causes of death, and cardiovascular disease currently constitutes the single most frequent cause of death of adults in the United States.

A number of large-scale prospective studies have identified a set of characteristics that distinguish groups of people who are vulnerable to developing coronary artery disease (CAD) from people who remain healthy. These so-called risk factors include elevated blood pressure, hyperlipidemia, a positive family history, and cigarette smoking (see Chapter 3).[1-3] These risk factors, however, have been disappointing in their ability to predict individuals who develop CAD and offer only a partial explanation of why a specific person develops CAD at a particular time. Moreover, these same risk factors have been even less useful in predicting subsequent mortality or morbidity once the disease has developed.[4] As a consequence, the role of psychologic, behavioral, and social factors has received growing recognition in the medical community and has been the subject of numerous scientific investigations. The purpose of this chapter is to provide a brief overview of the psychosocial aspects of cardiovascular disease.

A holistic perspective

It is important to develop a framework for understanding human behavior as it relates to health and illness. Even Hippocrates observed that "the mode in which the inhabitants live, and what are their pursuits, whether they are fond of drinking and eating to excess, and given to indolence, or are fond of exercise and labor"—in effect, people's total life-style—must be considered when studying disease. Although an extended discussion about the various models of human behavior is beyond the scope of this chapter, mention should be made of the *biopsychosocial* model that is currently gaining widespread recognition in medicine and the behavioral sciences.[5] This model incorporates a holistic view of human functioning, emphasizing the need to understand the patient and his or her disease in a psychosocial context. All disease is considered to have psychologic and social, as well as physical, aspects. This perspective represents a shift from the traditional biomedical model that focuses almost exclusively on the human organism as a physical object that can be completely understood by laws of physics and biochemistry. In contrast, the biopsychosocial model extends the notion of disease beyond purely somatic parameters. The term *illness* is perhaps more inclusive and implies a necessary consideration of the social, cultural, and psychologic factors that contribute to the etiology, manifestations, and subsequent outcome of the disease process. The biopsychosocial model does not ignore biochemical, genetic, or other biologic influences. Rather, to understand the determinants of disease and to arrive at a rational and effective treatment regimen, a holistic perspective is necessary. The patient, the social and cultural environment, and the complementary system devised by society to meet the patient's needs, that is, the health care system, all represent forces that influence the course of the disease.

THE ROLE OF LEARNING

The physician-patient relationship has typically been one in which the patient adopts a sick role and the physician adopts a professional role. These roles are learned behaviors that are transmitted by the culture. For the patient, sick behavior extends beyond the primary symptoms to include a set of behaviors that develop secondary to the disease. For example, the attention and sympathy a patient receives may serve to reinforce a pattern of illness behavior that may eventually be maintained independently of the disease itself.

Each role imposes certain responsibilities and obligations (Table 13-1). The patient must be motivated to get well, must seek help, and must accept the physician as acting in his or her best interest. As a result of adopting these principles, the patient is often exempted from certain obligations and personal responsibilities. For example, the patient may not have to return to work or perform routine household duties. Moreover, the patient is frequently not held responsible for symptoms or for the behaviors that may result from the disease.

The physician, on the other hand, is obligated to act in the patient's best interests and to be ethically and morally responsible. As a result, physicians claim

Table 13-1. Complementary roles of patient and physician

Patient	Physician
Sick role obligations	**Professional role obligations**
Be motivated to get well	Act in the welfare of the patient in facilitating recovery
Seek technically competent help	Be guided by the roles of professional behavior
Cooperate with the physician and treatment regimen	Acquire and use high technical competence
Privileges	Be affectively neutral and objective
	Engage in professional self-regulation
Exemption from normal social responsibilities	**Privileges**
Exemption from responsibility for one's own health	Access to physical and psychologic domains and to confidential information
	Professional authority and dominance

Modified from Parsons, T.: The social system, New York, 1951.

the privilege of having full access to patients' private lives and may assume control of the relationship with the patient as well as authority over other health care providers.

In the past 10 years the role of social learning in the development of *illness behavior* has received growing attention. For example, Mechanic[7] has described illness behavior as the different ways in which patients perceive and respond to illness. He attempted to account for the reasons why some people ignore their symptoms and do not seek medical help, whereas others tend to overreact to symptoms and place excessive demands on physicians and medical care facilities.

Chronic illness behavior represents a more longstanding pattern of response characterized by complaints of pain or dysfunction that seem disproportionate to objective medical evidence. Multiple somatic complaints, a constant search for diagnosis or more successful treatment, and behaviors designed to elicit attention from medical staff and family are typical chronic illness behaviors. Although there may be a physiologic basis for some symptoms, the perception of the symptoms and the resultant behaviors are considered to be subject to the laws of learning. Behavior that is followed by a desirable experience, and/or behavior that is followed by the discontinuation of a negative or aversive experience tends to be reinforced; that is, the *consequences* of behavior affect the likelihood of its recurrence. Typical social reinforcers include sympathy, attention, and avoidance of embarrassment or pain. For example, a patient who develops chest pain while performing housework and then experiences pain relief upon stopping makes an association of the behavior (resting) with the diminution of pain, which increases the likelihood of not performing such activities. When the patient also receives attention and sympathy for pain behaviors (such as verbal complaints, grimacing, or posturing), such social reinforcers may also serve to reinforce the pain behaviors. Furthermore, it is possible for a patient to avoid routine responsibilities that may be assumed by others such as family members. This situation is often referred to as *secondary gain*, that is, the social advantages of being ill. In this manner a patient may learn to function at a lower level than is appropriate given the purely physical, or organic, limitations of the condition. The sick role thus can become an ingrained style of behaving that is highly resistant to change.

Psychosocial and behavioral precursors

The psychologic and behavioral precursors of coronary disease have been observed for centuries. Dr. John Hunter, who suffered from angina pectoris, once observed, "My life is at the mercy of any rogue who chooses to provoke me."[8] Unfortunately, Dr. Hunter died after a heated board meeting at St. George's Hospital in London in 1793.[9] In 1897 Sir William Osler stated, "I believe the high pressure at which men live and the habit of working the machine to its maximum capacity are responsible [for arterial degeneration] rather than the excess of eating and drinking. . . ."[10]

In the past 50 years there has been a growing body of scientific data implicating a variety of social, psychologic, and behavioral factors in the pathogenesis and expression of clinical CAD.[11,12] For example, such factors as social mobility or social status incongruity (for example, the difference between aspiration and level of achievement), excessive life change, absence of social support, depression, and chronic tension have all been suggested as playing an etiologic role in the development of CAD. Moreover, overt life-style behaviors such as overeating, cigarette smoking, and sedentary living have received widespread recognition.

A constellation of behaviors receiving a great deal of attention is the type A (coronary-prone) behavior pattern. The type A behavior pattern is characterized by excessive competitive drive, extreme desire for recognition and achievement, a chronic sense of time urgency, motoric hyperactivity, and underlying hostility. The converse, type B, behavior pattern is defined as a relative absence of these characteristics.

The classification of individuals as type A or type B is usually determined by clinical judgments based on a series of specific questions. These questions are designed to elicit a particular *style* of response that is often displayed by type A individuals, as well as to acquire information regarding the individual's typical behavior based on self-reported attitudes and practices.[13] During the type A interview, the subject is asked approximately 20 to 25 questions dealing with feelings of ambition and competitiveness, past history of feelings of anger, sense of time urgency and impatience, and current feelings of irritation and frustration. *The manner in which the interview is conducted attempts to create a situation whereby type A behaviors can be observed.* For example, the interviewer purposefully interrupts the subject to elicit anger, asks questions rapidly to encourage a quick response, and slows a question, stumbling over words, to facilitate an interruption on the part of the respondent. Thus, assessment of the type A behavior pattern depends more on the basis of *observed overt behaviors* than on the self-reported habitual behavior of the patient.

A second, widely used measure of the type A behavior pattern is an objective, computer-scored questionnaire called the Jenkins Activity Survey for Health Prediction (JAS). The JAS yields an overall type A score and three factor-analytically derived subscales, called "Speed and impatience," "Job involvement," and "Hard driving."[14-16] Typical questions include the following:

1. Has your spouse or some friend ever told you that you eat too fast? Type A subjects often say, "Yes, often," whereas type B subjects say, "No, no one has told me this."
2. When you listen to someone talking, and this person takes too long to come to the point, do you *feel* like hurrying him along? Type A subjects usually say, "Frequently," and type B subjects say, "Almost never."
3. Do you ever set deadlines or quotas for yourself at work or at home? Type A subjects respond, "Yes, once a week or more often," and type B subjects usually respond, "No."

In a series of retrospective and prospective studies, individuals displaying the type A behavior pattern have been shown to have two to seven times the incidence of CAD seen in their type B counterparts.[17-19] For example, the Western Collaborative Group Study identified 3154 healthy men who were studied annually over a mean period of 8½ years.[20] The results of this study are shown in Fig. 13-1. Of the 257 men that developed CAD during this period (1960 to 1970), 178 were classified as type A by the interview method, whereas only 79 were classified as type B. When traditional risk factors such as age, serum cholesterol, blood pressure, and smoking habits were statistically controlled, the relative risk of CAD

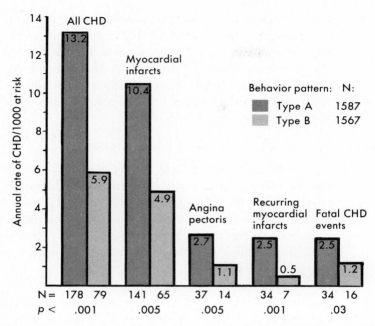

Fig. 13-1. Annual rate of CAD in 3154 subjects studied prospectively in the Western Collaborative Group Study over a mean period of 8.5 years. The higher incidence of all forms of CAD, including recurrent myocardial infarctions, in type A subjects is shown. *N*, number of cases. (From Friedman, M., and Rosenman, R.H.: Ann. Clin. Res.**3:**300, 1971.)

for type A was about twice that of type B. Furthermore, despite a relatively small sample, the fivefold greater rate of recurrent myocardial infarctions in type A subjects compared with type B subjects was highly significant. Comparable results have been obtained using the JAS.[19]

The National Heart, Lung, and Blood Institute recently assembled a review panel of scientists to evaluate critically the type A concept. They concluded[21]:

The review panel accepts the available body of scientific evidence as demonstrating that Type A behavior . . . is associated with an increased risk of clinically apparent coronary heart disease in employed middle-aged U.S. citizens. The risk is greater than that imposed by age, elevated values of systolic blood pressure, and serum cholesterol, and smoking, and appears to be of the same order or magnitude as the relative risk associated with the latter three of these other factors.

Subsequent research has confirmed the association between the type A behavior pattern and CAD in a variety of settings and cultures. Research is currently underway to determine the underlying psychophysiologic mechanisms responsible for this relationship. Several studies have documented increased coronary atherosclerosis among type A individuals,[22-24] although two studies have failed to confirm this finding.[25,26] Other studies have shown type A subjects to exhibit increased sympathetic and neuroendocrine response to challenging situations.[27,28] It is now believed that the increased risk of CAD observed in type A persons may be mediated by increased levels of epinephrine and cardiovascular hyperresponsivity (especially heart rate and systolic blood pressure) during stressful situations.

Further research is necessary to clarify the pathophysiology of CAD and the mechanisms by which type A behavior may influence the disease process. Moreover, it remains to be seen whether modification of type A behavior pattern results in reduced incidence of CAD. The Coronary Recurrence Prevention Program in California is currently investigating the possible impact of modification of type A behavior pattern on rates of recurrent myocardial infarction, but no data are available at this time.

Psychologic adjustment to coronary heart disease

The emotional, behavioral, and social impact of a heart attack is often profound and, for many patients, may be even more debilitating than the limitations imposed solely by the physical effects of the disease. Psychologic adaptation begins when symptoms are first noticed and continues throughout hospitalization and the subsequent return home. For the purposes of the present chapter, three phases of the illness will be discussed: prehospital, hospital, and posthospital.

PREHOSPITAL PHASE

Probably the most common reaction of the patient to the first signs of illness is simply to do nothing and hope that the symptoms go away. The average time between symptom onset and admission to a medical facility is about 3 hours, although patients may delay seeking help for more than 24 hours.[29]

Approximately 55%-65% of the time between symptom onset and hospital arrival involves what has been termed *decision time*. During this period patients become aware of their symptoms and may engage in various behaviors designed to provide themselves with relief: they may rest, take medication, or discuss the problem with spouse or friends. An additional 25% of the time between symptom onset and entry into the medical facility involves the period of *medical preparation*. It is during this time sequence that the physician is contacted and arrangements are made for subsequent hospital care. The remaining 10% is time required for transportation to the hospital and is typically referred to as *transportation time*.

Since more than half of all deaths following myocardial infarction occur within the first 4 hours, it is important that the interval between symptom onset and medical care be reduced. Longer time to respond to symptoms appears to be unrelated to demographic factors such as age, sex, or socioeconomic status. Psychologic factors appear to play a predominant role, especially in the decision time. Denial, that is, the tendency to ignore or minimize the true significance of the symptoms, seems to be the most common reaction and often leads to the incorrect attribution of symptoms to such noncardiac factors as indigestion or dysfunction in other organ systems.[30]

Probably the most important remedy to the lengthy delay in response to cardiac symptoms is education of patient, family, and physician. It is interesting to note that available data suggest that the subgroup of patients who delay appropriate response the most are individuals with a past history of cardiac problems. Cardiac patients should be instructed to consult their physicians when symptoms first develop rather than waiting to see if their medication is effective. Patients should not be falsely reassured if their symptoms have not progressed, and they should be encouraged to act quickly and decisively. Physicians are encouraged to get to know their patients so that they can better judge the significance of the patient's symptoms. Unfortunately, it is not uncommon for physicians to use the same maneuvers as their patients, blaming other organ systems or minimizing the symptoms perhaps, in the belief that the patient is exaggerating or overreacting to minor symptoms.

HOSPITAL PHASE

Admission to the hospital is an unmistakable sign to the patient that something is wrong and that medical intervention is required. The single most important emotional feature of patients in the initial acute phase of their illness is extreme fear and anxiety. The content of anxious thought usually focuses on the realization of the possibility of sudden death, concerns about being abandoned and out of control, and the conscious preoccupation with symptoms such as shortness of breath, chest pain, fatigue, or irregular heart rhythm. Depression, hostility, and agitation also are observed in many patients. Cassem and Hackett[31] have developed a model for the temporal sequence of emotional reactions in patients with CAD, based on the reasons for psychiatric referral on the CCU. The sequence is graphically displayed in Fig. 13-2. The patient feels heightened anxiety during the first 2 days of hospitalization and subsequently becomes depressed for a few days. Anxiety and depression both decline after 5 or 6 days as a result of the mobilization of defense mechanisms such as denial and repression. *Isolation of affect* is the third common defense mechanism that helps the patient cope with the illness. This process involves the acknowledgment of the reality of the situation, but the affective or emotional component of this awareness is uncon-

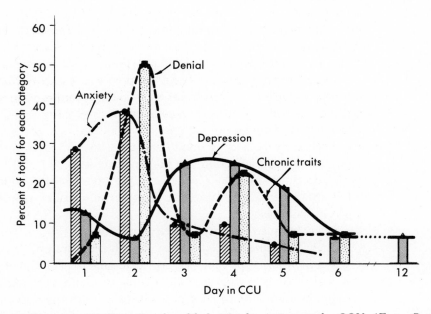

Fig. 13-2. Time course of emotional and behavioral reaction on the CCU. (From Cassem, N.H., and Hackett, T.: Ann. Intern. Med. **75**:9, 1971.)

scious. Although the majority of patients do not require formal psychiatric intervention, a substantial number do experience significant emotional distress. Many patients have confronted death for the first time; they are frightened and depressed over the perceived loss of physical health; worry about future employment, family relations, and personal finances are also common.

While patients with CAD often tend to avoid admitting fears and worries during brief interviews, more intensive contact in which the patient is given an opportunity and permission to discuss feelings and problems in a supportive, nonthreatening environment can be extremely therapeutic. Most patients will welcome a chance to "get things off their chest," and the process often promotes feelings of reassurance and relief.

Patient teaching is another important aspect of the acute, or hospital, phase. Frequently patients have trouble assimilating and retaining all the information presented to them. However, most want to know about their condition (in varying degrees of detail), so it is often useful to sit down with the patient and spouse to review the important aspects of cardiac care. It is imperative to *listen* as well as to talk with the patient. Patients will communicate what they know and desire to know if given an opportunity. Disguised fears and anxieties and misconceptions about their illness also can become apparent. For example, the statement "I guess this means I'll never go back to work" may reflect apprehension about remaining autonomous, anxiety about being dependent on others, and uncertainty about the realistic limitations of the illness. Such statements should be explored and discussed with the patient.

Although each patient is different and needs to be treated as an individual, specific issues should be reviewed with every patient before discharge. The following objectives based on the American Nursing Association Standards of Cardiovascular Nursing Practice have been suggested as guidelines for patient education[32]:

A. Demonstrate a knowledge level that will enable the patients to make appropriate therapeutic judgments and seek medical help when indicated.
   1. Accurately describe what to do if chest pain occurs.
   2. Describe the signs and symptoms that necessitate medical advice.
      a. Chest pain unrelieved by nitroglycerin and rest
      b. Increased shortness of breath
      c. Fainting
      d. Very slow or rapid heart rate
   3. Be able to accurately take own pulse.
   4. State time, date, place, and person(s) to be seen for follow-up care.
B. Maintain a pharmacologic regimen compatible with therapeutic and personal goals.
   1. State when to take each medication.
   2. Describe desired effects of each medication.
   3. Describe possible adverse reactions to each medication.
   4. Describe what to do if adverse reactions to medication occur.
C. Maintain a dietary intake compatible with therapeutic and personal goals.
   1. Describe dietary restrictions.
   2. Describe rationale for restrictions.

3. State examples of foods to avoid.
4. State that excessive body weight increases the work of the heart.
5. Describe the effects of alcohol on the heart.
6. Describe the effects of coffee on the heart.
D. Demonstrate a knowledge level that enables the patients to appropriately modify their life-styles.
1. Describe the pathophysiology of myocardial infarction and angina pectoris.
2. Identify risk factors and relate them to the development of coronary disease.
3. Identify the patients' own risk factors.
4. Indicate an understanding of the importance of providing the heart with adequate oxygen and rest by describing factors that decrease oxygen supply and/or increase work load.
   a. Digestion of food
   b. Cigarette smoking
   c. Emotional stress
   d. Very hot or cold weather
   e. Very hot or cold baths or showers
   f. Isometric exercises (give examples of these)
   g. Working with arms above shoulder level
   h. Sexual behavior
E. Participate in the planning of modification of patient's life-styles.
1. Describe own plan for the resumption of the following activities that is consistent with prescribed activity level.
   a. Activities of daily living
   b. Household tasks
   c. Sexual activity
   d. Vocational activities
   e. Driving a car
   f. Recreation
2. Discuss plans to decrease or stop cigarette smoking.
3. Discuss plans to minimize or eliminate sources of stress and tension.
4. Discuss and implement plan to screen children for risk factors.
F. Demonstrate coping mechanisms effective in adapting to patients' altered life-styles.
1. Ability to cope with anxiety as evidenced by the following:
   a. Sleep at least 6 uninterrupted hours in a 24-hour period.
   b. Relax body musculature during rest periods.
   c. Talk about events other than those related to self or own illness.
   d. Resume grooming behavior.
G. Maintain activity pattern that is compatible with therapeutic and personal goals.
1. Describe factors that should be taken into account when walking.
   a. Distance
   b. Speed
   c. Weather
   d. Incline

2. Discuss plan for walking, and outline stages of progression (see Chapter 14).

Patient teaching is an extremely important activity and has been shown to increase patients' knowledge and to improve subsequent psychologic employment, and medical adjustment. An excellent review of the importance of nursing staff and the stresses of the CCU experience can be found in a recent paper by Cassem, Nelson, and Rich.[32] It should be noted, however, that patients differ in their receptivity to health information, and that the amount of responsibility and information given to a patient must be carefully determined by taking into account the patient's ability to comprehend and use the information.

A number of research investigations have attempted to relate stressful experience on the CCU to subsequent recovery. In general, data suggest that the CCU equipment, activities, and procedures do not result in any long-term maladjustment in coronary patients.[33] However, at least one study[34] has shown that witnessing a coronary crisis in the CCU can result in physiologic arousal (that is, heightened systolic blood pressure) and an increased subjective anxiety.

The CCU is stressful for the staff as well as for the patients. Patients demand intense personal contact from staff whom they do not know and may never see again after discharge from the hospital. The CCU nurse must be capable of establishing rapport quickly with patients, providing expert medical care and emotional support, and then being able to maintain an emotional detachment and objectivity in making nursing decisions and in aiding the patients' release from the CCU.

Although emotional stresses require adjustment, the physical demands of work on the CCU can be equally challenging. For example, heavy lifting, unpredictable scheduling, and a hectic work pace are common conditions to which nurses are subjected. Regular group meetings can be extremely effective in helping staff cope more effectively with the intense job demands and deal more constructively with interpersonal conflicts.

POSTHOSPITAL PHASE

The patient is transferred from the CCU to a ward with less supervision after about a week but remains under intensive medical care for the next 1 to 2 weeks. The posthospital phase begins with the patient's discharge from the hospital and for all practical purposes continues indefinitely thereafter. During this phase the responsibility for the patient's care shifts from the hospital team of physicians, nurses, physical therapists, and others to the patient and family.

It has been widely documented that psychologic and behavioral factors affect the course of recovery, and that psychologic problems are seldom resolved during the acute period of hospitalization. For example, research has documented that at 6 months to 1 year after discharge from the hospital, as many as 88% of the patients sampled were anxious or depressed, 50% reported disturbed sleep, 20% did not return to work, and 83% complained of excessive weakness.[35] Heart disease also affects the family, and marital conflicts, often centering around medical instructions (concerning such areas as diet, medication, and activity), are not uncommon.[36]

Unlike the structured hospital setting, the return home often means that the patient is unsupervised and that no concrete, specific guidelines are made available to him. The patient may be uncertain about the extent to which physical activity is permissible, and the advice "take it easy" is too often misunderstood or so general as to be of no real value. Concern about sexual functioning, apprehensiveness about returning to work, and awareness of diminished energy and strength are not uncommon.

In general, emotional distress reaches its peak during the patient's convalescence. There appear to be at least five main problem areas that affect a substantial number of coronary patients: (1) excessive concerns about health, (2) organic problems, (3) emotional problems, (4) continuation of personality problems from the time before the illness, and (5) developmental issues and existential concerns.

EXCESSIVE CONCERNS ABOUT HEALTH

Once a person has experienced a myocardial infarction, good health can no longer be taken for granted. Many patients become sensitized to their bodily functioning. In extreme cases patients may become preoccupied with their health and overreact to even minor discomfort. Fear and anxiety are prominent: patients are afraid of death and fear being abandoned.

Cardiac neurosis is a term often used to describe the situation in which the patient has become completely debilitated by the illness. Fear of leaving home or anxiety over physical exertion may be present, and even minor symptoms are thought to be emergencies or precursors of a fatal cardiac event. Although some hypochondriacal patients are also depressed, the affective component is often minimal, whereas the behavioral and biologic components are pronounced. The possibility that the patients' overconcern about the integrity of their body may reflect a *masked depression* (physical complaints hiding or obscuring the depression) or a *depressive equivalent* (physical complaints reflecting the clinical manifestations of depression) should not be overlooked. On rare occasions hypochondriasis may also reflect a prepsychotic condition in which the patient's ability to test reality is significantly impaired. Most hypochondriacal patients, however, are afraid of having a disease but do not have the bizarre ideation characteristic of the psychotic patient.

Hypochondriacal patients share several basic characteristics. They are insecure, and their self-concept is vulnerable; they tend to feel incomplete, and their identity often is overly dependent on others; and they feel internal conflict about their need to depend on others. Encouragement and support, firm and concrete guidelines for progressive physical exercise, and regularly scheduled medical checkups appear to be very therapeutic for hypochondriacal patients.

ORGANIC PROBLEMS

Impaired cognitive functioning is present in a small but not necessarily insignificant proportion of patients with coronary disease.[37-39] For patients who undergo bypass surgery, cognitive changes appear to be even more common. *Pump time*, that is, time on the cardiopulmonary bypass pump, has been suggested as one mechanism by which patients sustain impairment of cognitive functioning. Patients with preexisting organic impairment may be especially vulnerable; surgical survivors may have exhibited less dysfunction than those who die after surgery. Typical symptoms that patients report are memory loss, decline in intellectual functioning, or occasional aphasic signs (such as difficulty remembering a name, decreased fine-motor control, or problems performing routine arithmetic tasks). Occasionally patients may display a labile mood, apathy, or psychomotor retardation. These latter symptoms may not reflect organic impairment but rather an underlying depression that may require careful evaluation.

In addition to the effects that the disease process may have on cognitive functions, advancing age contributes to a general decline in mental abilities. Old age is associated with a decline in cognitive functioning, and cardiac disease is most common in the latter half of the life cycle. Research has suggested that "crystallized" abilities, such as a person's vocabulary or fund of information, may remain intact, whereas "fluid" abilities, such as problem solving or verbal reasoning skills, may deteriorate more quickly, as a result of the combined effects of aging and organic damage.

Administration of neuropsychologic tests such as the Halstead-Reitan Neuropsychological Battery can be used to evaluate precisely the presence and extent of organic impairment. These procedures include a variety of behavioral tasks involving assessment of memory, reasoning and conceptual abilities, and psychomotor performance. Impaired functioning can often be inferred on the basis of patterns of scores or by the departure of scores from normative data. A comprehensive review of psychologic strategies for evaluating coronary patients is presented elsewhere.[40]

Postoperative psychosis is a related disorder that can be dramatic in its clinical manifestations. Estimates of the prevalence of delirium in postcardiotomy and coronary bypass patients range from 0.1% to as high as 30% to 40%, with the typical rate for any given hospital setting probably somewhere in between. The characteristic symptoms of the psychosis include perceptual distortions, visual and auditory hallucinations, delusions, and disorientation. Somatic concomitants of anxiety are also common, including hyperventilation, elevated heart rate and blood pressure, and sweating. Although the etiology of the psychosis is not known, current research suggests that organic factors, most likely cerebral ischemia, may be important. Patients whose psychologic defenses, especially those of repression and denial, deteriorate may be more likely to experience delirium than patients whose defenses remain effective.

Delirium is typically treated with the use of major tranquilizers such as chlorpromazine hydrochloride (Thorazine), chlordiazepoxide hydrochloride (Librium), or haloperidol (Haldol). Moreover, it has been suggested that a supportive environment in which patients are encouraged to talk about their fears and anxieties may reduce the frequency of postoperative psychosis and facilitate more rapid recovery.

EMOTIONAL PROBLEMS

As previously described, psychologic and behavioral factors affect the course of cardiac rehabilitation. Although available data are somewhat variable from one study to another, most studies report that the majority of patients experience anxiety and depression; yet there is also agreement that the extent of emotional distress declines substantially over the course of 1 to 2 years after the infarction. For an excellent review of the subject, the reader is referred to a recent paper by Doehrman.[33]

Depression is a common complaint and is often characterized by sadness, crying spells, sleep disturbance (such as early morning awakening), excessive fatigue and weakness, and low energy. Anxiety is also fairly common, although the defense mechanisms of repression, denial, and isolation of affect often protect the patient from consciously experiencing the discomfort associated with anxiety. Most patients do not suffer from significant and debilitating anxiety 1 year after myocardial infarction. For patients whose symptoms persist, however, antidepressant medication [such as doxepin hydrochloride (Sinequan)] is often helpful in reducing symptoms.

CAD may evoke feelings of vulnerability and worthlessness. The patient may become dependent or unconsciously allow himself to become passive as a result of the socially acceptable role as patient. Encouraging the patient to talk about feelings and to become more physically active are important aids to treatment. The importance of exercise therapy is now widely recognized and is discussed in Chapter 14.

PROBLEMS THAT HAVE CONTINUED FROM EARLIER YEARS

Most patients who develop CAD are not psychiatric patients. However, patients with significant emotional problems also develop heart disease. Problems that have developed over the course of a lifetime rarely improve after a heart attack. People who are prone to depression can be extremely affected by a sudden decline in their health. Similarly, people who tend to act impulsively or who show an inability to tolerate life's frustrations may exhibit a continuation of past behaviors: they may continue to overeat, overdrink, or overindulge themselves in ways that have a negative effect on themselves or on those around them.

In brief, those individuals who have problems before their illness are likely to have problems after their illness. Marriages are seldom improved when one member becomes sick, and often CAD may cause additional problems for couples and families.

DEVELOPMENTAL ISSUES AND EXISTENTIAL CONCERNS

Erik Erikson[41] has identified eight stages of human development. Each stage has its own salient issues that require resolution. The last stage, *ego integrity* implies an acceptance of life as it has turned out and death as the inevitable outcome of human life. He notes, "Wisdom then is detached concern with life itself in the face of death itself. It maintains and conveys the integrity of experience in spite of the decline in bodily and mental functions."[42]

Familial, cultural, and spiritual values become more important as one grows older, and illness often brings about a reevaluation of what is meaningful, not just in terms of what happens after death but what happens before death. A myocardial infarction may make a patient seek to avoid feelings of helplessness and hopelessness and may stimulate a renewed interest in people. It is not uncommon for patients to review their lives and to reflect on opportunities chosen and neglected. Some patients adopt a new philosophy about life and shift from material to more spiritual interests.

Patients with CAD are often in their middle years and must face developmental issues common to middle age. The most important issues facing middle-aged and older adults is how to cope with loss: for the myocardial infarction patient, the most obvious loss is that of physical prowess and functional abilities. This may threaten the individual's self-concept and marked loss of physical abilities may lead to forced dependence on others.

As one gets older, the experience of illness becomes more frequent, and it is more difficult to compensate for lost friends. Patients may feel lonely, isolated, and deserted and experience a loss of shared memories. Retirement also can be traumatic. It means an end of a phase of life, and with loss of work is often a loss of a sense of autonomy and power. Loss of relationships with co-workers, of social status, and of income is also experienced.

Talking about life requires someone who is willing to listen. Although professional help is often useful, a patient should also be encouraged to talk with spouse, relatives, and friends.

Treatment considerations

Most published research on the psychologic treatment of myocardial infarction patients has been about treatment in the form of group psychotherapy. To date, results have been mixed. Several studies have demonstrated improved psychologic well-being in the treatment group compared to a no-treatment control group, and at least one study[43] has reported a significantly lower mortality in the treated group. However, it has been noted that group treatment of cardiac patients does not follow a process similar to group treatment of psychiatric patients. (For a select review, see Blanchard and Miller.[44]) Educational and supportive groups appear to be preferable to self-exploratory or psychoanalytic groups.

Several recent studies have employed behavioral techniques including progressive muscle relaxation training and stress management techniques. The main behavioral treatments for patients with coronary disease appear to be those that attempt to reduce the deleterious effects of stress on the patient either by modifying the source of the stress or by modifying the patients' perceptions and reactions to stress. *Progressive muscle relaxation,* in which the patient is taught to tense and relax muscles, is an example of a technique counteracting the effects of a stressful environment. Other behavioral techniques for treating stress reactions include *cognitive restructuring,* in which the patient is taught to reinterpret events to make them less stressful, and *systematic desensitization,* in which the patient learns to relax to counteract the emotional or physical symptoms during exposures to situations that evoke symptoms. *Biofeedback,* a treatment designed to teach patients control of autonomic nervous system functions, has been used successfully to treat a variety of cardiovascular disorders including cardiac arrhythmias, hypertension, and peripheral vascular disease. However, the effectiveness of behavioral techniques in actually prolonging life in patients with coronary disease has not been established.

Recovery from heart attack is a complex process. Social, psychologic and medical factors are all important and interrelated. Successful treatment is most likely to be achieved by the collaborative efforts of nurses, physicians, psychologists, physical therapists, and vocational counselors. The key ingredient is an interest in and commitment to victims of a disease with important psychosocial as well as physical consequences.

REFERENCES

1. Epstein, F.: The epidemiology of coronary heart disease: a review, J. Chronic Dis. **18:**735, 1965.
2. Keys, A.: The individual risk of coronary heart disease, Ann. N.Y. Acad. Sci. **134:**1046, 1966.
3. Simborg, D.W.: The status of risk factors and coronary heart disease, J. Chronic Dis. **22:**515, 1970.
4. Blumenthal, J.A., and Califf, R.: Secondary prevention of coronary heart disease. In Surwit, R.S., and others, editors: Behavioral treatment of disease, New York, 1982, Plenum Publishing Corp.
5. Engel, G.L.: The need for a new medical model: a challenge for biomedicine, Science **196:**129, 1977.
6. Parsons, T.: The social system, New York, 1951, The Free Press.
7. Mechanic, D.: Social psychologic factors affecting the presentation of bodily complaints, N. Engl. J. Med. **286:**1132, 1972.
8. Kobler, J.: The reluctant surgeon: a biography of John Hunter, New York, 1960, Doubleday & Co., Inc.
9. Kligfield, P., and Hunter, J.: Angina pectoris and medical education, Am. J. Cardiol. **45:**367, 1980.
10. Osler, W.: Lectures on angina pectoris and allied states, New York, 1897, D. Appleton.
11. Jenkins, C.D.: Psychologic and social precursors of coronary disease, N. Engl. J. Med. **284:**244, 307, 1971.
12. Jenkins, C.D.: Recent evidence supporting psychologic and social risk factors for coronary disease, N. Engl. J. Med. **294:**987, 1033, 1976.
13. Rosenman, R.H.: The interview method of assessment of the coronary-prone behavior pattern. In Dembroski, T.M., and others, editors: Coronary-prone behavior, New York, 1978, Springer-Verlag New York Inc.
14. Jenkins, C.D., Rosenman, R.H., and Friedman, D.: Development of an objective psychological test for the determination of the coronary-prone behavior pattern in employed men, J. Chronic Dis. **20:**371, 1976.
15. Zyzanski, S.J., and Jenkins, C.D.: Basic dimensions within the coronary-prone behavior pattern, J. Chronic Dis. **22:**781, 1970.
16. Jenkins, C.D., Zyzanski, S.J., and Rosenman, R.H.: Progress toward validation of a computer-scored test for the Type A coronary-prone behavior pattern, Psychosom. Med. **33:**193, 1971.
17. Friedman, M., and Rosenman, R.H.: Association of specific overt behavior pattern with blood and cardiovascular findings, J.A.M.A. **169:**1286, 1959.
18. Rosenman, R.H., and others: A predictive study of coronary heart disease: the Western Collaborative Group Study, J.A.M.A. **189:**15, 1964.
19. Jenkins, C.D., Rosenman, R.H., and Zyzanski, S.J.: Prediction of clinical coronary heart disease by a test for the coronary-prone behavior pattern, N. Engl. J. Med. **290:**1271, 1974.
20. Rosenman, R.H., and others: Coronary heart disease in the Western Collaborative Group Study: final follow-up experience of 8½ years, J.A.M.A. **233:**872, 1975.
21. The Review Panel on Coronary Prone Behavior and Coronary Heart Disease: A critical review, Circulation **63:**1199, 1981.
22. Friedman, M., and others: The relationship of behavior pattern A to the state of the coronary vasculature: a study of fifty-one autopsy subjects, Am. J. Med. **44:**525, 1968.
23. Blumenthal, J.A., and others: Type A behavior pattern and coronary atherosclerosis, Circulation **58:**634, 1978.
24. Frank, K.A., and others: Type A behavior pattern and coronary angiographic findings, J.A.M.A. **240:**761, 1978.
25. Dimsdale, J.E., and others: Type A personality and extent of coronary atherosclerosis, Am. J. Cardiol. **42:**583, 1978.
26. Dimsdale, J.E., and others: Type A behavior and angiographic findings, J. Psychosom. Res. **23:**273, 1979.
27. Dembroski, T.M., and others: Effects of level of challenge on pressor and heart rate responses in Type A and B subjects, J. Appl. Soc. Psychol. **9:**209, 1979.
28. Blumenthal, J.A., and others: Task incentives and cardiovascular response in Type A and Type B individuals, Paper presented at the annual meeting of the Society for Psychophysiological Research, Washington, D.C., October 1981.
29. Gentry, W.D., and Haney, T.: Emotional and behavioral reaction to acute myocardial infarction, Heart Lung **4:**738, 1975.
30. Hackett, T.P., and Cassem, N.H.: Factors contributing to delay in responding to the signs and symptoms of acute myocardial infarction, Am. J. Cardiol. **24:**651, 1969.
31. Cassem, N.H., and Hackett, T.P.: Psychiatric consultation in a coronary care unit, Ann. Intern. Med. **75:**9, 1971.
32. Cassem, N.H., Nelson, K., and Rich, R.R.: The nurse in the coronary care unit. In Gentry, W.D., and Williams, R.B., editors: Psychological aspects of myocardial infarction and coronary care, ed. 2, St. Louis, 1979, The C.V. Mosby Co.

33. Doehrman, S.R.: Psychosocial aspects of recovery from coronary heart disease: a review, Soc. Sci. Med. **11**:199, 1970.

34. Bruhn, J.G., and others: Patients' reaction to death in a coronary care unit, J. Psychosom. Res. **14**:65, 1970.

35. Wishnie, H.A., Hackett, T.P., and Cassem, N.H.: Psychological hazards of convalescence following myocardial infarction, J.A.M.A. **215**:1292, 1971.

36. Cassem, N.H., and Hackett, T.P.: Psychological rehabilitation of myocardial infarction patients in the acute phase, Heart Lung, **2**:382, 1973.

37. Gilberstadt, H., and Sako, Y.: Intellectual and personality changes following open-heart surgery, Arch. Gen. Psychiatry **16**:210, 1967.

38. Kornfeld, D.S., Zimberg, S., and Malm, J.R.: Psychiatric complication of open-heart surgery, N. Engl. J. Med. **273**:287, 1965.

39. Heller, S.S., and others: Psychiatric complications of open-heart surgery: a reexamination, N. Engl. J. Med. **283**:1015, 1970.

40. Blumenthal, J.A.: Assessment of patients with coronary heart disease. In Keefe, F.J., and Blumenthal, J.A., editors: Assessment strategies in behavioral medicine, New York, 1982, Grune & Stratton, Inc.

41. Erikson, E.H.: Identity and the life cycle: psychological issues, Monograph 1, New York, 1959, International Universities Press.

42. Erikson, E.H.: Insight and responsibility: letters on the ethical implications of psychoanalytic insight, New York, 1964, W.W. Norton & Co.

43. Ibrahim, M.A., and others: Management after myocardial infarction: a controlled trial of the effects of group psychotherapy, Int. J. Psychiatry Med. **5**:253, 1974.

44. Blanchard, E.B., and Miller, S.T.: Psychological treatment of cardiovascular disease, Arch. Gen. Psychiatry **34**:1402, 1977.

14

REHABILITATION AFTER MYOCARDIAL INFARCTION

Elizabeth Wagner
R. Sanders Williams

Goals of the rehabilitation process and basic concepts

One can identify two basic goals in approaching the patient who has survived a myocardial infarction: first, to eliminate any physical or psychologic barriers that impede the patient's resumption of a satisfying and productive life; and second, to minimize the patient's risk for subsequent adverse cardiovascular events such as sudden cardiac death, progressive angina pectoris, and recurrent myocardial infarction. Although these same goals have served as a standard for medical management of the postinfarction patient for half a century, in the last 10 years some radical changes have occurred in the practices of physicians and nurses in their management of patients recovering from a heart attack.

For at least 30 years, from the 1930s until the late 1960s, tremendous restrictions were placed by physicians on the activities of their postinfarction patients. Standard medical practice recommended a month or more of hospitalization after an infarction, much of which was spent in complete bed rest. After discharge even moderate physical exercise, sexual activity, and return to full employment were often prohibited for periods up to a year or, in some cases, indefinitely. These recommendations were based on concerns that even routine activities constituted undue stress upon a damaged heart and exposed the patients to excessive risk of further life-threatening cardiac events. More often than not these restrictions were placed arbitrarily, without reference to the results of functional testing or other pertinent clinical variables in individual patients.

In the 1980s sudden arrhythmic death and recurrent infarction remain serious risks to individuals who have experienced an initial infarction. However, the restrictions formerly placed on all patients recovering from a myocardial infarction are currently viewed as generally excessive; for most individuals, a far more aggressive approach is not only safe but more likely to facilitate the patient's return to an active and productive mode of living.

Many major medical centers, as well as an increasing number of community hospitals, have instituted formal programs of cardiac rehabilitation for their patients surviving myocardial infarction. To address the two major clinical goals just stated, most cardiac rehabilitation programs have emphasized three basic principles: (1) early and repeated functional testing of the patient (generally,

501

graded treadmill exercise tests) to provide a rational basis for recommending or proscribing specific activities in the recovery period and to help identify patients in need of drug treatment or surgical treatment of complicating features such as arrhythmias or angina pectoris, (2) individually prescribed, graduated programs of exercise training to augment functional work capacity, and (3) a rehabilitation team approach involving health professionals skilled at psychologic, dietary, and vocational evaluation and counseling. The remainder of this chapter focuses on the specifics of cardiac rehabilitation programs organized around these three principles. Although quantitative data supporting the superiority of this approach to the management of the postinfarction patient over the more prevalent forms of physician-office management are just beginning to appear, there is a growing enthusiasm among clinicians for the special services offered through formal cardiac rehabilitation programs.[1-3]

Sequential steps in cardiac rehabilitation

It is important that the rehabilitation of the patient who has suffered a myocardial infarction be viewed as a continuous and logical process that begins in the CCU and extends to a lifetime program of prudent activity and risk-factor control. The efficacy of the rehabilitation team is greatly compromised when rehabilitation efforts are delayed until weeks or months after the patient has left the hospital. To provide a convenient framework for discussion, the management of the postinfarction patient can be divided into four phases (Fig. 14-1): inpatient management in the CCU and hospital ward, the transition period in the 3 to 6 weeks following hospital discharge, the active rehabilitation period commencing

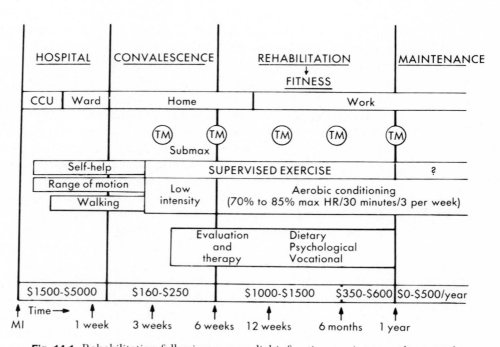

Fig. 14-1. Rehabilitation following myocardial infarction: an integrated approach.

approximately 6 weeks from the date of the infarction, and the maintenance phase, wherein the subject seeks to maintain the highest possible level of the functional capacity and risk-factor control achieved during the active rehabilitation phase. It should be emphasized, however, that this identification of "phases" is a somewhat arbitrary one; future research may dictate changes in the lengths of time subjects spend in each phase or in the activities that are deemed safe and effective in each time period. Likewise, the major emphasis should be placed on the continuity of care as the patient passes through the initial weeks and months of recovery rather than on peculiar features of each rehabilitation phase.

PHASE I: INPATIENT MANAGEMENT

Once the pain associated with acute infarction has been relieved and the patient has been stabilized and is free from its life-threatening complications, the rehabilitation process should begin.[4] For patients with no complications the use of bedside toilet facilities or short walks to a private bathroom, as well as other self-care activities such as shaving, dressing, and bathing, are appropriate even within the first 24 to 48 hours. Excessive dependence on the CCU staff for routine self-care activities should be strongly discouraged. Range of motion exercise or chair sitting minimizes the deleterious effects of bed rest[5] and forestalls the excessive and unwarranted fear of even minimal physical activity that persists in many patients for extended periods following their infarction. Early activity also minimizes the risk of venous thrombosis and pulmonary embolus.[6]

Gradually increasing periods of walking about the room or in the ward corridor can be started by the third hospital day for most patients. It is obvious that activity schedules must be curtailed in patients experiencing ventricular or atrial arrhythmias, postinfarction angina, or congestive heart failure. The walking performed by postinfarction patients in the inpatient phase is in no way designed to constitute aerobic training. Its purpose is to minimize physical deconditioning, to prevent venous thrombosis, and to foster a positive psychologic outlook. Walking sessions should be short (5 to 20 minutes) and of low intensity (heart rates <100 in most subjects), and multiple short walks during the day are probably preferable to a single longer walk.

Whenever possible the patient should be introduced during the hospital stay to the physicians and/or nurses who will be managing the postdischarge rehabilitation. This establishes continuity for postinfarction management and guards against the patient receiving conflicting instructions about postdischarge activities.

PHASE II: THE IMMEDIATE POSTDISCHARGE PERIOD

In many locales postinfarction patients with no complications are leaving the hospital 7 to 10 days after admission.[7] In the first few weeks after discharge patients are extremely vulnerable to fears about their future, anxiety over the safety of routine activities, and situational depressions. Although most patients are given extensive instructions about home activities prior to hospital discharge, their receptivity for understanding detailed activity schedules during their hospitalization is often low, unless instructions can be reinforced frequently when the patient returns home. Office visits to their physician cannot practically be frequent enough to reinforce previously delivered instructions (and to answer new questions), which many patients seem to require. Although many formal cardiac rehabilitation programs do not institute group exercise sessions for coronary patients until 6 weeks or more after their infarction, other centers enroll patients in group exercise classes within the first week after discharge. Beginning supervised exercise classes immediately after hospital discharge seems preferable for a number of reasons. Close contact with the patient is maintained by the rehabilitation team, allowing prompt identification of complicating medical events, facilitating proper interpretation of new symptoms, and providing reassurance to the patient and his family. Specific attention should be given to the adjustments of spouses in this difficult period. Getting the patient out of the home and into a group setting reinforces a positive outlook toward the eventual resumption of full activities, and daily exercise prescriptions can be more closely monitored.

An important feature of the immediate postdischarge period should be an evaluation of the patient's functional status. Whereas this evaluation may be as simple as the physician or nurse walking around the ward with the patient and checking the heart rate, rhythm, and blood pressure, many centers now obtain more quantitative data from a formal treadmill or bicycle exercise stress test within the first few weeks after the patient's infarction.[8,9] This early functional evaluation offers several advantages: it allows more rational recommendations regarding home activity, since they are based on individual patient data rather than dogmatic generalizations; it enhances identification of patients who are at high risk for early reinfarction or sudden death; and, when favorable results are obtained, it provides considerable reassurance to the patient and reduces anxiety over home activities. Research centers are currently evaluating the optimal use of exercise testing in the first few weeks after an infarction in identifying patients who may benefit from specific pharmacologic therapy or early coronary artery bypass surgery.

In addition to reducing patient anxiety and providing a component of group therapy, enrolling patients in supervised exercise classes during the first 3 to 4 weeks after hospital discharge has essentially the same rationale as that for the exercise prescribed during the inpatient phase: limiting the deleterious effects of physical deconditioning and maintaining a psychologic climate favorable for a return to normal activities. In contrast to physical training regimens described in the section entitled "Exercise prescriptions," medically supervised exercise in phase II is prescribed at rather low intensities, with no attempt to have patients exercising in an aerobic training range.

PHASE III: ACTIVE CARDIAC REHABILITATION: AEROBIC TRAINING AND RETURN TO WORK

The specific features of cardiac rehabilitation programs serving patients from 6 weeks to 1 year after infarction are detailed in the following sections of this chapter. The goals of phase III cardiac rehabilitation build on and extend the more limited goals of phases I and II. The patient needs a realistic reassessment of the limitations, if any, that are imposed on him by cardiac disease and a specific plan to reduce these limitations as much as possible. The specific goals of treatment continue to be to optimize drug therapy and to identify patients whose clinical outlook is likely to be improved by surgical interventions, to limit irrational or excessive anxiety in patients in whom such psychologic features impede functioning in vocational or leisure activities, and to minimize risk factors for recurrent catastrophic cardiac events.

The central focus of most cardiac rehabilitation programs is medically supervised aerobic exercise in a group setting. The psychologic benefits of this type of program have already been discussed in the comments on phase II rehabilitation. The additional physiologic benefits offered by aerobic conditioning in infarction patients are considerable and are well established by quantitative data from several centers. Functional work capacity is enhanced, and favorable changes occur in several major coronary risk factors including hypertension, hyperlipidemia, obesity, and diabetes mellitus. These results can be expected even in subjects with severely damaged ventricles or with postinfarction angina.[1-4,10,19]

Based on histologic studies of the time course of scar formation in infarcted myocardium, and on other rather poorly defined clinical observations, the convention of beginning aerobic training 6 to 8 weeks from the date of a myocardial infarction has become established. There are no firm data that earlier institution of vigorous exercise has deleterious effects, but it seems entirely reasonable to delay aerobic training to this date, since there is no compelling reason to begin earlier. For the patient who has undergone a submaximal exercise test at the ninth to twenty-first day, a symptom-limited exercise test is recommended 6 weeks after infarction to allow further individualized exercise prescription and to base the decision about return either to work or to specific leisure activities on pertinent physiologic data. Psychologic, dietary, and vocational evaluations should also be completed at this time. If either specific interventions for psychologic problems or major changes in dietary habits are to be recommended, they are often easier to implement before the patient returns to full-time employment.

Symptom-limited exercise tests are recommended to monitor the responses to exercise training and to identify patients with worsening myocardial ischemia; they should be administered after 6 weeks of aerobic training, after 6 months, and after 1 year. In addition to functional testing, monitoring of the patient's overall clinical condition by a medical history and a physical examination and the assessment of risk-factor control are recommended at these intervals.

PHASE IV: MAINTENANCE PROGRAMS

A number of criteria have been presented to define the patients who have been fully rehabilitated from their myocardial infarctions. These include (1) return to gainful employment if this is medically feasible, (2) achievement of an acceptable level of functional capacity that allows the patient to perform desired work or leisure activities (9 METs* is a conventional threshold); (3) optimal control of all risk factors for recurrent cardiac events, (4) successful patient

---

*An understandable and useful method of measuring the energy cost of certain activities is through the use of the unit called the MET, or metabolic equivalent of the task. A MET is defined as the rate of energy expenditure requiring an oxygen consumption of 3.5 ml/minute/kg body weight. One MET is equal to the energy cost of a person sitting quietly on a chair. Five METs therefore means that an activity of this level requires five times the oxygen costs of sitting quietly in a chair.

education regarding necessary restrictions on activity, proper medication usage, and continued risk-factor control. Some patients may meet these criteria within a few months after infarction, whereas other patients either have medical limitations that render rehabilitation to completely normal activity impossible or are unable to adhere to prescribed treatment regimens that would facilitate complete rehabilitation. Patients successfully achieving criteria for complete rehabilitation should be encouraged to continue a program of regular exercise and risk-factor control. Many patients are able to accomplish this on their own without further specialized assistance from the rehabilitation team. A more detailed discussion of medically unsupervised exercise training for coronary patients is included later. On the other hand, many other patients either enjoy participation in a group cardiac fitness program or lack the self-motivation to maintain an unsupervised exercise training program. Many rehabilitation programs offer low-cost, minimally supervised, "maintenance" programs for these types of individuals.

Progressive activity programs
THE PHYSIOLOGIC RATIONALE FOR EXERCISE TRAINING IN PATIENTS WITH CAD

Medically supervised physical training sessions constitute the central focus of most programs of comprehensive management of myocardial infarction survivors. The rationale for this emphasis on exercise training is twofold: such programs clearly lead to substantial augmentation of functional work capacity in coronary patients, in the presence or absence of angina pectoris, and such programs induce favorable changes in psychologic function and in risk factors for recurrent cardiac events.[1-4,10-22]

A consideration of some basic concepts of exercise physiology illustrates the effects of physical conditioning on exercise performance. Fig. 14-2 depicts the heart rate response to treadmill exercise in a subject who had experienced a myocardial infarction that produced considerable ventricular damage. The resting left ventricular ejection fraction of 20% determined from radionuclide angiography is considerably reduced from the normal range of 50% or greater. At 2 months after this patient's infarction and prior to beginning an aerobic conditioning program, his heart rate rose rapidly with only minimal exertion, and he was forced to discontinue exercise because of shortness of breath. After 2 months of exercise training he again was forced to discontinue exercise because of shortness of breath and had the same heart rate as on the pretraining study; but he was able to exercise to a peak work load comparable to that of most healthy males in his age group. Note also that his heart rate was considerably lower on the posttraining treadmill test than on his base-line test at any given level of work. Since heart rate is the major factor determining the oxygen requirements of the heart itself, the occurrence of this "training bradycardia" means that trained subjects can perform any task with lower myocardial oxygen costs and at reduced coronary blood flows. This effect of physical training can produce substantial, sometimes dramatic, changes in the level of activity coronary patients can perform before the onset of angina pectoris or fatigue.

In most normal subjects exercise training produces increased exercise capacity and training bradycardia both by increasing the maximal pumping capacity

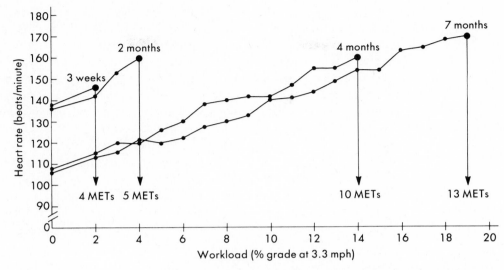

Fig. 14-2. Heart rate as a function of work load during serial treadmill exercise tests in a 43-year-old patient who suffered an extensive anterior myocardial infarction. Tests were performed at the stated intervals following his infarct. The exercise test performed 3 weeks after infarct was a submaximal test. Following 5 more weeks of low-level exercise (*2 months*), a symptom-limited (dyspnea) test revealed no conditioning effect and a persistently low exercise capacity. The patient then participated in a carefully graduated aerobic training program. Subsequent treadmills at *4 months* and *7 months* after infarct demonstrate major cardiovascular conditioning effects: increased work capacity and bradycardia at submaximal workloads. He returned to full-time employment *6 months* following his infarct. The vertical arrows point to the MET equivalent of his treadmill performance at each testing interval. The left ventricular ejection fraction is 20%.

of the heart (peak cardiac output during exercise) and by increasing the ability of the exercising skeletal muscle to extract and utilize oxygen from the blood. In preliminary data from our institution, many cardiac patients achieve this same kind of training response without any change in the maximal cardiac output. This observation that the training effect in myocardial infarction patients may be predominantly caused by effects of exercise training on skeletal muscle rather than on the heart itself has encouraged investigators to use exercise training as a form of therapy for patients with severely damaged ventricles. Clearly, even these subjects can increase their exercise capacity and develop training-induced sinus bradycardia.

The manner in which exercise training may improve the quality of life in infarction patients is illustrated in Fig. 14-3, *A*, which depicts the maximal work capacity in METs of 11 patients before and after 6 months of exercise training. The arrow to the right illustrates the approximate work capacity required for common activities such as light gardening or doubles tennis. Since most persons cannot sustain activities requiring greater than 85% of maximal work capacity for more than a few minutes, the majority of these subjects would have been unable to perform even these simple activities before the training program. However, following training most of these subjects would perform these types of activities without difficulty.

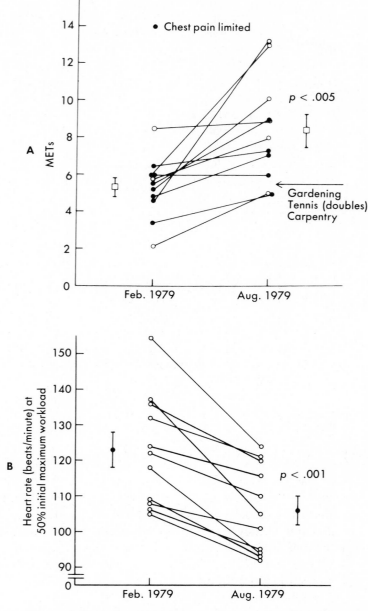

Fig. 14-3. A, Effects of physical conditioning on functional work capacity in patients following myocardial infarction. Each circle represents the results of symptom-limited treadmill testing prior to *(left)* and following *(right)* 6 months of physical conditioning in an individual patient. The squares depict mean values (±S.E.M.). The horizontal arrow demonstrates the approximate oxygen demands required for the indicated activities. Most subjects cannot perform sustained work requiring more than 85% of their maximal work capacity. **B,** Heart rates at a standard treadmill submaximal work load (50% of the initial maximum) prior to and following physical conditioning in the same subjects shown in **A.** It is important to note that all these subjects demonstrated training bradycardia (and therefore would be expected to perform routine activities with lower myocardial oxygen requirements), although several did not elevate their maximum work capacities.

Fig. 14-3, *B* shows the effects of physical training on exercise heart rate at a standard work load in the same subjects depicted in Fig. 14-3, *A*. Even those subjects who failed to augment their maximal work capacities developed training-induced sinus bradycardia.

In addition to these effects on work capacity the "physical training effect" includes favorable changes in a number of medical problems that are prevalent in myocardial infarction patients. Physical training aids in the management of hypertension[12,16] and obesity[13] and improves glucose tolerance in subjects with diabetes mellitus.[17] By most reports it lowers plasma triglycerides and low-density lipoprotein cholesterol levels and increases levels of high-density lipoprotein cholesterol,[15] the concentration of which has a strong inverse correlation with risk of cardiac events in large-scale population studies. Exercise training may also enhance the fibrinolytic activity of blood plasma,[22] perhaps reducing the risk of intravascular thrombus formation.

Despite extensive evidence linking physical activity to reduced cardiac mortality in population studies,[23-28] it has not been demonstrated conclusively that exercise training and risk-factor control indeed reduce the incidence of further major cardiac events in patients who have experienced a previous myocardial infarction.[1-4,29-31] However, even in the absence of conclusive data regarding the effects of exercise training on longevity in infarction survivors, a persuasive case can be made for physical conditioning programs purely on the basis of the well-documented improvements in exercise capacity and for the less quantifiable but widely substantiated psychologic benefits of this type of intervention. It is perhaps pertinent to note that conclusive evidence for beneficial effects on patient survival is also lacking for two other widely prescribed cardiac treatment modalities: antiarrhythmic drug therapy for ventricular arrhythmias and coronary artery bypass grafting for coronary occlusive disease (except for left main coronary stenosis).

EXERCISE PRESCRIPTIONS

To achieve the goal of cardiovascular fitness or conditioning in the cardiac patient, an exercise prescription geared to the need and capabilities of the individual must be formulated.[1-4,32] In large measure, exercise prescription is based on careful analysis of the graded exercise test. The duration of the test and the maximum heart rate attained by the patient, as well as the blood pressure response, and signs of ischemia, arrhythmias, and other problems must be evaluated before the prescription is formulated. The level of activity in the first few weeks of aerobic training should be kept at a low level to prevent undue muscle soreness, to decrease orthopedic problems, and to allow a safe adaptation period with minimum risk. Another important feature is regular review (often weekly) of the exercise prescription, with changes recommended on the basis of observation of the subject during the training sessions and of the results of repeat exercise testing performed at the previously stated intervals in the activity program.

The exercise prescription for the cardiac patient has four main characteristics, which need to be analyzed individually: type, intensity, duration, and frequency of physical activity.

Type of activity. The exercises selected for physical conditioning in the cardiac patient should generally be repetitive, rhythmic, low-resistance contractions of the large muscle groups of the body.[1-4,32,33] Activities that may be categorized in this group are brisk walking, jogging, stationary and regular cycling, stair climbing, swimming, and other selected exercises. Whichever activity is selected, it should be pleasurable to the patient and not produce prolonged fatigue or discomfort. Highly competitive activities are to be avoided by cardiac patients, except carefully selected, low-risk individuals.

Intensity of activity. The work intensity of the cardiac patient during the exercise session must be determined by the most recent stress test. Studies in both normal subjects and coronary patients suggest that the previously described exercise training effects occur most readily if the intensity of the training stimulus is sufficient to increase oxygen consumption to 60% to 75% of maximum oxygen consumption. Since heart rate increases linearly with increases in oxygen consumption,[5] simple measurements of heart rate during exercise constitute a readily available measure of the adequacy of the training stimulus. One can approximate 60% to 75% of maximum oxygen consumption by adding 60% to 75% of the increment between resting heart rate and maximum heart rate to the resting heart rate. For example, if the resting heart rate is 80 beats/minute and the peak exercise heart rate is 180 beats/minute, 60% of maximal oxygen consumption will occur at a heart rate of 140 beats/minute (60% of (180 − 80) + 80) and 75% of maximum oxygen consumption will occur at 155 beats/minute: 75% of (180 − 80) + 80. A proper training range for a patient limited by angina at a heart rate of 130 beats/minute would likewise be 110 to 118. In practice we have patients count their pulses for 10-second intervals and multiply by 6; the training ranges are therefore rounded off to the nearest multiple of 6.

To ensure against the occurrence of potentially dangerous myocardial ischemia during training sessions, exercise is limited to heart rates of 10 to 15 beats/minute below the heart rates at which angina or other signs of myocardial hypoperfusion are evident during stress testing.

A previously sedentary patient should probably begin his exercise plan at a low level of work intensity, gradually increasing the intensity level over several weeks to the calculated training range. Signs of excessive fatigue, breathlessness, and other adverse symptoms must be watched for and carefully avoided. The use of the concept of the maximum safe heart rate limit and target heart rate zones during the conditioning activity is probably the safest way of calculating the work of the heart and thus the intensity of the exercise prescription.

Duration of activity. Any activity chosen by the cardiac patient should be begun slowly at a low intensity for several minutes. Following this warm-up phase of 5 to 10 minutes, a stimulus period of 20 to 40 minutes with the patient's heart rate in his target zone has been shown to be effective in producing aerobic training effects in cardiac patients. Several minutes should also be allowed for cooling down at the end of the stimulus activity, when a gradual return of the metabolic and circulatory systems to base-line activity occurs. The warm-up and cool-down periods have been shown to be the most likely times for exercise-related ventricular fibrillation to occur and should therefore take place in close physical proximity to the medical staff and emergency equipment.

Frequency of activity. An endurance activity must be continued on a regular basis to achieve the proper conditioning response. Usually three times per week is sufficient and may limit the risk of orthopedic injury. At lower levels of activity or if a more rapid achievement of training effects is desired, a schedule of 5 days per week is preferable. Rapid achievement of training effects may be a motivational stimulus to continue regular activity in the cardiac rehabilitation program.

In composing an exercise prescription for use by the cardiac patient, individual preferences, goals, and personal safety must be taken into consideration. Getting the patient involved in the planning phases can be useful and educational and may ensure greater adherence by and pleasure for the patient.

SUPERVISED VERSUS UNSUPERVISED EXERCISE

The preferred setting for the conditioning or training of the cardiac patient is the supervised setting of the cardiac rehabilitation program. This setting allows for close observation and facilitates patient education and the initiation of the conditioning response in the individual. These effects in turn should produce a more favorable compliance rate. Although the risk of controlled exercise in myocardial infarction survivors[34] appears to be very small (less than 1 death per 100,000 patient-hours in supervised programs), serious problems such as ventricular fibrillation and myocardial infarction do occur rarely. Over 75% of cardiac arrest victims in medically supervised exercise programs are successfully resuscitated, whereas such events are almost uniformly lethal when they occur outside of medical supervision.

Economically and logistically a supervised program is not feasible for all cardiac patients. Williams and co-workers[35] have formulated the following guidelines to identify patients who may be at particularly high risk during unsupervised exercise:
1. Patients with low maximal functional capacity (<6 METs)
2. Those with severely depressed left ventricular function
3. Those with complex ventricular arrhythmias
4. Those with QT prolongation on the ECG
5. Those with exercise-induced hypotension
6. Those unable to perform effective self-monitoring of their exercise heart rate

These authors recommend that patients with CAD who lack these high-risk features may perform conditioning exercises in an unsupervised setting if they have demonstrated a clear understanding of the principles of safe physical conditioning. The patients should demonstrate knowledge of their maximum safe heart rate limit and their target heart rate zone prescribed for them at the most recent treadmill test; and they should be reliable observers of their own heart rates during exercise. Many patients, regardless of the issue of safety, require the structure of a supervised exercise program to achieve and maintain physiologic training effects and are unlikely to adhere to an unsupervised program.

ENERGY REQUIREMENTS OF COMMON ACTIVITIES

Some cardiac rehabilitation programs allow participants to perform certain activities depending on the MET expenditure of the exercise (see footnote on p. 505) in relation to the patient's own functional capacity. This is a rational method, but allowances should be made[33] for the skill level of the individual in sports

Table 14-1. Common activities and MET expenditure

Utility as a conditioning stimulus	Activity	MET expenditure
Too intermittent and below threshold for conditioning except for most severely limited patients	Light housework	1½ METs
	Walking 1 mile/hr	2-2½ METs
	Walking 2 miles/hr	2-3 METs
	Golf (using motorized cart)	2-4 METs
Low level conditioning for most patients	Walking 3 miles/hr	3-4 METs
	Moderate housework	3-4 METs
	Cycling 6 miles/hr	3-4 METs
	Golf (pulling cart)	3-4 METs
Adequate conditioning if not too intermittent and carried out for 20-30 min	Heavy housework	4-5 METs
	Walking 3½ miles/hr	4-5 METs
	Cycling 8 miles/hr	4-5 METs
	Golf (carrying clubs)	4-5 METs
	Tennis (doubles)	4-5 METs
	Calisthenics	4-5 METs
Good conditioning exercises if continuous for 20-30 min	Swimming 20 yards/min	5 METs
	Walking 4 miles/hr	5-6 METs
	Cycling 10 miles/hr	5-6 METs
	Dancing	5-6 METs
Good conditioning exercises	Walking 5 miles/hr	6-7 METs
	Cycling 11 miles/hr	6-7 METs
	Singles tennis	6-7 METs
	Jogging 5 miles/hr	7-8 METs
	Cycling 12 miles/hr	7-8 METs
Excellent conditioning exercises, but competitive sports should be avoided by patients unless careful evaluation predicts a low risk for such endeavors	Running 5½ miles/hr	8-9 METs
	Cycling 13 miles/hr	8-9 METs
	Running 6-8 miles/hr	<10 METs
	Competitive singles tennis, handball, squash, racquetball	<10 METs

activities, environmental conditions, body size, amount of rest periods, and other factors. Some common activities and their MET expenditure are listed in Table 14-1.[36]

Health education programs

At least part of the educational aims of the cardiac rehabilitation program are focused on attempting to modify reversible risk factors for progression of atherosclerosis and further cardiac events. The framework of this educational process begins in the early in-hospital phase of the program, with individual instruction and counseling continuing during the outpatient phases of cardiac rehabilitation. Most cardiac rehabilitation programs use the exercise component as the nucleus, with educational efforts concentrated on the exercise prescriptions. However, dietary modifications to control hyperlipidemia, hypertension, and obesity, psychologic aspects, and smoking cessation assume major importance in many subjects. Other educational goals should be the clear understanding by the patient of proper medication usage (especially proper use of sublingual nitroglycerin) and knowledge of the danger signs that merit immediate medical attention.

Physicians and nurses who manage patients recovering from myocardial infarction should be aware of the special contributions that other allied health professionals may make to the rehabilitation effort. Cardiac rehabilitation centers incorporate exercise physiologists, clinical nutritionists, clinical psychologists, and vocational specialists, along with physicians and nurses, into a rehabilitation team. By this approach, specialists from each of these areas assist in the evaluation of the patient and provide reports to the managing physician. Moreover, they often have specific roles in the educational aspects of the rehabilitation program. The high prevalence of adverse life-style habits, of maladaptive responses to environmental stresses, and of acute or chronic emotional distress in coronary patients provides the reason for including these types of allied health specialists in the rehabilitation process on a nearly routine basis.

Adherence to a prudent life-style sometimes requires changes in ingrained habits. Individual instruction and formal classes geared to understanding the principles of physical conditioning and the personal limits of each patient's performance are important educational elements of the cardiac rehabilitation program. Environmental influences affecting exercise, especially if outdoor exercise is utilized, are components the patient needs to know thoroughly. Recognition of limiting symptoms during physical activity must be thoroughly explained by staff members and understood by patients.

DIETARY EDUCATION

Several of the risk factors for CAD are amenable to dietary modification.[2,37] Most noteworthy of these are lipid abnormalities, hypertension, obesity, and diabetes. The dietary education therefore centers around reducing the intake of saturated fats, cholesterol, and simple sugars, restriction of sodium ingestion, and limiting total caloric consumption to that required to maintain ideal body weight.

A skilled dietitian is often important to help analyze each patient's dietary habits and to make specific suggestions that allow the diet to remain palatable to the individual, affordable, nutritionally adequate, and yet achieve the desired effects.

The dietary change of most importance for many cardiac patients is restricting total calories to control obesity. In addition to the deleterious effects obesity may have on diabetes, hypertension, and lipoprotein levels, excessive body weight may greatly impair functional work capacity in subjects limited by angina pectoris or congestive heart failure.

The group setting of the supervised exercise program along with specialized dietary counseling can help the individual adjust to reduced caloric intake until the ideal body weight is achieved and maintained. Ideal body weight can be calculated from standard nomograms or from body density determinations with the goal of 15% body fat composition in adult men and 20% in adult women. This information can be best ascertained by underwater weight determinations (if the facilities are available) or by use of the skin calipers to estimate body fat composition. The reduction diet chosen for the patient must be reasonable and allow for increasing activities, such as regular exercise and return to work. A weight loss of 1 to 3 pounds per week without symptoms of ketosis can be expected for most subjects consuming 700 to 1000 calories daily. Family involvement is important, and emphasis on the prevention of CAD for the entire family and the generalized use of the prudent diet—limited in sodium, saturated fats, and cholesterol and high in complex carbohydrates—should be stressed.

CIGARETTE SMOKING

Continued cigarette smoking is a major risk factor for secondary cardiac events and thus cannot be overlooked in any multifactorial approach to this problem. The program for smoking cessation starts with instruction from the physician about the deleterious effects of smoking. Individual and group counseling, including the use of behavior modification techniques, may prove useful in many instances. By these methods up to 50% of subjects can successfully discontinue smoking on a permanent basis.

PSYCHOLOGIC ASPECTS OF CARDIAC REHABILITATION

Patients respond to a cardiac event with a large diversity of coping mechanisms. Some patients appear to deny the gravity of the situation, whereas others exaggerate the problem and may never return to routine activities despite minimal limitations on physiologic cardiac function. Situational depression is almost uniformly present to some degree. For an understanding of these varied responses and adaptations a thorough psychologic evaluation when the patient initially enters a supervised cardiac rehabilitation program is useful (see Chapter 13). The medical evaluation conducted by physicians or nurses should specifically address psychologic issues, and psychologic test procedures and individual interview sessions with a psychologist can often contribute a great deal to patient management. Attention is usually given to the patient's reaction to environmental stresses, basic personality traits, present level of anxiety and depression, and other behavioral characteristics. Appropriate recommendations concerning stress management and behavioral modification may be made, and referral for psychiatric intervention or psychotropic medication may be advised.

Sexual activity

A point of great concern to patients after a cardiac event is the resumption of sexual activity.[38] Although sudden death during sexual intercourse has been reported and is greatly feared, the risk of sexual activity for cardiac patients with familiar sexual partners has probably been overemphasized. Most patients free from angina at heart rates up to 130 beats/minute during exercise testing can safely resume sexual activity soon after hospital discharge, but individual counseling with the physician is desirable after the patient's functional capacity has been evaluated. The patient should be encouraged to report any symptoms experienced during intercourse. It may be encouraging to the patient entering a cardiac rehabilitation program to know that exercise training or conditioning may enhance sexual performance,[39] especially if an increased angina threshold and reduced anxiety over other activities can be achieved. Adjustments in medications such as prophylactic nitroglycerin also may decrease symptoms during sexual activity.

Return to work

Another area of great concern to infarction patients is when and if they should return to work. This decision, of course, is made by the personal physician and the patient with the assistance of a vocational counselor after the patient's functional capacity has been properly evaluated by treadmill or other tests.[1-4] The vocational counselor is usually able to offer valuable suggestions after collecting data about the patient's present job. In addition to the functional capacity of the patient and the demands of the job, other variables to consider are age, skill, emotional tension, and environmental factors. Vocational recommendations should also consider the specific nature of work activities requiring physical labor. The capacity of a subject to perform an occupation requiring work with the arms may not be directly assessable by treadmill exercise testing only. Also, since most cardiac rehabilitation programs achieve cardiovascular conditioning with motion involving the large muscles of the legs and hips, the fitness of the arms and shoulders may not be improved.[5] Individualized programs designed to increase the endurance of the upper body may need to be developed for these patients.

Long-term patient adherence to rehabilitation programs

Despite the favorable physiologic adaptations that occur with exercise conditioning and despite the best efforts of the rehabilitation team, a sizable proportion of infarction patients fail to continue dietary and exercise habits that have been prescribed for them. In recent data from Duke University's Cardiac Rehabilitation Program, Blumenthal and co-workers[40] demonstrated that noncompliers could be distinguished from compliers by a certain set of physical and psychologic parameters obtained at the time of entry into the program. Compliers were those who attended 75% of the sessions over a 1-year period, whereas noncompliers were those who ceased attending the rehabilitation program during this period of time. Dropouts had greater cardiac disability with lower left ventricular ejection fraction as evaluated by radionuclide angiography. However, no other risk factors such as obesity, hypertension, or elevated serum lipids distinguished these noncompliers. The psychologic factors common to the individuals who dropped out of the program indicated that this group was experiencing more psychologic stress. These individuals were most concerned with their health, had higher scores on anxiety and depression, and were socially introverted. Their ego strength was lower, and testing indicated inadequate coping mechanisms. Efforts to identify strategies to increase compliance in patients with these characteristics are underway.

Summary

The rehabilitation of the patient recovering from a myocardial infarction has two major goals: to eliminate any potentially reversible physical or psychologic barriers that impede resumption of a satisfying and productive life, and to minimize risk for subsequent catastrophic cardiac events. Modern concepts of cardiac rehabilitation emphasize early functional testing to facilitate rational, individualized patient management, progressive exercise conditioning programs, and intensive and repeated patient education and counseling regarding psychologic, social, sexual, and vocational aspects of the recovery from myocardial infarction and addressing modification of risk factors for subsequent adverse events.

For greater depth regarding specific issues in cardiac rehabilitation than that provided by this chapter the reader is referred to several recent textbooks and reviews.[1-3,10,41]

REFERENCES

1. Amsterdam, E.A., and others: Exercise in cardiovascular health and disease, New York, 1977, Yorke.
2. Pollock, M.L., and Schmidt, D.H.: Heart disease and rehabilitation, Boston, 1979, Houghton Mifflin Co.
3. Wenger, N.K.: Exercise and the heart, Philadelphia, 1978, F.A. Davis Co.
4. Wenger, N.K.: Research related to rehabilitation, Circulation **60**:1636, 1979.
5. Astrand, P., and Rodahl, K.: Textbook of work physiology, New York, 1970, McGraw-Hill Book Co.
6. Miller, R.R., and others: Prevention of lower extremity venous thrombosis by early mobilization, Ann. Intern. Med. **84**:700, 1976.
7. McNeer, J.F., and others: Hospital discharge one week after myocardial infarction, N. Engl. J. Med. **298**:229, 1978.
8. Markiewicz, W., and others: Exercise testing soon after myocardial infarction, Circulation **56**:26, 1977.
9. DeBusk, R.F., and others: Cardiovascular responses to dynamic and static effort soon after myocardial infarction, Circulation **58**:368, 1978.
10. Clausen, J.P.: Circulatory adjustments to dynamic exercise and effect of physical training in normal subjects and in patients with coronary artery disease, Prog. Cardiovasc. Dis. **18**:459, 1976.
11. Clausen, J.P.: Effect of physical training on cardiovascular adjustments to exercise in man, Physiol. Rev. **57**:815, 1977.
12. Black, H.R.: Nonpharmacologic therapy for hypertension, Am. J. Med. **66**:837, 1979.
13. Bjorntorp, P.: Exercise in the treatment of obesity, Clin. Endocrinol. Metab. **5**:431, 1976.
14. Blumenthal, J.A., and others: The effects of exercise on the Type A (coronary-prone) behavior pattern, Psychosom. Med. **42**:289, 1980.
15. Hartung, G.H., and others: Relation of diet to high-density-lipoprotein cholesterol in middle-aged marathon runners, joggers, and inactive men, N. Engl. J. Med. **302**:357, 1980.
16. Mau, H.S., and Wagner, E.D.: Cardiovascular rehabilitation: effects of exercise and diet on blood pressure, Circulation **62**:111, 1980.
17. Pedersen, O., and others: Increased insulin receptors after exercise in patients with insulin-dependent diabetes mellitus, N. Engl. J. Med. **302**:886, 1980.
18. Redwood, D.R., and others: Circulatory and symptomatic effects of physical training in patients with coronary artery disease and angina pectoris, **286**:959, 1972.
19. Williams, R.S., and others: Reduced epinephrine-induced platelet aggregation following cardiac rehabilitation, J. Cardiol. Rehab. **1**:127, 1981.
20. Mann, G.V., and others: Exercise to prevent coronary heart disease: an experimental study of the effects of training on risk factors for coronary disease in men, Am. J. Med. **46**:12, 1969.
21. Conn, E., and others: Physical conditioning in patients with severely depressed left ventricular function, Am. J. Cardiol. **49**:296, 1982.
22. Williams, R.S., and others: Physical conditioning augments endothelial release of plasminogen activators in healthy adults, N. Engl. J. Med. **302**:987, 1980.
23. Leon, A.S., and Blackburn, H.: The relationship of physical activity to coronary heart disease and life expectancy, Ann. N.Y. Acad. Sci. **301**:561, 1977.
24. McNeer, J.F., and others: The role of the exercise test in the evaluation of patients for ischemic heart disease, Circulation **57**:64, 1978.
25. Morris, J.N., and others: Vigorous exercise in leisure-time and the incidence of coronary heart disease, Lancet **1**:333, 1973.
26. Paffenbarger, R.S., Jr., and others: Physical activity as an index of heart attack risk in college alumni, Am. J. Epidemiol. **108**:161, 1978.
27. Paffenbarger, R.S., Jr., and Hale, W.E.: Work activity and coronary heart mortality, N. Engl. J. Med. **292**:545, 1975.

28. Rose, C.L., and Cohen, M.L.: Relative importance of physical activity for longevity, Ann. N.Y. Acad. Sci. **301**:671, 1977.

29. Naughton, J.: The national exercise and heart disease project: development, recruitment, and implementation. In Wenger, N.A., editor: Exercise and the heart, Philadelphia, 1978, F.A. Davis Co.

30. Rechnitzer, P.A., and others: A controlled prospective study on the effect of endurance training on the recurrent rate of myocardial infarction, Am. J. Epidemiol. **102**:358, 1975.

31. Coronary Drug Project Research Group: Implications of findings in the coronary drug project for secondary prevention trials in coronary heart disease, Circulation **63**:1342, 1981.

32. American College of Sports Medicine: Guidelines for exercise testing and exercise prescription, Philadelphia, 1980, Lea & Febiger.

33. Fletcher, G.F., and others: Oxygen consumption and hemodynamic response of exercises used in training of patients with recent myocardial infarction, Circulation **60**:140, 1979.

34. Haskell, W.K.: Cardiovascular complications during exercise training on cardiac patients, Circulation **57**:920, 1978.

35. Williams, R.S., and others: Guidelines for unsupervised exercise in patients with ischemic heart disease, J. Cardiol. Rehab. **1**:213, 1981.

36. The Committee on Exercise: Exercise testing and training of individuals with heart disease or at high risk for its development: a handbook for physicians, Dallas, 1975, American Heart Association.

37. Turpeinen, O.: Effect of cholesterol-lowering diet on mortality from coronary heart disease and other causes, Circulation **59**:1, 1979.

38. McLane, M., and others: Psychosexual adjustment and counseling after myocardial infarction, Ann. Intern. Med. **92**:514, 1980.

39. Stein, R.A.: The effect of exercise training on heart rate during coitus in the post myocardial infarction patient, Circulation **55**:738, 1977.

40. Blumenthal, J.A., and others: Determinants of exercise compliance in coronary rehabilitation: a prospective study, Psychosom. Med. **43**:93, 1981.

41. Oberman, A.: Key references: cardiac rehabilitation, Circulation **62**:909, 1980.

15

DEATH AND DYING

Frederic W. Hafferty

The history of concern over death and dying in the United States in the past 2 decades largely reflects a preoccupation with a particular disease, cancer. Associated with this preoccupation has been a similar focus on a particular course of dying, the lingering and often painful terminal illness. Much of the literature on death and dying, either overtly or covertly, therefore focuses on the cancer patient. Many of the themes addressed in the literature, involving such effects as pain and disfigurement, are grounded in the field of oncology. Even the largest single health care movement to arise within the death and dying movement, the hospice,* heavily focuses on care of the terminally ill cancer patient. Conversely, relatively little attention has been paid to the thanatologic† implications of cardiovascular disease even though it is and has been the leading cause of death in the United States.

Even with that qualification in mind it is important to recognize that there has been a considerable amount of change during the past 20 years in the public's awareness of issues involved in death and dying. Courses and workshops have sprung up by the thousands, television specials have been aired, and national news media routinely carry articles and commentary on a topic that was once taboo. This growing attention has not, however, occurred in a social vacuum. Major changes in American society have both fostered and supported this new focus.[1] The civil rights movement, an increased concern with issues of equal opportunity and quality of life, is one such development. A more critical and skeptical view of the role of science and technology and an increased awareness of diminishing resources, both economic and material, are two more. Other changes include a decreasing emphasis on religious paradigms in the consideration of social and ethical issues, the rise of consumer rights advocacy, and continuing shifts in morbidity and mortality patterns resulting in an expanding elderly population. Thus the emphasis on candor, humanism, and self-determination now so visible in the death and dying circles has been nurtured and supported by a host of broader social developments. These broader shifts in the nation's social fiber will continue both to influence and in turn be influenced by issues in medical care as they relate to the themes of critical care, death, and dying.

---

*For a more extended discussion of this term see p. 533 of this chapter.
†From the Greek work "thanatos," which means death.

The rapid rise in prominence of thanatologic issues was not without negative consequences. As we "discovered" this national taboo, many people rushed in to provide improved care for the terminally ill. Almost literally overnight solutions were being generated for what were, essentially, ill-defined problems. Fear of death seemed accorded the status of a national disease, something to be attacked and conquered. Ironically, this push for immediate solutions to the "death and dying problem" can be interpreted as yet another indicator of its taboo status rather than as a rational response to it. A case in point was early data that identified physicians as either unwilling or unable to disclose a terminal prognosis to their patients. These data were often accompanied by findings that patients often really knew or preferred to know their diagnosis. It seemed to matter little that much of these latter data were anecdotal, impressionistic, or methodologically suspect. Healthy people were asked if they would like to be told, informed patients were asked if they were glad that they were told, but no uninformed terminally ill patients were asked if they were pleased not to have been told. In short, drawing conclusions about patients' desire to know from people who are either not patients or who have already been told is suspect. Similarly, it seems methodologically and ethically untenable to ask uninformed patients about whether they would prefer to be told or not. Thus the cry was raised, grounded more in some sense of moral or ethical outrage than in appropriate methodologies, that terminally ill patients *should* be told and had a *right* to know of their terminal prognosis. This mixing of ethical and empiric orientations resulted in a rush to tell the truth, and in some cases institutional policies mandating that all patients receive such information.[2] Lost for the moment was the understanding that a situation where virtually all patients are told and one where none or few are told are ironically equivalent: neither one is truly patient centered. Authority and autonomy remain in the hands of health professionals. Often left equally unaddressed is that the specific act of telling a patient his prognosis is in no way synonymous with the difficult and complicated task of establishing a relationship or context in which death and dying can be discussed.

Life-threatening versus terminal illness

Patients who have a cardiovascular disease can be expected to perceive and react to the threat of disease differently from patients with cancer because of a number of factors. First, there exists a host of signs and symptoms that discriminate between the two. For example, cancer symptoms are often more nonspecific and vague and often more gradual in onset than those of many cardiovascular diseases. Similarly, there is more specificity of diagnosis with cardiovascular disease. Pain and the control of pain are more predominantly featured in the disease course of the cancer patient. Conversely, the absence of symptoms may be problematic in an individual whose life is soon to be threatened by a massive coronary. Surgery for the patient who has coronary artery disease is more reconstructive than ablative; the reverse is true for the patient with cancer. For the patient facing cardiovascular surgery, the treatment itself inherently involves a potential life threat, a life threat made more ominous because of its temporal immediacy.[3,4]

Not only does the onset of the two diseases differ, but their courses of dying may be radically different. Death from cancer is usually expected and occurs over time. Death from cardiovascular disease can assume a similar profile but may also be unexpected and sudden, with little or no forewarning. Finally, from attitudinal and behavioral perspectives cardiovascular disease and cancer are viewed and reacted to differently within both medical and lay circles. There exists a sense of optimism and hope in the treatment of cardiovascular disease that is lacking in that of cancer. In part this may be owing to the rapid development of surgical techniques and technologic breakthroughs in the area of cardiovascular disease; the proliferation of coronary bypass operations, heart valve replacements, and even complete transplants are cases in point. Heart disease has emerged with an image of being more curable. Thus attitudes in approaching the disease are more positive, less hopeless, but also more aggressive. As phrased by Eys, "The cardiologist frequently requires last-ditch efforts because recovery is the expected norm, even if the mortality is very high."[5] In summation, the label *terminally ill* is less contextually appropriate in the case of cardiovascular patients than in the area of oncology. The particular etiology and course of cardiovascular illness experienced by patients and perceived by their caregivers indicate that the label *life threatened* seems much more appropriate than its counterpart, *terminally ill.*

Attitudes toward death and dying

The classification of an individual as dead or dying has profound implications not only for the individual so labeled but for society in general. It is therefore distressing to note that the concepts themselves are not at all clearly defined. Although it seems obvious to contend that virtually any rational adult can differentiate between someone who is alive and someone who is dead, the traditional medical criteria used to distinguish the living from the dead have been rendered more, not less, obtuse in recent years. Delineating between dying and not dying is even a more nebulous task. What are the attitudinal, behavioral, or biophysical characteristics that distinguish a dying individual from one who is not? When does dying start? Similarly, when does it stop? Although an obvious and partially correct answer to this last question would be, "with death," the question has particular importance (and not so obvious an answer) for the life-threatened individual who has, for example, suffered a heart attack that is not fatal. If we consider dying as a status, the question, "How does one stop dying?" or "How does one exit from this status?" is the most critical for the caregiver to address. At what point, using what cues, and for what reasons do caregivers cease to perceive a patient as "dying"? We may ask the same question of family, friends, and even the patient. Underlying these questions is a perspective stressing the process of dying as a psychosocial event accompanied by sometimes vaguely defined and often arbitrary and capricious biologic correlates. An individual's status is changed, sometimes quite abruptly, when he is labeled as dying. Roles are altered, and autonomy is diminished. As Mauksch[6] points out, the entrance into patient status, particularly that of a hospitalized patient, is a stripping process. One relinquishes clothing, control over environment, and freedom of movement, to name but a few. These restrictions are often justified by a medical system with an either implicit or explicit promise of cure. For the terminally ill or life-threatened patient such restrictions lose much of their recuperative rationale. Often, terminally ill or life-threatened individuals find that to others their illness over-shadows all other aspects of their being.[7] People view the individual not as, for example, a salesman with a life-threatening condition but as a dying father or a dying salesman. The terminal or life-threatened condition becomes paramount in the eyes of others, with all other roles or characteristics viewed in that light. The resulting behavior is not necessarily marked by obvious avoidance of dis-tancing. As Trillin most cogently illustrates[8]:

> Unconsciously, even with a certain amount of kindness [people] regarded me as someone who had been altered irrevocably. . . . Their distance from me was marked most of all by their inability to understand the ordinariness, the banality of what was happening to me. They marveled at how well I was "coping with cancer." I had become special, no longer like them.

Once again we return to the fact that *dying* is a socially generated and maintained label, a status, with profound implications for the living.

A second important distinction is that the often-used phrase, "death and dying" is not a singular concept. There is an obvious relationship, in that death can be viewed as the end of a process we label dying. There are, however, major differences. For example, one's attitudes toward death may scarcely reflect one's attitudes toward dying. Furthermore, as Lester[9] has pointed out, attitudes toward death can be differentiated into attitudes toward death of self and attitudes toward death of others. Attitudes toward dying are similarly differentiated. Finally, we must recognize that attitudes toward death or dying are not static but change and evolve over time. In short, it is a mistake to view an individual as possessing a single attitude toward death and dying. For each person, the concepts of death and dying will take on a broad variety of meanings depending not only on such obvious variables as personal contact history and social, cultural, or religious backgrounds, but also on the situational influences of present contact with, or distance from, a situation of death or dying. It is therefore not necessary, and in fact highly unlikely, that the hospitalized terminally ill patient, his family, and the caregivers will share similar frames of reference. For caregivers dying may represent failure and frustration, for the patient pain and isolation, and for the family economic hardship. Each stands in a different place relative to the others in the dying process, and for each person a different orientation emerges as predominant. That these frames of reference may come into conflict is a reality of the terminal or life-threatening illness that must be recognized and dealt with.

The role that a "fear of death" or a "death anxiety" plays in the overall anxiety experienced by a life-threatened cardiovascular patient is an important issue. Investigators such as Hackett and co-workers[10] have identified anxiety as the predominant attribute in the majority of such patients. Other authors, such as Gentry and co-workers,[11] have correlated the degree of anxiety experienced to the degree of denial utilized by patients. Research as exemplified by that of Gentry and Haney[12] has extended this theme by attempting to identify the underpinnings of anxiety in cardiovascular patients. Their findings identified death concern as a major variable. More specifically, a high concern with death resulted at a prehospital stage with less delay in seeking care and a perception of self as more sick. In the hospital CCU an increase in death concern paralleled increases in subjective anxiety, physiologic stress, and levels of reported pain. The authors also reported that patients with a high level of death fear displayed a higher level of functional stress than patients who expressed less concern over dying. Foster[13] found myocardial infarction patient communication to center around feelings of "living under the spectre of death." Blacher[14,15] proposes that death concerns have much to do with postcardiotomy psychosis.

Whether the fear and anxiety experienced and/or displayed by the life-threatened cardiovascular patient is at root a fear of death is an empiric question that has not yet been adequately answered. However, there are further delineations, which should be made on a more clinical level. The following discussion of types of coping reactions to the threat of death and dying serves as an exploration.

The reality of dying is multifaceted, involving the patient in a social, psychologic, and biologic web of influencing factors. "Fear of dying" is largely meaningless, since it describes nothing contextually. The phrase is essentially a label, a descriptive handle. As a process, dying may involve pain, isolation, existential crises, or the exploration and attainment of new and more meaningful relationships. It can be good *and* bad, freeing *and* confining, fear *and* ecstasy inducing. It is therefore better that we ask of ourselves and our patients what it is about dying that is anxiety provoking. It has been proposed by Freud and others that fear of death (which again should not be confused with dying) is universal. This frame of reference can be extremely problematic. An eagerness to identify the fear of death that is present in all persons often is accompanied by a tendency for caregivers to move from the descriptive to the prescriptive. Rather than using concepts descriptively to better understand patient care situations, caregivers can sometimes use them prescriptively, that is, come to expect the behavior described. As with the phrase "fear of dying," simply labeling a patient as having a fear of death involves yet another empty diagnostic category. A fear of death cannot be addressed. A fear of the unknown, a fear of losing body or self-control, a fear of losing identity, or a fear of losing family and friends can be both specifically identified and addressed.[16] Finally, self-fulfilling prophecies may occur in which patients prematurely, inadequately, or inaccurately labeled come to manifest the behaviors or attitudes expected of them.

Reactions to the threat of dying or death
STAGES OF DYING

The most widely known of the behavioral/attitudinal descriptions of reactions to dying are the five stages described by Kübler-Ross. Detailed in her familiar book, *On Death and Dying*, these stages can be summarized as (1) denial—"No, not me," (2) Rage and anger—"Why me?" (3) bargaining—"Yes me, but . . . ," (4) depression—"Yes . . . me," (5) acceptance—"It's all right." Although Kübler-Ross has on occasion stated that these not be considered literal stages, she has consistently described them as if they occur in a linear, sequential, and developmental manner. This facet of Kübler-Ross's work has generated criticism because other field investigators and researchers have not been able to duplicate her orderings. This is not to say that terminally ill patients do not display anger, denial, or bargaining but that, for example, bargaining is not necessarily sequentially or causally linked to anger.

The popularity of Kübler-Ross's writings has created not only an expectation that this is the way things are, but also a belief that this is the way things should be. The result is a host of normative expectations that evidence themselves in both the patient and provider populations. A patient exhibiting bargaining, for example, may be evaluated by others as being closer to accepting death than one who exhibits rage or anger. Health care providers who note anger in a patient may see denial as over and bargaining on the way. Patients who exhibit bargaining after a period of observed depression may be seen as having regressed or moved further away from a state of acceptance. It is more appropriate and clinically accurate to consider such behavioral responses to the threat of dying as types, not stages, in which individuals may exhibit all or none of these modalities, in combination or separately, without reference to order or sequence. In this context the normative orientation *can* prove to be clinically helpful, for now it allows the health care provider to view such reactions as normal, expectable, and therefore (it is hoped) acceptable. This frame of reference also parallels Shneidman's[17] critique of Kübler-Ross in noting that the first four of her stages have negative affective connotations and may therefore be perceived as things that must be worked through, or otherwise conquered on the road to acceptance. In short, the stages concept is an inaccurate model, which when used as either a descriptive or prescriptive tool results in at the least an ineffective and at the worst a detrimental approach to patient care.

It should also be emphasized that patients are not the only ones who experience normal reactions to the threat of dying and death. Family and staff also may experience a multitude of feelings concerning the dying of a patient or loved one. The recognition that all parties involved react psychologically to a life-threatening situation allows us to recognize the possibility that different individuals may be in conflicting or competing psychologic states. If a patient is manifesting denial and the family rage and anger "No, not him!" or even "No, not me!", there is little sense of sharing or mutual support. This, or course, decreases the probability of resolution and in many cases exacerbates the situation.

Finally, for caregivers it should be emphasized that each of these five reaction types has direct and important implications for the organization and delivery of health care. For example, the expression of rage and anger, particularly that directed toward health care providers, can be extremely disruptive to the staff's mood as well as its work organization.[18] It is the cooperative, appreciative, and not overly demanding individual that is often viewed as a "good patient" by staff. The patient displaying rage or anger is none of these. Bargaining, when transacted with staff, can be troublesome because it strikes at the very core of the superordinate-subordinate relationship, which is grounded in the hospital authority structure. The patient who says, "Yes, but . . . " does not display an unwavering allegiance to what the caregiver has decided is a necessary course of therapeutic action. The withdrawal that accompanies depression can be troublesome for staff in that it represents yet another form of the unappreciative or perhaps uncooperative patient. Even a state of acceptance can be stressful and provoke anxiety for health care providers. Acceptance is marked by a withdrawal from the world of the social,[19] and although it is psychodynamically much different from denial, behaviorally it may be virtually indistinguishable. Ironically, the reaction that can be least troublesome or threatening for staff is denial. For those staff members unwilling to work with or talk to dying or life-threatened patients about their fears or concerns, whether this be in general, or at some specific time, the possibility of initiating and/or reinforcing denial in the patient is an all too frequent event in the world of clinical medicine.

DENIAL

The coping mechanism of denial during a life-threatening illness involving coronary care deserves particular attention because of the multifaceted role that denial plays in the course of illness for a coronary patient. Three important themes should be emphasized. First, denial may be viewed as functional or dysfunctional, depending on the context. For example, when considering the onset of chest pains in the case of a patient who has suffered a myocardial infarction, denial may be viewed as dysfunctional and in fact dangerous. The interpretation of these chest pains as indigestion, or the delay, fostered by denial, in seeking health care are obvious examples.[20] Assuming survival at this phase of the illness, several authors have observed the beneficial aspects of denial among newly hospitalized patients,[21-23] for whom the goals are recovery from the initial insult and stabilization of the condition. The reduction of anxiety and the bolstering of hope fostered by denial play an important role. That cardiac patients are essentially asymptomatic after hospitalization is unfortunate and possibly precurses a third phase, in which denial once again becomes dysfunctional: the patient, unencumbered by symptoms, may neglect or refuse to follow posthospitalization treatment protocols. This tendency, supported by the mutually reinforcing lack of symptoms and denial, is a serious health problem. Medications not taken and physical activities too vigorously pursued are but two of many examples.

Denial may be viewed in terms of gradations. On the most general level caregivers may notice denial of what Weisman[24] terms *primary facts*. Here a patient may deny the nature of the disease itself. ("I'm not sick, just run down.") On another level a patient may acknowledge the facts of the disease but not its implications. Finally, a life-threatened patient may acknowledge both facts and implications but deny the outcome—extinction or death.

It is most important that caregivers recognize that denial is not in and of itself a defense but rather a label describing what defenses do. Unfortunately, the term *denial* has been so broadened in meaning that it now covers virtually any and all situations involving an alteration or avoidance of reality. Rather than locate denial in the mind or behavior of an individual, clinical health care providers would be more therapeutic and structurally realistic to view denial as manifested and maintained within the context of social interaction. As pointed out by Weisman, an individual's use of denial is selective and does not occur with all individuals with whom he is in contact. At root, therefore, denial has the primary purpose of protecting a significant relationship. For the life-threatened patient such an individual is a physician or nurse. In fact, the more significant the relationship is, the more likely is the appearance of denial. Thus denial should be viewed not as a frame of mind, or general psychologic state, but as a dimension of human interaction; and it should therefore be addressed as such. The provider of clinical care who perceives denial in a patient should not blithely assume that the altering of reality observed is also being manifested by the patient in interactions with others. Such a perspective locates the denial outside of the particular interaction in question and distances the labeler from any responsibility or connection with the behavior observed and labeled. This frees the labeler from any feeling of connection with or responsibility for the identified denial. Denial is an evaluation and label based on a discrepancy between the reality testing of the observer and that of the patient. That it also serves to protect a relationship, particularly one based on paternalism or subordinate-superordinate dimensions, places a certain responsibility on the caregiver to explore ways in which denial may be minimized *within its specific context*.

Dying trajectories and social death

It is a major thesis of this chapter that the process of dying, the state of death, and even the treatment of critically ill patients cannot be adequately understood from a purely biomedical perspective. The decision to treat and the treatment itself of critically ill patients have been consistently found to be grounded in evaluations of patients in both physiologic and social terms.[25]

The concept of social death is particularly cogent in this context. In a general sense social death may be viewed as the absence of behaviors normally directed toward living people and/or the presence of behaviors normally directed toward the dead. Within this framework the concept of social death can be applied to a broad spectrum of situations, ranging from literally treating the alive as dead to various forms of isolationism and ostracism. In examining the behavior of emergency room staff toward patients brought in dead on arrival, Sudnow[26,27] and Simpson[28] found that is was social and not strictly medical factors that were primary in the decision to resuscitate, the efforts made at resuscitation, the decision to suspend resuscitation efforts, and the treatment of the body after death. Factors found as influencing either the presence of absence of intensive resuscitation efforts included age, social background (often inferred from appearance), apparent sobriety, and the presence or absence of inferred social deviancy or perceived moral character.

Both Sudnow and Simpson found that the older the patient was, the more readily the physician accepted a dead on arrival status, the more cursory the examination and the less intensively the resuscitation efforts. Similarly, the perceived or inferred moral character of the patient, particularly of "those who refuse to care for themselves," has impact. Also, the handling of the body after death, its use as a teaching tool or for the practice of various skills, is tied to the social status of the patient before death. Conversely, the younger, the "innocent," and the famous may take significantly longer to be pronounced dead. The resuscitation efforts made at the death of President Kennedy is an example of the last.

A phenomenon related to these extreme examples of social death involves the well-documented avoidance and isolation of the terminally ill patient by caregivers and family. This kind of behavior can range from ostracism as a form of social annihilation to more informal exclusionary types of behavior, including avoidance of eye contact, exclusion from conversations, or omission of certain conversational topics (references to the future, for example). The loss of a "fully live" status for an elderly patient has already been mentioned but needs to be continuously emphasized. The phrase "He has lived a full life" is a commonly heard reflection at the death of elderly person. However innocently intended it may also be viewed as evidence that we evaluate the life of an elderly person in a sense categorically different from that used for a younger person.

The importance of the concept of social death and its parallel phenomenological death[29] coronary care of life-threatening illness is apparent in several ways. The concepts ask us to examine critically factors that influence decisions to code or not code, or decisions to initiate or abandon aggressive therapies. Certainly we can use the concept of social death to view the informal "slow code," in which the initiation of or response to a code order is carried out with less than the greatest of haste. Likewise, between a full code and no code there exist a number of intervention possibilities organized around a triadic hierarchy of intervention. Usually perceived in terms of invasiveness, from least to most, the attending physician can communicate to his colleagues the need for any one or combination of (1) chemicals, (2) shock (DC cardioversion), and (3) intubation, depending on how energetically the code is to be pursued. The specification that the patient should be administered chemicals but not intubated accomplishes a number of latent purposes. First, it allows a physician who feels uncomfortable about doing nothing to do something. Second, for those patients for whom it is felt that some action short of pulling out all stops is warranted, such an option is available. Finally, it provides caregivers with specific treatment recommendations that are also indirect indications of how aggressively a code situation should be pursued.

A second concept critical to understanding the phenomenon of death and dying from both biologic and social contexts is that of dying trajectories. Most fully developed in the writings of Glaser and Strauss,[30-32] this concept allows us to explore a full range of dying behaviors and, more important, to focus on the particular problems associated with both the type and timing of deaths and dying commonly found in coronary care.

First it is important to note that various hospital services house different types and amounts of dying. These different modes and courses are reflected by differences in work organization and coping strategies used by staff. On some wards there is little dying, on others a great deal. In some service units the dying most often encountered is quick, in others the dying process extends over a longer period of time. It is this course of dying that Glaser and Strauss refer to as the *dying trajectory*. It has two basic properties: duration and shape. Shape refers to the seriousness of the condition and how biologically close or far away the patient is from death. Although the authors point out that dying trajectories are perceived rather than the actual courses of events, it is helpful to view them from both frames of reference: anticipated and actual. This duality allows for a matching of anticipated with actual and, or course, a prediction of the medical and social consequences of situations where the two trajectories do not conform.

Although in viewing the coronary care patient any of Glaser and Strauss's types of trajectories can be identified, it is quick dying, and in particular the unexpectedly quick trajectory, that is of notable importance in the world of coronary care.

In service units such as intensive care units, CCUs, and emergency rooms an abrupt trajectory is a relatively common course of dying. These services are both technologically and organizationally structured to intervene quickly in the case of a patient who is dying quickly. When a death is anticipated and in fact expected, the staff's emotional equilibrium need not be severely taxed. The death is planned for emotionally and organizationally. Extenuating circumstances are certainly not ruled out. The patient, for example, may have a high social value to certain staff members. The family may not have expected or accepted the death in quite the same way as either the staff or the patient and thus may cause scenes, which must be dealt with by the staff. As will be touched on in a later section, the *mere availability of methods of intervention puts tremendous pressures on staff to utilize such equipment, particularly in an environment where moral, ethical, and normative aspects of critical care are not routinely examined.*

An unexpectedly quick trajectory may take several shapes. On the one hand death may not be expected at all. In other cases death is anticipated but not at the time or manner in which it actually occurs. The basic component of an unexpectedly quick trajectory is, of course, surprise, and this element of the unexpected gives rise to several stressful consequences for those involved. One of the most severe is the possibility of clinical incompetence. The question of why patients died, particularly "when they were not supposed to," is a painful, threatening, and clinically serious issue. Questions about errors of commission and omission may be raised, and review and accountability may be challenged. Other stressful consequences of an unexpectedly quick trajectory include informing the family. Often these individuals had not only expected the patient to live but had been led to believe that it had been expected by the staff themselves. In many cases an autopsy must be performed and permission for it sought from already shocked and grieving survivors. As opposed to a longer trajectory, particularly one that is unfolding as expected, an unexpectedly quick trajectory finds relationships abruptly terminated. Anticipatory grief[33] may either be interrupted or not undergone at all; family or personal affairs may not have been attended to or resolved. In short, death preparation, leave-takings, working through "stages," and progress toward acceptance are either blunted or altogether absent. Since there is little or no expectation of "impending" death, the staff may be similarly unprepared; thus, when an unexpected death does occur, it can be an occasion for much recrimination and guilt over what could or should have happened.

An important quality of dying trajectories is that they can be manipulated. As advances in medical technology and knowledge improve our ability to intervene in the matter of life and health, so they do in the matter of death. More than ever before the term *natural death* is a euphemism for situations in which medical intervention has proven ineffectual. As our ability to mechanically mimic and biochemically duplicate body processes increases, so do our abilities to alter the course and timing of death. In short, the transition from life to the absence of life can be shortened or prolonged by a variety of strategies and mechanisms. For whatever motives (although usually viewed as humanitarian) the fact remains that substantial control of the dying process has in fact passed from the hands of nature to those of medical technology and its practitioners.

As with any power the ability to manipulate a dying trajectory is not without liabilities and negative consequences. In addition to the present and potential ethical, moral, legal, and professional issues raised, staff may encounter a series of potentially upsetting situations, the solutions for which sometimes call for a more extensive use of the same mechanisms (in this case, purposeful alteration of the trajectory) that originally caused the problem. One example involves the fact that patients disconnected from respirators may manifest physical signs such as sudden body movements or gasping for breath. They may visibly die. These physiologic responses have the potential to undermine greatly the sentimental order of the staff. This contrasts with a relatively benign death in which the transition appears to be from a state of temporary sleep to one of permanent sleep. Staff are less prone to upset when a transition is accompanied by as few visual cues as possible. One consequence of this is the employment of what might be termed "thanatologic fine tuning," the adjustment of fluid intake and chemicals so that the patient is brought to a close-to-death state of biologic equilibrium, in which a discontinuance of respiratory assistance results in a death showing only minimal change in overall body physiology. Thus not only does the discontinuance of the respirator result in a purposeful trajectory change, but it may be accompanied by other purposeful actions or nonactions designed to minimize its visual and physiologic impact. In such a case even manipulations must be manipulated.

Communicating with the critically ill

No task is more difficult and yet so seminal to the care of critically ill patients as establishing and maintaining open lines of communication. Unfortunately thanatologic research and education have tended to oversimplify grossly what is an extremely complex issue. The result has been less than adequate patient care and a continued source of stress for staff.

A case in point is the frequently made observation that most patients want to be told of their terminal condition. It has already been argued that this contention rests on dubious methodologic grounds. Moreover, this contention obscures the simple fact that an individual's orientation toward information about his life-threatening condition varies over time. Most patients have times when information is desired and times when it is not; similarly, most patients seek information at certain times and not at others. To assume a unilateral "patients want to know" perspective ignores this reality.

In attempting to bring some form of order to the problems involved in communicating with patients, health care professionals can be found advocating some form of two distinct themes. One position, normative in orientation, argues for a structure, rule, or policy that might be uniformly applied to issues of patient communication. Such a position usually arises in reaction to patient avoidance and interstaff conflicts over what constitutes appropriate levels of candor with patients. A second position, highly visible in medicine and highly critical of the first camp as overly restrictive, argues that each patient should be individually handled depending on the circumstances and informed not according to rules but according to individual needs. However flexible and patient centered this orientation might sound, the method, when subjected to empirical scrutiny, does not operate as contended. All human beings, whether they be caregivers or not, prefer patterned and stereotypic ways of dealing with others, particularly in situations involving stress. Nurses and physicians behave no differently when it comes to informing patients of their prognoses or diagnoses. Furthermore situational flexibility is in reality almost always based on some second-level rules or generalized norms for interpreting the behavior of others. The beliefs that a life-threatened patient who asks about his condition is seeking reassurance and that a patient who does not ask questions does not want answers are two examples.

Where does this leave us? How then do we best consider the issue of patient-caregiver communication? First, although there are and can be no rules for *what* to say (content), there are ways of viewing interactions with patients and other staff (structure) that can prove beneficial in shaping what is said in individual situations. Staff should place a priority on viewing communication as a process and not an event. Arguments about candor, honesty, or truth telling, quite frankly, direct attention away from this critical point. The most important question for a caregiver is not "How do I inform my patient of a terminal prognosis?" but rather, "How do I establish and support an ongoing dialogue with my patient so that issues involved in dying may be raised and discussed in an atmosphere of mutual respect and trust?" Of course, the latter question represents an often unattainable ideal, but is also represents a qualitatively different way of viewing the patient-caregiver relationship and the nature of patient-caregiver communication. To contend that patients be told *the* truth implies that there is *a* truth to be told, and that once told it has been communicated. Nothing could be more wrong or more detrimental to establishing and maintaining a good patient-caregiver relationship. Health care providers need to remember that there is a distinct difference between what is said (the meaning intended by the speaker) and what is heard (the meaning received by the listener). Patients may need to discuss issues involving their prognosis on several different occasions. Once is hardly ever enough! A second problem with this orientation is that it fails to provide a proper emphasis to the goal of establishing an atmosphere of dialogue between the patient and caregiver. It portrays communication as a monologue, with the patient the one lacking information and the caregivers the holders of critically important information. Although it is true that providers possess important information regarding diagnosis and prognosis, the prominence that this type of information plays in "to tell or not to tell" debates distorts what should be the goal of patient-caregiver communication: an ongoing, mutually beneficial, and supportive dialogue. Any model or portrayal of the issue that locates all relevant and important knowledge in the hands of one party sadly undermines this goal. Patients have a great deal to tell caregivers. In fact, it is only through the process of being receptive to patient needs that caregivers render truly caring care.

A corollary can also be made in response to those who argue for some form of limited disclosure, as representing a median ground between total candor and actual deception. Although advocates point to such laudable motives as the need to preserve hope or the desire not to emotionally overwhelm already ill patients, the assumption underlying a limited disclosure position is that the message itself (usually diagnostic or prognostic information) is so terrifying that it must be altered or muted. If this is an assessment generated while working with a specific patient, it may be warranted. To anticipate such a prescription for patients outside of any specific interaction is not only prejudicial but also indicative of staff rather than patient attitudes and fears.

The concept of limited disclosure can also be criticized because, practically speaking, it is extremely difficult to maintain over time. Such a strategy involves an entangling degree of coordination, and thus stress, for the participants.[34] Often, rather than someone attempting to undertake the arduous task of coordinating who tells what to whom, all communication is vested in one individual (usually the physician), with others (usually nurses) instructed to say nothing that would contradict whatever information arises from that designated source. This strategy results in distancing the most visible and physically present patient care provider, the nurse, from the patient. It stifles communication, promotes deception, and also places inordinate stress on the physician-nurse relationship. It is an unfortunate consequence of the structured care in tertiary care centers that many physicians, because of their relatively minimal contact with patients (as compared with nurses), are frequently unaware of the consequences of such a policy.

A final point, which underscores the complexity of the issue of patient-caregiver communication, is the caution to caregivers against being too understanding of a patient's life-threatened status. This point was made earlier in the chapter in reference to the Trillen article but needs to be reemphasized. Paradoxically, for example, a sympathetic acknowledgement of the appropriateness of anger or depression in a patient may inadvertently be used by caregivers as yet another way of avoiding the patient and his situation. One can be so accepting of a patient's feelings that they are never explored, challenged, or confronted.

The decision to treat critically ill patients

It seems ironic that as increasingly sophisticated technology has increased medicine's ability to intervene more frequently and successfully, conflicts among the moral, ethical, and normative considerations have increased and become more complicated. One result of this state of affairs has been an increase in potentially stressful situations encountered by staff.

The search for causes of this state of affairs is complex. Some explanation can be found in the juncture of a medical educational system that continues to be dominated by tertiary care settings and ready access to high-technology medicine both developed and housed in these locations. Students educated on the forefront of medical technology—the cutting edge of medical science—come to view the use of such modern medical techniques and technology as synonymous with good medicine. This orientation, coupled with access to such resources, creates a technologic imperative, in which the utilization of technology is generated as much or more by its availability than by rational therapeutics. Relevant also is the concept of cultural lag, which points to the historical discrepancy between social and technologic change. By definition, the development of social mechanisms to deal with changes rendered by technologic change must lag behind such innovations. Examples abound in the area of medicine. The legal and social uproar that was and is being generated over recent breakthroughs in transplant technology is but one small example; the call for new definitions of death and changes in social value systems constitutes the social response. On an individual level evidence of cultural lag can best be seen in interpersonal and individual stress and anomie.

The solution for some types of problems lies in improved staff communication.

Other types of problems, however, are more embedded in traditional ways of perceiving or defining situations and will remain troublesome until fundamentally different orientations are developed. It is unrealistic to expect the legal process to develop these new orientations. In many court decisions it has struggled simply to locate decision-making power within the hands of the medical profession without expanding on the broader social, ethical, or moral principles involved.[35-41] Indeed, it is highly questionable whether social, ethical, and moral principles should lie within its purview.

A more promising direction lies in the field of philosophy and ethics. There seems to be little reservation within medical circles in acknowledging the presence of ethical issues. There is, however, much resistance within these same circles to the methodologies and structure of ethical and philosophic analysis.[42-43] This is indeed unfortunate. Debates involving, for example, distinctions between active and passive euthanasia have circulated in medical centers for decades and remain essentially unresolved.[44-59] Although resolution is not imminent, a few principles may be outlined for consideration.

First, with the attention currently being given issues involving "brain death" in both legal and medical circles, it is critically important for caregivers to remember that a definition of death is not the same thing as criteria for recognition or measurement of when that state is reached. Health care providers frequently confuse the two. Such a melding is even evident in the now-famous Harvard University Report "A Definition of Irreversible Coma."[60] In general, what has been confused is the fact that although issues pertaining to measurement are indeed in the domain of science and medicine, issues pertaining to definition are not.[61] Instead, this latter question type belongs most appropriately and can be answered most satisfactorily when treated as a social and philosophic question.

On an individual level caregivers faced with or involved in decisions about the termination of life supports should attempt to address a few critical questions. First, what is so essentially significant about life that its loss is considered tragic?[62] Second, what is the quality whose absence in an entity means that entity should no longer be considered human? These are not easy questions, nor can their answers be concise and totally unambiguous. The fact remains, however, that physicians and nurses are undertaking critical care decisions without overt articulation of these issues. As incongruous as it may seem, patients often *acquire* the right to die.[63] What we are dealing with, then, is often not the unambiguous application of clear criteria to clinical cases but rather the evolution of an illness trajectory in which at some perhaps arbitrary point a status transformation occurs, and the right to die is attained. It seems reasonable to assume that social factors are prominently featured in such a status shift. Their context and content, however, have yet to be delineated.

Near-death experiences

Near-death experience has been one of the latest in a long line of topics to emerge in the death and dying literature. Patients who have undergone an unexpectedly quick trajectory and survived, particularly survivors of cardiac arrest and other cardiovascular insults, have had their experiences widely publicized in recent years.

The range of phenomena, both physical and psychic, that have come to be included under the label of *near-death experience* is extensive. They include a sense of peace and well-being, a passage from one world to another, usually accompanied by darkness, an appearance of light, an entering into a world of light, a life review, an encounter with a "presence," an encounter with deceased loved ones, an experience of "making the decision" to return to life, and the now relatively popularized "tunnel of darkness" and out-of-body experiences.[64-66] The obvious parallels that this topic has with psychic phenomena and parapsychology casts, for some people, a heavy pall of suspicion over it. For others the claims that near-death experiences offer proof of both the existence of an afterlife and a supreme being are a dampening agent. The convergence of this topic with the overall growth, development, and direction of the work of Kübler-Ross is a case in point. Originally a self-described nonbeliever in life after death,[67] she developed as a result of her work a belief in the existence of God, a belief that was soon augmented by belief in the existence of a specific form of afterlife, out-of-body experiences, and spirit guides.[68] For some Kübler-Ross exemplifies the tragedy of science run astray. For others she represents hope, the promise of a blissful death, and a secular promise of an eternal afterlife.

The major criticism of near-death experience as proof of an afterlife[69-70] can be found in those using a psychoanalytic frame of reference.[71-75] This perspective relies on concepts such as isolation of affect, denial, and displacement to explain the reactions of patients to a near-death experience. Patients are viewed as unable to face the full implications (death) of, for example, their cardiac arrest.

Whatever the relative merits of psychoanalytic and spiritualistic orientations, two facts remain unescapable. First, both frames of reference expend much of their interpretive efforts attempting to explain why individuals report the experiences they do. In fact, for some the relationship of near-death experiences to the question of survival after death is the predominant issue.[76] The second fact, corollary commonly overlooked, is that neither camp seeks to deny the phenomenologic reality of the experiences reported. It is this focus on the experience itself, *the what* as contrasted with *the why*, that has immediate and direct clinical relevance for the health care provider who works with life-threatened individuals.

Two points need to be emphasized. First, a health care provider need not believe in a supreme being, heaven, or even the reality of near-death experiences to acknowledge, as a subjectively based experience, a patient's reported near-death encounter. Second, the published accounts relate the subjective realities of only a small fraction of the individuals who are conscious of having undergone a near-death experience. Embarrassment and a fear of appearing foolish or crazy are some of the reasons explaining the reluctance of many patients to communicate their experiences to others. It also seems reasonable to assume that individuals may experience much anxiety and consternation over the ontologic meaning of these experiences.[77] If the health care provider can resist the impulse to intrude with an interpretation, much can be done to support the patient in his own search for meaning. The critical element in this case, as in all communication with patients, is to differentiate between what a person says and what a person means. In the end, a patient with a near-death experience who asks caregivers, for example, if they believe in God or raises questions about the existence of God is not interested as much in the caregivers' personal beliefs as in determining whether that bright-light experience was God or that calm serenity was the presence of heaven. A sharing of your personal spiritual beliefs may be in some cases altogether appropriate; however, this does not undercut the fact that a caregiver's beliefs cannot establish the ontologic reality of that patient's experiences. For argument's sake, suppose a caregiver believes both in the existence of God and in a totally complete and accurate recollection of near-death experiences by the patient; a conclusion by that caregiver that a patient-reported meeting of a presence was in fact a meeting with God is inappropriate on two levels. First, there is actually no epistemologic basis on which to argue that the God in our beliefs and the God in the near-death experience are one and the same. Second, and more relevant to a clinical care perspective, a professional's quick pronouncement as to the meaning of things may stifle a patient's exploration of what could have been a profoundly important and rich experience. When dealing with issues such as near-death experiences health care professionals may be well advised to adopt a general rule of thumb, and assume nothing. An encounter with God may induce euphoria on one day and depression the next. An encounter with long-deceased relatives may not be a meeting with dearly loved and treasured individuals. Rather than provide the patient with a ready-made frame of reference, it is much more appropriate to avoid such a temptation and encourage and support the patient's own search for meaning. There is every reason to anticipate ambivalence in a patient who has had a near-death experience and therefore every reason to approach the patient with as little paternalism and prejudgment as possible.

In conclusion, the patient who undergoes a near-death experience should receive optimal care in an environment where he can both discuss and explore his experiences. This care is compromised when the health care providers allow their own beliefs, fears, or questions to dictate how to handle in a clinical situation and interpret near-death experiences.

Alternative resources

Over the past 2 decades but particularly in the last 10 years a number of resources have been established to better address the particular needs of the terminally ill and life-threatened patient. Some of these have been hospital based, and some have been located in the community, whereas others still lack any geographic referent at all.

The most notable has been the hospice movement.[78] More appropriately thought of as a philosophy of care rather than as a literal physical structure there currently exist over 150 formally organized hospice programs in this country.[79] Although largely focused on the terminally ill cancer patient, its emphasis on comprehensive and coordinated care and its willingness to address the medical, psychoemotional, social, and spiritual needs of patients are applicable to all terminally ill patients. A special emphasis of hospice programs is the development and utilization of resources so as to provide patients with alternatives to inpatient hospital care, care that is increasingly expensive and synonymous with the utilization of high-technology medicine. Affording patients the opportunity to spend all or part of their remaining days at home is a special goal of a hospice program. Hospice programs are also designed, through the use of specially trained medical staff and auxiliary personnel, to address issues of abandonment, loss of self-management, control over environment, control of pain, and bereavement.

In addition to hospices, a number of patient-run and directed self-help groups have sprung up around the country. Some, such as Make Today Count (for terminally ill patients) and the Society of Compassionate Friends (for bereaved parents), have assumed a national presence. Many other groups exist, unnamed, focusing around either specific diseases (such as end-stage renal disease) or social states (such as widow or widower groups). Sometimes these groups are affiliated with and supported by resources of hospital outpatient clinics. Others exist independently of any organized medical entity.

A third "resource," which has gained increased attention over the past decade, has been the concept of the living will.[80] Generically, a living will is a written statement, directed from patient to physician, requesting that certain medical procedures usually referred to as life sustaining not be employed in a situation in which death is inevitable. Although it carries no legal mandate, the will itself, in whatever its written form, carries a strong symbolic message: that dying can, under certain circumstances, be unduly and unreasonably prolonged, that the process of dying is too frequently removed from the control of the patient, and that in situations of imminent death caregivers may not be routinely expected to act in accordance with patient desires.

Since a living will may carry a moral but no legal mandate, a movement has generated to develop legally binding provisos. Spurred on by the precedent-setting California Natural Death Act in California, which was passed into law in 1977, over half the United States have passed or have pending similar legislation.[81] Actively opposed by right-to-life groups and largely unsupported by organized medicine, most of this type of legislation, as typified by the California act, is so restrictively written as to be often inapplicable to virtually all of the patients it is drafted to aid. Such acts, however, whatever their detractions and shortcomings, do provide symbolic evidence of public concern for the issues of personal control, dignity, and autonomy in life-threatening and terminal situations.

Conclusions

Working with terminally ill and life-threatened patients is an extremely stressful but also potentially rewarding undertaking. Providing care for such patients is a challenge because it embodies the need for coordinated and comprehensive medical care delivery. It leads to frustration because, in part, hospitals, as structural units of care delivery, are not currently organized to facilitate the delivery of such care.

Two main themes run throughout the material presented in this chapter. First is the premise that it is through a critical understanding of issues involved in the care of the life-threatened patient that health care providers may become more *responsive* to their own and patient needs and thus less *reactive* to the situational pressures that surround them. Second is a perspective on patient care that stresses *relationship*. Providing care for life-threatened patients goes beyond simply talking to or being with patients. The overall goal is to develop and maintain an atmosphere in which needs and awareness can be encouraged, nurtured, and communicated. At root, patient care must be viewed from a transactional perspective. Health providers who think of care as something done to or for someone rather than with someone has misconstrued the mission of medicine.

A corollary of this second theme is a perspective that the providing of care is a process, which over time, by its very nature, undergoes shifts and modifications in needs, goals, and the very meaning of what is being transacted. Thus the establishment of a mutually collaborative and supportive system is a major goal in structuring patient care activities. Care for the critically ill involves a great deal of flexibility, sensitivity, knowledge, and skills on the part of the caregiver. In this context the caregiver may be viewed as a therapeutic facilitator whose goal is to support the patient in adapting within the context of an ever-changing and always complex illness picture.[82]

REFERENCES

1. Hingson, R., and others: In sickness and in health: social dimensions of medical care, St. Louis, 1981, The C.V. Mosby Co.
2. Alsop, S.: Stay of execution, Philadelphia, 1973, J.B. Lippincott Co.
3. Eys, V.: To die from cancer or from a heart attack. In Reiffel, J., and others, editors: Psychosocial aspects of cardiovascular disease, New York, 1980, Columbia University Press, p. 204.
4. Williams, R.R.: Cardiovascular disease and cancer: comparisons and contrasts. In Reiffel, J., and others, editors: Psychosocial aspects of cardiovascular disease, New York, 1980, Columbia University Press.
5. Eys, V.: To die from cancer or from heart attack. In Reiffel, J., and others, editors: Psychosocial aspects of cardiovascular disease, New York, 1980, Columbia University Press, p. 207.
6. Mauksch, H.O.: The organizational context of dying. In Kübler-Ross, E., editor: Death: the final stage of growth, Englewood Cliffs, N.J., 1975, Prentice-Hall, Inc.
7. Goffman, E.: The presentation of self in everyday life, Garden City, N.Y., 1959, Doubleday & Co., Inc.
8. Trillin, A.S.: Of dragons and garden peas, N. Engl. J. Med. **304:**699, 1981.
9. Lester, D.: Experimental and correlational studies of the feat of death, Psychol. Bull. **67:**27, 1967.
10. Hackett, T.P., Cassem, N.H., and Wishnie, H.A.: The coronary care unit, N. Engl. J. Med. **279:**1365, 1968.
11. Gentry, W.D., Foster, S., and Haney, T.: Denial as a determinant of anxiety and perceived health status in the coronary care unit, Psychosom. Med. **34:**39, 1975.
12. Gentry, W., and Haney, T.: Emotional and behavioral reaction to acute myocardial infarction, Heart Lung **4**(5):738, 1975.
13. Foster, S.B.: Effect of interpersonal communication on urinary sodium potassium ratio (a stress indicator), master's thesis, Washington, D.C., 1971, Catholic University of America.
14. Blacher, R.S.: The hidden psychosis of open-heart surgery: with a note on the sense of awe, J.A.M.A. **222:**3, 1972.
15. Blacher, R.S.: Heart disease, heart surgery, and death. In Reiffel, J., and others, editors: Psychosocial aspects of cardiovascular disease, New York, 1980, Columbia University Press.
16. Pattison, E.M.: The experience of dying, Am. J. Psychother. **21:**32, 1967.
17. Shneidman, E.S.: Death wish and stages of dying. In Shneidman, E.S., editor: Death: current perspectives, Palo Alto, Calif., 1976, Mayfield Publishing Co.
18. Glaser, B.G., and Strauss, A.L.: Awareness of dying, Chicago, 1965, Aldine Publishing Co.
19. Kübler-Ross, E.: On death and dying, New York, 1969, Macmillan, Inc.
20. Olin, H.S., and Hacket, T.P.: The denial of chest pain in 32 patients with acute myocardial infarction, J.A.M.A. **190:**977, 1964.
21. Blacher, R.S., and Joseph, E.D.: Psychological reaction to a cardiac monitor, Mt. Sinai J. Med. **39:**4, 1972.
22. Weisman, A.D., and Hackett, T.F.: Predilection to death, Psychosom. Med. **23:**232, 1961.
23. Hackett, T.P., Cassem, N.H., and Wishnie, H.A.: The coronary care unit, N. Engl. J. Med. **279:**1365, 1968.
24. Weisman, A.D.: On dying and denying: a psychiatric study of terminality, New York, 1972, Behavioral Publications.
25. Crane, D.: The sanctity of social life: physicians' treatment of critically ill patients, New York, 1975, Russell Sage Foundation.
26. Sudnow, D.: Passing on: the social organization of dying, Englewood Cliffs, N.J., 1967, Prentice-Hall, Inc.
27. Sudnow, D.: Dead on arrival, Trans-Action. (5) Nov. 36, 1973.
28. Simpson, M.A.: Brought in dead, Omega **7**(3):243, 1976.
29. Kastenbaum, R.J.: Death, society, and human experience, ed. 2, St. Louis, 1981, The C.V. Mosby Co.
30. Glaser, B.G., and Strauss, A.L.: Awareness of dying, Chicago, 1965, Aldine Publishing Co.
31. Glaser, B.G., and Strauss, A.L.: Time for dying, Chicago, 1968, Aldine Publishing Co.
32. Glaser, B.G., and Strauss, A.L.: Anguish: a case history of a dying trajectory, Mill Valley, Calif., 1970, The Sociology Press.
33. Fulton, R., and Fulton, J.: A psychosocial aspect of terminal care: anticipatory grief, Omega **2:**91, 1971.
34. Glaser, B.G., and Strauss, A.L.: Awareness of dying, Chicago, 1965, Aldine Publishing Co.
35. Superior Court of New Jersey: In the matter of Karen Quinlan, an alleged incompetent. In Weir, R.F., editor: Ethical issues in death and dying, New York, 1977, Columbia University Press.

36. Curran, W.J.: The Saikewicz decision, N. Engl. J. Med. **298**:499, 1978.
37. Schram, R.J., Kane, J., and Roble, D.T.: "No code" orders: clarification in the aftermath of Saikewicz, N. Engl. J. Med. **299**:875, 1978.
38. Paris, J.J.: Court intervention and the dimunition of patients' rights: the case of Brother Fox, N. Engl. J. Med. **303**:876, 1980.
39. Paris, J.J.: The New York Court of Appeals rules on the rights of dying incompetent patients: the conclusion of the Brother Fox case, N. Engl. J. Med. **304**:1424, 1981.
40. Curran, W.J.: Court involvement in the right to die cases: judicial inquiry in New York, N. Engl. J. Med. **305**:75, 1981.
41. New York Court of Appeals, No. 658: In the matter of John Storar, March 31, 1981.
42. Ingelfinger, F.J.: Bedside ethics for the hopeless case, N. Engl. J. Med. **289**:914, 1973.
43. Pinkus, R.L.: Medical foundations of various approaches to medical-ethical decision-making, J. Med. Philos. **6**:295, 1981.
44. Ruddick, W.: Can doctors and philosophers work together? Hastings Center Report **11**(2):12, 1981.
45. Gillick, M.: The ethics of cardiopulmonary resuscitation: another look, Ethics Sci. Med. **7**:161, 1980.
46. Dunphy, J.E.: On caring for the patient with cancer, N. Engl. J. Med. **295**:313, 1976.
47. Epstein, F.H.: Responsibility of the physician in the perservation of life. In Reiffel, J., and others, editors: Psychosocial aspects of cardiovascular disease, New York, 1980, Columbia University Press.
48. American Heart Association: Medical considerations and recommendations, J.A.M.A. **227**:864, 1974.
49. Spencer, S.S.: "Code" or "no code": a nonlegal opinion, N. Engl. J. Med. **300**:138, 1979.
50. Duff, R.S., and Campbell, A.G.M.: Moral and ethical dilemmas in the special care nursery, N. Engl. J. Med. **289**:980, 1973.
51. Brown, N.K., and others: The preservation of life, J.A.M.A. **211**:76, 1970.
52. Veatch, R.M.: Caring for the dying person—ethical issues at stake. In Barton, D., editor: Dying and death: a clinical guide for caregivers, Baltimore, 1977, The Williams & Wilkins Co.
53. Rachels, J.: Active and passive euthanasia, N. Engl. J. Med. **292**:78, 1975.
54. Montague, P.: The morality of active and passive euthanasia, Ethics Sci. Med. **5**:39, 1978.
55. Kary, C.: A moral distinction between killing and letting die, J. Med. Philos. **5**(4):326, 1980.
56. Fletcher, J.: Elective death in ethical issues in medicine. In Torrey, E.F., editor: Ethical issues in modern medicine, Boston, 1968, Little, Brown & Co.
57. Steinbock, B.: The intentional termination of life, Ethics Sci. Med. **6**:59, 1979.
58. Correspondence, N. Engl. J. Med. **292**:863, 1975.
59. Ladd, J.: Positive and negative euthansia. In Bayles, M.D., and High, D.M., editors: Medical treatment of the dying: moral issues, Cambridge, Mass., 1978, Schenkman Publishing Co., Inc.
60. A definition of irreversible coma, 1968, Report of the ad hoc committee of the Harvard Medical School to examine the definition of brain death, J.A.M.A. 205:6:337, 1968.
61. Veatch, R.M.: Death, dying, and the biological revolution, New Haven, Conn., 1976, Yale University Press.
62. Veatch, R.M.: Caring for the dying person—ethical issues at stake. In Barton, D., editor: Dying and death: a clinical guide for caregivers, Baltimore, 1977, The Williams & Wilkins Co.
63. Duff, R.S., and Campbell, A.G.M.: Moral and ethical dilemmas in the special care nursery, N. Engl. J. Med. **289**:890, 1973.
64. Ring, K.: Life at death, New York, 1980, Coward, McCann & Geoghegan, Inc.
65. Moody, R.A., Jr.: Life after life, Atlanta, 1975, Mockingbird Books.
66. Moody, R.A., Jr.: Reflections on life after life, Atlanta, 1977, Mockingbird Books.
67. Kübler-Ross, E.: Questions and answers on death and dying, New York, 1974, MacMillan Inc.
68. Kübler-Ross, E.: Interview, Playboy, p. 69, May 1981.
69. Moody, R.A., Jr.: Life after life, Atlanta, 1975, Mockingbird Books.
70. Rawlings, M.: Beyond death's door, Nashville, 1978, Thomas Nelson Inc.
71. Druss, R.G., and Kornfeld, D.S.: The survivors of cardiac arrest: a psychiatric study, J.A.M.A. **201**:75, 1967.
72. Ehrenwald, J.: Out-of-body experiences and the denial of death, J. Nerv. Ment. Dis. **159**:227, 1974.
73. Noyes, J., Jr., and Klett, R.: The experience of dying from falls, Omega **3**:45, 1972.
74. Noyes, J., Jr., and Klett, R.: Depersonalization in the face of life-threatening danger: a description, Psychiatry **39**:19, 1972.
75. Hunter, R.C.H.: On the experience of nearly dying, Am. J. Psychiatry **124**:122, 1967.
76. Stevenson, I., and Greyson, B.: Near-death experiences: relevance to the question of survival after death, J.A.M.A. **242**:265, 1979.
77. Ring, K.: Life at death, New York, 1980, Coward, McCann & Geoghegan, Inc.
78. Cohen, K.P.: Hospice prescription of terminal care, London, 1979, Aspen Systems Corp.
79. Garfield, C.A., Larson, D.G., and Schuldberg, D.: Mental health training and the hospice community: a national survey, Berkeley, Calif., 1980, The Weight Institute.
80. Veatch, R.M.: Death and dying: the legislative options, Hastings Cent. Rep. **7**:5, 1977.
81. Relman, A.: Michigan's sensible "living will," N. Engl. J. Med. **300**:1280, 1979.
82. Barton, D., editor: Dying and death: a clinical guide for caregivers, Baltimore, 1977, The Williams & Wilkins Co.

INDEX

A